CW00662878

Textbook of Rabbit Medicine

Commissioning editor: Mary Seager
Development editor: Caroline Savage
Production controller: Anthony Read
Desk editor: Jackie Holding
Cover designer: Alan Studholme

Textbook of Rabbit Medicine

Frances Harcourt-Brown

With illustrations by Nigel Harcourt-Brown

BUTTERWORTH HEINEMANN

OXFORD AUCKLAND BOSTON JOHANNESBURG MELBOURNE NEW DELHI

Butterworth–Heinemann
Linacre House, Jordan Hill, Oxford OX2 8DP
225 Wildwood Avenue, Woburn, MA 01801-2041
A division of Reed Educational and Professional Publishing Ltd

A member of the Reed Elsevier plc group

First published 2002

© Reed Educational and Professional Publishing Ltd 2002

All rights reserved. No part of this publication may be reproduced in any material form (including photocopying or storing in any medium by electronic means and whether or not transiently or incidentally to some other use of this publication) without the written permission of the copyright holder except in accordance with the provisions of the Copyright, Designs and Patents Act 1988 or under the terms of a licence issued by the Copyright Licensing Agency Ltd, 90 Tottenham Court Road, London, England W1P 0LP. Applications for the copyright holder's written permission to reproduce any part of this publication should be addressed to the publishers

British Library Cataloguing in Publication Data
Harcourt-Brown, Frances
Textbook of rabbit medicine
1. Pet medicine 2. Rabbits – Diseases 3. Rabbits
I. Title II. Harcourt-Brown, Nigel H.
636.9'322'0896

ISBN 0 7506 4002 2

For information on other veterinary publications
visit our website at www.bh.com/veterinary

Printed and bound in the United Kingdom

Transferred to Digital Print 2010

PLANT A TREE
BTCV
British Trust for Conservation Volunteers
FOR EVERY VOLUME THAT WE PUBLISH, BUTTERWORTH-HEINEMANN WILL PAY FOR BTCV TO PLANT AND CARE FOR A TREE.

Contents

Acknowledgements

The publishers and author would like to acknowledge the support of Burgess Supafeeds in the production of this book.

Foreword

The huge increase in the popularity of rabbits as pets has taken the veterinary world by surprise. Practitioners have experienced an ever-growing number of clients demanding the highest standards of care for their rabbits, and this has led to a demand for more and better information on the veterinary treatment of this species. Until relatively recently, much of the information on rabbit health and diseases related primarily to those animals bred for meat, or kept in research laboratories. This new publication represents a major advance in meeting the needs of those practitioners seeking comprehensive clinical information on pet rabbits. Not only does it provide detailed coverage of the diseases of this species, it includes extensive information on the basic biology of the rabbit. An understanding of the normal anatomy, physiology and behaviour of this species is an essential prerequisite to the successful management of its disease problems, and readers will find these sections of the book an invaluable resource.

Although the general approach of the book is similar to texts which deal with diseases of more familiar species, the author reminds us throughout of the need to consider the 'whole rabbit', and to appreciate that the effects of disease in one organ system can result in serious problems in other systems. The information on diseases is also presented in sections dealing with specific disease agents, and this is cross-referenced with those chapters dealing with the different body-systems.

The book is filled with helpful summary tables and flow charts that the busy practitioner can use for rapid reference. There are comprehensive dose rate tables, based both on what limited published data exists, but also on the author's own extensive experience. It is the inclusion of such first hand information that makes this book so special – Frances Harcourt-Brown not only has extensive clinical experience in dealing with rabbits, she also keeps rabbits as pets and has a genuine and deep enthusiasm for this species. This is not to imply that the book contains too much that is anecdotal. The author cites numerous references, and makes clear which of her recommendations are based on published data, and which on current 'best practice'. The references given also highlight her own many contributions to the field of rabbit medicine and biology. Some of the conclusions drawn and recommendations made may be controversial, but that is to be expected in this rapidly growing field, and the author always makes clear the basis for her opinions. The enthusiasm of the author for her subject is also shown by the inclusion of line-drawings, together with a good selection of colour images of specific disease conditions.

The completion and publication of this text represents a tremendous achievement. It provides comprehensive coverage of our current knowledge of the veterinary care of pet rabbits. It is destined to become essential reading for all veterinarians dealing with these animals, and will have a very significant influence on our ability to manage disease in this species.

Paul Flecknell

Preface

In 1986, when my eldest daughter was nine, we bought a Netherland Dwarf rabbit. My daughter studied her books and asked me if her rabbit would 'get malocclusion' as this seemed to be such a problem in pet rabbits, especially Netherland Dwarfs. After some consideration, I realised that I could not reassure her and started to wonder how pet rabbits acquired dental problems. I tried to find out the answer to this question plus any other information about clinical diseases of pet rabbits but discovered that reliable answers to my questions were not to be found in the literature. This was because most of the information was related to diseases of rabbits kept in colonies for commercial or laboratory purposes. So, I set about discovering as much as I could for myself by piecing together published information and relating it to the diseases that I was seeing in individual pet rabbits presented for treatment at our practice. I tried to learn as much from each case as possible. Times have changed since 1986; rabbits are becoming increasingly popular as companion animals and there is a rising demand from the general public for a high standard of veterinary treatment. Many pet rabbits are now insured against veterinary treatment. Although information on diseases of pet rabbits can now be found in books, magazines and on the Internet, much of it is anecdotal. In order to meet the need for a comprehensive text, the 'Textbook of Rabbit Medicine' has been written for the veterinary surgeon when faced with a pet rabbit to treat. Common ailments, such as dental disease, abscesses and ophthalmic conditions are covered in detail and wherever possible, the book is based on proven facts taken from peer-reviewed journals. The text also includes a large number of anatomical drawings and radiographs. The drawings have been provided by my husband Nigel and most of these have been made from original dissections. They represent many months of hard work.

Among the many authors whose work has provided the building blocks for this book, three people have stood out. All three are professors. Firstly, Professor Robert Barone, who with his co-authors C. Pavaux, P.C. Blin, and P. Cuq produced 'Atlas d'anatomie du lapin', published in 1973. The discovery of this book was an exciting moment. It is a comprehensive collection of wonderful anatomical illustrations of the rabbit. This book has now been superseded by a collection of comparative anatomy books, *Anatomie comparée des mammifères domestiques*. The second professor, Peter Cheeke, has written many books and articles. His book 'Rabbit Feeding and Nutrition' is a comprehensive treatise on rabbit nutrition. It is easy to read and gives valuable insight into the complexity of the rabbit's digestive system and the importance of diet to the health of the individual. The third professor is Paul Flecknell. Paul's extensive publications, especially on anaesthesia and analgesia, have raised awareness in the veterinary profession and have greatly improved the chances of successful treatment for all small mammals, including rabbits.

Many people have helped with the preparation of this book. Professor Anthony King was an inspirational teacher during my undergraduate days at Liverpool University. More recently, he has given me encouragement and constructive criticism of some of the anatomical aspects of the text. Friends and relatives have translated French and German references and, for this, I thank Michael and Ulrike Lierz, Abigail Rouse and my nephew and niece Tim and Amanda Strong. My thanks also go to John Hird, Nick Carmichael and Heather Holloway for their scrutiny of the Anaesthesia and Clinical Pathology chapters. I am indebted to my professional colleagues Allison Gleadhill and Gill Howard for reading through the text, correcting mistakes and for their continued interest in rabbit related topics. I am grateful to the nurses and other members of our practice who have endured my obsession with rabbits and have helped me to treat and nurse these patients with dedication and commitment. Our four children deserve thanks for their forbearance during my preoccupation with rabbit diseases over the last few years. Lastly, and most importantly, I would like to thank my husband Nigel who has helped and encouraged me throughout every stage. He has been my mentor, scrutineer and anatomical illustrator as well as housekeeper, cook and professional partner.

Frances Harcourt-Brown

1

Biological characteristics of the domestic rabbit (*Oryctolagus cuniculi*)

1.1 Origins of the domestic rabbit

Domestic rabbits are descended from the European rabbit, *Oryctolagus cuniculus*, that belongs to the order *Lagomorpha*, which are characterized by the presence of a second small pair of upper incisors or peg teeth. Lagomorphs were once considered to be a suborder of the *Rodentia*, which is divided into *Sciuromorpha* (squirrel-like rodents), *Myomorpha* (mouse-like rodents) and *Hystricomorpha* (porcupine-like rodents) that includes guinea pigs and chinchillas. Current opinion suggests that *Rodentia* and *Lagomorpha* have no fundamental similarities and on the basis of structural features and serological data, *Lagomorpha* show more affinity to *Artiodactyla* (hoofed mammals) (Nowak, 1999).

Other lagomorphs include hares and pikas. All members of the lagomorph order are terrestrial and eat only vegetation. Fossil records show that the European rabbit, *Oryctolagus cuniculus*, was confined to the Iberian peninsula and Southern France following the Pleistocene. Since that time, the species has been introduced to many parts of the world with the exception of North America, where the native wild rabbit is either *Sylvilagus floridanus* (Cottontail) or *Sylvilagus bachmani* (Brush Rabbit). The North American Jackrabbit, *Lepus californicus*, is from the hare genus.

It is not clear when the European rabbit was introduced into Great Britain. The Romans brought many food animals with them, such as pheasant and quail and it is believed that they not only introduced rabbits but also kept them in cages, thereby starting the process of domestication. The modern pet rabbit still retains many of the characteristics of its wild counterparts despite changes in size, colour, coat texture and temperament.

1.2 Wild rabbits

The behavioural characteristics of lagomorphs differ between species. For example, cottontails (*Sylvilagus* spp.) do not dig burrows, although they may use burrows made by other animals. Females dig holes to make nests and sit over the hole to suckle the young. Vegetation is used to cover the fur-lined nest between feeds. Cottontails are solitary animals in contrast with *Oryctolagus cuniculus* that live in groups with a defined social hierarchy (Nowak, 1999).

The European rabbit, *Oryctolagus cuniculus* prefers a sandy, hilly terrain with shrubs and woody plants and is not found at altitudes above 600 m. It often digs complex burrows or warrens that can be 3 m deep and 45 m long. The tunnels are about 15 cm in diameter and the living chambers 30–60 cm high. The main surface entrances are usually indicated by mounds of earth but there are numerous other small openings that lack these mounds. *Oryctolagus cuniculus* is essentially nocturnal, leaving the burrow in the early evening and returning in the morning, although it can be seen grazing or basking during the day. The home range is rarely larger than 20 hectares (Nowak, 1999).

Wild rabbits live in groups of two to eight adults plus juveniles with a defined social hierarchy (McBride, 1988). The group's territory is defended by the males, while the females dig out deep burrows to nest in. Male rabbits within the group will establish a dominance hierarchy with the older heavier males at the top. Aged males that have been usurped by younger, fitter rabbits are driven from the group to become solitary satellite males (Lockley, 1978). Young male rabbits are also often driven from the group when they reach puberty either to join another warren or to lead solitary lives in the hedgerows. The females tend to remain within the original group. Female rabbits are less aggressive towards each other than males, but will defend a chosen nesting site ferociously. Territories are scent marked with pheromones from the scent glands on the chin and genital area or by urine marking. Dominant males will continually scent mark their territory by rubbing their chins on branches and bushes and leaving piles of strategically placed faeces. They also mark territory by spraying urine, sometimes on to other individuals.

When wild rabbits emerge from their burrows at dusk, they begin to feed. Initially, they graze grass and vegetation, raising their heads at intervals to survey the surroundings, perhaps chewing through a long stalk or blade of grass at the same time. After half an hour or so, they will start to look around for other palatable plants to nibble. They are constantly on the look out for danger and will readily bolt back to their burrow. Hard faecal pellets are always voided above ground, never in the burrow and soft caecotrophs are usually consumed during periods of rest underground, although occasionally rabbits exhibit this behaviour above ground (Lockley, 1978). The only vocal sounds that are made are a loud high-pitched scream of terror or a range of growls and hums that denote pleasure or defence. Apprehensive or frightened rabbits will thump the ground with their hind feet. The loud thumping sounds acts as an alarm signal to other rabbits in the vicinity.

Many of the behavioural characteristics of their wild ancestors are still present in the modern day pet rabbit. Domestication has resulted in rabbits that are far tamer than their wild counterparts and easy to handle. Although some domestic rabbits still retain the tendency to dig holes and live underground, many do not, with the result that domestic rabbits that escape or are released do not survive for long in the wild. Conversely, wild rabbits seldom become tame in captivity, although the occasional individual will overcome its fear of humans. Hand-reared orphans usually grow into fearful adults. Even rabbits that are born as a result of egg transfer from a wild rabbit to a domesticated tame host retain their shy nature (Adams, 1987).

1.3 External characteristics

Rabbits have a thin skin and dense fur that consists of a soft undercoat and stiff guard hairs. They do not have footpads; instead the feet are covered with thick fur. The skin on the neck is loose and pendulous and forms a pronounced dewlap in females of some breeds. The nostrils are sensitive with large numbers of tactile vibrissae. Scent glands are situated in the deep inguinal spaces that are found on either side of the anus immediately dorsal to the urogenital opening. In the male rabbit, the testicles are found in hairless scrotal sacs on either side of the penis. The inguinal canal remains open and the testicles can be retracted into the abdomen. Retraction occurs during periods of sexual inactivity or during periods of insufficient food. Male rabbits have rudimentary nipples.

1.4 Reproduction

Rabbits are well known for their ability to reproduce quickly. Puberty occurs at 4–9 months with smaller breeds maturing earlier than larger breeds. Like the cat and the ferret, rabbits are induced ovulators. Although they do not show a regular oestrus cycle, they do vary in receptivity and a cyclic rhythm exists.

Follicle stimulating hormone (FSH) stimulates ovarian follicles to develop and produce oestrogens that cause the female to be receptive. Follicular development occurs in waves with five to 10 follicles on each ovary being at the same stage of development at any one time. When the follicles reach maturity they produce oestrogen for about 12–14 days. If ovulation has not occurred during this period, the follicles degenerate with a corresponding reduction in oestrogen level and sexual receptivity. After about 4 days a new wave of follicles begins to produce oestrogen and the doe becomes receptive again. Many factors influence this cyclic rhythm including nutrition, light, temperature, sexual stimulation and individual variation. In general, the receptive period lasts 14–16 days with a period of non-receptivity for 1–2 days (Patton, 1994). Mating stimulates ovulation approximately 10 hours *post coitus* (Harkness, 1987). Ovulation can also be induced by proximity of an entire male, mechanical stimulation of the vagina or by the act of being mounted by another female.

Gestation is maintained by progesterone that is produced exclusively by the ovarian *corpora lutea*. In the absence of fetuses, pseudopregnancy can occur after ovulation and is maintained by corpora lutea that degrade after approximately 17 days (Fekete and Huszenicza, 1993). In the wild, unfavourable winter conditions or lack of food suppress follicular activity. Does can be mated soon after giving birth and may be lactating and pregnant at the same time. Litter sizes vary and larger breeds generally have larger litters (Sandford, 1996). Average litter size is five to eight, the length of gestation is 30–32 days so it is possible for a doe to have six litters in a year and produce 40–50 offspring. The nest is made out of hay or other bedding material and lined with fur plucked from the doe's abdomen and flanks. Parturition usually takes place in the morning and is completed in less than half an hour although, occasionally, young can be born hours or even days apart (Adams, 1987). The young are born bald, blind and helpless. Most passive immunity is obtained before birth, although some antibodies are present in the colostrum (Brewer and Cruise, 1994). In the wild, newly born rabbits or 'kits' are cleaned and nursed by the doe before she leaves the nest and blocks the entrance. She will stay in the vicinity of the nest but only returns once or twice daily to feed the kits for a period of 3–5 minutes during which time a baby rabbit can drink 20% of its bodyweight (Donnelly, 1997). Rabbit milk is concentrated, containing 13–15% protein, 10–12% fat and 2% carbohydrate. The young rabbits emerge from the nest at about 18 days, start nibbling grass or hay at 3 weeks and are weaned at about 25 days of age.

Key points 1.1

- Domestic rabbits are descended from the European rabbit, *Oryctolagus cuniculus* and retain many behavioural characteristics of their wild ancestors
- Wild rabbits live in groups of 6–8 with a well defined social hierarchy. Males fight for dominance and females aggressively defend their nesting site
- Wild rabbits seldom become tame in captivity even if they are hand-reared
- Rabbits are induced ovulators without a defined oestrus cycle. Females show a cyclic rhythm of sexual receptivity
- Pseudopregnancy is the result of ovulation without fertilization. Ovulation can be stimulated in the absence of mating by the close proximity of a male, mechanical stimulation or mounting by another female
- Lactating does remain in the vicinity of their nest and defend it but only return once or twice daily to suckle the young.

1.5 Digestive physiology

The alimentary tract of the rabbit is adapted for the digestion of large quantities of fibrous food (Figure 1.1). Rabbits are hindgut fermenters and rely on microbial fermentation of food within the caecum to provide nutrients. In the stomach and small intestine, digestion and absorption of nutrients is similar to monogastric mammals. The end-products of the digestive processes are separated in the colon into indigestible material and substances that can be metabolized by caecal microorganisms. Separation of the ingesta depends on particle size. The proximal colon of the rabbit is specially adapted for the separation of large particles of

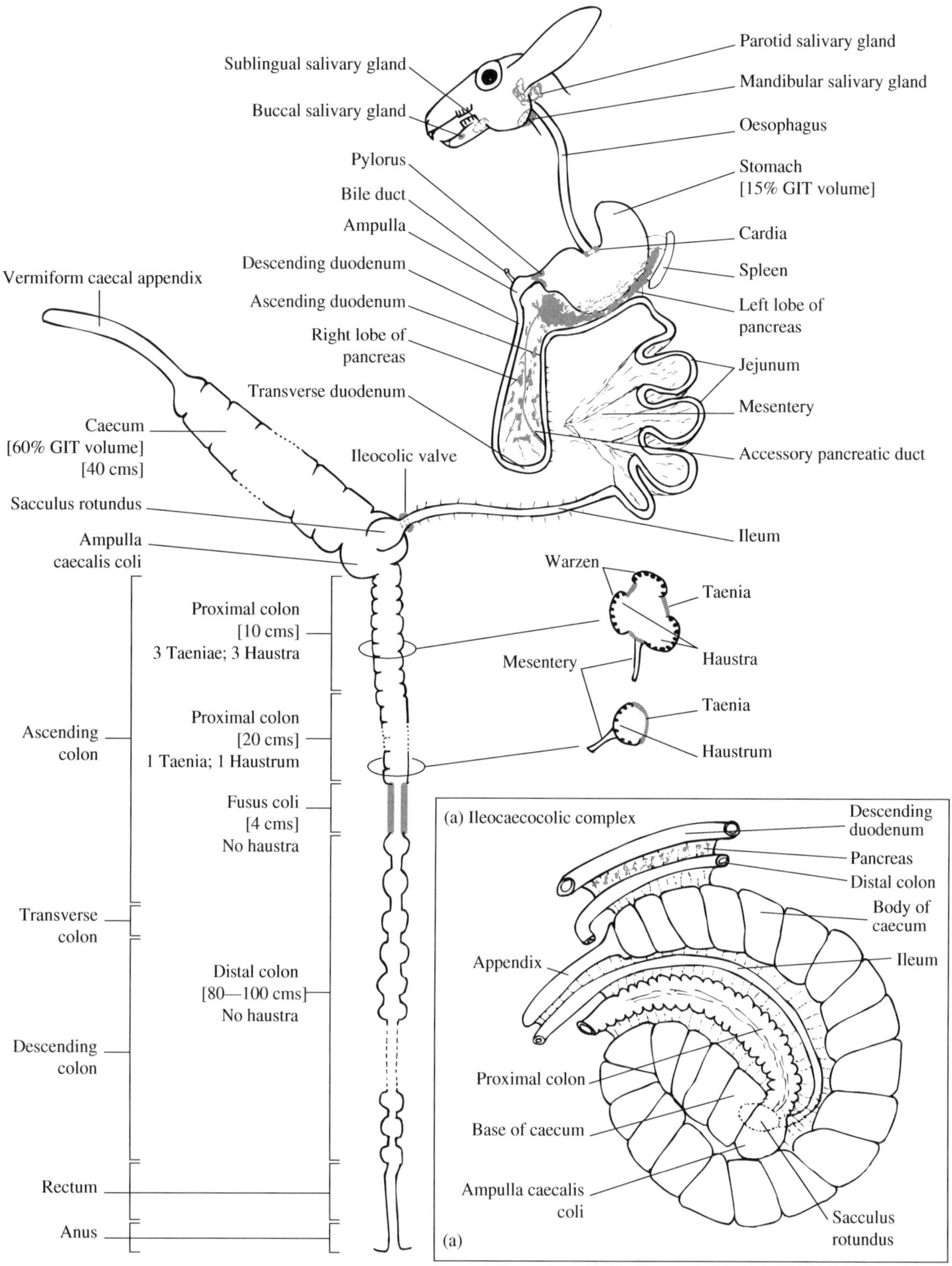
Sublingual salivary gland
Buccal salivary gland
Parotid salivary gland
Mandibular salivary gland
Oesophagus
Stomach
[15% GIT volume]
Pylorus
Bile duct
Ampulla
Descending duodenum
Ascending duodenum
Right lobe of pancreas
Transverse duodenum
Cardia
Spleen
Left lobe of pancreas
Jejunum
Mesentery
Accessory pancreatic duct
Vermiform caecal appendix
Caecum
[60% GIT volume]
[40 cms]
Ileocolic valve
Sacculus rotundus
Ampulla caecalis coli
Ileum
Warzen
Taenia
Haustra
Mesentery
Taenia
Haustrum
Proximal colon
[10 cms]
3 Taeniae; 3 Haustra
Proximal colon
[20 cms]
1 Taenia; 1 Haustrum
Fusus coli
[4 cms]
No haustra
Distal colon
[80—100 cms]
No haustra
Ascending colon
Transverse colon
Descending colon
Rectum
Anus
(a) Ileocaecocolic complex
Descending duodenum
Pancreas
Distal colon
Body of caecum
Ileum
Appendix
Proximal colon
Base of caecum
Ampulla caecalis coli
Sacculus rotundus
(a)

Figure 1.1.

Figure 1.1. Schematic diagram of the anatomy of the alimentary tract of the rabbit. The alimentary tract of the rabbit is adapted for the digestion of large quantities of fibrous food. The teeth continually grow and wear against each other to maintain their shape. The incisors are worn to a fine cutting edge that can be used to slice through vegetation or gnaw hard substances such as bark or wood. The occlusal surfaces of the cheek teeth are worn to an effective grinding surface that is used to reduce food particles to a small enough size to be swallowed. There are a number of well-developed salivary glands. The cardia and pyloric sphincter are muscular and well-developed. The relatively voluminous stomach is simple in type and always contains food. The stomach contents comprise approximately 15% of the contents of the gastrointestinal tract.

The duodenum forms a loop with descending, transverse and ascending parts. It has an extensive mesentery. The duodenum begins with a slight enlargement approximately 1 cm from the pylorus that receives the bile duct. The right lobe of the pancreas is widely dispersed in the mesoduodenum as many isolated lobules. The main body and left lobe of the pancreas run in the mesentery that attaches the transverse colon to the stomach and spleen (see Figure 10.4). A single accessory pancreatic duct opens into the junction between the descending and transverse duodenum.

The jejunum is long, convoluted and relatively free of attachments. It occupies the dorsal half of the left flank and the caudal half of the abdomen (see Figures 3.3–3.5). The ileum is closely associated with the mesentery that connects part of the ascending colon to the caecum to form the ileocaecocolic complex (see 1.1a). The end of the ileum is expanded into a thick walled *sacculus rotundus*.

The caecum and appendix are shown as a straight tube, but are in fact a coiled spiral (see 1.1a). The thin-walled caecum is a large organ that ends in an appendix that is heavily endowed with lymphoid tissue. The ascending colon of the rabbit can be divided into four sections. The first section is approximately 10 cm long and has three longitudinal flat bands of muscular tissue or *taeniae* that separate rows of *haustra* or sacculations. Small protrusions, 'warzen' (warts), approximately 0.5 mm in diameter, can be seen on the mucosa in this section of colon. The second section of ascending colon is approximately 20 cm in length and has a single *taenia* and fewer, smaller *haustra*. The third portion of the ascending colon is termed the *fusus coli* and is a muscular area about 4 cm long. The *fusus coli* opens into the fourth section of ascending colon that is histologically indistinguishable from the transverse and descending colon. Because the *fusus coli* forms such a natural division between two morphologically and functionally distinct sections of the rabbit colon, the terms 'proximal' and 'distal' colon are sometimes used instead of ascending, transverse and descending colon (Snipes *et al.*, 1982). The proximal colon includes the three *taeniae* section, the single *taenia* section and the *fusus coli*. The distal colon is 80–100 cm long and runs from the *fusus coli* to the rectum.

1.1a Ileocaecocolic complex. (Figure shows a ventral view of the ileocaecocolic complex, which occupies more than half of abdomen, mainly on the right side (see Figures 3.3–3.5)). The complex has been slightly unrolled in order to illustrate its component parts. There are mesenteric attachments between the caecum, appendix, proximal colon, ileum, distal colon and descending duodenum. These organs form a complex three-dimensional structure in rabbits. The term 'ileocaecocolic complex' is used to describe the structure in this text.

The body of the caecum has a spiral form consisting of one and a half turns, ending in an appendix that extends to the right flank. The axis of the spiral is the base of the caecum that receives the end of the ileum in the form of the *sacculus rotundus.* The ileum lies between the concavity of the body of the caecum and the convexity of the upper ascending colon and is attached to these two structures by peritoneal folds. Because of their peritoneal attachments to the spiral caecum, the ileum and upper ascending colon are also arranged in a spiral, and are integral components of the ileocaecocolic complex. The upper ascending colon begins as a smooth oval dilation, the *ampulla coli,* that forms the junction with the *sacculus rotundus* and the caecum. Parts of the descending colon and descending duodenum are attached to the distal end of the caecum by peritoneal folds. The left lobe of the pancreas lies in the peritoneal fold between the descending duodenum and descending colon.

indigestible fibre from smaller particles that can be degraded and used as a substrate for bacterial fermentation in the caecum. The two components are simultaneously sent in opposite directions.

Indigestible fibre passes down the colon to be rapidly eliminated as hard, dry faecal pellets. Smaller particles and fluids pass into the caecum where bacterial fermentation releases volatile fatty acids and synthesizes proteins and vitamins. Pellets of soft caecal contents (caecotrophs) are periodically expelled from the anus and re-ingested as a source of nutrients. This digestive strategy utilizes bacterial fermentation to synthesize nutrients and avoids the need to store large volumes of food in the digestive tract. Vegetation can be efficiently digested below ground without the need to spend long periods grazing and exposed to predators.

The rabbit's characteristic of consuming caecotrophs directly from the anus is known as 'caecotrophy', although the term coprophagia is still used in some texts. Coprophagia is defined as 'the ingestion of dung or faeces' (Blood and Studdert, 1999). Faeces are defined as 'body waste discharged from the intestine' and so, strictly speaking, faecal material is not the substance that is ingested by rabbits as it is not waste material but nutritionally rich caecal contents. The terms 'soft faeces' or 'night faeces' are sometimes used to describe the capsules of caecal material known as caecotrophs. The term 'night faeces' is misleading. Caecotrophs are produced during the day in wild rabbits. They are produced several hours after feeding during a quiet undisturbed period, which is during the day for a wild rabbit in its burrow but can be during the night or early morning for a domestic or laboratory rabbit in its cage or hutch.

1.5.1 Ingestion of food

The rabbit has a wide visual field that allows it to watch for predators while it is grazing. The visual field does not include the area immediately under the nose. Food selection and ingestion is based on smell and from tactile information gained from the sensitive vibrissae around the nose and lips.

The teeth are adapted for the ingestion of a fibrous diet. All the teeth are open rooted and grow continuously. The incisors are adapted to cut through vegetation. The two large upper incisors have two tiny secondary incisors situated immediately behind them. The two lower incisors occlude just behind the upper primary incisors and wear against them to form a sharp cutting edge. There is a thick layer of enamel on the anterior aspect of the upper primary incisors but no enamel on the posterior aspect. (Hirschfeld *et al.*, 1973). The enamel on the lower incisors is evenly distributed on all aspects. The distribution of enamel in combination with the occlusal positioning of the upper and lower incisors allows the teeth to be constantly sharpened. Wild rabbits are capable of chewing through aluminium (Adams, 1987). The rate of growth of the upper incisors is approximately 2 mm per week (Shadle, 1936). Canine teeth are absent and there is a wide diastema between the incisors and the premolars and molars which are grossly indistinguishable from each other. The premolars and molars form a row of five or six cheek teeth that are used for grinding the food before it is swallowed. The food is ground between the cheek teeth with jaw movements of up to 120 per minute (Brewer and Cruise, 1994).

Saliva is continuously secreted and contains amylase. Hunger is stimulated by a dry mouth and contractions of an empty stomach or by a decrease in blood levels of metabolites such as glucose, amino acid, lactic acid or volatile fatty acids (Fekete, 1989).

1.5.2 Anatomy and digestion in the stomach and small intestine

The stomach comprises about 15% of the volume of the gastrointestinal tract (Cruise and Brewer, 1994). It has a well-developed cardiac sphincter that prevents vomiting, and a muscular pyloric area. There is always food material in the stomach. Together, the caecum and the stomach contain over 80% of the digesta (Lang, 1981) and the amount of material in them is dependent on age, breed, diet and time of day. Water and large quantities of acid are secreted into the stomach. The postprandial pH can fall to 1–2, which effectively sterilizes ingesta before it passes into the small intestine. The stomach pH of suckling rabbits is higher at approximately

5–6.5, which permits the passage of bacteria through the stomach to the hindgut to colonize the caecum. During the digestion of caecotrophs the stomach pH rises to 3.0 (De Blas and Gidenne, 1998). Transit time of food through the stomach is approximately 3–6 h (Carabaõ and Piquer, 1998).

The duodenum begins with a slight enlargement that receives the bile duct. The right lobe of the pancreas is diffuse and is situated in the mesoduodenum of the duodenal loop. The body and the left lobe of the pancreas are much denser than the right lobe. The left lobe lies between the stomach and the transverse colon and extends as far as the spleen. A single pancreatic duct opens at the junction of the transverse and ascending loops of the duodenum (see Figure 1.1). This is the accessory pancreatic duct. The terminal part of the main pancreatic duct disappears during embryonic development. The accessory pancreatic duct communicates with both pancreatic lobes. The jejunum is long and convoluted. The end of the ileum is expanded into a spherical thick walled enlargement known as the *sacculus rotundus* that forms the junction between the ileum, caecum and proximal colon. The *sacculus rotundus* is unique to the rabbit and has abundant aggregations of lymphoid tissue and macrophages in the lamina propria and submucosa. An ileocolic valve controls movement of digesta from the ileum into the *sacculus rotundus* and also prevents reverse flow into the small intestine. Motilin, a polypeptide hormone secreted by enterochromaffin cells of the duodenum and jejunum, stimulates gastrointestinal smooth muscle. Fat stimulates and carbohydrate inhibits its release. In the small intestine, motilin activity is decreased aborally. It disappears in the caecum and reappears in the colon and rectum (Brewer and Cruise, 1994).

Digestion and absorption of nutrients in the stomach and small intestine are similar to other monogastric animals. Caecotrophs are digested in this section of the gastrointestinal tract. Caecotrophs are pellets of caecal material that contain microorganisms and the products of microbial fermentation such as amino acids, volatile fatty acids and vitamins. They are encapsulated in a gelatinous mucous coating that protects them from the acidity of the stomach. Some fermentation takes place within the caecotrophs as they lie in the gastric fundus for 6–8 hours before being digested. Lysozyme is secreted by the colon and incorporated into the caecotroph during its passage through the large intestine (Camara and Prieur, 1984). The bacteriolytic activity of lysozyme enables microbial protein to be degraded and absorbed from the small intestine in addition to the amino acids and vitamins that are present in the caecotrophs. Amylase is produced by bacteria within the caecotroph that converts glucose into carbon dioxide and lactic acid, which is absorbed from the stomach and small intestine (Fekete, 1989).

Hydrochloric acid and pepsin initiate digestion in the stomach that continues in the small intestine in a manner similar to other mammals. Pancreatic amylase production is relatively modest. There are alternative sources of amylase such as saliva and caecotrophs. In rabbits, ligation of the pancreatic duct does not result in pancreatic insufficiency (Brewer and Cruise, 1994). Proteolytic enzymes and chymotrypsin can be found in the intestinal lumen within a few weeks of the operation. It is thought that small pancreatic ducts that connect directly with the duodenum are the source of the enzymes. Bicarbonate is secreted into the duodenum and neutralizes the acidic digesta as it leaves the stomach. In the jejunum bicarbonate is absorbed rather than secreted. Transit time through the small intestine is fast. Estimated retention times in the jejunum and ileum are 10–20 and 30–60 minutes respectively (Carabaõ and Piquer, 1998).

1.5.3 Anatomy of the hindgut

The anatomy of the rabbit's digestive system is illustrated in detail by Barone *et al.* (1973) and Barone (1997). A schematic representation of the rabbit's digestive system is given in Figure 1.1. The ileocaecocolic segment is illustrated in Figure 1.1a and the topographical anatomy of the small intestine and colon is described in Figure 10.2.

The *sacculus rotundus* opens into the *ampulla caecalis coli* that forms a T-junction between the ileum, caecum and proximal colon. The *ampulla caecalis coli*, caecum and proximal colon are specially adapted for mixing and

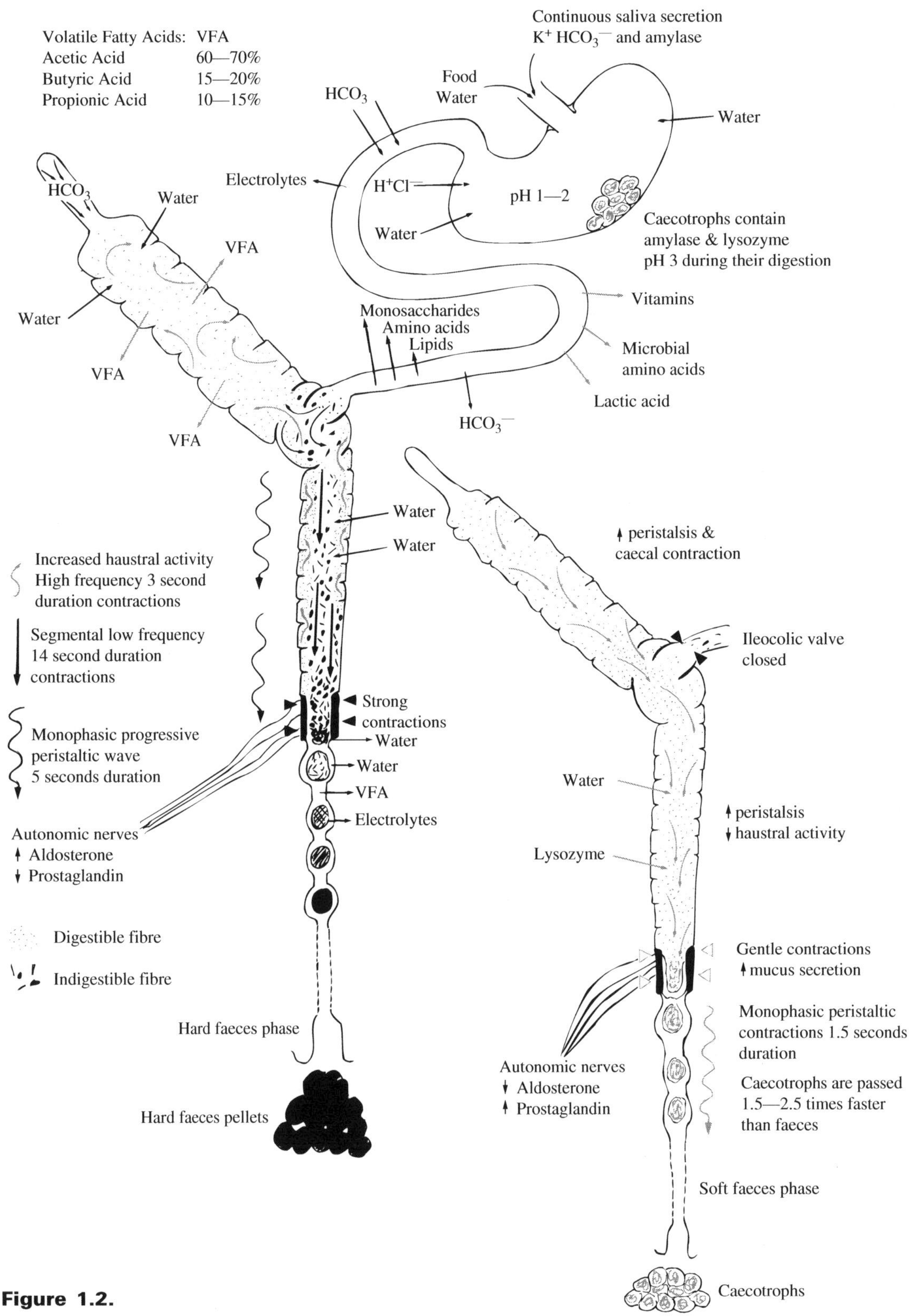
Volatile Fatty Acids: VFA
Acetic Acid 60—70%
Butyric Acid 15—20%
Propionic Acid 10—15%
Continuous saliva secretion
K+ HCO3− and amylase
Food
Water
HCO3
Water
Electrolytes
H+Cl−
pH 1—2
Water
Caecotrophs contain
amylase & lysozyme
pH 3 during their digestion
Vitamins
Microbial
amino acids
Lactic acid
Monosaccharides
Amino acids
Lipids
HCO3−
HCO3
Water
VFA
Water
VFA
VFA
Water
Water
Increased haustral activity
High frequency 3 second
duration contractions
Segmental low frequency
14 second duration
contractions
Monophasic progressive
peristaltic wave
5 seconds duration
Strong
contractions
Water
Water
VFA
Electrolytes
Autonomic nerves
↑ Aldosterone
↓ Prostaglandin
Digestible fibre
Indigestible fibre
Hard faeces phase
Hard faeces pellets
↑ peristalsis &
caecal contraction
Ileocolic valve
closed
Water
↑ peristalsis
↓ haustral activity
Lysozyme
Gentle contractions
↑ mucus secretion
Monophasic peristaltic
contractions 1.5 seconds
duration
Caecotrophs are passed
1.5—2.5 times faster
than faeces
Autonomic nerves
↓ Aldosterone
↑ Prostaglandin
Soft faeces phase
Caecotrophs

Figure 1.2.

separating large quantities of food. Large particles of indigestible fibre are separated from small fermentable particles and fluid. The large particles are sent distally along the colon while the small particles and fluid are sent proximally into the caecum where bacterial fermentation takes place (Figure 1.2). The thin walled caecum ends in a narrow blind appendix that is heavily endowed with lymphoid tissue. The appendix is often described as 'vermiform' due to its worm-shaped appearance. The gut-associated lymphoid tissue (GALT) of the rabbit is predominantly in the hindgut and represents over 50% of the total lymphoid tissue, which may account for the relatively small spleen of rabbits (Percy and Barthold, 1993).

The ascending colon of the rabbit is divided into four sections. At the proximal end, the *ampulla caecalis coli* opens into the first section that is approximately 10 cm long and has three longitudinal flat bands of muscular tissue or taeniae separating rows of haustra or sacculations. Small protrusions, approximately 0.5 mm in diameter, can be seen on the mucosa in this section of colon. These cauliflower-like protrusions have been termed *'warzen'* (warts) and are believed to be unique

Figure 1.2. The activity of the digestive system during excretion of hard and soft faeces. The motility and function of the hindgut gut can change depending on the type of faeces that are formed within the colon. The formation of hard faeces is known as the **hard faeces phase** and the expulsion of caecotrophs is known as the **soft faeces phase**. The phases of excretion follow a marked circadian rhythm. The hard faeces phase is shown in black. The soft faeces phase is shown in green. Exchange of water, electrolytes and nutrients across the intestinal epithelium alter with the phase of faeces excretion. The direction of water and electrolyte exchange is indicated by arrows.

The proximal part of the ascending colon is able to separate digesta into two fractions that are simultaneously sent in opposite directions. During the hard faeces phase, water is secreted into the proximal colon and the intestinal contents are thoroughly mixed by contractions of the caecum and colon. Large indigestible particles (> 0.5 mm) tend to accumulate in the lumen of the proximal part of the ascending colon and are moved distally, whereas smaller particles accumulate at the circumference in the sac-like *haustra. Haustrum* is the latin term for a pump. Haustral activity sends the small particles and fluid proximally into the caecum where bacterial fermentation takes place. The indigestible fraction, composed of large particles, is moved rapidly through the proximal colon to the *fusus coli* and distal colon where it is formed into hard, round, dry pellets that are excreted from the anus. Rhythmic caecal contractility is greatest during the hard faeces phase.

Periodically, the motility of the caecum and proximal colon alters completely. Haustral activity ceases, the caecum contracts sending caecal material swiftly along the large intestine. In the *fusus coli* the material is formed into soft pellets that become encapsulated in mucus (see Plate 22). This is the soft faeces phase of excretion when caecotrophs pass through the colon to be expelled from the anus. Expulsion of caecotrophs coincides with a decrease in rhythmic motility of the caecum and proximal colon, and increase in motility of the distal colon. Soft faeces or caecotrophs are expelled one or twice daily, at least four hours after feeding, usually during periods of rest.

The transit time for soft faeces through the colon is 1.5–2.5 times faster than for hard faeces. Motility in the upper gastrointestinal tract remains the same during the hard and soft faeces phases. The differences in colonic motility during the hard and soft faeces phase of excretion are most pronounced in the second section of proximal colon that has a single row of *haustra*.

The *fusus coli* is a specially adapted area of the colon that acts as a differential pacemaker for the initiation of peristaltic waves in the proximal and distal colon that alter with the phase of faeces excretion. The *fusus coli* is highly innervated and is influenced by hormones such as aldosterone and prostaglandins. During the hard faeces phase, the intestinal contents lose considerable quantities of water, potassium and sodium during their passage through the *fusus coli.* Water is mechanically squeezed out of the fibrous material before it passes to the distal colon where absorption of water, volatile fatty acids and electrolytes continues leaving the residue of dry, indigestible matter that is expelled as hard faecal pellets.

to lagomorphs. They represent an increase in the surface area of the colon that would favour increased absorption. The protrusions may also assist mechanical separation of intestinal contents. Histologically, the muscular layers of the taenia contain many autonomic fibres that are part of the myenteric plexus (Snipes *et al.*, 1982). The second section of ascending colon is approximately 20 cm in length and has a single taenia and fewer, smaller haustra. There is an abundance of myenteric plexus in this region. The third portion of the ascending colon is termed the *fusus coli* and is a muscular area about 4 cm long (see Plate 22). This area is highly innervated and vascular. The mucosal surface of the *fusus coli* is distinguished by prominent longitudinal folds and contains numerous goblet cells. The *fusus coli* opens into the fourth section of ascending colon that is histologically indistinguishable from the transverse and descending colon. Because the *fusus coli* forms such a natural division between two morphologically and functionally distinct sections of the rabbit colon, many physiological texts have abandoned the traditional description of ascending, transverse and descending colon and use the terms 'proximal' and 'distal' colon instead (Snipes *et al.*, 1982). The proximal colon includes the three taeniae section, the single taenia section and the *fusus coli*. The distal colon is 80–100 cm long and runs from the *fusus coli* to the rectum. The mucosa of the distal colon is smooth with no surface specialization. The tunica mucosa possesses short crypts with numerous goblet cells reaching into the base. This section of the colon is thin walled and usually contains hard faecal pellets.

1.5.3.1 Motility of the hindgut

The motility and function of the hindgut gut can change depending on the type of faeces that are formed within the colon. The formation of hard faeces is known as the hard faeces phase and coincides with feeding activity. The expulsion of caecotrophs is known as the soft faeces phase. The phases of excretion follow a marked circadian rhythm. In caged rabbits with *ad lib* access to food, feed intake increases from 15.00 to 18.00 h and remains high until midnight. Intake then reduces until 02.00 when a new phase starts with a maximum at 06.00 ending at 08.00 when the soft faeces phase begins. This natural pattern of feeding behaviour and faecal excretion can be seen in pet rabbits, although it may be altered by type and availability of food, age, pregnancy and lactation (Carabaõ and Piquer, 1998).

During the hard faeces phase, water is secreted into the proximal colon, which aids the process of mixture and separation. Intestinal contents are thoroughly mixed by contractions of the caecum and colon that separate the digesta into large indigestible particles, and small particles including bacteria and water-soluble components. The indigestible fraction is moved rapidly through the proximal colon to the *fusus coli* and distal colon before being excreted from the anus. The fermentable fraction is moved in a retrograde direction back into the caecum. The large indigestible particles (> 0.5 mm) tend to accumulate in the lumen of the proximal part of the ascending colon and are moved distally, whereas smaller fermentable particles accumulate at the circumference in the sac-like haustra. Haustral activity sends the small particles proximally into the caecum. Caecal contractility is greatest during the hard faeces phase when the liquid intestinal contents are mixed and separated in the proximal colon. Periodically, the motility of the caecum and proximal colon alters completely. Haustral activity ceases and caecal material is moved swiftly along the large colon. In the *fusus coli* the material is then separated into pellets that become encapsulated in mucus. This is the soft faeces phase of excretion. Soft faeces or caecotrophs are expelled at least 4 h after feeding, usually during periods of rest.

The *fusus coli* is a specially adapted area of the colon that acts as a differential pacemaker for the initiation of peristaltic waves in the proximal and distal colon (Ruckesbusch and Fioramonti, 1976). The nature and direction of the peristaltic waves alter with the phase of faeces excretion. The *fusus coli* is highly innervated and is influenced by hormones such as aldosterone and prostaglandins. During hard faeces production aldosterone levels are high, but they fall during the soft faeces phase of excretion. Prostaglandins inhibit motility of the proximal colon and stimulate the distal colon aiding the elimination of soft faeces or caecotrophs (Pairet *et al.*, 1986).

Three types of contractions occur in the proximal colon. Haustral activity results from high frequency repetitive contractions of the haustral walls that last about 3 seconds and coincide with orally migrating shallow annular constrictions. Segmental activity is the result of low frequency deep annular constrictions that move aborally and last about 14 seconds. The third type of contraction of the proximal colon is a monophasic progressive wave of peristaltic contractions. These peristaltic contractions last about 5 seconds during the hard faeces phase and 1.5 seconds during the soft faeces phase (Ehrlein *et al.*, 1982). Expulsion of caecotrophs coincides with a decrease in motility of the caecum and proximal colon and increase in motility of the distal colon. The transit time for caecotrophs through the colon is 1.5–2.5 time faster than for hard faeces (Fiaromonti and Ruckesbusch, 1976). Motility in the upper gastrointestinal tract remains the same during the hard and soft faeces phases with slow contractions of the small intestine occurring every 10–15 minutes (Ruckesbusch *et al.*, 1985). The differences in colonic motility during the hard and soft faeces phase of excretion are most pronounced in the second section of proximal colon that has a single layer of haustra.

During the hard faeces phase, the intestinal contents lose considerable quantities of water, potassium and sodium during their passage through the *fusus coli* (Snipes *et al.*, 1982). The compression of intestinal contents into faecal pellets during the hard faeces phase can be correlated with the strong muscular wall of the *fusus coli* and its dense innervation. Water is mechanically squeezed out of the fibrous material before it passes to the distal colon where absorption of water, volatile fatty acids and electrolytes continues, leaving a residue of dry, indigestible matter that is expelled as hard, dry faecal pellets.

1.5.3.2 Caecal fermentation

The end products of digestion in the stomach and small intestine are separated in the colon into two components: small particles that can act as a substrate for caecal microorganisms and large particles of indigestible lignified material. Small particles are propelled into the caecum, which acts as a huge bacterial fermentation chamber to which nutrients and water are continually added. Studies of the enzymatic activities of the caecal microflora indicate that ammonia use, ureolysis, proteolysis, and cellulysis take place in that order. Xylanolysis and pectinolysis also occur (Carabaõ and Piquer, 1998). The intestinal contents that reach the hindgut are composed of undigested food, excretion products and substances produced by the digestive tract itself. Small particles of complex carbohydrates such as oligosaccharides, cellulose, hemicellulose and pectins that are not digested in the small intestine reach the caecum for bacterial degradation. Plant proteins that are bound to cell wall constituents are also degraded in the caecum to form ammonia that is metabolized to amino acids by the caecal microflora. Products of intestinal cellular desquamation and digestive enzymes act as a nitrogen source for protein synthesis (Fraga, 1998). Soluble ions such as urea are osmotically transferred across the caecal wall to be metabolized. High protein diets increase blood urea levels and increase caecal ammonia levels (Fraga, 1998). During periods of protein deprivation, urea from catabolism passes into the caecum to provide a nitrogen source for bacterial amino acid synthesis (Fekete, 1989). Mucopolysaccharides secreted from goblet cells in the mucosa serve as a significant carbohydrate source for caecal fermentation. *Bacteroides* spp. ferment mucopolysaccharides (Cheeke, 1987).

In healthy rabbits, high numbers of large anaerobic metachromatic bacteria are present in the caecum (Lelkes and Chang, 1987). Non-pathogenic, gram-negative *Bacteroides* spp. predominate in a flora composed of a wide variety of gram-positive and gram-negative rods, cocci, filaments, coccobacilli and spirochaetes. Species such as *Bifidobacterium, Endophorus, Clostridium, Streptococcus* and *Acuformis* have been identified (Cheeke, 1987; Carabaõ and Piquer, 1998). Over 74 strains of anaerobic bacteria have been isolated from the caecal mucosa and many of these species have not been identified (Straw, 1988). *Lactobacillus* and *E. coli* spp. are usually absent from the normal gut flora of adult rabbits but may be found in rabbits fed on a high carbohydrate, low fibre diet. The intestinal flora contains many non-pathogenic protozoa. *Entamoeba cuniculi* is a large sluggish amoeba that is found in large numbers in the lumen of the large intestine. The flagellate, *Giardia duodenalis* can be found in the duodenum but does not cause clinical disease. *Eutrichomastix, Enteromonas* and *Retortamonas* spp. are non-pathogenic protozoa found in the caecum (Owen, 1992).

Volatile fatty acids are produced by the caecal microflora and absorbed across the caecal epithelium as an energy source for the rabbit. Caecal contents contain 60–70% acetic acid, 15–20% butyric acid and 10–15% propri-onic acid, although the ratios of volatile fatty acids can change in relation to the fibre content of the diet. The caecal epithelium has a high electrolyte transport capacity suited to the absorption of the large quantities of electrolytes that are present in the luminal fluid (Clauss *et al.*, 1989). The appendix secretes an alkaline fluid rich in bicarbonate ions that buffer volatile fatty acids produced by caecal fermentation. The appendix also contains lymphoid tissue.

The composition of the caecal microflora does not remain constant and is affected by time of day, age and diet. Caecal pH shows a diurnal rhythm similar to feeding behaviour and is most alkaline in the morning and most acid in mid afternoon (Brewer and Cruise, 1994). Fluctuations in caecal pH have an effect on the population of caecal microorganisms. Ammonia and volatile fatty acids produced by caecal degradation and fermentation affect caecal pH. Like any continuous culture system, there are a number of homeostatic mechanisms in place. Bicarbonate secreted from the appendix acts as a buffer. Other substances such as fibre also have a buffering capacity dependent on the carboxyl, amino and hydroxyl groups (Gidenne *et al.*, 1998). The rate of production and absorption of volatile fatty acids is dependent on type and availability of substrate. Gut motility affects the supply of nutrients and water for microbial fermentation and the absorption of nutrients. Energy appears to be the most limiting factor for optimum microbial activity (Fraga, 1998).

1.5.3.3 Expulsion and ingestion of caecotrophs

Bacterial fermentation within the caecum results in synthesis of amino acids, volatile fatty acids and water-soluble vitamins. Some nutrients produced by the caecal microflora are absorbed across the caecal wall. The remaining contents of the caecum form a soft, dark-coloured paste rich in bacteria, amino acids, vitamins and minerals. The paste is expelled as soft faeces or caecotrophs. Caecal contents pass into the colon rapidly without mechanical separation of solids and liquid and the faecal masses are divided in the *fusus coli* (see Plate 22). Lysozyme is secreted into the lumen of the distal colon during the soft faeces phase (Camara and Prieur, 1984) and incorporated into caecotrophs. The glandular portion of the *fusus coli* is instrumental in lubricating the intestinal surface of the colon facilitating the rapid transport of intestinal contents. Goblet cells secrete mucus which encapsulates the pellets and inhibits the diffusion of electrolytes. In this way, large masses of pelleted caecal contents are produced which are expelled as intermittent bunches of caecotrophs.

In healthy rabbits, caecotrophs are consumed straight from the anus and are swallowed whole. Stimulation of rectal mechanoreceptors, the perception of the specific odour of the soft faeces and the blood concentrations of various metabolites and hormones trigger the ingestion of caecotrophs from the anus (Fekete, 1989). When food is scarce, all caecotrophs are consumed. When food is available *ad libitum*, the protein and fibre content of the ration influence the amount of caecotrophs consumed. Increased levels of fibre increase caecotrophy whereas high protein levels reduce it.

Key points 1.2

- The gastrointestinal system of the rabbit is adapted for the digestion of large quantities of fibrous food
- Rabbits are hindgut fermenters with a large caecum that periodically expels its contents into the colon. Microbial fermentation in the caecum results in the formation of a soft paste containing amino acids, volatile fatty acids, microorganisms and vitamins
- Mucous encapsulated pellets of the soft caecal material or 'caecotrophs' are ingested as they emerge from the anus and subsequently digested to supply an additional source of nutrients. This process is known as caecotrophy

- Digestion in the stomach and small intestine is similar to other monogastric animals
- The colon of the rabbit is adapted to mix and separate large indigestible fibre particles from small digestible fragments and fluid
- The indigestible and digestible fibre components of the diet are simultaneously propelled in opposite directions in the proximal colon
- Periodically, the pattern of motility in the large intestine and caecum changes completely to expel caecal contents as caecotrophs
- A specially adapted area of the colon, the *fusus coli*, acts as a pacemaker to control colonic motility. The *fusus coli* is highly innervated and vascular and is influenced by blood metabolites and hormones such as prostaglandins and aldosterone
- Small particles and fluid are directed in a retrograde direction from the proximal colon to the large caecum where bacterial fermentation takes place. Volatile fatty acids are the products of bacterial fermentation
- The substrate for caecal fermentation is composed of undigested food that reaches the colon plus excretion products, and substances such as mucopolysaccharides and desquamated cells from the digestive tract
- Urea can diffuse into the caecum from the bloodstream to act as a nitrogen source for the caecal bacteria
- The population of microorganisms within the caecum is finely balanced and changes with the time of day, caecal pH, and dietary substrate
- Long particles of undigested fibre are propelled through the distal colon and expelled as hard faeces. Absorption and secretion of water, electrolytes and volatile fatty acids in the large intestine alter according to the type of faeces that is passing through
- Indigestible fibre stimulates intestinal motility.

1.6 Metabolism

1.6.1 Energy metabolism

Volatile fatty acids provide an energy source for herbivorous species, such as rabbits, that utilize bacterial fermentation as part of the digestive process. The proportion and type of volatile fatty acids that are produced depend on the substrate that is metabolized and the species of bacteria that are present. In ruminants, the predominant volatile fatty acid is proprionate, which is produced by *Lactobacillus* species that are present in the rumen but are absent from the rabbit caecal microflora (Cheeke, 1987). In rabbits, acetates predominate followed by butyrate and proprionate with small quantities of isobutyrate, isovalerate and valerate. Increased amounts of fibre in the diet increase the proportion of acetate that is produced. Lactate is produced by bacterial fermentation within the caecotroph in the stomach and is subsequently absorbed during digestion of the caecotroph in the small intestine.

Considerable energy is required by the hindgut for the metabolism and absorption of volatile fatty acids, electrolytes and other nutrients. This energy is mainly supplied by butyrate produced by *Bacteroides* spp. that predominate in the caecal microflora. Rabbit caecal-colonic epithelial tissue metabolizes butyrate without the production of ketone bodies. Volatile fatty acids absorbed from intestinal tract provide a regular energy source for the rabbit. Lactate enters the portal circulation from the stomach and small intestine while volatile fatty acids originate from the hindgut. Net absorption from the digestive tract is greatest during the hard faeces phase, which is matched by increased hepatic metabolism and the removal of propionate and butyrate from the circulation, leaving acetate and lactate available for extra-hepatic tissue metabolism (Carabaõ and Piquer, 1998). Due to alterations in hepatic metabolism, arterial concentrations of volatile fatty acids remain constant during both hard and soft phases of excretion, although their absorption and metabolism follow a circadian rhythm parallel to the activity of the adrenal gland (Vernay, 1987).

1.6.2 Water metabolism

Rabbits normally drink 50–100 ml/kg/24 h (Brewer and Cruise, 1994) although this quantity is affected by the water content and composition of the diet. The complex digestive processes of the rabbit require water to be continually absorbed and secreted along the gastrointestinal tract. Saliva is continuously secreted into the mouth and water is secreted into the stomach. In the caecum, water is absorbed from the contents, which contain 20–25% dry matter (Fekete, 1989). In the colon, absorption or secretion of water varies in each section of the colon and depends on whether hard or soft faeces are being formed. During the soft faeces phase, caecal contents pass through the colon with relatively little change in composition. During the hard faeces phase water is secreted into the proximal colon and mixed with intestinal contents. The water content of the digesta is highest immediately before the *fusus coli* and decreases sharply during the passage through the fusus and along the distal colon (Snipes *et al.*, 1982). The complex exchange of water across the intestinal wall permits changes in hydration status without obvious fluid loss.

The rabbit kidney differs from other mammalian species. In common with neonates and amphibians, there is a wide variation in the number of glomeruli that are active at any one time. Hydration, uncomplicated by vasoconstriction, leads to a marked increase in glomerular activity. As much as a 16-fold increase in water diuresis is possible without significant change in glomerular filtration rate. When blood pressure is increased, there is little or no change in renal plasma flow (Brewer and Cruise, 1994).

1.6.3 Electrolyte exchange

The absorption and secretion of electrolytes along the intestinal tract of the rabbit is complex. Saliva is continually formed by a two-stage process in which an isotonic fluid with a constant, plasma-like electrolyte composition is modified in the salivary glands (Fekete, 1989). Sodium and chloride are resorbed and potassium and bicarbonate are secreted.

Bicarbonate is secreted into the duodenum and absorbed from the jejunum in which there is an inter-relationship between bicarbonate secretion and sodium and chloride absorption. The caecal appendix secretes an alkaline fluid rich in bicarbonate that is also secreted in the proximal colon to moderate the rising pH due to volatile fatty acid production (Fekete, 1989).

The transport of electrolytes across the colonic wall is regulated by aldosterone and is related to the type of faeces that is being produced. During the soft faeces phase, aldosterone concentrations are at their lowest and water, sodium and chloride are secreted while potassium is conserved. During the hard faeces phase, water and bicarbonate are secreted into the proximal colon and water, volatile fatty acids, sodium, potassium and chloride are absorbed from the distal colon thereby conserving water and electrolytes (Cheeke, 1987).

1.6.4 Acid–base balance

The renal regulation of acid–base balance is different in rabbits in comparison with other domestic species. Rabbits have a limited ability to transfer hydrogen or bicarbonate ions between blood and urine because some metabolic pathways that are present in other species are absent or restricted. The enzyme carbonic anhydrase is absent from the thick ascending limb of the renal tubule of rabbits (Dobyan *et al.*, 1982; Brewer and Cruise, 1994). In other species such as humans, monkeys and rats, carbonic anhydrase is present in the ascending tubule epithelial cells in large amounts. The enzyme is required for the rapid formation of carbonic acid that is an important step in the excretion of hydrogen ions and conservation of bicarbonate.

In other mammals, ammonia is produced in the kidney by glutamine deamination in response to a fall in plasma pH or a decreased concentration of bicarbonate. Ammonia acts as part of the buffering system in the renal tubule by combining with hydrogen ions before being excreted in the urine as ammonium ions. In rabbits, glutamine deamination only takes place in response to reduced serum bicarbonate concentrations but not a drop in plasma pH, which compromises the rabbit's response to metabolic acidosis. In other species there are alternative biochemical pathways that result in ammonia synthesis but these pathways appear to be absent in the rabbit (Brewer and Cruise, 1994).

The rabbit also has problems correcting alkalosis. A large bicarbonate load can reach the kidney of rabbits as a result of bacterial fermentation in the gut and from tissue metabolism of acetate. In other species, bicarbonate is neutralized by the products of ureagenesis and alkalosis is avoided. In rabbits, insufficient ammonium may be available from tissue metabolism to neutralize bicarbonate, especially during periods of protein deficit (Brewer and Cruise, 1994). Alkaline secretion into the gut increases in response to metabolic alkalosis (Vattay *et al.*, 1989).

1.6.5 Calcium metabolism

Rabbits have an unusual calcium metabolism. It is characterized by total serum calcium concentrations that vary over a wide range and are 30–50% higher than other mammalian species (Buss and Bourdeau, 1984). Total serum calcium concentrations can reflect dietary calcium intake (Chapin and Smith, 1967a, b). Hypocalcaemia is rare, although lactation tetany can occur in nursing does (Barlet, 1980). Experimentally, hypocalcaemic tetany can be induced by parathyroidectomy (Tan *et al.*, 1987) or by feeding diets deficient in calcium or vitamin D (Chapin and Smith, 1967a; Bourdeau *et al.*, 1986).

It is not clear why rabbits have higher blood calcium levels than other species. Their calcium metabolism has been studied extensively. Experimentally, hypocalcaemia or hypercalcaemia can be brought about by the infusion of EDTA or calcium gluconate. Reciprocal elevations in PTH or calcitonin in response to EDTA or calcium gluconate infusion indicates that these hormones regulate serum calcium concentrations in rabbits as in other species (Warren *et al.*, 1989; Bourdeau *et al.*, 1986). However, rabbits appear to differ from humans in the level at which serum ionized calcium is set to initiate a parathyroid hormone (PTH) response (Warren *et al.*, 1989). An analogy has been made with the syndrome of benign familial hypercalcaemia in humans that is a genetic condition characterized by hypercalcaemia without changes in renal function, blood pressure or any other potential sequels to chronic hypercalcaemia such as soft tissue mineralization.

Not only do rabbits have higher total serum calcium concentrations than other species but they are also different in the way calcium is absorbed from the gut and excreted by the kidney. Calcium can be absorbed from the intestinal tract either by passive diffusion or by active transport across the mucosa. Active transportation involves a carrier protein that is synthesized in the intestinal mucosa in response to 1,25-dihydroxyvitamin D_3, the active metabolite of vitamin D. A drop in serum calcium concentration stimulates PTH release which, in turn, stimulates the conversion of biologically inert 25-dihydroxyvitamin D_3 to 1,25-dihydroxyvitamin D_3 in the kidney, thereby indirectly increasing the absorption of calcium from the intestine.

Calcium is not only absorbed from the gastrointestinal tract, it is also secreted into the gut across the intestinal mucosa. This process is independent of serum calcium concentrations and can take place in a hypocalcaemic animal. It has been demonstrated that secretion of calcium into the gut continues during periods of calcium deprivation in rabbits (Barr *et al.*, 1991).

In rabbits, passive intestinal absorption of calcium is efficient. If dietary calcium concentrations are adequate, it appears that vitamin D is not required for calcium absorption (Bourdeau *et al.*, 1986; Kamphues, 1991). However, vitamin D increases intestinal absorption of calcium and is required if dietary calcium levels are low (Brommage *et al.*, 1988). Because it is absorbed passively, there is no feedback mechanism and calcium is absorbed in proportion to the dietary calcium concentration (Cheeke and Amberg, 1973). Blood calcium concentrations increase if dietary calcium levels are elevated.

The rabbit kidney is capable of excreting or conserving calcium according to metabolic need. Responses are mediated by PTH and 1,25-dihydroxyvitamin D_3 (Bourdeau *et al.*, 1988). Tubular reabsorption of calcium by the kidney increases during periods of calcium deprivation (Bourdeau and Lau, 1992). During periods of high calcium intake the rabbit kidney is capable of increasing the fractional excretion of calcium into the urine considerably (Whiting and Quamme, 1984).

The excretion rates of calcium are proportional to dietary intake (Kennedy, 1965). Calcium precipitates as calcium carbonate in the alkaline urine of rabbits and high dietary calcium intake results in large amounts of urinary sediment. Normal rabbit urine is turbid due to the presence of calcium carbonate. Pregnant, lactating or growing rabbits or those that are anorexic or on a calcium deficient diet can excrete clear urine.

There appears to be a difference in calcium metabolism in immature and mature rabbits. Serum calcium concentrations are not as variable in growing rabbits as in mature rabbits (Kamphues *et al.*, 1986; Gilsanz *et al.*, 1991). Immature rabbits on forced high dietary calcium concentrations do not develop soft tissue calcification like their adult counterparts (Kamphues *et al.*, 1986).

1.7 Thermoregulation

Rabbits are unable to sweat or pant effectively to dissipate body heat. The main thermoregulatory mechanism is by heat exchange in the ears that have a large arteriovenous anastomotic system. In the nose, the nasal glands moisten inspired air, which also has a role in thermoregulation. Rabbits are unable to tolerate high ambient temperatures, which can prove fatal.

1.8 Diurnal rhythms

Many behavioural and physiological processes of rabbits show a marked diurnal rhythm. In the late afternoon wild rabbits emerge from their burrows to feed, explore, socialize and mate. Grazing resumes during the early morning before the rabbit returns to the warren. Hard faecal pellets are voided during these periods above ground. During the day, caecotrophy takes place while the rabbit is resting in the burrow, typically between 08.00 and 17.00 h. Female rabbits give birth in the morning and feed their young at night (McBride, 1988). Domesticated rabbits also follow a natural daily rhythm. Laboratory rabbits that are fed *ad lib* consume little food between 06.00 h and midday and increase their intake between 17.00 h and midnight, eating most food during the night. Caecotrophs are expelled during periods of minimal feed intake in the morning and sometimes during the evening. If food is restricted, caecotrophs are excreted approximately 5 h after a meal. If a collar is fitted to prevent the ingestion of caecotrophs, feeding still ceases during caecotroph excretion suggesting that cessation of food intake is not associated with gastric filling (Hörnicke *et al.*, 1984).

The diurnal feeding pattern affects digestive processes and caecal motility which also follow a circadian rhythm. Ingestion of food is associated with increased caecal motility and the excretion of hard faeces. Caecotrophy is associated with a decline in caecal contractions so caecal contractions are at a maximum when the animal is feeding. If food is withheld completely, the circadian rhythm of caecal contractions is maintained, but at a lower frequency that does not correlate with soft or hard faeces production (Hörnicke *et al.*, 1984). Absorption of volatile fatty acids and their metabolism in the liver shows a circadian rhythm parallel to the activity of the adrenal gland. Volatile fatty acid absorption into the portal circulation is greatest during the hard faeces phase of digestion, although arterial levels remain remarkably constant (Vernay, 1987). Bile acid production shows a circadian rhythm (Fekete, 1989). There is a diurnal variation in haematological values (Fox and Laird, 1970) with lowest total white blood cell and lymphocyte counts occurring in the late afternoon and evening in association with increased neutrophil counts. Eosinophil counts peak during the afternoon with the lowest values occurring in the morning. Blood urea nitrogen shows a diurnal variation that is linked with feeding patterns. Even body temperature follows a 24-h cycle (Lazurus-Balow, 1928).

Key points 1.3

- Some metabolic processes in rabbits differ from other mammalian species
- The absorption and secretion of water and electrolytes along the intestinal tract is complex
- Some of the metabolic pathways that correct acid–base disorders are absent from the rabbit kidney
- In rabbits, calcium homeostasis is mainly regulated by the kidney, which is capable of both conserving calcium

and excreting large amounts of calcium into the urine

- Calcium is absorbed readily from the intestine in proportion to dietary concentrations
- Blood calcium levels in rabbits are higher and not as closely homeostatically maintained as in other species
- Excreted calcium forms calcium carbonate precipitates in the alkaline urine of rabbits. Normal rabbit urine is turbid. Growing, lactating, pregnant or acidotic rabbits may excrete clear urine
- Serum calcium concentrations of growing rabbits are not as variable as in mature rabbits
- Rabbits cannot dissipate heat efficiently and are susceptible to heat stroke
- Many behavioural and physiological processes of rabbits show a marked diurnal pattern.

References

Adams, C.E. (1987). The laboratory rabbit. In *The UFAW Handbook on The Care and Management of Laboratory Animals*, 6th edn. pp 415–436. Longman Scientific and Technical.

Barlet, J.P. (1980). Plasma calcium, inorganic phosphorus and magnesium levels in pregnant and lactating rabbits. *Reprod Nutr Develop.*, **20**, 647–651.

Barone, R., Pavaux, C., Blin, P.C., Cuq, P. (1973). *Atlas d'anotomie du lapin*. Masson et Cie.

Barone, R. (1997). *Anatomie comparée des mammifères domestiques*. (French text). Vigot.

Barr, D.R., Sadowski, D.L., Hu, J., Bourdeau J.E. (1991). Characterisation of the renal and intestinal adaptations to dietary calcium deprivation in growing female rabbits. *Miner Electrolyte Metab.*, **17**, 32–40.

Blood, D.C., Studdert, V.P., (1999). *Ballieres Comprehensive Veterinary Dictionary*, 2nd edn. Balliere Tindall.

Bourdeau, J.E., Shwer-Dymerski, D.A., Stern, P.A., Langman, C.B. (1986). Calcium and phosphorous metabolism in chronically Vitamin D-deficient laboratory rabbits. *Miner Electrolyte Metabol.*, **12**, 176–185.

Bourdeau, J.E., Bouillon, R., Zikos, D., Langman, C.B. (1988). Renal responses to calcium deprivation in young rabbits. *Miner Electrolyte Metabol.*, **14**, 150–157.

Bourdeau, J.E., Lau, K. (1992). Regulation of cystosolic free calcium concentration in the rabbit connecting tubule: a calcium absorbing renal epithelium. *J Lab Clin Med.*, **119**, 650–662.

Brewer, N.R., Cruise, L.J. (1994). Physiology. In *The Biology of the Laboratory Rabbit*, 2nd edn. (P.J. Manning, D.H. Ringler, C.E. Newcomer, eds). pp 63–70. Academic Press.

Brommage, R., Miller, S.C., Langman, C.B. *et al.* (1988). The effect of chronic vitamin D deficiency on the skeleton in the adult rabbit. *Bone*, **9**, 131.

Buss, S.L., Bourdeau, J.E. (1984). Calcium balance in laboratory rabbits. *Miner Electrolyte Metabol.*, **10**, 127–132.

Camara, V.M., Prieur. D.J. (1984). Secretion of colonic isozyme of lysozyme in association with cecotrophy of rabbits (Abstract). *Am J Physiol.*, **247**, G19–23.

Carabaõ, R., Piquer, J. (1998). The digestive system of the rabbit. In *The Nutrition of the Rabbit*. (C. de Blas and J. Wiseman, eds). pp 1–16. CABI Publishing.

Chapin, R.E., Smith, S.E. (1967a). Calcium requirement of growing rabbits. *J Anim Sci.*, **26**, 67–71.

Chapin, R.E., Smith, S.E. (1967b). The calcium tolerance of growing rabbits. *Cornell Vet.*, **57**, 492–500.

Cheeke, P.R. (1987). *Rabbit Feeding and Nutrition*. Academic Press.

Cheeke, P.R., Amberg, J.W. (1973). Comparative calcium excretion by rats and rabbits. *J Anim Sci.*, **37**, 450.

Clauss, W., Hoffmann, B., Schafer, H., Hornicke, H. (1989). Ion transport and electrophysiology in rabbit cecum (Abstract). *Am J Physiol.*, **256**, G1090–G1099.

Cruise, L.J., Brewer, N.R. (1994). Anatomy. In *The Biology of the Laboratory Rabbit*, 2nd edn. (P.J. Manning, D.H. Ringler, C.E. Newcomer, eds). pp 47–60. Academic Press.

De Blas, E., Gidenne, T. (1998). Digestion of starch and sugars. In *The Nutrition of the Rabbit*. (C. de Blas and J. Wiseman, eds). pp 17–38. CABI Publishing.

Dobyan, D.C., Magill, L.S., Friedman, P.A. *et al.* (1982). Carbonic anhydrase histochemistry in rabbit and mouse kidneys (Abstract). *Anat Rec.*, **204**, 185–197.

Donnelly, T.M. (1997). Basic anatomy, physiology and husbandry. In *Ferrets, Rabbits and Rodents, Clinical Medicine and Surgery*. (E.V. Hillyer, K.E. Quesenberry, eds). pp 147–159. W.B. Saunders.

Ehrlein, H.J., Reich, H., Schwinger, M. (1982). Physiological significance of the contractions of the rabbit proximal colon (Abstract). *Q J Exp Physiol.*, **67**, 407–417.

Fekete, S. (1989). Recent findings and future perspectives of digestive physiology in rabbits: a review. *Acta Vet Hung.*, **37**, 265–279.

Fekete, S., Huszenicza, G. (1993). Effects of T-2 toxin on ovarian activity and some metabolic variables of rabbits. *Lab Anim Sci.*, **43**, 646–649.

Fioramonti, J., Ruckesbusch, Y. (1976). Caecal motility in the rabbit. III Duality of faecal excretion (Article in French, English summary). *Ann Rech Vet.*, **7**, 281–295.

Fox, R.R., Laird, C.W. (1970). Biochemical parameters of clinical significance in rabbits. II. Diurnal variations. *J Hered.*, **61**, 261–265.

Fraga, M.J. (1998). Protein requirements. In *The Nutrition of the Rabbit*. (C. de Blas and J. Wiseman, eds). pp 133–144. CABI Publishing.

Gidenne, T., Carabaõ, R., García, J., de Blas, C. (1998). Fibre Digestion. In *The Nutrition of the Rabbit*. (C. de Blas, J. Wiseman, eds). pp 69–88. CABI Publishing.

Gilsanz, V., Roe, T.F., Antunes, J., Carlson, M. *et al.*

(1991). Effect of dietary calcium on bone density in growing rabbits. *Am J Physiol.*, **260**, E471–E476.
Harkness, J.E. (1987). Rabbit husbandry and medicine. *Vet Clin N Am: Small Anim Pract.*, **17**, 1019–1044.
Hirschfield, Z., Weinrab, M.M., Michaeli, Y. (1973). Incisors of the rabbit: morphology, histology and development. *J. Dent. Res.*, **52**, 377–384.
Hörnicke, H., Ruoff, G., Vogt, B. *et al.* (1984). Phase relationship of the circadian rhythms of feed intake, caecal motility and production of soft and hard faeces in domestic rabbits. *Lab Anim.*, **18**, 169–172.
Kamphues, J. (1991). Calcium metabolism of rabbits as an etiological factor for urolithiasis. *J Nutr.*, **121**, S95–S96.
Kamphues, V.J., Carstensen, P. Schroeder, D. *et al.* (1986). Effect of increasing calcium and Vitamin D supply on calcium metabolism in rabbits (Article in German. English summary) *J Anim Physiol Nutr.*, **50**, 191–208.
Kennedy, A. (1965). The urinary excretion of calcium by normal rabbits. *J Comp Path.*, **75**, 69–74.
Lang, J. (1981). The nutrition of the commercial rabbit. Part 1. Physiology, digestibility and nutrient requirements. *Nutr abstr rev, Series B*, **51**, 197–217.
Lazarus-Balow, P. (1928) The temperature of normal rabbits. *J Pathol Bacteriol.*, **31**, 517–524.
Lelkes, L., Chang, C.L. (1987). Microbial dysbiosis in rabbit mucoid enteropathy. *Lab Anim Sci.*, **36**, 757–764.
Lockley, R.M. (1978). *The Private Life of the Rabbit.* Andre Deutsch Ltd.
McBride, A. (1988) *Rabbits and Hares.* Whittet Books Ltd.
Nowak, R.M. (1999). Order Lagomorpha. In *Walker's Mammals of the World. Volume II,.* 6th edn. pp 1715–1738. The Johns Hopkins University Press.
Owen, D.G. (1992). *Parasites of Laboratory Animals. Laboratory Animal Handbooks No 12.* Royal Society of Medicine Services Ltd.
Pairet, M., Bouyssou, T., Ruckesbusch, Y. (1986). Colonic formation of soft feces in rabbits: a role for endogenous prostaglandins. (Abstract). *Am J Physiol.*, **250**, G302–G308.
Patton, N.M. (1994). Colony husbandry. In *The Biology of the Laboratory Rabbit.* 2nd edn. (P.J. Manning, D.H. Ringler, C.E. Newcomer, eds). pp 28–44. Academic Press.
Percy, D.H. and Barthold, S.W. (1993). Rabbit. In *Pathology of Laboratory Rodents and Rabbits.* pp 179–223. Iowa State University Press.
Ruckesbusch, Y., Fioramonti, J. (1976). The *fusus coli* of the rabbit as a pacemaker area. *Experientia*, **32**, 1023–1024.
Ruckesbusch, Y., Pairet, M., Becht, J.L. (1985). Origin and characterization of migrating myoelectric complex in rabbits (Abstract). *Dig Dis Sci.*, **30**, 742–748.
Sandford, J.C. (1996). *The Domestic Rabbit*, 5th edn. Blackwell Science.
Shadle, A.R. (1936). The attrition and extrusive growth of the four major incisor teeth of domestic rabbits. *J Mammol.*, **17**, 15–21.
Snipes, R.L., Clauss, W., Weber, A., Hörnicke, H. (1982). Structural and functional differences in various divisions of the rabbit colon. *Cell Tissue Res.*, **225**, 331–346.
Straw, T.E. (1988). Bacteria of the rabbit gut and their role in the health of the rabbit. *J Appl Rabbit Res.*, **11**, 142–146.
Tan, S.Q, Thomas, D, Wellington, J.A.O. *et al.* (1987). Surgical thyroparathyroidectomy of the rabbit. *Am J Physiol.*, **252**, F761–E767.
Vattay, P., Wenzl, E., Feil, W. *et al.* (1989). Role of acid base balance and mucosal blood flow in alkaline secretion of rabbit duodenum (Abstract). *Acta Physiol Hung.*, **73**, 81–87.
Vernay, M. (1987). Origin and utilisation of volatile fatty acids and lactate in the rabbit: influence of the faecal excretion pattern. *Br J Nutr.*, **57**, 371–381.
Warren, H.B., Lausen, N.C., Segre, G.V. *et al.* (1989). Regulation of calciotropic hormones *in vivo* in the New Zealand White rabbit. *Endocrinology*, **125**, 2683–2689.
Whiting, S.J., Quamme, G.A. (1984). Effects of dietary calcium on renal calcium, magnesium and phosphate excretion by the rabbit. *Mine. Electrolyte Metab.*, **10**, 217–221.

Diet and husbandry

2

2.1 Housing

The quiet docile nature of the rabbit combined with its fertility and rapid growth rate has led to its intensive production for commercial and laboratory purposes. Units housing several thousand does are found in countries such as China, Hungary or the USA. At the other end of the scale, in the developing world, a few rabbits are often kept as 'biological refrigerators', i.e. a source of small quantities of meat that is fresh and readily available (Cheeke *et al.*, 1982). The social and behavioural needs of such animals are ignored when they are housed individually in small, wire mesh cages or confined to tiny hutches. There are many welfare implications associated with keeping rabbits in cages, as they are not able to follow their natural instincts. Abnormal behaviour patterns such as stereotypies and restlessness have been recorded. Perpetual wire biting and pawing behaviour has been described in rabbits confined to small cages and does provided with an open nesting box and no bedding material to cover the young (Stauffacher, 1992). A proven link has been established between small cage size and painful conditions such as skeletal disorders or ulcerative pododermatitis in intensively reared rabbits (Drescher, 1993; Drescher and Loeffler, 1996). Morphological differences have been observed in the adrenal glands of rabbits kept in wire cages and those kept in group housing conditions on solid floors (Drescher and Breig, 1993).

In recent years, conditions have improved for many laboratory rabbits. They can be kept in social groups of four to eight animals with no detriment to their health (Turner *et al.*, 1997). It has been proven that rabbits prefer to be in proximity with each other and 'interact with enrichment objects' such as wooden sticks, parrot toys or balls designed for cats (Huls *et al.*, 1991). Keeping rabbits in this way not only benefits the rabbits but also the people looking after them. Love (1994) described the response of animal technicians to group housing by saying they 'found it more agreeable to work with rabbits that came to the front of the cage when they heard the sounds of people, rather than cowering away' and 'it was a pleasure to see the rabbits interact with each other'. Stauffacher (1992) describes in detail many ways in which housing for rabbits can be constructed to permit natural behaviour patterns. Despite these advances, most breeding and exhibition rabbits still live their entire life confined to small cages. Some breeders still insist that rabbits should be kept singly in small cages and that large hutches and runs lead to aggression and behaviour problems (Sandford, 1996). At last, the pet owning fraternity is becoming aware of the rabbit's social nature and need for exercise. There has been a steady increase in the number of house rabbits and the status of the rabbit has shifted from the child's pet to a member of the family. A rabbit can be a satisfactory companion for adults that are out at work all day and find the needs of a dog or cat too demanding. Hopefully the days of keeping pet rabbits in solitary confinement in a barren hutch at the bottom of the garden are now coming to an end. There is legislation governing the welfare of rabbits that is summarized in Box 2.1.

Box 2.1 Legislation governing the welfare of rabbits

There is legislation governing the welfare of farmed rabbits in the UK. The advice also applies to pet rabbits kept in hutches although they are not technically covered by the legislation. Separate legislation governs the transport and slaughter of rabbits. A guide to the legal requirements for farmed rabbits has been produced by UFAW (Universities Federation for Animal Welfare) and can be summarized as follows:

Rabbits must be provided with:
- Adequate lighting to enable the inspection of the animals at any time.
- Wholesome food that is appropriate and in sufficient quantity to maintain good health and satisfy nutritional needs.
- A daily supply of fresh drinking water.
- Suitable accommodation with a suitably bedded floor for the isolation of a sick or injured rabbit.
- Cages of sufficient size to allow the rabbits to move around, feed and drink without difficulty, and allow all the rabbits kept in them to be able to lie on their sides at the same time.
- Cages of sufficient height to allow rabbits to sit upright on all four feet without their ears touching the top of the cage.
- Shelter from bad weather including direct sunlight.
- Daily inspection of all automatic equipment, such as drinkers, by a competent person.
- An alarm on automatic ventilation systems that is independent of the mains electricity and will give warning when the system fails to function properly.
- Daily inspection of stock and the prevention of unnecessary suffering or distress.
- Veterinary care. Prescription only medicines (POM) including antibiotics and vaccines can only be supplied by the veterinary surgeon that has the rabbits in his/her care.

Rabbits have been used as foster mothers for ostrich chicks with benefits for both ostriches and rabbits (Madeiros, 1997). The ostrich chicks and rabbits have a strong affinity for each other. The rabbit provides a mother figure for the ostrich that is introduced as a day old hatchling. By 6–8 weeks the ostrich chick becomes independent.

2.2 Hutches for pet rabbits

Traditionally, pet rabbits are kept in hutches in the garden, shed or garage. Hutches are a convenient method of housing rabbits, but it is important to provide time for exercise each day. At least 4 h daily exercise is required (Richardson, 2000). Longer periods or unrestricted exercise are preferable.

The hutch should be as big as possible, especially if two rabbits are housed together. It needs to be situated in a dry, cool, well-ventilated site protected from wind and rain. Poor ventilation and ammonia build-up predispose to conjunctivitis and respiratory tract infections. It is preferable to situate the hutch against a sheltered wall outside, rather than in an enclosed, stuffy shed or garage. Rabbits are tolerant of cold conditions and can withstand winter weather provided they have shelter and plenty of bedding material. Thin rabbits with no body fat are more susceptible to the effects of cold and need extra protection on cold nights. Hot conditions and direct sunlight with no shade are distressing for rabbits as they cannot sweat or pant effectively. The optimum temperature range for rabbits is 15–20°C, which can be checked with a maximum and minimum thermometer.

Rabbits produce copious quantities of urine and faeces, which are usually deposited in one part of the hutch that should be cleaned once or twice daily. A litter tray, which can be washed and cleaned easily, can be placed in that area of the hutch. Most rabbits will use a litter tray. Many free-range rabbits will return to an open hutch or covered area especially to use their tray. Bedding that is not fouled and remains clean and dry can be left in the hutch. Many types of material can be used as bedding. Garden peat has been recommended to neutralize ammonia and reduce irritation to the eyes and respiratory tract (Malley, 1995). An economical bedding material is a layer of newspaper covered in hay. This can be rolled up for disposal. The hay provides *ad lib* high fibre food in addition to a soft bed that is kind to the hocks.

2.3 Exercise

Exercise is of paramount importance for the physical and mental health of rabbits. Immobile rabbits are at increased risk of ulcerative pododermatitis, osteoporosis and spinal fractures. There is a proven association between confinement and the development of spinal deformities (Drescher and Loeffler, 1996). Exercise improves blood circulation and prevents pressure sores. The opportunity to explore is mentally beneficial. All methods of providing exercise should be escape proof, although escapees instinctively remain close to their home territory and can usually be found providing they have not been carried off by a predator or are in search of a receptive mate.

Grass and natural vegetation is the ideal diet for rabbits. Access to a garden, enclosure or pen outside has much to commend it. Natural daylight is the best way of providing the correct amount of vitamin D for the animal's needs. Rabbits enjoy basking in the sun. However, their destructive and burrowing instincts, along with a taste for bedding plants makes free access to the garden impractical for most pet owners. Free rabbits are also prey to neighbours' dogs, cats and other animals such as foxes so a well-fenced area or mesh pen is required. Ideally this should be a permanent structure that allows the rabbit to establish a familiar territory and feel secure. An area of approximately 3 m^2 (10 square feet) is sufficient, although larger areas are preferable. Branches, drainpipes, boxes and other enrichment objects can be placed in the enclosure to provide cover and recreation.

It is possible to train rabbits to return to their hutch at specified times of the day by rewarding them with food. Many pet rabbits are tame enough to be picked up, especially if they have been handled daily from an early age are regularly stroked and spoken to. These animals can be given free access to a garden during the day, perhaps under supervision, and returned to the hutch at night. Alternatively, portable wire mesh runs can be used. There are many designs, some of which are can be moved around the lawn allowing the rabbits to keep the grass down. Enclosed yards are an acceptable alternative to a garden. Rabbits can also be allowed to exercise in the house.

2.4 Burrowing

The opportunity to dig its own burrow is appreciated by many rabbits but not by their owners. Once they have dug out and established a burrow, most rabbits appear satisfied and do not start another. Females are more likely to dig burrows than males as their instinct is to dig out new nesting sites, especially during the spring. Pregnant or pseudopregnant does exhibit marked burrowing behaviour, although it can still be exhibited by spayed females.

2.5 Companionship

Rabbits are social creatures that benefit from companionship, preferably from another rabbit. A bonded pair becomes inseparable. They spend time grooming each other and there are many benefits to mutual grooming, such as reducing parasite numbers in the fur and cleaning inaccessible places such as the face or back of the neck. Occasionally, a dominant rabbit will barber the fur of its companion. Neutering rabbits that are kept together is necessary to prevent fighting and unwanted pregnancies. Guinea pigs can be kept as companions for rabbits, although this arrangement is not as satisfactory as two rabbits together. There is a small risk of the guinea pig contracting *Bordetella bronchiseptica*, which is asymptomatic in rabbits but can cause pneumonia in guinea pigs. Neutering is required to prevent bullying and constant sexual harassment of the guinea pig.

Rabbits have distinctive personalities and strong individual likes and dislikes of other rabbits. It is not possible to predict accurately whether newly introduced rabbits will form an instant rapport or attack each other. Neutered rabbits of the opposite sex are most likely to bond, although it is possible to keep same sex pairs together. Pairs of male rabbits need to be castrated to prevent fighting.

Ideally, rabbits should be introduced on neutral territory with plenty of room for escape and hiding places to retreat into. If this is not possible, introducing the female to the male on his territory is more likely to be successful than the reverse. When they are first introduced, most rabbits spend a period chasing each other around and pulling some hair out, but will settle down eventually. A rabbit that has spent its entire life confined to a hutch may not realize that it can run around and is daunted by both the great outdoors and its new companion. It is not unusual for such rabbits to remain quiet and immobile for several days before they gain confidence and start to explore. If possible, a period of separated proximity is advisable to allow rabbits to become accustomed to each other's presence before they are introduced. Adjacent pens separated by wire mesh allow rabbits to sniff each other. It is a promising sign when the two are found lying side by side on either side of the mesh. Some rabbits never bond, others accept any new companion readily.

2.6 Winter housing

The advice is often given that rabbits should be given shelter from the winter weather by bringing the hutch into a shed or garage. As a result, many rabbits do not come out of their hutch for 6 months of the year because owners fear their pet will 'catch a chill'. It is important to provide exercise during the winter as well as the summer. Free-range rabbits that are kept outside all year round often choose to sit in the rain and snow despite having a hutch full of warm bedding to go into if required. They seem impervious to cold and as long as they have access to shelter, plenty of food and protection from predators, rabbits can be kept outside during the winter. Thin or ill rabbits or those that have not been acclimatized cannot be kept in this fashion and need to be given extra protection indoors or in a hutch or shed during inclement weather. They can be allowed outside if the weather is good. If rabbits are not exposed to natural daylight during the winter months, vitamin D deficiency can occur. Undetectable vitamin D levels have been found in blood samples taken from pet rabbits during the spring, especially from those rabbits housed in hutches (Figure 2.1) (Fairham and Harcourt-Brown, 1999).

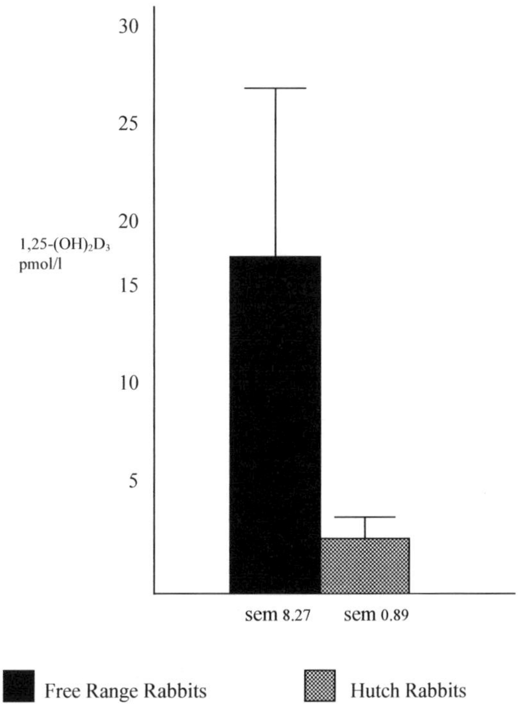

Figure 2.1. Mean (sem) plasma vitamin D (1,25-$(OH)_2D_3$ concentration in pet rabbits. During the spring, blood samples were taken from seven rabbits that lived in hutches and four rabbits that had been kept under free-range conditions with unlimited access to natural daylight through the winter months. The samples were spun and the plasma frozen immediately before shipping in a frozen state to a laboratory for 1,25-$(OH)_2D_3$ assay. Four rabbits, one from the free-range group and three from the hutch group had undetectable plasma 1,25-$(OH)_2D_3$ concentrations (< 2.5 pmol/l) indicating that vitamin D deficiency can be present in pet rabbits, especially after the winter. The rabbits were kept in North Yorkshire where winter sunshine is minimal. In laboratory rabbits kept without exposure to ultraviolet light and fed on a vitamin D deficient diet, it takes approximately 5 months for serum concentrations of 25-OH-D and 1,25-$(OH)_2D_3$ to become undetectable. (From Fairham and Harcourt-Brown (1999), reprinted with permission from *Veterinary Record*).

2.7 Free-range rabbits

Stauffacher (1992) described the behaviour of rabbits in 'near-to-nature' or free-range conditions. The rabbits were kept in an open-air turfed enclosure with several trees and bushes. They were kept in groups of up to 30 animals and their daily activities followed a double diurnal rhythm with periods of rest alternating with periods of activity around dusk and dawn. During periods of rest, the rabbits sought out places with a good overview of the enclosure under bushes or near trees where they would huddle together and engage in mutual grooming. This method of husbandry permits natural behaviour patterns, encourages grazing and normal caecotrophy and allows animals to groom themselves and each other thoroughly thereby removing skin debris, dead hair and parasites from the coat. In a study by Harcourt-Brown and Baker (2001) blood samples from rabbits kept under free-range conditions had higher red cell and lymphocyte counts than rabbits kept in hutches, suggesting that they were healthier (see Figure 6.1).

2.8 House rabbits

In recent years, there has been a trend to give pet rabbits the run of the house. House rabbits make good companions and can be trained to use a litter tray. They are usually provided with some sort of sleeping accommodation to which they can retreat and can be confined while their owners are out at work. Most house rabbits are neutered, especially males, to reduce territory marking by spraying or defaecating outside the litter tray. Rabbits can bond closely with human owners and make entertaining responsive pets. They will play with toys, beg for treats and follow their human companion around the house. Dogs and cats can learn to tolerate rabbits as companions.

2.9 Litter trays

Large cat litter trays or gravel trays from the garden centre can be used for rabbits to urinate and defaecate in. Hay, straw, cat litter, peat, soil or 'natural' litters made from hemp, corn cobs or reclaimed wood pulp are all used as litter materials for rabbits. Clay litters are not advisable as some rabbits will eat the litter which can impact the caecum (Brown, 1997). Organic solvents in litter materials derived from preserved pine wood shavings or cedar chips have been reported to cause hepatotoxicity and are therefore inadvisable (*Rabbit Health News*, 1991). Hay or clean, chopped straw can be used in rabbit litter trays.

2.10 Breeds of rabbits

Domestication has resulted in a wide range of breeds with different attributes. They can be roughly divided into two groups; fancy breeds and fur breeds (Sandford, 1996). The fur breeds include Rex, Angoras and Satin rabbits with their beautiful coat textures. Fancy breeds include the Belgian Hare, Lop and Dwarf rabbits with their varying physical characteristics. Most pet rabbits belong to the smaller breeds such as Dwarf lops, Dutch or English. Pedigree rabbit breeders often sell surplus stock to the pet trade and occasionally one of the more obscure breeds may turn up as a pet. Pedigree stock is identified by aluminium rings slipped over the hock when the rabbit is 8–10 weeks old. The rings are supplied by the British Rabbit Council in a range of sizes. Each ring has the year of birth and a unique number from which the rabbit can be identified. Many pet rabbits are the result of interbreeding between pets and are cross breeds. As with other domestic animals, there are breed predispositions to disease. For example, Dwarf rabbits are prone to congenital incisor malocclusion (Fox and Crary, 1971). Dutch, Havana and Tan rabbits have a high incidence of uterine neoplasia (Greene, 1941).

2.10.1 Angoras

Angoras have been bred for wool production for hundreds of years. The wool is plucked or sheared and either spun on its own or mixed with sheep's wool. Plucked wool is superior to shorn wool. Commercial Angoras are kept in a specialized manner to prevent staining and matting of the fur. After defleecing, woollen jackets can be worn for 2–3 weeks to reduce heat loss or a strip of fleece can be left along the back (Lebas *et al.*, 1998). Commercial Angoras are not provided with bedding but are kept on wire mesh floors and hay is provided in a rack. The long fine coat is a definite disadvantage for the pet animal as it difficult to keep the rabbit free from knots and mats. It is not surprising that a high number of Angoras arrive at rescue shelters for rehoming. The breed is prone to intestinal obstruction by felts of ingested hair.

Key points 2.1

- Hutches are not suitable for rabbits to be kept in all the time
- Daily exercise is vital for physical and mental health of rabbits. At least 4 h exercise daily is recommended, including during the winter months
- Rabbits benefit from companionship and form close bonds. The ideal companion is another rabbit, preferably of the opposite sex. Neutering is required
- Rabbits each have their own character. Some individuals are sociable, others are not
- Laboratory rabbits are often group-housed. It is possible to keep social groups of up to eight animals
- Most rabbits naturally use a litter tray
- Angoras do not make easy pets due to the demands of grooming their long, fine coat.

2.11 Nutrition

Rabbits are strict herbivores with a digestive system that is adapted to the ingestion of a high fibre diet. Digestive physiology is described in Section 1.5. Briefly, indigestible fibre is separated from fermentable components in the proximal colon and is rapidly eliminated in hard faecal pellets. The fermentable components, which consist of small particles and fluid, are moved back into the caecum where bacterial fermentation takes place to release volatile fatty acids that are absorbed as an energy source. Caecal contents are expelled periodically as mucous encapsulated caecotrophs that are reingested and digested as a source of amino acids and vitamins. This strategy permits the digestion of large volumes of fibrous foods without storage in the gastrointestinal tract. Digestion can take place when the rabbit is below ground and not vulnerable to predation.

Since their domestication, rabbits have been fed on a variety of diets. During the last war in the UK, when food was scarce, backyard rabbits were kept as a source of protein that could survive on weeds, household scraps and foods that the producer could grow himself. This still occurs in many developing countries where rabbits are fed on a range of forage materials. Large-scale rabbit production has led to the development of pelleted foods of known analysis suitable for commercial rabbits. The nutritional requirements for pregnancy, lactation, growth and fur production have been well researched but the requirements for long-term maintenance of unproductive rabbits has been overlooked. Nutritional disease is common in rabbits kept as pets. For owners, providing food that is eaten readily and enjoyed is one of the most rewarding aspects of keeping a rabbit. The visual appearance of food influences the owner when choosing a product, so pelleted diets have become unpopular and a wide range of visually attractive, highly coloured cereal mixes have evolved as 'rabbit food' in the UK. These diets are cheap to produce and many are put together by food compounders that normally make rations for farm animals. The choice of ingredients is based on general nutritional principles combined with cost and availability of ingredients. Scientific, long-term feeding trials are not carried out. The nutrient value, vitamin and mineral content of a diet is calculated by extrapolating figures taken from data tables of ingredients rather than analysing the food itself. The recent trend towards convenience foods for both humans and their pets has resulted in owners purchasing rabbit food from the local supermarket or pet shop rather than preparing their own. There are many myths and old wives' tales about feeding rabbits that unnerve the owner and dissuade them from home-produced diets and drive them to the apparent safety of commercial rabbit foods. Unfortunately, most commercial foods do not provide the ideal diet for a pet rabbit. Dietary recommendations for pet rabbits are described in Box 2.7.

2.12 Appetite

Hunger is stimulated by a drop in blood glucose, lactic acid, amino acids and volatile fatty acids. Dryness of the mouth and contractions of the stomach stimulate eating (Fekete, 1989). The volume of food that is eaten is influenced by its composition and texture and by the individual likes and dislikes of the rabbit. Increasing the fibre content of the diet increases the total volume that is consumed (Bellier and Gidenne, 1996). Rabbits will eat a variety of foods but show a preference for fibre and may eat hay or straw in preference to their compound feed. It can be difficult to persuade rabbits to eat new foods once they have become accustomed to a particular diet. New batches of food may be refused despite it appearing to be exactly the same to the owner. Sweet foods are generally palatable. Molasses are used in many commercial rabbit foods to improve palatability (Cheeke, 1994). Bitter tastes such as the saponins in alfalfa are well tolerated (Cheeke, 1987).

Most rabbits enjoy leafy plants. A whole variety of plants can be eaten including many garden weeds and ornamental plants (see Box 2.7). Sunflower leaves were found to be most palatable in a study by Harris *et al.* (1983). Rabbits appear to enjoy foods of different textures. Pellets are preferable to ground meal. Biscuits or hard pieces of breakfast cereal are accepted readily. Bark is stripped from young trees or shrubs. All parts of the plant may be eaten including the stem and roots, although the growing tips are usually nibbled off first. Tree leaves are eaten, especially in the autumn when the leaves fall.

Like many activities in rabbits, appetite follows a diurnal pattern. Wild rabbits feed at dusk and dawn. Pet rabbits may not be hungry during the day and are most likely to eat in the early evening or overnight.

2.13 Dietary requirements of rabbits

2.13.1 Carbohydrate

Carbohydrates are compounds of carbon, hydrogen and oxygen with the empirical formula of $(CH_2O)_n$ where n is >3. Some molecules contain phosphorus, nitrogen or sulphur and not all follow the $(CH_2O)_n$ rule, e.g. deoxyribose $C_6H_{10}O_4$. Carbohydrates can be classified according to the complexity of their structure, i.e. monosaccharides, oligosaccharides, polysaccharides and complexed carbohydrates such as glycoproteins. Alternatively, they can be categorized into sugars, starches and fibre. Fibre is expelled undigested (indigestible fibre) or fermented in the caecum to produce volatile fatty acids (digestible or fermentable fibre).

Carbohydrates are an important energy source. They can be digested and absorbed from the stomach and small intestine or degraded and fermented by the caecal microflora. Simple monosaccharide sugars such as glucose, fructose and galactose are absorbed from the small intestine in a similar manner to other species. Starches are polysaccharides that are abundant in seeds, fruits, tubers and roots and are broken down to simple sugars during digestion. The reaction is catalysed by amylase that is secreted by the salivary glands and pancreas and is also present in caecotrophs as a result of bacterial synthesis. The age of the rabbit, dietary levels and the type of starch influence digestion and absorption in the small intestine. For example, cereal starches are more fermentable than those found in roots or tubers. Starch is found in plants as granules that are insoluble in cold water, but when a suspension of starch in water is heated, the granules swell and eventually gelatinize. Gelatinized starches can form complexes with proteins that reduce the digestibility of both starch and protein (Cheeke, 1987). Feed manufacturing processes and exogenous enzymes supplements also affect starch digestibility (De Blas and Gidenne, 1998). Starch that is not digested and absorbed in the small intestine passes into the caecum as a substrate for bacterial fermentation.

Residual starch that reaches the caecum or 'carbohydrate overload' is thought to be a predisposing factor in the development of enterotoxaemia in young rabbits. *Clostridium spiroforme* requires glucose as a substrate for iotatoxin production and glucose is yielded during bacterial fermentation of carbohydrate (Cheeke, 1987). In commercial units, enterotoxaemia is seen in young rabbits in association with high carbohydrate, low fibre diets. However, the situation is different in the adult pet rabbit where the sensitivity to high starch diets is controversial (Lowe, 1998). Recent work has indicated that there is a difference in starch digestibility between young and adult rabbits. Adult rabbits appear to digest starch more efficiently than young ones. Very small amounts of starch reach the caecocolic segment of adults. Even in lactating rabbits that consume high quantities of carbohydrate, almost all the starch is hydrolysed before it reaches the caecum (De Blas and Gidenne, 1998). Therefore the role of starch as a predisposing factor for imbalances of the caecal microflora and the development of enteric disorders remains unclear. Experimental work has given conflicting results (Cheeke, 1987; De Blas and Gidenne, 1998). However, the general consensus of opinion is that overload of rapidly fermentable carbohydrates in the large intestine increases the likelihood of digestive disorders, at least in susceptible, recently weaned rabbits. Dietary starch has no influence on the chemical composition of caecal contents or on the production or composition of soft and hard faeces (Carabaõ *et al.*, 1988).

2.13.2 Fibre

2.13.2.1 Digestible (fermentable) and indigestible fibre in rabbits

Dietary fibre is an important component of the diet for rabbits (see Box 2.2). Fibre is defined as 'that portion of ingested foodstuffs that cannot be broken down by intestinal enzymes and juices of monogastric animals and therefore passes through the small intestine and colon undigested' (Blood and Studdert, 1999). This definition is confusing in ruminants and hindgut fermenters because the gut flora breaks down and 'digests' some fibre molecules by microbial fermentation. Therefore, in herbivores, fibre can be either 'digestible' or 'indigestible' and digestibility varies with species and their digestive physiology. The term 'fermentable' fibre can also be used to describe 'digestible' fibre that is broken down by microbial fermentation. In rabbits, fibre is separated in the proximal colon into large and small particles. Particles larger than 0.5 mm do not enter the caecum and are swiftly expelled undigested. This is the 'indigestible fibre' component of the diet. Particles smaller than 0.3 mm are moved into the caecum where they are digested by bacterial fermentation. This component of the diet is known as 'digestible' or 'fermentable' fibre. Within the caecum the digestibility of fibre depends on the chemical composition and size of the particle. The ease with which bacteria can degrade fibre particles depends on the molecular structure and chemical properties of the fibre and the surface area that the bacteria can adhere to.

Fibre is composed of plant cell walls. Plant cell walls consist of complex carbohydrates such as polysaccharides, oligosaccharides, cellulose, hemicellulose, gums and pectins, which are embedded in a lignin matrix. Most

Box 2.2 The importance of dietary fibre to rabbits

Dietary fibre can be divided into *indigestible* fibre that passes straight through the alimentary tract without entering the caecum and *fermentable* (digestible) fibre that is directed into the caecum and provides a substrate for bacterial degradation and fermentation by the caecal microflora.

Indigestible fibre is important to:
- Stimulate gut motility that moves digesta and fluid into the caecum for fermentation
- Provide forage material to prevent boredom and behavioural problems such as fur chewing
- Provide dental exercise and optimal dental wear
- Stimulate appetite and ingestion of caecotrophs

Fermentable fibre is important to:
- Provide a substrate for caecal microflora
- Provide optimal caecal pH and volatile fatty acid production
- Prevent proliferation of pathogenic bacteria in the caecum
- Increase fibre content of caecotrophs so they are of firm consistency

of these molecules can be broken down and 'digested' by caecal fermentation. Some components such as oligosaccharides are water soluble, whereas most components such as pectins, cellulose and hemicellulose are insoluble. Hemicelluloses and pectins are the substances that glue plant cells together. Cellulose is a linear polymer of glucose that forms the skeleton of most plant structures and plant cells in which it can be closely associated with lignin. Lignin is not a carbohydrate but a complex cross-linked structure made up of many phenylpropanoid units (McDonald *et al.*, 1996). Lignin and cellulose combine to provide structural rigidity to plants. Strong chemical bonds exist between lignin and plant polysaccharides and cell wall proteins that reduce the digestibility of these compounds. Lignin is almost completely indigestible and the lignin content of plants increases with age. Lignin is present in large quantities in wood, hulls and straw.

Therefore, in rabbits, fibre can be classified as either 'indigestible' or 'fermentable'. Indigestible fibre is composed of particles that are bigger than 0.3–0.5 mm. Their chemical composition is not important although these particles are mostly made up of lignin and cellulose. 'Fermentable' fibre is composed of particles smaller than 0.3–0.5 mm and the digestibility is greatly affected by their chemical composition (see Figure 2.2).

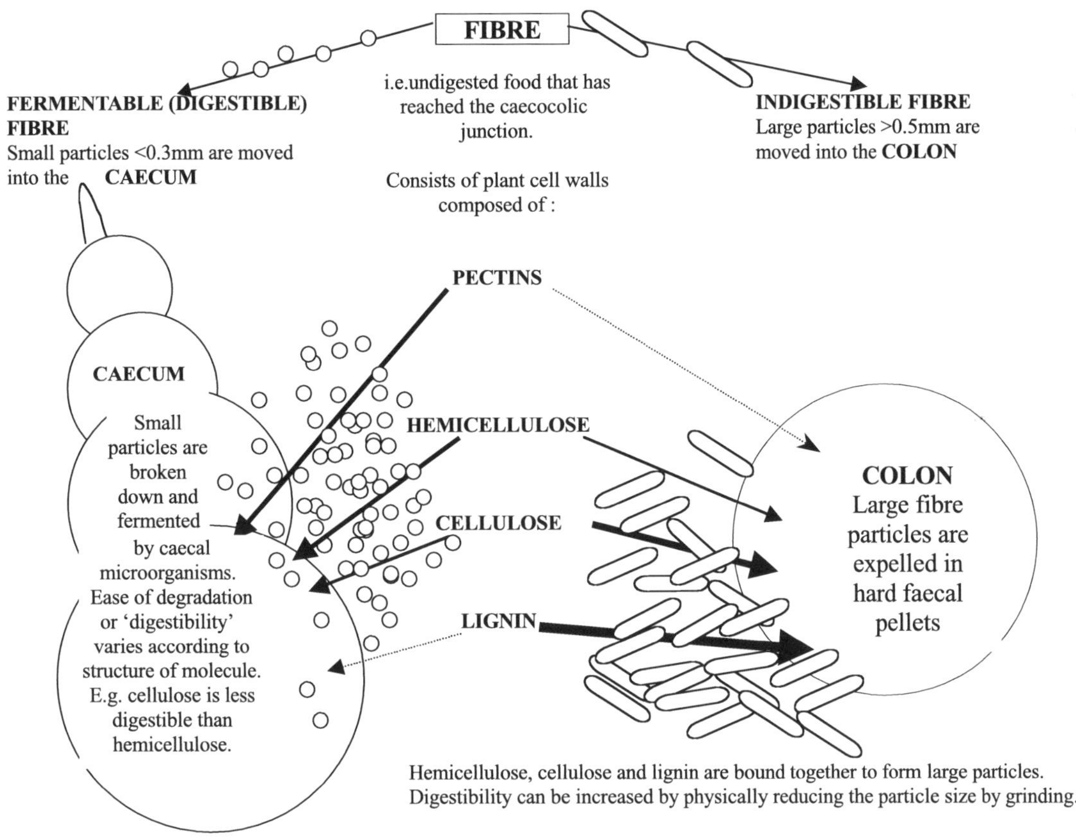

Figure 2.2. Digestion of fibre in rabbits. Some precaecal digestion of fibre takes place by enzymes in the stomach and small intestine. Fibre that reaches the hindgut is either degraded by caecal microflora or expelled undigested. The proximal colon is adapted to separate indigestible fibre from fibre that can be fermented in the caecum. Large undigestible fibre particles pass into the colon and are expelled rapidly. Small particles pass into the caecum to undergo bacterial fermentation. Indigestible fibre promotes gut motility but does not have any nutrient value. Digestible (fermentable) fibre provides nutrients but has no direct effect on gut motility.

2.13.2.2 Digestion of fermentable fibre within the caecum

In rabbits, there is evidence that partial digestion of fibre can take place in the stomach and small intestine by the action of enzymes such as pectinases and xylanases (Gidenne *et al.*, 1998). However, most digestion of fibre takes place by the microbial flora within the caecum. Digestibility within the caecum depends on the nature of the plant material and, to a lesser extent, processing procedures. Hemicelluloses and pectins are broken down more easily than cellulose, which requires degradation by cellulolytic bacteria and requires time for attachment of the bacteria to the cell wall before degradation starts. Degradation of cellulose takes longer than hemicellulose because of its linear polymer structure (Gidenne *et al.*, 1998), so it is less fermentable than hemicellulose. Cellulose can be closely associated, both chemically and physically, with other compounds such as hemicellulose and pectin and affect their digestibility. It can also be combined with lignin that is almost completely indigestible. The digestibility of fibre within the caecum affects the rabbit's appetite and growth rate. Grinding down lignin so that it passes into the caecum depresses voluntary food intake in comparison with cellulose that is more fermentable (Chiou *et al.*, 1998).

The chemical structure of fibre molecules gives them a buffering capacity that is dependent on the concentration of carboxyl, amino and hydroxyl groups (Gidenne *et al.*, 1998). The type of fibre has an effect on caecal pH which, in turn, can affect the balance of caecal microflora. For example, wheat straw tends to increase caecal pH, whereas beet pulp decreases it. Balanced sources of fibre such as alfalfa do not modify caecal pH (Gidenne *et al.*, 1998).

Particle size within the caecum affects retention time for microbial fermentation (Gidenne *et al.*, 1998). Small particles have a larger surface area for bacteria to adhere to. The particle length of fibre depends on the plant source and processing procedures. Digestibility of lignified material can be increased by alkali treatment to dissolve lignin and release cellulose and other compounds for microbial degradation. Grinding down lignin to small particles allows it to be retained in the caecum where it cannot be digested. The degree of grinding is an important consideration as it alters the way in which fibre is separated in the proximal colon. Grinding fibre to particles small enough to be moved into the caecum rather than colon detracts from the beneficial effect of indigestible fibre on intestinal motility. There is general agreement that screen sizes for production of complete compound feeds should be 2 mm. Screen sizes of 1 mm induce digestive upsets (Lowe, 1998).

Some cell wall constituents, such as pectins and gums, are hydrophilic and tend to form gels in solution. This property is used to produce bulk laxatives in humans because the compound takes up water in the digestive tract and increases the volume of faeces and promotes peristalsis. In rabbits, these compounds are moved into the caecum where they absorb water and increase retention time. Caecal impactions have been associated with the use of bulk laxatives in rabbits.

2.13.2.3 The importance of indigestible fibre

Rabbits have a natural appetite for fibrous foods. They will strip and eat bark, chew roots and dried fibrous vegetation and may eat hay in preference to fresh green foods. Indigestible fibre plays an important role in maintaining good health in rabbits. Chewing and grinding food wears the teeth and helps to maintain normal dental occlusion. A diet deficient in fibrous material has been implicated in cheek tooth overgrowth (Crossley, 1995). Diets low in indigestible fibre predispose to gastrointestinal hypomotility and the retention of food and hair in the stomach, which forms trichobezoars (hairballs). Slow gut motility and increased food retention time in the hindgut can result in alterations in gut flora and the development of enterotoxaemia. The provision of a diet high in indigestible fibre to house rabbits reduces the ingestion of non-food items such as carpet fibres or plastic litter trays. Fur chewing and barbering is also linked to low fibre diets (Quesenberry, 1994). Diets containing low dietary fibre depress voluntary food intake (Bellier and Gidenne, 1996).

Fibre has an effect on caecotrophy. The amount of fibre in the diet affects the time that digesta is retained in the caecum for microbial fermentation. Carabaõ *et al.* (1988) measured the weight of soft faeces that were produced by rabbits fed varying levels of fibre. The weight of soft faeces was then compared to the weight of caecal contents. They found that a relatively small amount of the caecal contents were removed each day in rabbits fed diets containing less than 14% fibre. In rabbits consuming a diet of greater than 14% fibre, the caecal material was almost entirely removed each day. Diets high in indigestible fibre increase the rabbit's appetite for caecotrophs (Fekete and Bokori, 1985). The fibre content of caecotrophs is proportional to the crude fibre level of the diet, although their dry matter content is unaffected by changes in dietary fibre content (Carabaõ *et al.*, 1988). Indigestible fibre has no effect on the composition of caecotrophs because large fibre particles do not enter the caecum and are excreted in the hard faecal pellets.

2.13.2.4 Recommended dietary fibre for rabbits

The fibre content of a diet is often expressed as 'crude fibre'. This term refers to the percentage of the original food that remains after boiling in acid and alkali alternately. Crude fibre is mainly a measurement of the lignin and cellulose component of the diet and does not include other fermentable fibre components. Neither does crude fibre analysis give an indication of particle length or the effect on gut motility.

An alternative measurement of fibre is 'neutral detergent fibre' (NDF) and 'acid detergent fibre' (ADF). The NDF is made up of cell wall constituents – pectins, cellulose, hemicellulose, lignin etc. ADF is the residue of NDF after acid extraction of the feed sample and is mainly indigestible lignocellulose complex. Digestible hemicellulose is the difference between NDF and ADF. ADF gives a better indication of indigestible fibre content than crude fibre.

Recommended dietary fibre levels for rabbits vary between texts. In many cases, crude fibre figures are given that are not particularly helpful. Dietary fibre requirements have been determined for commercial rabbits but not for pet ones. Rabbits that are used for meat production need to grow rapidly and convert food efficiently. The digestibility of the fibre content of the diet is an important consideration for peak performance. The importance of indigestible fibre is often overlooked. It is known that less than 10% crude fibre results in caecal acidosis and results in a high incidence of enteritis. Crude fibre levels of 10–15% are recommended for commercial rabbits for optimal growth rates (Cheeke, 1987).

In contrast to commercial rabbits, pet rabbits are not growing and do not need to convert food efficiently. The indigestible fibre component of the diet is of greater importance than fermentable fibre. In pet rabbits, it is important to promote intestinal motility and prevent obesity. Lowe (1998) recommends crude fibre levels of 13–20% for pet rabbits with a level of 12.5% indigestible fibre. Jenkins (1991) recommends a level of 18–24% fibre for pet rabbits, although the type of fibre is not specified. The fibre analysis of some ingredients of rabbit foods is summarized in Table 2.1. For pet rabbits, a permanent source of indigestible fibre such as *ad lib* grass or hay will ensure adequate fibre levels as long as the rabbit actually eats it. Soiled, unpalatable hay or underlying dental disease can substantially reduce indigestible fibre intake.

2.13.2.5 Sources of fibre for pet rabbits

Concentrated foods usually include a fibre source, such as grass or alfalfa. The fibre has to be processed in some way to incorporate it into the food, which can affect its digestibility and its effect on gut motility. Grass and hay are good sources of fermentable and indigestible fibre for rabbits. Hay can be provided in addition to, or instead of grass. It is not only a source of fibre but also enriches the environment and prevents abnormal behaviour (Berthelsen and Hansen, 1999). Alfalfa is a source of fibre that is used in commercial rabbit diets in many countries. Alfalfa hay not only provides fibre but has a high calcium content. Alfalfa hay is not generally available in the UK. Instead, meadow hay suitable for feeding to pet rabbits is available from most pet shops. Meadow hay is preferable to alfalfa for pet rabbits. Fresh grass is the ideal food and

Table 2.1 Fibre analysis of some rabbit foods

Analysis on dry matter basis

Crude fibre: The crude fibre content is determined by boiling an ether extracted food sample in dilute acid and alkali alternately before burning in a furnace. The difference in weight before and after burning is the crude fibre fraction. This is not an accurate measurement as many cell wall components are destroyed during process. Historically, this is the measurement that is included in food analysis tables (Cheeke, 1987).

Neutral detergent fibre (NDF) is the percentage of food remaining after boiling in neutral detergent that leaves most components of cell wall intact.

Acid detergent fibre (ADF) is the percentage of neutral detergent fibre (NDF) that remains after boiling in acid which removes the hemicellose component.

Indigestible fibre is represented by ADF.

Hemicellulose is represented by difference between NDF and ADF. Hemicellulose is fermented in the caecum.

Ingredient	*Crude fibre (%)*	*NDF (%)*	*ADF (indigestible fibre guide) (%)*	*NDF-ADF (hemicellulose content) (%)*	*Comments*
Alfalfa	30.2	49.3	37.5	11.8	
Beet, sugar	20.3	32.1	17.9	14.2	High in starch and sugars
Beans	8	16.8	12.3	4.5	
Bran	11.4	47.5	13.7	33.8	
Cabbage	17	24.4	13.6	10.8	
Carrots	9.4		13.4		
Grass, dried	21	54.1	28.2	25.9	
Grass growing	13	57.7	29.6	28.1	Fibre content varies with stage of growth
Hay (poor quality)	38	74.1	45.2	28.9	
Hay (good quality)	29.8	65	36.4	28.6	
Kale	17.9	24.3	19.7	4.6	
Maize	2.4	11.7	2.8	8.9	High in starch
Oats, rolled	10.5	31	14.9	16.1	High in starch
Oats, naked	4.5	11.4	4.2	7.2	High in starch
Peas	6.3	11.6	7.6	4	
Straw (Wheat)	41.7	80.9	50.2		
Swedes	10.0	14	12.5	1.5	High in starch

Reference sources:
Rabbit Feeding and Nutrition (1987) Cheeke, P. Academic Press. San Diego.
Animal Nutrition 5th Edition (1995) McDonald, P. *et al.*, Longman Ltd.

rabbits have evolved to live on it. Garden weeds are also a source of fibre and give variety to the diet. Pet rabbits that are allowed free access to a garden will browse on a selection of plants. They have their own individual likes and dislikes and will eat tough fibrous vegetation as well as soft new shoots. Tree leaves are eaten, especially in the autumn when the leaves have fallen and are within easy reach. Leaves from apple and hazel are especially enjoyed by rabbits (Richardson, 1999). Bark may be stripped from branches and from the base of trees. Exposed roots may be chewed through. Young docks, brambles, raspberry leaves, sow thistle, chickweed, groundsel, dandelions, clover, plantain, goose grass, ground elder and vetches are among a host of plants that are enjoyed by pet rabbits. Unfortunately, annual bedding plants, herbs and other decorative garden shrubs will also be enjoyed and destroyed by a rabbit that is given the run of the garden.

Fresh fruit and vegetables can be fed as an additional source of fibre, especially when natural vegetation is scarce. Broccoli, brussels sprouts, cabbage, spring cabbage, carrots, carrot tops, celery, cauliflower leaves, maize plants, pea pods, swedes, corncobs, spinach, kale, culinary herbs are all enjoyed by rabbits. Although there can be problems if a single item is fed all the time, a mixed diet including three different items each day is safe. Fruit and succulent salad items such as lettuce, tomatoes and cucumber are poor fibre sources and can lead to transient uneaten soft caecotrophs.

2.13.3 Oligosaccharides

Oligosaccharides are molecules with a low degree of polymerization that are not digested by enzymes in the digestive tract but are rapidly degraded and fermented by caecal microflora (De Blas and Gidenne, 1998). Oligosaccharides can be classified as 'soluble fibre' as they are water soluble. The type of oligosaccharide is important in its effect upon the microbial population. A diet containing gluco-oligosaccharides that release glucose after hydrolysis in the caecum causes diarrhoea in young rabbits, whereas fructo- or galacto-oligosaccharides do not have the same effect (Lebas *et al.*, 1998). Currently, there is considerable interest in fructo-oligosaccharides because they are reputed to be beneficial in the human gastrointestinal tract by providing the correct substrate for the proliferation of desirable bacterial species such as *Bifidobacteria*. (Campbell *et al.*, 1997). Certain plants such as chicory, asparagus, bananas and artichokes contain fructo-oligosaccharides that stimulate the growth of *Bifidobacteria* spp. in the human colon, hence the term 'bifidogenesis', which may be used to describe this effect. Fructo-oligosaccharides have been called 'prebiotics', as the principle of their beneficial effects is similar to probiotics, i.e. to encourage the growth of beneficial bacteria and inhibit pathogenic species. Fructo-oligosaccharides are utilized by *Bacteroides* spp. that prevail in healthy caecal microflora of rabbits. Fructo-oligosaccharides increase calcium, magnesium and iron absorption from the colon and rectum of rats (Ohta *et al.*, 1995a, b) and reduce serum triglyceridaemia in humans (Roberfroid, 1997). In rabbits, a reduction in morbidity after the introduction of pathogenic *E. coli* has been reported in rabbits fed on a fructo-oligosaccharide supplemented diet (Maertens and Villamide, 1998). Fructo-oligosaccharides are now included in many proprietary rabbit foods.

2.13.4 Protein

Proteins are made up of essential and non-essential amino acids. Essential amino acids are those that are not synthesized by the animal and must be ingested in the diet. The requirement for essential amino acids is affected by growth, lactation, pregnancy and wool production. Certain amino acids can be partly replaced by other amino acids. For example, methionine can be replaced by cystine, and tyrosine can partly replace phenylalanine. Although rabbits have an essential amino acid requirement (see Box 2.3), the situation is complicated by caecotrophy. Microorganisms within the caecum synthesize amino acids that are absorbed from the caecotroph during digestion. The amino acid composition of soft faeces is affected by the microbial population and the digestibility of dietary protein.

Box 2.3 Essential amino acid requirement of rabbits (From Lang, 1981)

Arginine
Glycine
Histidine
Isoleucine
Leucine
Lysine
Sulphur amino acids:
Methionine + cystine
Phenylalanine + tyrosine
Threonine
Tryptophan
Valine

Herbivores such as wild rabbits obtain their protein entirely from plants, although animal protein such as fish, meat or bone meal has been used in commercial feeds for rabbits (Cheeke, 1987). Plant proteins can be divided into two major classes – seed and leaf proteins. Seed proteins are contained in the endosperm and in the outer bran layer. The proteins of forage plants are concentrated in the leaves, tightly bound to cellulose in the cell wall. The digestibility of protein varies according to its source and is also influenced by the age of the animal. Dietary protein levels are important to produce good growth rates and performance in commercial rabbits and are a major consideration for commercial rabbit feeds. High protein levels are not required for maintenance of non-productive pets.

Grass is a source of protein and amino acids for rabbits. The protein content of grass decreases with maturity, although the relative proportions of amino acids do not alter greatly and are similar between plant species (McDonald *et al.*, 1996). Grass is rich in arginine, glutamine and lysine but methionine and isoleucine are limiting. Cereal proteins are deficient in certain amino acids, particularly lysine and methionine. Legume seeds such as peas and beans are good sources of protein and their high lysine content is often used to balance the lysine deficiency of cereals in mixed rations. Supplementation with sulphur-containing amino acids such as methionine and cysteine is required for wool production by Angora rabbits (Lebas *et al.*, 1998).

The optimum dietary protein level for maximum growth is 16% and 18–19% for lactation (Cheeke, 1994). This level of protein is excessive for the maintenance of a non-productive pet rabbits that are prone to obesity. High dietary protein reduces the rabbit's appetite for caecotrophs. Excess dietary protein alters the caecal microflora and increases the pH thereby predisposing the proliferation of pathogenic bacteria (Cheeke, 1994). High dietary protein also increases ammonia production and excretion and reduces air quality in poorly ventilated housing thereby contributing to the development of upper respiratory tract and conjunctival infections.

Insufficient dietary protein or essential amino acid deficiency results in impaired protein synthesis and poor tissue regeneration. Excessively low protein diets should be avoided and some consideration of the protein quality is important for the pet rabbit (Lowe, 1998). Rabbits that do not eat their caecotrophs or selectively eat a restricted diet can suffer from essential amino acid deficiency. Lysine and methionine are most likely to be the limiting essential amino acids. Protein levels of 12–16% are adequate for pet rabbit rations (Lowe, 1998).

Key points 2.2

- Large numbers of rabbits are reared for meat in many countries. As a result, rabbit nutrition has been extensively researched. Rabbits are able to utilize a wide range of foods
- Most nutritional data relate to the growing, pregnant, lactating or breeding animal with a short life span
- The nutritional requirements of the non-productive pet rabbit are completely different from the commercial rabbit
- Incorrect feeding causes many diseases of pet rabbits
- Owners are often confused by conflicting advice that is given by breeders, pet shops or food manufacturers. The advice may be based on legend, marketing material or data obtained from commercial production that is not relevant to the pet animal
- Digestion of starch in the small intestine is affected by the age of the rabbit. Adults digest starch more efficiently than young animals. Undigested starch that reaches the caecum can act as a substrate for bacterial fermentation and predispose to the development of enterotoxaemia
- Fibre is important to maintain optimum digestion and a healthy caecal microflora. Digestible fibre provides a substrate for bacterial fermentation in the caecum. Indigestible fibre stimulates gut motility
- The amount of indigestible fibre in the diet is very important. Too little results in reduced gastrointestinal motility and digestive disorders. Too much results in malnutrition
- Grass and good quality meadow hay are ideal sources of digestible and indigestible fibre. Wild plants and garden weeds are also good sources of fibre
- It is possible to transmit infectious or parasitic disease from wild animals by feeding contaminated grass or hay
- High levels of dietary protein are not necessary for pet rabbits although they do have an essential amino acid requirement.

2.13.5 Fats

The digestion and absorption of fats in rabbits is similar to monogastric animals. Fat globules are emulsified by the action of bile salts before being broken down by pancreatic lipase and absorbed from the small intestine. Fats and oils have been used in rabbit rations to provide an energy source that avoids carbohydrate overload of the hindgut. Dietary fat reduces intestinal absorption of calcium due to the formation of calcium soaps in the gut. Fat stimulates gastrointestinal motility and improves palatability of the diet. Vegetable oils are more digestible than animal fats (Cheeke, 1987). The fat content affects the keeping quality of pellets and the cost of production.

For pet rabbits, high dietary levels of fats and oils are disadvantageous due to the propensity of rabbits to become obese. High fat diets increase the risk of hepatic lipidosis by altering lipid metabolism and promoting ketogenesis and hypoglycaemia during periods of starvation (Jean-Blain and Durix, 1985). Obese animals with a fatty liver are at great risk of developing fatal fatty degeneration of the liver and kidneys if they become anorexic.

Most commercial diets contain 2.5–4.0% fat, but treat foods such as chocolate drops or sweet biscuits contain higher amounts.

2.13.6 Vitamins

2.13.6.1 Vitamin A

Vitamin A, or retinol, is a fat-soluble, organic alcohol formed in animal tissues from caretenoid pigments in plants of which β-carotene is the most important. β-carotene is converted to vitamin A primarily in the intestinal mucosa and is stored in the liver, from which it is transported, protein bound, to cells according to metabolic need.

Vitamin A is necessary for vision, bone development, maintenance of epithelial integrity, reproduction and immunological response. Retinol makes up part of a retinal pigment, rhodopsin, which is necessary for vision, especially in dim light. Vitamin A is required by epithelial tissue and deficiency results in squamous metaplasia and keratinization. Vitamin A also plays an important role in combating infection and has been termed the 'anti-infective vitamin'. In several species, vitamin A deficiency is accompanied by low levels of immunoglobulins, although the exact function of the vitamin in the formation of these proteins is unknown (MacDonald *et al.*, 1996). Growth and reproduction are affected by vitamin A deficiency. Excessive quantities of vitamin A lead to toxicity with symptoms similar to those of deficiency.

The vitamin A content of plants varies considerably. The long hydrocarbon chain is easily oxidized especially when exposed to heat, light, moisture and heavy metals (McDonald *et al.*, 1996). Exposure to sunlight during the curing process destroys much of the vitamin A in hay or alfalfa. Storage and rancidity of feeds also reduces vitamin A content, although the addition of antioxidants can reduce the loss. Cereals, with the exception of yellow maize, are poor sources of vitamin A.

Grazing animals generally obtain more than adequate amounts of vitamin A from pasture and build up liver reserves. Deficiency is rare in farm animals that are fed on silage and well preserved hay over the winter months, although vitamin A deficiency has been reported in cattle housed indoors on high cereal rations (McDonald *et al.*, 1996).

Rabbits housed indoors or in hutches and fed on cereal mixtures and poor quality hay are candidates for vitamin A deficiency if they do not eat the parts of the diet that contain the vitamin and mineral supplement. Because of the role of vitamin A in the maintenance of epithelial tissues and mucous membranes, deficient animals are susceptible to disease and infection. A high incidence of enteritis occurs in vitamin A deficient rabbits (Cheeke, 1994).

Experimental vitamin A deficiency has been studied in rabbits. Retarded growth and weight loss occur in growing animals with the development of neurological symptoms in severe cases. Hydrocephalus and cerebellar herniation can occur in immature rabbits (Phillips and Bohstedt, 1937). In the adult, eye lesions can be the first sign of deficiency with the development of keratitis that progresses to iridocyclitis, hypopyon and permanent blindness (Hunt and Harrington, 1974). Lacrimal gland tissue and the bone surrounding the optical foramen has found to be unaffected by vitamin A deficiency, although these tissues are affected in other species (Fox *et al.*, 1982; Ubels and Harkema, 1994). Reproductive problems such as fetal malformations, low fertility and abortions have been associated with both vitamin A deficiency and excess (Cheeke, 1987). Intercurrent disease such as hepatic coccidiosis due to *Eimeria steidae* infection can interfere with vitamin A metabolism and therefore increase dietary requirement.

Vitamin A activity is expressed in international units (IU) and the dietary requirement for rabbits appears to be 10 000–18 000 IU/kg (Lowe, 1998). Fresh green foods and grass are good sources of vitamin A.

2.13.6.2 Vitamin D

Vitamin D is a fat-soluble vitamin that is also a hormone, which plays an important role in calcium and phosphorus metabolism. A vitamin is defined as 'an organic substance found in foods that is essential in small quantities for growth, health and survival' (Blood and Studdert, 1999). A hormone is defined as 'a chemical transmitter substance produced by cells of the body and transported by the bloodstream and other means to the cells and organs which carry receptors for the hormone and on which it has a specific regulatory effect' (Blood and Studdert, 1999). Therefore vitamin D is both vitamin and hormone and has a range of physiological effects in addition to its role in calcium metabolism. Vitamin D receptors are found in many tissues including the stomach, brain, pituitary gland, gonads, parathyroid glands, epidermis, dermis, monocytes and activated T and B lymphocytes, although the exact physiological action in these tissues is unclear (Holick, 1990).

There are several metabolites of vitamin D that are either ingested in the diet or synthesized in the body. The number of terms and abbreviations that refer to vitamin D and its metabolites can be confusing. These terms are defined in Box 2.4.

Ultraviolet light is required to convert an endogenous vitamin D precursor, 7-dehydrocholesterol, to pre-vitamin D_3 in the skin. Further conversion to vitamin D_3 (cholecalciferol) takes place before it is transported to the liver, bound to plasma protein. Plants contain a different vitamin D precursor, ergosterol, which is also converted by ultraviolet light to produce ergocalciferol or vitamin D_2. This process takes place in the plant when vegetation, such as hay, dries in the sunshine. Ergocalciferol is transported, protein bound, from the gut to the liver where, like vitamin D_3 (cholecalciferol), it is hydroxylated to form 25-hydroxycholecalciferol (25-OH-D) which is, in turn, converted to the active vitamin D metabolite 1,25-dihydroxycholecalciferol (1,25$(OH)_2$D) in the kidney. Conversion of 25-OH-D to 1,25$(OH)_2$D is stimulated by parathyroid hormone (PTH) released from the parathyroid gland in response to low serum calcium concentrations.

Box 2.4 Definition of terms relating to vitamin D

Vitamin D: A group of closely related steroids with anti-rachitic properties
Vitamin D_2 (Ergocalciferol, calciferol): An exogenous provitamin formed from ergosterol in plants when they are exposed to ultraviolet light. Vitamin D_2 is converted to 25-OH-D in the liver
Vitamin D_3 (Cholecalciferol): An endogenous provitamin that is converted to 25-OH-D in the liver
Vitamin D_4 and D_5: occur naturally in the oils of some fish*
Ergosterol: A sterol that occurs in plants. It is converted to vitamin D_2 under exposure to ultraviolet light
7-dehydrocholesterol: A derivative of chlolesterol that is metabolized to vitamin D_3 in skin exposed to ultraviolet light
25-OH-D (25-hydroxycholecalciferol, calcifediol, 25-dihydroxyvitamin D): a metabolite of vitamin D that is formed and stored in the liver. There is a negative feedback controlling the conversion of provitamins (vitamin D_2 and D_3) to 25-OH-D
1,25(OH_2)D (1,25-dihydroxycholecalciferol, calcitriol, 1,25-dihydroxyvitamin D): The active metabolite of vitamin D that is formed in the kidney from 25-OH-D under the influence of parathyroid hormone (PTH) that is released in response to low serum calcium concentrations.

*From Blood, Henderson and Radostits (1979).

The main function of vitamin D is to maintain serum calcium levels within the normal range. This is achieved by its effects on the intestinal absorption of calcium, mobilization of calcium to and from bone and renal regulation of calcium excretion. $1,25(OH)_2D$ stimulates intestinal absorption of calcium and osteoclastic activity in bone. High quantities of vitamin D causes bone resorption and raise blood calcium levels. Low quantities of vitamin D reduce intestinal absorption and renal conservation of calcium and result in a drop in blood calcium, which stimulates PTH release. PTH stimulates bone resorption to release calcium and restore blood levels. Therefore, osteomalacia can result from both deficiency and excess of vitamin D. Elevated PTH concentrations stimulate the kidney to conserve calcium.

Vitamin D toxicity can be the result of excessive dietary intake. Intestinal absorption of calcium and osteoclastic activity are increased and result in blood levels that exceed the renal capacity for excretion. This leads to deposition of calcium in soft tissue such as the aorta and kidney.

Vitamin D deficiency can arise from inadequate dietary intake of exogenous precursors, or inadequate exposure to ultraviolet light that is required for conversion of endogenous precursors. Deficiency of vitamin D results in rickets in growing animals and osteomalacia in adults. In humans, vitamin D deficiency is now recognized as a major cause of metabolic bone disease in elderly people (Holick, 1996).

The role of vitamin D in calcium regulation in rabbits differs from other species. Vitamin D does not appear to play the same regulatory role in intestinal absorption as in other mammals. Studies into chronic vitamin D deficiency in adult rabbits indicate that intestinal absorption of calcium is passive and efficient and does not require vitamin D (Bourdeau *et al.*, 1986). However, vitamin D increases intestinal absorption of calcium and is required if dietary levels are low (Tvedegaard, 1987; Brommage *et al.*, 1988).

In rabbits, vitamin D plays an important role in phophorus metabolism. Vitamin deficiency results in a reduction in intestinal absorption of phosphorus. Experimental studies have shown that chronic vitamin D deficiency can result in hypophosphataemia and osteomalacia (Brommage *et al.*, 1988).

Photosynthesis of vitamin D takes place in the skin of fur and fleece bearing animals such as horses and sheep, although it is absent from some carnivorous species such as cats which obtain vitamin D from prey (How *et al.*, 1994). Sunlight is required for endogenous vitamin D synthesis by rabbits. Rickets can be induced in growing rabbits by keeping them in the dark or under artificial light (Kato, 1966; Curry *et al.*, 1974). It takes approximately 5 months for serum concentrations of 25-OH-D and $1,25(OH)_2D$ to become undetectable in rabbits on a vitamin D deficient diet (Nyomba *et al.*, 1984; Brommage *et al.*, 1988).

Undetectable serum concentrations of $1,25(OH)_2D$ have been found in pet rabbits during the spring after they were confined to hutches for the winter (see Figure 2.1). Pet rabbits kept in free-range conditions with unrestricted access to natural daylight through the winter had significantly higher $1,25\text{-}(OH)_2D3$ concentrations (Fairham and Harcourt-Brown, 1999). Vitamin D deficiency may be a contributory factor in the development of dental disease (see Section 7.5.1.1).

Vitamin D is rare in foods. Liver and animal fats are a source of vitamin D for carnivorous species but not for an obligate herbivore such as a rabbit. Instead, vitamin D must be metabolized endogenously or obtained from a dietary source such as sun-dried vegetation or a vitamin supplement. Irradiated plant sterols with anti-rachitic potency occur in the dead leaves of plants or sun-cured hays rather than in the green leaves of growing plants. Variation in the vitamin D content of hay can occur with different methods of curing. Exposure to irradiation by sunlight for long periods causes a marked increase in anti-rachitic potency of cut fodder, whereas modern hay making techniques with its emphasis on rapid curing tends to keep vitamin D levels at a minimum (Blood *et al.*, 1979). Rabbits enjoy eating dried vegetation such as fallen tree leaves in the autumn and will often eat them in preference to grass. There is also an interaction between vitamin A and vitamin D. Vitamin A appears to intensify the severity of rickets and inhibit the ability of vitamin D to cure the disease. Vitamin A administration to rats produced a decrease in total bone ash, increased the epiphyseal bone width and eliminated the ability of vitamin D to elevate serum calcium levels in a study by Rohde *et al.* (1999).

Commercial rabbit pellets are supplemented with vitamin D. In a study by Warren *et al.* (1989) rabbits from a breeding farm were found to have blood levels of 25-OH-D ten times higher than their laboratory counterparts despite comparable 1,25(OH_2)D values. The diet of the farmed rabbits contained 2200 IU/kg of vitamin D, yet PTH and serum total and ionized calcium values were not statistically different from the laboratory rabbits. Vitamin D toxicity has caused soft tissue mineralization in rabbits that were erroneously fed excessive quantities of supplement (Zimmerman *et al.*, 1990). Dietary levels above 2300 IU/kg appear to be toxic (Cheeke, 1987). A level of 800–1200 IU/kg is recommended for pet rabbits (Lowe, 1998). In view of the risk of inducing vitamin D toxicity by dietary administration, it seems sensible to expose rabbits to sunshine so they can synthesize their own vitamin D rather than rely on dietary supplementation. Sunlight has many beneficial physiological and psychological effects.

2.13.6.3 Vitamin E

Vitamin E is a fat-soluble vitamin that acts synergistically with selenium in most animals and prevents peroxide damage to tissues. Peroxides are formed during normal metabolic processes and are detoxified during a process catalysed by glutathione peroxidase, which contains selenium. Vitamin E is a natural antioxidant that inactivates the peroxides that cause widespread tissue damage. Vitamin E and/or selenium deficiency classically results in nutritional muscular dystrophy, which has been described in rabbits (see Section 12.6.1.4).

Green forages and cereals are good sources of vitamin E. Young grass contains more vitamin E than mature herbage. Leaves contain 20–30 times as much vitamin E as stems and up to 90% can be lost during haymaking, although losses are lower during artificial drying. Similarly, the vitamin E activity of cereal can decline rapidly if the grain is kept in moist conditions (McDonald *et al.*, 1996).

In rabbits, intercurrent liver disease caused by *Eimeria steidae* infection affects the metabolism of fat-soluble vitamins and predisposes to the development of muscular dystrophy. The requirement for vitamin E increases with dietary levels of polyunsaturated fatty acids and vegetable oils. A dietary level of 40–70 mg/kg has been suggested for pet rabbits (Lowe, 1998)

2.13.6.4 Vitamin K

Vitamin K is a clotting factor. Deficiency causes impaired blood clotting. Vitamin K is produced by caecal microorganisms and is a constituent of caecotrophs. Grass also contains vitamin K. Deficiencies are unlikely to occur in pet rabbits.

2.13.6.5 B-complex vitamins

Caecotrophs are a rich source of the B vitamins, niacin, riboflavin, pantothenic acid and vitamin B_{12}. Primary deficiencies of these vitamins are unlikely to occur in rabbits, as most diets contain sufficient quantities, in addition to the amounts that are synthesized by the caecal flora. Niacin and choline deficiencies have been induced under experimental conditions. Vitamin B_{12} requires cobalt, which could be a limiting factor in the diet.

2.13.6.6 Vitamin C

Vitamin C or ascorbic acid is synthesized from glucose in the liver by most mammals. It is required for the maintenance and repair of connective tissue. Ascorbic acid is stored in tissues with high metabolic activity such as adrenal glands, hypophysis and leucocytes (Verde and Piquer, 1986). Rabbits can synthesize vitamin C. However, there is evidence that the vitamin C requirements of rabbits increase during periods of stress when plasma ascorbic acid has been shown to decrease significantly (Verde and Piquer, 1986). Administration of vitamin C in conjunction with vitamin E prevented an increase in liver enzymes in rabbits experimentally infected with *Trypanosoma brucei brucei* (Umar *et al.*, 1999).

Key points 2.3

- Intercurrent disease such as coccidiosis increases the requirement for vitamins such as A or E
- Vitamin A deficiency can occur in housed rabbits on cereal diets and poor quality hay
- In most species, vitamin D is required for active transport of calcium from the gut to the bloodstream but in rabbits with sufficient dietary concentrations, calcium is absorbed efficiently and passively from the gut in the absence of vitamin D
- Passive calcium absorption is dependent on a diffusion gradient across the gut wall. Low dietary calcium results in a lower gradient and less absorption
- In rabbits, the regulatory role of vitamin D is due to its interaction with PTH and its effects on renal excretion and conservation of calcium
- If dietary calcium is low, active vitamin D dependent calcium absorption may be required because the passive diffusion gradient is low
- Vitamin D deficient rabbits develop rickets
- Sunlight is required for endogenous vitamin D synthesis
- Rabbits enjoy basking in the sun
- Undetectable vitamin D levels have been recorded in pet rabbits
- Cereal mixes contain supplements that contain calcium and vitamin D. Rabbits that selectively feed may leave the portion of the diet containing the vitamin and mineral supplement uneaten
- Vitamin D can be obtained in the diet from sun dried vegetation such as hay. Modern techniques can dry hay without the need for sunshine and, therefore, hay may be vitamin D deficient
- Vitamin D toxicity has been recorded in rabbits and causes mineralization of soft tissues, especially the kidneys and aorta
- Rabbits can synthesize vitamin C
- Caecotrophy provides a source of vitamins B and K.

2.13.7 Minerals

2.13.7.1 Calcium

Calcium is the most abundant mineral in the body. In combination with phosphorus it forms the dense, hard material of bone and teeth. It is an important cation in intracellular and extracellular fluid and is essential to blood clotting, muscle contractions, nerve cell activity, hormone regulation and the maintenance and stability of cell membranes. Rabbits require a constant supply of calcium for their teeth that continually erupt at a rate of approximately 2 mm per week. Calcium metabolism and its unusual aspects in rabbits are discussed in Section 1.6. Briefly, rabbits absorb calcium readily from the diet and do not homeostatically maintain blood levels as closely as other species. Total serum calcium levels vary across a wide range and are higher than in other mammals. Increased dietary calcium levels bring about an increase in serum calcium (Chapin and Smith, 1967a) which is excreted in the urine in the form of calcium carbonate, which give the urine a thick creamy appearance (Cheeke and Amberg, 1973). Urinary calcium levels are also related to dietary calcium intake (Kennedy, 1965).

Absorption of calcium across the intestinal mucosa is achieved by two parallel processes: active vitamin D dependent transcellular transport and passive paracellular diffusion (Breslau, 1996). In the rabbit, the main mechanism of calcium absorption appears to be passive diffusion, although active transport is important if dietary levels are low. Passive diffusion is bidirectional and depends on the concentration gradient between the intestinal lumen and the blood. Calcium is absorbed primarily in its ionic form and compounds that bind with calcium to form insoluble complexes reduce its availability (Breslau, 1996). The solubility of minerals such as calcium, magnesium and phosphorus in intestinal contents is affected by pH. For example, calcium absorption is increased in horses fed a high fibre diet due to lower stomach pH and increased saliva and pancreatic secretions that increase the solubility of calcium in the gut (Meyer *et al.*, 1992). It is not known if an analogous situation exists in the rabbit. Phytates, oxalates and acetates form complexes with calcium and other minerals and can prevent absorption (Fowler, 1986). Phytic acid (inositolhexaphosphoric acid) is present in high quantities in grains and beans. Oxalates are present in a number of plants including swede, spinach and alfalfa in which

Table 2.2 Mean calcium (Ca) and phosphorus (P) content (%) of three randomly selected brands of mixed rations sold as rabbit food

Samples of rabbit food were taken from batches of mixed rations bought from the same three pet shops on three different occasions. 1 lb (0.45 kg) of food was sent for analysis. The remainder of the batch was picked over to remove the whole grain and the pellets, which are the ingredients most likely to be rejected by pet rabbits (see Figure 2.3). 1 lb (0.45 kg) of the remaining ration (without pellets and grain) was sent for analysis.

Sample	*Food A*	*Food A (no pellets or grain)*	*Food B*	*Food B (no pellets or grain)*	*Food C*	*Food C (no pellets or grain)*
1 Ca (%)	0.70	**0.26****	0.56	0.46	0.79	**0.16******
P (%)	0.35	**0.28**	0.39	0.30	0.32	**0.26**
2 Ca (%)	0.63	**0.28****	0.51	0.38**	0.87	**0.11******
P (%)	0.41	**0.34**	0.39	0.32	0.36	**0.27**
3 Ca (%)	0.65	0.39**	0.49	0.48	0.98	**0.14******
P (%)	0.41	0.29	0.39	0.32	0.36	**0.29**

Figures in **bold** denote an inverse calcium:phosphorus ratio.
** Calcium levels below the 0.4% minimum level recommended for rabbits by National Research Council (1977) Nutrient Requirements of Rabbits.
**** Calcium level below the 0.22% minimum dietary requirement for rabbits determined by Chapin and Smith (1967).
NB. A level of at least 0.44% calcium has been determined for maximum bone ash and bone density (Chapin and Smith, 1967).
(Reprinted from Harcourt-Brown (1996) with permission from the *Veterinary Record*).

20–30% of the calcium is in the form of calcium oxalate that reduces its availability. In a study by Cheeke *et al.* (1985), 49% of the calcium in calcium oxalate was available to rabbits. Low oxalate, high calcium vegetables include kale, broccoli, turnip, collard and mustard greens (Breslau, 1996). Calcium can also bind with long-chain unsaturated fatty acids in the intestine to form insoluble soaps.

Calcium absorption can be enhanced by certain dietary factors. Soluble complexes can be formed with certain amino acids such as lysine and arginine and antibiotics such as chloramphenicol and penicillin. The soluble complexes prevent the formation of insoluble complexes and therefore facilitate calcium absorption. Lactose also increases the absorption of calcium from the gut (Breslau, 1996).

Many ingredients of rabbit food have a low calcium content that decreases the concentration gradient for passive diffusion from the gut into the blood. Vitamin D may not be available for active calcium transport across the gut wall. Undetectable vitamin D levels have been recorded in pet rabbits (Fairham and Harcourt-Brown, 1999). Calcium deficiency can be a contributory factor to poor tooth and bone quality and dental disease in pet rabbits.

The selection of cereals and legumes from mixed rations results in a diet containing less in calcium than the amount required for bone calcification (Table 2.2) (Harcourt-Brown, 1995, 1996). Excessive dietary calcium may contribute to the development of urolithiasis (Kamphues *et al.*, 1986). Therefore, the dietary level of calcium is important. The calcium requirement for rabbits has been determined (Chapin and Smith, 1967a). A minimum of 0.22% is required to support normal growth but a level of 0.44% is required for bone calcification. A level of 0.6–1.0% is recommended for pet rabbits (Lowe, 1998). The calcium and phosphorus content of some ingredients of rabbit food is summarized in Table 2.3.

2.13.7.2 Phosphorus

Phosphorus has many physiological functions. It is closely associated with calcium and forms a major constituent of bone. Phosphorus occurs in phosphoproteins, nucleic acids and phospholipids and plays a vital role in energy metabolism. Absorption and excretion is regulated by vitamin D. Dietary phosphorus levels affect calcium absorption as calcium binds with phosphorus to form insoluble

Table 2.3 Calcium and phosphorus content of some common foods for rabbits

Type of food	*Water (%)*	*Dry matter (%)*	*Calcium (% of dry matter)*	*Phosphorus (% of dry matter)*	*Calcium: phosphorus ratio (approx.)*	*High, medium or low source of calcium*
Alfalfa	10	90	1.5	0.30	5:1	High
Apple	79	21	0.06	0.06	1:1	Low
Barley (grain)	11	89	0.07	0.39	1:6	Low
Banana	76	24	0.03	0.11	1:36	Low
Beans e.g. kidney	10	90	0.14	0.46	1:3	Low
Bran	11	89	0.16	0.14	1:1	Low
Bread	36	64	0.09	0.16	1:17	Low
Cabbage	78	12	0.64	0.35	2:1	Moderate
Carrot tops	83	17	1.94	0.19	10:1	High
Carrots	88	12	0.37	0.325	1:1	Moderate
Celery	94	6	0.66	0.47	1:1	Moderate
Chickweed			0.8	0.6	1:1	Moderate
Clover	80	20	1.4	1.30	1:1	High
Dandelion	85	15	1.3	0.46	3:1	High
Grass	80	205	0.50	0.37	1:1	Moderate
Goosegrass			1.5	0.4	4:1	High
Kale	85	15	1.60	0.50	3:1	High
Lettuce	95	5	0.86	0.46	2:1	Moderate
Maize	88	12	0.04	0.28	1:7	Low
Oats	10	90	0.03	0.33	1:11	Low
Peas	11	89	0.12	0.41	1:3	Low
Pineapple	75	15	0.14	0.07	2:1	Low
Shepherd's purse			2.0	0.6	3:1	High
Sunflower seeds	8	92	0.22	0.68	1:3	Low
Sowthistle			1.5	0.5	3:1	High
Spear thistle			1.8	0.4	4:1	High
Swede	88	12	0.36	0.32	1:1	Moderate
Turnip	91	9	0.56	0.28	2:1	Moderate
Wheat	11	89	0.16	1.14	1:7	Low

Reference sources:
The Nutrient Requirements of Farm Livestock (1976) No. 4.
Composition of British Feedingstuffs. Technical Review and Tables. Agricultural Research Council. London.
Rabbit Feeding and Nutrition (1987) Cheeke, P. Academic Press. San Diego.
Animal Nutrition 5th Edition (1995) McDonald P. *et al.*, Longman Ltd.

calcium phosphate in the gut. Phytates that are found in many plants, especially grains, contain phosphorus that is released into the digestive tract of some species due to the action of ruminal or caecal fermentation. Investigations have shown that phytate phosphorus is available to rabbits (Cheeke, 1987). Phytates or oxalates can bind with calcium in the gut and affect the calcium:phosphorus ratio. The availability to rabbits of phosphorus in alfalfa is low (Cheeke *et al.*, 1985).

Phosphorus deficiency results in rickets in growing animals and osteomalacia in adults. In some areas the soil is deficient in phosphorus and grazing animals show symptoms of 'pica' (depraved appetite) where they chew wood, bones and other foreign material. Growing parts of plants are richer in phosphorus (McDonald *et al.*, 1996). In rabbits, dietary restriction of phosphorus causes hypophosphataemia and an increase in urinary excretion of calcium.

The calcium:phosphorus ratio in the diet affects bone density. In rabbits, a low calcium: phosphorus ratio of 1:2 or 1:3 does not affect bone calcification or growth rate unless dietary phosphorus levels are high. If dietary phosphorus concentrations increase to more than 1%

then bone density decreases if the calcium:phosphorus ratio falls below 1:1. Many cereals have phosphorus levels greater than 1% and a calcium:phosphorus ratio that is less than 1:1 and can therefore affect bone density. Rabbits are tolerant of a high calcium:phosphorus ratio. Growth rate and bone density are not affected by increasing calcium concentrations to a ratio of 12:1 (Chapin and Smith, 1967b).

The minimum requirement of phosphorus for optimum bone strength in growing rabbits is 0.22% (Mathieu and Smith, 1961). A nutritional requirement of phosphorus for maintenance of adult rabbits has not been determined. A dietary level of 0.4–0.8% has been suggested for pet rabbits (Lowe, 1998). The phosphorus content of grass and hay is less than 0.4% (McDonald *et al.*, 1996).

2.13.7.3 Other minerals

The nutritional requirement of magnesium, manganese, iron, zinc, copper and cobalt have been determined for rabbits. The precise role of magnesium in rabbit nutrition is largely unknown but deficiency has been linked with alopecia and alterations in fur texture. Experimentally induced magnesium deficiency results in poor growth, hyperexcitability and convulsions (Cheeke, 1987). Theoretically, excessive quantities of goitrogenic vegetables such as cabbage and brussels sprouts could result in iodine deficiency. These vegetables contain glucosinolates that convert to thiocyanate which can cause iodine deficiency and goitre. Suggested dietary levels of trace elements are given in Box 2.5.

Key points 2.4

- The correct amount of dietary calcium is important for rabbits
- Rabbits teeth grow at approximately 2 mm per week and require a constant supply of calcium
- Calcium deficiency results in poor mineralization of the bones and teeth. Excessive amounts of dietary calcium result in large amounts of calcium carbonate sediment in the urine, and predisposes to sludgy urine and cystitis
- A minimum level of 0.44% calcium is required for bone calcification
- Rabbits that select cereals and legumes from cereal mixes will be on a low calcium diet
- Poor quality hay can be deficient in either calcium or vitamin D or both
- Some fruit and root vegetables such as apples and carrots are deficient in calcium
- Alfalfa contains a high level of calcium
- Grass, weeds and hay contain the correct dietary level of calcium for rabbits
- Factors such as pH, phytates, phosphates, oxalates and fats in the intestinal lumen can influence calcium uptake from the gut
- Phytate phosphorus is available to rabbits.

2.14 Salt licks and mineral blocks

Salt licks are sold for rabbits and are available from most pet shops. They attach to the cage bars or wire mesh. There is little evidence that additional salt is required but some rabbits like the taste. Mineral blocks are also unnecessary as there is no need to supply extra minerals to a rabbit on a balanced diet. Some blocks contain high levels of calcium that could be harmful if the rabbit gnaws and eats them in large amounts. A rabbit confined to a hutch may destroy and eat the mineral block as a displacement activity, not because it has a need for additional minerals.

2.15 Grass and hay for pet rabbits

The natural food of rabbits is pasture grass. Grass is a balanced source of vitamins, minerals, fermentable and indigestible fibre. Rabbits have evolved to live on grass, which they find palatable and enjoyable. Ideally, pet rabbits should be given the opportunity to graze for several hours a day. If a predator-free enclosure cannot be provided, then fresh grass can be picked daily throughout the summer months to feed to pet rabbits. Clippings from the lawn mower are not suitable as they ferment rapidly. There is a small risk of transmitting parasites from wild rabbits, dogs and foxes through grass collected from contaminated pasture. Viral haemorrhagic disease vaccination is advisable. If fresh grass is unavailable, then hay can be provided as a substitute. Hay and grass can be offered together.

Natural grasslands are made up of a number of grass species and include legumes and other wild plants. The chemical composition of the pasture alters throughout the year. Grass grows rapidly during warm, wet weather and dries out as the herbage matures, leaving a feed resource that is sometimes referred to as 'standing hay' (McDonald *et al.*, 1996). The crude protein content of pasture grass can vary from 0.3% in mature herbage to 3% in young heavily fertilized grass. The fibre content tends to increase as the protein levels decrease. The water-soluble carbohydrates of grass include glucose, fructose and sucrose and vary with the species. The cellulose content is generally 20–30% and hemicelluloses vary from 10 to 30% (McDonald *et al.*, 1996). Lignin content increases with age and affects the availability of other nutrients except the water-soluble carbohydrates. The lipid composition is low and rarely exceeds 0.6%. The mineral content varies with species, stage of growth, soil type, cultivation conditions and fertilizer application. Green herbage is a rich source of vitamin A, vitamin E and many B vitamins, especially riboflavin. The vitamin D content increases as grass matures and is present in greater quantities in sun-dried hay than in young grass.

The species of grass depends on the type of pasture. In the UK, perennial ryegrass (*Lolium perenne*) is the most important species of sown pastures, but Italian ryegrass (*Lolium multiflorum*), timothy (*Phleum pratense*) and the fescues (*Festuca* spp.) are all common. In older pastures, these are accompanied by 'weed' grass species, particularly meadowgrass (*Poa pratensis*), Yorkshire fog (*Holcas lanatus*), and the bents (*Agrostis* spp.). In moorland pastures other species such as mat grass (*Nardus stricta*) and purple moor grass (*Molinia caerulea*) are found.

The digestibility of perennial ryegrass, Italian ryegrass and timothy are similar although hay made from timothy is slightly higher in crude fibre (34.1%) than ryegrass (30.5%). The protein content of timothy is lower than other grasses (McDonald *et al.*, 1996).

Traditional haymaking is dependent on a period of fine weather, which cannot be relied upon in the UK. The ideal haymaking weather is dry and sunny with a mild breeze. Rapid drying techniques using field machinery and barn drying equipment have recently been introduced to overcome some of the problems associated with unpredictable weather. The aim of haymaking is to reduce the moisture content of the green crop to a level low enough to inhibit the action of plant and microbial enzymes. Valuable nutrients are lost during the drying process due to the action of enzymes, oxidation, leaching and mechanical damage. The vitamin content of hay depends on the manner in which it was dried and the length of exposure to sunlight. Prolonged exposure to sunlight increases the vitamin D content, whereas rapid drying preserves the vitamin A content. Increased drying time allows bacterial fermentation to take place and rain on a partly dried crop leaches out minerals and encourages the growth of moulds (McDonald *et al.*, 1996). Ideally, good quality, sweet smelling, dust-free fresh hay that is suitable for feeding to horses should be selected for rabbits.

Lucerne or alfalfa (*Medicago sativa*) is a leguminous plant found in warm temperate areas and is grown as a forage crop. In the USA, alfalfa is used for grazing and for artificial drying to make hay. In the UK, some alfalfa is grown and harvested for silage or for artificial drying to make hay. The drying process can affect the vitamin D content. Dried alfalfa is approximately 25% crude fibre and is also rich in protein, calcium and vitamin A. It is high in oxalate that binds with calcium in the gut and affects absorption. Alfalfa can easily be grown in dry conditions and has proven to be a useful feed for rabbits in many parts of the world. In the UK, although alfalfa is recognized as a useful foodstuff for rabbits, it is not universally available and is only incorporated into a few types of rabbit foods. Some breeders use a high fibre horse food made from alfalfa to feed to rabbits. Alfalfa is retained in the digestive tract for longer than plain cellulose suggesting that it is digested to some degree in the caecum (Chiou *et al.*,1998).

Problems associated with feeding hay include the risk of transmitting infections and parasites to rabbits from vermin which have inhabited the crop prior to purchase. In the USA skunks and raccoons harbour ascarids, *Baylisascaris* for which rabbits act as paratenic hosts. Visceral larva migrans can result in tissue damage to a variety of organs including brain, heart and liver. Hay that has been contaminated with raccoon or skunk faeces is a potential source of infection. *Baylisascaris* eggs require 30 days outside the host to become infective.

Seeds and stems of hay can cause foreign body reactions and are a common cause of disease in pet rabbits. A number of conditions including tracheitis, rhinitis, abscesses, malocclusion, conjunctivitis and skin irritation are caused by stalks or seeds penetrating the oral and pharyngeal mucosa. They can also lodge in the nasal passages, nasopharynx or larynx. Grass seeds may become entangled in the fur and work their way into the dermis causing irritation and infection. Dusty hay can cause conjunctival and respiratory tract irritation and predispose secondary *Pasteurella* infections. Overhead feeders and hayracks increase the likelihood of dust and fragments of hay entering the nose or eyes.

2.16 Types of commercial rabbit food

A suggested food analysis for adult pet rabbits is summarized in Box 2.5.

Box 2.5 Suggested food analysis for adult pet rabbits

- Crude fibre: > 18%
- Indigestible fibre: > 12.5%
- Crude protein: 12–16%
- Fat: 1–4%
- Calcium: 0.6–1.0%
- Phosphorus: 0.4–0.8%
- Vitamin A: 10 000–18 000 IU/kg
- Vitamin D: 800–1200 IU/kg
- Vitamin E: 40–70 mg/kg
- Trace elements: Magnesium 0.3%, Zinc 0.5%, Potassium 0.6–0.7%

NB. It is especially important to ensure that growing rabbits receive sufficient calcium. Mixed rations are not suitable for young rabbits that are kept in groups where it is impossible to ensure that each individual is eating a balanced diet.

There is a variety of rabbit foods available in the UK. The owner's choice is often based on advice from the pet shop or breeder or on marketing and advertising literature. There are

Box 2.6 Labelling requirements for rabbit food

In the UK there are legal requirements covering the information that is given to purchasers of rabbit food (North Yorkshire County Council, Trading Standards and Regulatory Service; personal communication).

- Commercially prepared feeds are considered to be complete, complementary or a food supplement and this information should be displayed on the packaging. Complete feeds should provide all the nutrients required by the animal in the correct quantities. Complementary feeds require additional foods to be included in the diet. Feed supplements are concentrated sources of nutrients such as vitamins and minerals that are used to supplement other diets
- Labelling should include the name and address of the person guaranteeing that the information is accurate and the name and description of the feed plus a list of ingredients
- There must be directions for use and a 'best before' date
- For food sold loose, the pet shop should display a statutory notice indicating the nutritional properties of the feed and the species of animal for which the product is intended. The statutory statement should be displayed in close proximity to the feed. The minimum requirements, which must be displayed, are protein, oil, fibre and ash
- For pre-packed food the statutory notice should be displayed on the packaging or on a label attached to the packaging of the feed itself
- Despite the requirement to display information, there is no requirement to produce feeds to certain compositional standards
- The stated composition of the feed should not vary although small variation (± 20%) may be acceptable.

Producers that make false claims are liable for prosecution under the Trades Description Act 1968 but only statements pertaining to some measurable parameter can be proved to be false. Therefore phrases such as 'for a happy, healthy pet' or 'for the rabbit that has everything' are unlikely to be challenged although such statements can be misleading.

Box 2.7 Feeding recommendations for pet rabbits

- Introduce new foods gradually
- Good quality hay or grass should be available at all times, unless a complete diet is provided that specifically states that no other food is needed. Even with a complete diet, additional hay, grass or vegetables will not be harmful
- Feed a wide range of green foods and vegetables every day. Fruit and succulent vegetables such as lettuce and tomatoes should be given in moderation
- Follow manufacturer's instructions when feeding proprietary rabbit food. If the rabbit does not eat all the mixture, change the diet
- If possible, allow rabbits outside to exercise in natural daylight. Care is needed to prevent them escaping or being attacked by neighbours' dogs. Rabbits can be very destructive in the garden
- Feed small amounts of concentrated food, such as pellets, cereal mixes or extruded diets, only once a day and remove the bowl after a couple of hours. If there is food left in the bowl, feed less food the next day. Hay or grass is available if the rabbit feels hungry
- No more than 2–3% of the rabbit's bodyweight of cereal mixes, pelleted or extruded rations should be fed daily.

Safe plants for rabbits

- Grass of any type is safe, palatable and ideal for rabbits. Vaccination against viral haemorrhagic disease (VHD) is advisable due to the risk of transmission from wild rabbits
- Wild plants that are safe include: agrimony, brambles, chickweed, clover, coltsfoot, cow parsnip (hogweed), dandelion, young docks, goosegrass, ground elder, groundsel, knapweed, mallow, mayweed, plantain, raspberry, sea beet, shepherd's purse, sow-thistle, trefoil, vetch, wild strawberry and yarrow (NB: Many of these plants are illustrated in Virginia Richardson's book *Rabbit Nutrition*)
- Safe cultivated plants include: artichoke leaves, apple, beetroot, broccoli, brussels sprouts, cabbage, carrots and carrot tops, celery, cauliflower leaves, chicory, coriander, corncobs, green beans, kale, kohl rabi, lettuce (in moderation), parsley, peapods, pear, parsnip, radish, spinach, spring greens (spring cabbage), sprout peelings, sunflowers plants, swedes, sweetcorn plants, turnips, watercress. Turnips and spinach should be fed occasionally (not more than once a week) due to their oxalate content
- Tree leaves can be eaten by rabbits, especially from fruit trees and hazel.

legal requirements for the labelling of rabbit food that are summarized in Box 2.6. Commercial feeds are divided into complementary and complete diets. Complementary diets are meant to be fed as part of a diet that includes other foods, usually hay. Complete diets do not require any supplementary food items.

The visual appearance of the food is important to the owner but probably not to the rabbit. The rabbit has a wide visual field that enables it to observe surrounding predators while it is eating. The visual field does not include the area below the mouth, so food selection is based on odour and tactile information from the vibrissae. Feeding recommendations for pet rabbits are summarized in Box 2.7.

2.16.1 Pelleted diets

Pelleted food consists of small cylinders of ingredients that have been ground and compressed together with a binding agent. Vitamins and minerals can be incorporated into the pellet along with sweetening agents such as molasses to improve palatability. Particle size of the ingredients is important, as it affects the digestibility of the ration and its rate of passage through the digestive tract (Lang, 1981). Small particles tend to accumulate in the caecum and lead to an increased incidence of enteritis (Sanchez *et al.*, 1984). Pelleted diets can be complete or complementary. They vary in quality. Coccidiostats are usually incorporated into the pellet to reduce the incidence of coccidiosis in intensive rabbit units. The actual pelleting process does not kill any oocysts that may be contaminating the feed (Owen, 1978).

The advantages of pelleted diets are that they are convenient, easy to store and do not allow the rabbit to select out certain ingredients. Different formulations can be pelleted to provide diets for rabbit that are pregnant, lactating or growing. Fibre can be incorporated into the pellet but processing reduces some of its beneficial properties and tends to make the pellets friable. Pellet binders can be used to overcome this problem. Substances such as magnesium lignosulphate, which is a byproduct of the wood pulp industry, or a clay mineral binder such as sodium betonite can be used (Lang, 1981). Disadvantages of pelleted diets are their low palatability in comparison with mixed cereal rations and the owners' perception that they look boring. As a complete diet, pellets provide little in the way of dental exercise and are not a good source of indigestible fibre. Supplementary hay is required.

2.16.2 Extruded or expanded diets

Expanded diets are produced by blending and heating the raw ingredients to a high temperature, before being extruded and dried. The basic ingredients are ground and mixed prior to steam heating. A paste is formed that is forced through a shaped die and cooled. The result is a lightweight biscuit that can be any size or shape. It stores well and is virtually sterile. Long fibre particles can be incorporated without the pellets becoming friable and disintegrating. Vitamins are partly denatured by the processing and need to be added to the initial mixture in higher quantities to allow for this. Heat treatment increases starch digestibility (Cheeke, 1987) and reduces carbohydrate overload of the hindgut. Extruded diets are more palatable and digestible than pelleted rations (Tobin, 1996). They do not allow the animal to eat an unbalanced diet by selecting out favourite ingredients. Although extruded pellets can be made in a variety of sizes, shapes and colours, they still look less attractive than mixed rations to the owner and do not provide high quantities of indigestible fibre.

2.16.3 Mixed rations

The composition of mixed rations varies between sources. They can be complete or complementary. Most mixed rations are complementary and are designed to be fed with hay to provide indigestible fibre. Feed companies decide on the formulation according to cost, availability of ingredients and the experience of the nutritionist. Nutritional data are obtained from analysis tables and extrapolated to formulate a feed based on the requirements of commercial rabbits. Mixed rations are often sold loose from pet shops with no labelling information. Owners are encouraged to leave a bowl full of food with the rabbit permanently. The rations usually consist of flaked, micronized or rolled cereals and legumes mixed with highly coloured extruded 'biscuits' and pellets. Stems of alfalfa can be incorporated as a source of calcium and fibre. The colour of the extruded portions in combination with green flaked peas and yellow flaked maize make these mixtures visually appealing to the owner. Molasses or liquid sweetening agents can be added along with other ingredients such as locust beans or compressed linseed. Some rations contain byproducts from the human food industry, such as stale breakfast cereals. Whole grains are incorporated to prevent the rabbit picking out the kernel and leaving the fibrous husk. However, most rabbits are able to separate and eat the kernel and leave the husk uneaten. Wheat has a tendency to be pasty (Lowe, 1998) and is usually extruded into a coloured biscuit that is included in mixed rations. Pellets are added to the mixture as a vehicle for a powdered vitamin and mineral supplement. Some brands now incorporate the supplement into the extruded wheat portion or spray the whole mixture with a supplemented coating.

The advantages of mixed rations are that they are universally available, palatable, cheap, convenient and visually attractive to the owner. They are available from pet shops, supermarkets, agricultural suppliers, garages, garden centres and wholesalers under the universal name of 'rabbit food'. Apart from the general problems associated with feeding *ad lib* concentrated foods (obesity, insufficient dietary fibre, dental exercise and foraging), mixed cereal rations have the additional disadvantage of allowing rabbits to select out their favourite ingredients and leave the rest uneaten (see Figure 2.3). Discarded food is generally taken away by the owner and replaced with a fresh bowlful for the rabbit to select from. Owners worry about their pets being bored or hungry and sometimes refill

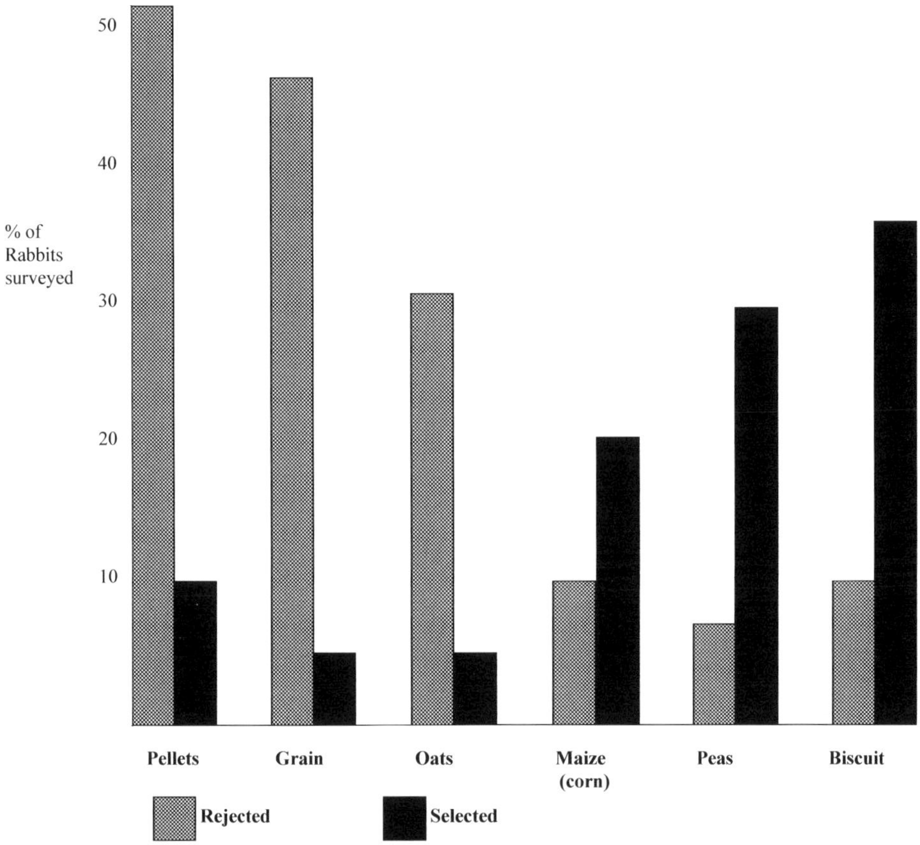

Figure 2.3. Selective feeding in rabbits. Results of owner questionnaire: food preference of pet rabbits. Ninety rabbit owners completed a questionnaire about the feeding habits of their pet. All the rabbits were fed on mixed rations purchased as 'rabbit food'. Hay was offered to all the rabbits in the survey although they did not always eat it. Some rabbits were given additional vegetables or allowed to graze in a run periodically through the summer months.
In nearly every case, a bowl of 'rabbit food' was left with the rabbit permanently. Discarded food was thrown away and the bowl topped once or twice daily. This feeding practice allowed rabbits to select their favourite food items and eat nothing else. Some rabbits existed on one or two ingredients. The low calcium cereals and peas were the rabbits' favourite part of the ration. The pellets that contain a vitamin and mineral supplement were the least palatable part of the mixture. However, some rabbits would eat the entire mixture and a minority would select the pellets. (From Harcourt-Brown (1996), reprinted with permission from *Veterinary Record*).

the bowl several times a day so the rabbit may exist on only one or two favourite ingredients. The pellets, which contain the vitamin and mineral supplement, are often left uneaten. The most palatable portions of these diets are the flaked peas and flaked maize which are deficient in calcium and have a low calcium to phosphorus ratio. Selection of these ingredients results in a diet with calcium concentrations below the rabbit's known dietary requirement (Harcourt-Brown, 1996). Demineralization of the bones and teeth results in dental problems (see Section 7.5.1.1). A balanced diet is especially important to juvenile rabbits that are growing rapidly and therefore susceptible to metabolic bone disease. Selection of low calcium cereals and legumes from mixed rations at this stage can have life-long detrimental effects on bones and teeth.

Key points 2.5

- Grass is a balanced source of vitamins, minerals, fermentable (digestible) and indigestible fibre for rabbits
- The digestibility of the species of grasses that are found in UK pastures are similar although timothy (*Phleum pratense*) has a slightly higher crude fibre and lower protein content
- Alfalfa (lucerne, *Medicago sativa*) is used for grazing and haymaking in warm countries. It is an unusual crop in the UK
- Alfalfa has a high fibre and calcium content
- Infections may be transmitted to pet rabbits from hay that has been contaminated by vermin
- Seeds and stems of hay can become lodged in the eye, mouth, nose, nasopharynx or larynx and are an underdiagnosed cause of clinical disease
- Commercial rabbit foods for rabbits are composed of pelleted, extruded or mixed rations
- Pelleted diets consist of ingredients that have been ground and compressed
- Extruded foods are ground, blended and cooked to form a lightweight biscuit that is sterile, palatable and stores well
- Mixed rations vary between sources and contain a range of ingredients including flaked, micronized, rolled or whole grains such as corn, wheat, oats or barley plus legumes such as peas and beans. Dried vegetables such as carrots and leeks may be added. Most mixed rations also contain pellets and/or extrusions
- Mixed rations that are available in countries outside the UK contain other ingredients such as sunflower seeds, peanuts, corn kernels or dried peas.

2.17 Problems associated with feeding

2.17.1 Locust beans and dried pulses

Locust beans are pods of either the Mediterranean carob tree (*Ceratomia siliqua*) or the African locust bean (*Parkia filicoidea*). The pod consists of a woody husk that is sweet and palatable to rabbits and contains hard shiny beans. The beans are used for the manufacture of gums and oils in the cosmetic industry. Crushed locust bean husks are sometimes included in rabbit foods and occasionally a hard bean can make its way into the mixture along with the husk. Unfortunately, these beans are too hard for rabbits to chew and can be swallowed whole. They pass through the stomach undigested and can lodge in the small intestine causing an acute obstruction and death. Dried peas and sweetcorn carry the same risk. Because of the risk of intestinal obstruction, many leading rabbit food manufacturers no longer use locust beans in their rations.

2.17.2 Toxic plants

Owners are often worried about the possibility of plant toxicity if they pick natural vegetation or give their rabbit the freedom of the garden. Rabbits will eat almost anything, including plants known to be toxic to other species and so it is not easy to reassure owners that their pet will not suffer any adverse effects. Toxicity varies and depends on a number of factors, such as the amount ingested, the part of the plant that is eaten and the frequency of ingestion. Drying can cause an increase or decrease in toxicity or have no effect at all.

Many plants that contain toxic compounds are acrid and unpalatable. Irritant compounds cause oral discomfort and are unlikely to be ingested in large quantities. Many plant poisons are not fatal and so the knowledge that a pet rabbit has eaten a known poisonous plant does not necessarily mean it will die. Conversely, plants that are considered safe can be toxic if ingested in large quantities or daily over a period of time. Examples in other species include apples or clover both of which can cause digestive upsets in ruminants. In general, if no ill effects are observed within 6 h of the ingestion of a potentially poisonous plant, then it is unlikely that signs will develop (Veterinary Poisons Unit, personal communication).

There are few definite reports of plant toxicity in rabbits. Instead, rabbits are reported to be resistant to the effects of pyrrolizidene alkaloids, which are found in plants such as ragwort and comfrey (Cheeke *et al.*, 1982).

Key points 2.6

- Although owners worry about plant toxicity in rabbits, there are few confirmed reports
- Rabbits appear to be resistant to many plant toxins such as ragwort, deadly nightshade, comfrey and laburnum
- Some agrochemicals used as weedkillers are toxic to rabbits
- Rabbits are sensitive to mycotoxins, such as aflatoxin.

Amaranthus species (*A. retroflexus*; Pigweed, Red Wheat, *A. viridis*; Green Amaranthus) causes ascites with lemon yellow serous fluid (Lorgue *et al.*, 1996). Although *Amaranthus* species are not native to the UK, garden escapes may be found on waste ground (Fitter *et al.*, 1974). *Amaranthus retroflexus* has been used in rabbit feeds with poor results (Cheeke, 1987). *Amaranthus albus* is the common garden plant 'Love Lies Bleeding'.

A condition known as 'head down disease' is caused by ingestion of Woolly Pod Milkweed (*Asclepias eriocarpa*) in the USA. Affected animals develop paralysis of the neck muscles and loss of coordination. Drooling, rough hair coat, subnormal temperature and tarlike faeces occur. Recovery is possible (see Section 12.6.1.2). The toxic principal is a resinoid. Woolly milkweed does not grow in Great Britain.

The houseplant, *Dieffenbacchia* is reputed to be poisonous to rabbits. Avocado leaves are also toxic to rabbits although the toxicity of the plant varies with the variety. Mexican avocados are less toxic than Guatemalan varieties. *Post-mortem* examination shows lung congestion (Craigmill *et al.*, 1984).

Daffodil bulbs and horse chestnuts are poisonous to dogs if they are eaten in quantities (Campbell, 1998) and many other garden plants can cause toxic symptoms, such as gastrointestinal effects, although they are not necessarily fatal. Examples include cotoneaster, honeysuckle and pyracantha. Plants used for Christmas decorations, i.e. holly, ivy and mistletoe are all known to be toxic in other species. The houseplants Leopard Lily and Christmas Cherry cause vomiting and diarrhoea in dogs (Campbell, 1998).

Long-term, continuous ingestion of certain vegetables can cause toxicity. Although the effects of goitrogenic vegetables such as cabbage, spring greens and brussels sprouts have not been documented in rabbits, there is a theoretical risk associated with feeding large amounts of these vegetables. Similarly oxalates in spinach, alfalfa and turnips can affect the absorption of some minerals such as calcium or magnesium. Problems with toxic principals in vegetables can be avoided by offering two or three types daily and changing the range each day. Grass is safe and can be given *ad lib*. Plants that may be toxic to rabbits are listed in Table 2.4 overleaf.

2.17.3 Chemicals

Cultivated crops do not cause the same amount of owner anxiety as natural vegetation, and yet there are health implications for rabbits fed on treated vegetation. Although rabbits appear relatively resistant to plant toxins, they are susceptible to some agrochemicals. For example, nitrophenols, which are used as herbicides, fungicides or antisprouting agents on potatoes, can make the plants extremely toxic to rabbits (Lorgue *et al.*, 1996). Ingestion of the toxin occurs by eating recently treated vegetation. The compounds stimulate tissue respiration while simultaneously impairing adenosine triphosphate (ATP) synthesis. Hyperthermia, methaemoglobinaemia, jaundice and pulmonary oedema are among the clinical signs. Ingestion of hay grown from a monoculture sprayed with a selective herbicide such as a triazine can cause poisoning. Treated, triazine-resistant weeds are dried and eaten in contaminated hay. Symptoms of poisoning in other species are non-specific and include anorexia, weight loss, depression, salivation, muscle atonia, weakness and paraplegia or hyperexcitability, Treatment is symptomatic and the prognosis generally good. Garden fungicides that are used to treat lawns also belong to the triazine group. Herbicides such as glycosate and substituted ureas are unlikely to be poisonous to rabbits.

2.17.4 Mycotoxins

Mycotoxins are toxic metabolites of fungi such as *Aspergillus* spp. that causes a range of

Table 2.4 Potentially toxic plants for rabbits

Rabbit owners are often concerned about the safety of feeding naturally growing plants and weeds to their rabbits. During an extensive search of the literature, few definite reports of plant toxicity in rabbits could be found although many plants were cited as potentially poisonous. There are anecdotal reports of bizarre behaviour in rabbits after presumed ingestion of some species of wild mushrooms. The following table is a list of potentially toxic plants for rabbits although in many cases, extrapolations have been made from other species.

The following plants can be bought as vegetables or grow in gardens and hedgerows in the UK. Poisonous plants from other countries are not included.

Plant	*Toxic principal*	*Comments*
Amaranthus: *A. retroflexus* (Red wheat) *A. viridis* (Green amaranthus)	Oxalic acid	Red wheat is known to be toxic to rabbits. *A. albus* is the garden plant Love-Lies-Bleeding
Antirrhinums		Known to be poisonous in other species
Arum	Calcium oxalate and other irritants	Can cause swelling and discomfort of the oral cavity in other species
Buttercups(fresh)	Protoaneminin	Causes irritation to mucous membranes including GI tract in other species
Bracken	Thiaminase	Toxic in cattle, sheep and horses + bone marrow suppressant
Bryony	Irritant substance and histamine	Berries and rhizomes are poisonous
Cabbage	Glucosinolate	Goitrogenic if fed in large quantities
Celandines	A variety of alkaloids	Unpalatable Irritant effects. Purgative
Charlock		Poisonous in other species
Comfrey	Pyrrolizidine Alkaloids	Hepatotoxic (rabbits appear to be resistant to toxic effects)
Convolvulus		Poisonous in other species
Crotalaria	Pyrrolizidine Alkaloids	Hepatotoxic (rabbits appear to be resistant to toxic effects)
Dahlia		Known to be poisonous in other species
Evergreens(except conifers)		Known to be poisonous in other species
Figwort		Reputed to be poisonous
Foxglove	Cardiac glycoside (digitalis)	Known to be poisonous in other species
Hellibore	Variety of alkaloids	Known to be poisonous in a range of species
(Christmas rose)		Whole plant is toxic especially during flowering
Hemlock	Variety of alkaloids	Whole plant is toxic Unpalatable
Henbane	Anticholinergic	Seeds are most toxic part of the plant Unpalatable
Horsetails	Thiaminase Alkaloids Silica	Toxic to other species (horses) if ingested over long periods. Remains toxic after drying, i.e. hay
Irises		Reputed to be poisonous
Ivy	Unidentified	Whole plant, including berries poisonous Large quantities need to be ingested.
Kale	Thiocyanates S-methyl-cysteine-sulfoxide Nitrates Antithyroid	Toxicity reported in ruminants Needs to be ingested large quantities Can cause haemolytic anaemia in other species
Laburnum	Alkaloids	Seeds especially are known to be poisonous in other species Rabbits may be resistant to toxic compounds

Lily of the valley	Variety of alkaloids	Variety of symptoms
Linseed	Cyanogenetic Heteroside	Ingestion of > 400 g/100 kg of oil-seed cake can be toxic in other species
Lupins	Quinolizidene Alkaloids	Most cultivated lupins are of low toxicity
Milkweed	Cardiac glycoside	
Monkshood (aconite)	Alkaloid	Unpalatable, irritant
Nightshade	Atropine	Many rabbits are resistant to poisoning due to presence of atropinesterase
Oleander	Cardiac glycoside	
Poppies	Opium alkaloids	Entire plant is toxic even after drying
Potato plants	Solanines	Can cause haemolysis in other species (cattle and pigs) if large quantities of leaves or stems are fed or small quantities over a long period
Potatoes	Nitrophenol	Potatoes may be sprayed with nitrophenols to prevent sprouting. The spray can be toxic to rabbits
Privet	Tannins Heteroside	Can be fatal in other species
Ragwort	Pyrrolizidine Alkaloids	Hepatotoxic Rabbits appear to be resistant to toxic effects
Scarlet pimpernel		Reputed to be poisonous
Speedwell		Reputed to be poisonous
Spurges	Alkaloids	Cause intense local irritation to mucous membranes in other species
Toadflax		Reputed to be poisonous
Tomato plants	Solanines	Can cause haemolysis in other species (cattle and pigs) if large leaves or stems are fed or small quantities over a long period
Travellers joy (Clematis vitalba)		Reputed to be poisonous
Wild celery		Reputed to be poisonous
Yew	Taxine	Cut branches more toxic than when fresh Very toxic in other species Can cause sudden death Probably toxic to rabbits

There are other toxic plants not included in this list that are wise to avoid, e.g. acorns, box hedging, laurel, cypress, verbena, potentilla, rhododendron, water dropwort. In general, plants that grow from bulbs can be considered to be potentially poisonous.
Reference sources: Lang, J. (1981); Cheeke, P.R. (1987); Sandford, J. (1996); Lorgue, G. *et al.*, (1996); Gfeller, R.W., Messonier S.P. (1998); Richardson, V. (1999).

diseases in many species. Aflatoxin is produced by *Aspergillus flavus* and may be found in mouldy feeds, especially peanuts. Subclinical aflatoxicosis affects natural defence mechanisms and immunogenesis. Rabbits are susceptible to aflatoxin toxicity, which causes gastroenteritis and liver damage. It is not known how widespread this problem is in pet rabbits that consume cereals and grains of uncertain age and quality. In a study by Fekete and Huszenicza (1993), rabbits did not refuse grain that contained sufficient aflatoxin to cause immunosuppression and fatal secondary bacterial infection.

References

Bellier R., Gidenne T. (1996). Consequences of reduced fibre intake on digestion, rate of passage and caecal microbial activity in the young rabbit (Abstract). *Br Vet J.*, **75**, 353–363.

Berthelsen, H., Hansen, L.T. (1999). The effect of hay on the behaviour of caged rabbits (Oryctolagus cuniculus) *Animal Welfare*, **8**, 149–157.

Blood, D.C., Henderson, J.A., Radostits O.M. (1979). *Veterinary Medicine*, 5th edn. p. 910. Balliere Tindall.

Blood, D.C., Studdert, V.P. (1999). *Ballieres Comprehensive Veterinary Dictionary*. Balliere Tindall.

Bourdeau, J.E., Shwer-Dymerski, D.A., Stern, P.A., Langman, C.B. (1986). Calcium and phosphorous metabolism in chronically vitamin D-deficient laboratory rabbits. *Miner Electrolyte Metab.*, **12**, 176–185.

Breslau, N.A. (1996). Calcium, magnesium and phosphorus: Intestinal absorption. In *Primer on the Metabolic Bone Diseases and Disorders of Mineral Metabolism.* (M.J. Favus, ed.) pp 49–56. Lippincott-Raven.

Brommage, R., Miller, S.C., Langman, C.B. *et al.* (1988). The effect of chronic Vitamin D deficiency on the skeleton in the adult rabbit. *Bone*, **9**, 131.

Brown, S.A. (1997). Rabbit gastrointestinal physiology and disease. *Proceedings of Atlantic Coast Veterinary Conference*, Atlantic City.

Campbell, A. (1998). Poisoning in small animals from commonly ingested plants. *In Practice*, **20**, 587–591.

Campbell, J.M., Fahey, G.C, Wolf, B.W. (1997). Selected indigestible oligosaccharides affect large bowel mass, cecal and fecal short-chain fatty acids, pH and microflora in rats (Abstract). *J Nutr.*, **127**, 130–136.

Carabaõ, R., Fraga, M.J., Santoma, G., de Blas, J. (1988). Effect of diet on composition of cecal contents and on excretion and composition of soft and hard feces of rabbits. *J Anim Sc.*, **66**, 901–910.

Chapin, R.E., Smith, S.E. (1967a). Calcium requirement of growing rabbits. *J Anim Sci.*, **26**, 67–71.

Chapin, R.E., Smith, S.E. (1967b). The calcium tolerance of growing rabbits. *Cornell Veterinarian*, **57**, 492.

Cheeke, P.R. (1987). *Rabbit Feeding and Nutrition.* Academic Press.

Cheeke, P.R. (1994). Nutrition and nutritional diseases. In *The Biology of the Laboratory Rabbit*, 2nd edn. (P.J. Manning, D.H. Ringler, C.E. Newcomer, eds). pp 321–333. Academic Press.

Cheeke, P.R., Amberg, J.W. (1973). Comparative calcium excretion by rats and rabbits. *J Anim Sci.*, **37**, 450.

Cheeke, P.R., Patton N.M., Templeton G.S. (1982). *Rabbit Production.* Interstate Publishers.

Cheeke, P.R., Bronson, J., Robinson, K.L., Patton N.M. (1985). Availability of calcium, phosphorus and magnesium in rabbit feeds and mineral supplements. *J Appl Rabbit Res.*, **8**, 72–74.

Chiou, P.W., Yu, B., Lin, C. (1998). The effect of different fibre components on growth rate, nutrient digestibility, rate of digesta passage and hindgut fermentation in domestic rabbits. *Lab Anim.*, **32**, 276–283.

Craigmill, A.L., Eide, R.N., Shultz, T.A., Hedrick, K. (1984). Toxicity of avocado (*Persea americana*, Guatamalan var.) leaves: Review and preliminary report. *Vet Hum Toxicol.*, **26**, 381–383.

Crossley, D.A. (1995). Clinical aspects of lagomorph dental anatomy: The rabbit (*Oryctolagus cuniculus*). *J Vet Dent.*, **12**, 137–140.

Curry, O.B., Basten, J.F., Francis, M.J.O., Smith, R. (1974). Calcium uptake by sarcoplasmic reticulum of muscle from vitamin D deficient rabbits. *Nature*, **249**, 83–84.

De Blas, E., Gidenne, T. (1998). Digestion of starch and sugars. In *The Nutrition of the Rabbit.* (C. de Blas and J.Wiseman, eds). pp 17–38. CABI Publishing.

Drescher, B. (1993). Zusammenfassende Betrachtung über den Einflub unterscheidlicher Haltungsverfahren auf die Fitness von Versuchs- und Fleischkaninchen. *Tierärzl Umschau*, **48**, 72–6.

Drescher, B., Breig, P. (1993). Einflub unterscheidlicher Haltungs-verfahren auf die Nebennien von Kaninchen. (Article in German, English abstract). *Tierärzl Umschau*, **48**, 30–34.

Drescher, B., Loeffler, K. (1996). Scoliosis, lordosis and kyphosis in breeding rabbits. *Tierärzl Prax*, **24**, 292–300.

Fairham, J., Harcourt-Brown, F.M. (1999). Preliminary investigation of the vitamin D status of pet rabbits. *Vet Rec.*, **145**, 452–454.

Fekete, S. (1989). Recent findings and future perspectives of digestive physiology in rabbits: a review. *Acta Vet Hung.*, **37**, 265–279.

Fekete, S., Bokori, J. (1985). The effect of the fibre and protein level of the ration upon cecotrophy of rabbit. *J Appl Rabbit Res.*, **8**, 68–71.

Fekete, S., Huszenicza, G. (1993). Effects of T-2 Toxin on ovarian activity and some metabolic variables of rabbits. *Lab Anim Sci.*, **43**, 646–649.

Fitter, R., Fitter, A., Blamey, M. (1974). *The Wild Flowers of Britain and Northern Europe.* Collins.

Fowler, M.E.,(1986). Metabolic bone disease. In *Zoo and Wild Animal Medicine,* 2nd edn. (M.E. Fowler, ed.) pp 69–90. W.B. Saunders.

Fox, R.R., Crary, D.D. (1971). Mandibular prognathism in the rabbit. *J Hered.*, **62**, 163–169.

Fox, R.R., Eaton, H.D., Crary, D.D. (1982). Vitamin A, beta carotene, and hereditary bupthalmus in the rabbit (Abstract). *J Hered.*, **73**, 370–374.

Gfeller, R.W., Messonier S.P. (1998). *Small Animal Toxicology and Poisonings.* Mosby.

Gidenne, T., Carabaõ, R., Garcia J., de Blas, C. (1998) Fibre digestion. In *The Nutrition of the Rabbit.* (C. de Blas and J. Wiseman, eds). pp 69–88. CABI Publishing.

Greene, H.S.N. (1941). Uterine adenomata in the rabbit. *J Exp Med.*, **73**, 273–292.

Harcourt-Brown, F.M. (1995). A review of clinical conditions in pet rabbits associated with their teeth. *Vet Rec.*, **137**, 341–346.

Harcourt-Brown, F.M. (1996). Calcium deficiency, diet and dental disease in pet rabbits. *Vet Rec.*, **139**, 567–571.

Harcourt-Brown, F.M., Baker, S.J. (2001). Parathyroid hormone, haematological and biochemical parameters in relation to dental disease and husbandry in pet rabbits. *J Small Anim Pract.*, **42**, 130–136.

Harris, D.J., Cheeke, P.R., Patton, N.M. (1983). Feed preference studies with rabbits fed fourteen different greens. *J Appl Rabbit Res.*, **6**, 120–121.

Holick, M.F. (1990). The use and interpretation of assays for Vitamin D and its metabolites. *J Nutr.*, **120**, 1464–1469.

Holick, M.F. (1996). Vitamin D and bone health. *J Nutr.*, **126**, 1159S–1164S.

How, K.L., Hazewinkel, H.A.W., Mol, J.A., (1994). Photosynthesis of vitamin D3 in cats. *Vet Rec.*, **134**, 384.

Huls, W.L., Brooks, D.L., Bean-Knudsen, D. (1991). Response of adult New Zealand white rabbits to enrichment objects and paired housing. *Lab Anim Sci.*, **41**, 609–612.

Hunt, C.E., Harrington, D.D. (1974). Nutrition and nutritional diseases of the rabbit. In *The Biology of the Laboratory Rabbit*, 2nd edn. (P.J. Manning, D.H. Ringler, C.E. Newcomer, eds). pp 403–428, Academic Press.

Jean-Blain,C., Durix, A. (1985). Effects of dietary lipid level on ketonaemia and other plasma parameters related to glucose and fatty acid metabolism in the rabbit during fasting. *Reprod Nutr Dev.*, **25**, 345–354.

Jenkins, J.R. (1991). Nutrition and nutrition related diseases of rabbits. *J Small Exotic Anim Med.*, **1**, 12–14.

Kamphues, V.J., Carstensen, P. Schroeder, D *et al.* (1986). Effect of increasing calcium and Vitamin D supply on calcium metabolism in rabbits (Article in German with an English Summary). *J Anim Physiol Nutr.*, **50**, 191–208.

Kato, J. (1966). Effects of the administration of vitamin D2, D3, parathyoid hormone and calcium on hypocalcification of rabbit dentine and on changes in blood constituents caused by experimental rickets. *Gunma J Med.*, **15**, 174–193.

Kennedy, A. (1965). The urinary excretion of calcium by normal rabbits. *J Comp Path.*, **75**, 69–74.

Lang, J. (1981). The nutrition of the commercial rabbit. Part 1. Physiology, digestibility and nutrient requirements. *Nutrition abstr rev. Series B*, **51**, 197–217.

Lebas, F., Gidenne, T., Perez, J.M., Licois, D. (1998). Nutrition and pathology. In *The Nutrition of the Rabbit.* (C. de Blas, J. Wiseman, eds). CABI Publishing pp. 197–213.

Lorgue, G., Lechenet, J., Rivière. (1996). *Clinical Veterinary Toxicology. English Edition.* (M.J. Chapman, ed.) Blackwell.

Love, J.A. (1994). Group housing: Meeting the physical and social needs of the laboratory rabbit. *Lab Anim Sci.*, **44**, 5–11.

Lowe, J.A. (1998). Pet rabbit feeding and nutrition. In *The Nutrition of the Rabbit.* (C. de Blas and J. Wiseman, eds). CABI Publishing.

Madeiros, C.A. (1997). Use of rabbits in ostrich rearing. *Vet Rec.*, **140**, 668.

Malley, A.D. (1995). The pet rabbit in companion animal practice: 1. A clinician's approach to the pet rabbit. *Irish Vet J.*, **47**, 9–15.

Maertens, L., Villamide, M.J. (1998). Feeding systems for intensive production. In *The Nutrition of the Rabbit.* (C. de Blas and J. Wiseman, eds). CABI Publishing pp. 255–271.

Mathieu, L.G., Smith, S.E. (1961). Phosphorus requirements of growing rabbits. *J Anim Sci.*, **20**, 510–513.

McDonald, P., Edwards, R.A., Greenhalgh, J.F.D., Morgan, C.A. (1996). *Animal Nutrition*, 5th edn. Longman.

Meyer, H., Stadermann, B., Schnurpel, B., Nehring, T. (1992). The influence of type of diet (roughage or concentrate) on the plasma level, renal excretion and apparent digestability of Ca and Mg in resting and exercising horses. *ProcEquine Nutr Physiol Soc.*, 12th Symposium, **12**, 233–239.

Nyomba, B.L., Bouillon, R., De Moor, P. (1984). Influence of vitamin D status on insulin secretion and glucose tolerance in the rabbit. *Endocrinology*, **115**, 191–197.

Ohta, A., Ohtsuki, M., Baba, S. *et al.* (1995a). Calcium and magnesium absorption from the colon and rectum are increased in rats fed fructooligosaccharides (Abstract). *J Nutr.*, **125**, 2417–2424.

Ohta, A., Ohtsuki, M., Baba, S. *et al.* (1995b). Effect of fructooligosaccharides on the absorption of iron, calcium and magnesium in iron-deficient anemic rats (Abstract). *J Nutr Sci Vitaminol (Tokyo)*, **41**, 281–291.

Owen, D. (1978). Effects of pelleting sterilisation of diet on 2 strains of rabbit coccidia. *Lab Anim.*, **12**, 49–50.

Phillips, P.H., Bohstedt, G. (1937). Studies on the effects of a bovine blindness-producing ration upon rabbits. *J Nutr.*, **15**, 309–319.

Quesenbery, K.A. (1994). Rabbits. In *Saunders Manual of Small Animal Practice.* (S.J. Birchard, R.G. Sherding, eds). pp 1345–1363. W.B. Saunders.

Rabbit Health News (1991). Volume 4, p. 2. Published by House Rabbit Society, PO Box 3242, Redmond WA 98073, USA.

Richardson, V. (1999). *Rabbit Nutrition.* Coney Publications.

Richardson, V. (2000). Rabbit husbandry and nutrition. *UK Vet*, **5**, 1–3.

Roberfroid, M.B. (1997). Health benefits of non-digestible oligosaccharides (Abstract). *Adv Exp Med Biol*, **427**, 211–219.

Rohde, C.M., Manatt, M., Clagett-Dame, M., DeLuca, H.F. (1999). Vitamin A antagonises the action of vitamin D in rats. *J Nutr.*, **129**, 2246–2250.

Sanchez, W.K., Cheeke, P.R., Patton N.M. (1984). The use of chopped alfalfa rations with varying levels of molasses for weanling rabbits. *J Appl Rabbit Res.*, **7**, 13–16.

Sandford, J.C. (1996). *The Domestic Rabbit*, 5th edition. Blackwell Science.

Stauffacher, M. (1992). Group housing and enrichment cages for breeding, fattening and laboratory rabbits. *Anim Welfare*, **1**, 105–125.

Tobin, G. (1996). Small pets – Food types, nutrient requirements and nutritional disorders. In *Manual of Companion Animal Nutrition and Feeding.* (N. Kelly, J. Wills, eds). British Small Animal Veterinary Association pp. 208–225.

Turner R.J., Held S.D., Hirst J.E. *et al.* (1997). An immunological assessment of group housed rabbits. *Lab Anim.*, **31**, 362–372.

Tvedegaard, E. (1987). Arterial disease in chronic renal failure. An experimental study in the rabbit. *Acta Pathol Microbiol Immunol Scand.. Section A. Suppl 290*, **95**, 3–28.

Ubels, J.L., Harkema, J.R. (1994). The rabbit lacrimal gland in vitamin A deficiency (Abstract). *Invest Ophthalmol Vis Sci*, **35**, 1249–1253.

Umar, I.A., Wuro-Chekke, A.U., Gidado, A., Igbokwe, I.O. (1999) Effects of combined parenteral vitamins C and E administration on the severity of anaemia, hepatic and renal damage in Trypanosoma brucei brucei infected rabbits (Abstract). *Vet Parasitol.*, **85**, 43–47.

Verde, M.T., Piquer, J.G. (1986). Effect of stress on the cortisone and ascorbic acid content of the blood plasma of rabbits. *J Appl Rabbit Res.*, **9**, 181–182.

Warren, H.B., Lausen, N.C., Segre, G.V. *et al.* (1989). Regulation of calciotropic hormones *in vivo* in the New Zealand White rabbit. *Endocrinology*. **125**, 2683–2689.

Zimmerman, T.E., Giddens, W.E., DiGiacomo, R.F., Ladiges, W.C. (1990). Soft tissue mineralization in rabbits fed a diet containing excess vitamin D. *Lab Anim Sci.*, **40**, 212–215.

3

The rabbit consultation and clinical techniques

3.1 Basic information about rabbits

Biological data are summarized in Box 3.1.

3.1.1 Stress

The effects of stress upon rabbits are significant (see Box 3.2). Catecholamines are released in response to stress and can initiate a number of problems. In extreme cases,

Box 3.1 Basic biological data for rabbits

Life span:	6–13 years
Urine volume:	20–250 ml/kg/24 h. Usually about 130 ml/kg/24 h
Water intake:	50–100 ml/kg/24 h
Optimum environmental temperature:	15–20°C (65–70°F)
Rectal temperature: Subnormal: Raised:	38.5–40°C (103.3–104°F) 38.0°C (100.4°F) 40.6°C (105°F)
Heart rate:	130–325 bpm
Respiratory rate:	32–60 bpm
Erythrocyte life span:	50 days
Blood volume:	55–65 ml/kg
Tidal volume:	20 ml (4–6 ml/kg)
Gastrointestinal transit time:	4–5 h
Intraocular pressure:	5–23 mmHg
Reproductive data	
Puberty:	4–5 months in small breeds 5–8 months in large breeds
Descent of testicles:	10–12 weeks
Age at which to neuter:	>3 months for males; >5 months for females
Interval between castration and infertility:	4 weeks
Pregnancy diagnosis:	Palpation: 10–12 days Radiologically after 11 days
Gestation:	30–32 days
Litter size:	Average 5–8
Milk composition:	13–15% protein, 10–12% fat and 2% carbohydrate
Birth weight:	40–100 g
Eyes open:	7 days
Weaning:	4–6 weeks

Box 3.2 Stress in rabbits

Causes of stress of rabbits
- Pain and disease
- Unfamiliar surroundings
- Transport
- Rough handling
- Proximity of potential predators: dogs, cats, ferrets, birds of prey and, for wild rabbits, humans
- A dominant companion and no means of escape
- Inability to exhibit natural behaviour patterns, e.g. to forage, make a nest or interact socially
- Poor husbandry: insufficient food, water and indigestible fibre, excessively high or low environmental temperature

Effects of stress in rabbits
Many of the effects of stress are linked to the release of catecholamines or corticosteroids and can be life-threatening:

- Catecholamine release can cause heart failure and death. Stress due to overcrowding has been used to induce cardiomyopathy in laboratory rabbits
- Stimulation of the sympathetic nervous system inhibits activity of the gastrointestinal tract. Gut motility is reduced, which can have a knock-on effect. Gut stasis, trichobezoar formation (hairballs), enterotoxaemia and mucoid enteropathy can all be linked with stress
- Stress in rabbits causes a marked decrease in urine flow, renal plasma flow and filtration rate. Oliguria can last from 30 to 120 minutes
- Stress can increase gastric acidity and cause gastric ulceration in rabbits
- Stress is immunosuppressive. Rabbits suffering from dental disease have significantly lower lymphocyte counts than healthy rabbits
- Stress affects carbohydrate metabolism. Handling alone can cause an increase in blood glucose to the order of 8.5 mmol/l. Blood glucose levels can be very high (20–25 mmol/l) in association with intestinal obstruction and other stressful diseases
- Stress causes anorexia that, in combination with disruption to normal carbohydrate metabolism, can lead to hepatic lipidosis, liver failure and death

Ways to minimize stress in rabbits undergoing veterinary treatment
- Use analgesics in any situation where the rabbit may be experiencing pain
- Use quiet, gentle handling and sedate or anaesthetize rabbits for painful or uncomfortable procedures
- Wrap rabbits in a towel for examination or procedures such as blood sampling
- Keep rabbits away from the sight, sound and smell of predators, e.g. barking dogs, ferrets
- Provide hay as bedding material for rabbits awaiting or recovering from surgery. Hay smells familiar and provides security for timid animals. It is also a source of indigestible fibre and foraging material
- Consider hospitalizing a bonded companion with a sick rabbit
- Minimize stressful procedures or devices, e.g. Elizabethan collars or nasogastric tubes

catecholamine release can cause heart failure and death. Stress due to overcrowding has been used to induce cardiomyopathy in laboratory rabbits (Weber and Van der Walt, 1975).

Stimulation of the sympathetic nervous system inhibits activity of the gastrointestinal tract. Gut motility is reduced, which can have a knock-on effect on caecal microflora and digestive function. Enterotoxaemia or gut stasis can result from any stressful situation. Mucoid enteropathy is associated with stressful situations such as weaning, parturition or re-homing.

Stress reduces renal blood flow in rabbits. In a study by Kaplan and Smith (1935) into the effects of diuresis and urine flow, a single dose of 50 ml/kg of water was given to rabbits before subjecting them to unpleasant or painful stimuli. The rabbits were subjected to electric shocks, loud bangs or being tied in a supine position on an animal board for long periods of time. In all cases the disturbing stimuli were immediately followed by a marked decrease in urine flow, renal plasma flow and filtration rate. Oliguria was frequently severe, lasting from 30 to 120 minutes. Some rabbits died in convulsions.

The control group of rabbits that were not stimulated and remained undisturbed could withstand diuresis by increasing urine flow.

Stress increases gastric acidity. Gastric ulcers are a common *post-mortem* finding in rabbits, especially in those that have been anorexic prior to death. In a survey of 1000 *post-mortem* examinations by Hinton (1980), 7.3% were found to have ulceration of the gastric mucosa that was related to the stress of the associated illness. Experimental stress ulcers have been induced in the gastric mucosa of laboratory rabbits by administering intraperitoneal injections of adrenaline (Behara *et al.*, 1980).

Stress can alter the differential white cell count in any species. Rabbits are particularly susceptible to the effects of stress. A car journey to the surgery, a period in the waiting room next to a barking dog or the excitement of handling can be reflected in the blood picture. Adrenaline and cortisol affect the distribution of lymphocytes throughout the body. Administration of exogenous adrenaline to rabbits results in redistribution of lymphocytes from spleen and bone marrow to peripheral blood, lungs and liver (Toft *et al.*, 1992a). Conversely, exogenous corticosteroid administration results in a redistribution of lymphocytes from the peripheral blood, bone marrow and spleen to the lymphatic tissue in rabbits (Toft *et al.*, 1992b). Prolonged periods of stress cause lymphopaenia. Rabbits suffering from clinical symptoms of dental disease have significantly lower lymphocyte counts than healthy rabbits kept under free-range conditions (Harcourt-Brown and Baker, 2001) (see Figure 6.1).

Carbohydrate metabolism is affected by stress. Handling alone can cause an increase in blood glucose to the order of 8.5 mmol/l. Blood glucose levels can rise to 20–25 mmol/l in critically ill rabbits, such as those with an intestinal obstruction. Disruptions in carbohydrate metabolism have potentially serious knock-on effects that can result in hepatic lipidosis, liver failure and death.

As a prey species, rabbits have many physiological and behavioural responses to adrenal hormones. The response to danger is either to 'freeze' or to jump and flee. Although the majority of pet rabbits are used to being handled by their owners and are not particularly stressed by clinical examination, there is always potential for them to suddenly spring up and attempt to escape. Broken bones or fractured teeth can be the consequence of a leap off the consulting table. Struggling rabbits can inflict injury by scratching with the hind legs or, very occasionally, biting.

Owners are often unaware of the stressful effect or the physical danger that is posed to their rabbit if it is sitting on their knee in full view of other animals in the waiting room. They may be next to potential predators such as ferrets, dogs, cats or birds of prey. Even the sound or smell of predators such as ferrets can be stressful. Loud noises, unfamiliar surroundings and car journeys all add to the stress levels of rabbits that are visiting the surgery. The effects of stress can be minimized by encouraging owners to leave their rabbits in the carrier in the waiting room, quiet gentle handling in the consulting room and the routine use of analgesics to all animals that may be in pain.

Key points 3.1

- Rabbits are a prey species and susceptible to the effects of adrenal hormones. Stress can allow the flare up of latent infections and cause gastrointestinal hypomotility, reduce renal blood flow and increase gastric acidity
- Pain, unfamiliar surroundings, loud noises and the proximity of predators can stress rabbits that are brought to a veterinary surgery
- The effects of stress can be minimized by gentle handling and routine use of analgesics.

3.1.2 Reproduction

Rabbits are induced ovulators without a defined oestrus cycle, although females vary in sexual receptivity and a cyclic rhythm exists (see Section 1.4). Full sexual receptivity occurs every 18 days and is manifested by restlessness and increased chin rubbing. Does are fertile immediately after kindling, especially during the summer months. Breeders usually take females to the buck for mating rather than vice versa as they can be territorial and attack the buck if he is put in her hutch. Sometimes the two are introduced on neutral territory. In general, females are mated for the first time at approximately 5 months old and are not bred from over the age of 3 years (Sandford, 1996). Mating takes place within a few minutes and can be accompanied by a scream from either party, which is deemed to be normal. Mating may be repeated after a couple of hours to improve the conception rate. Artificial insemination is a recognized technique in rabbit breeding. Pregnancy can be detected by abdominal palpation. The best time for pregnancy diagnosis is 10–14 days after mating when the fetal units can be felt as olive-sized masses. Fetal resorption can take place up to 20 days post-coitus. Mammary development occurs in late pregnancy. Radiographically, pregnancy can be detected after the 11th day.

Gestation takes 31–32 days. Some does remain sexually receptive during pregnancy and will continue to be mated by a male companion. During late pregnancy the doe may be seen carrying bedding material into her chosen nesting site. The nest is built from hay, straw or other bedding material. The quality of the nest varies between individual does and has a strong influence on the survival of the young. The doe will defend her chosen nesting site against potential intruders, especially if she is pregnant or lactating and can become aggressive towards owners, other rabbits or pets. Hair is pulled from the hip, dewlap and mammary glands to line the nest. She may consume less food at this point and should be tempted to eat, as pregnancy toxaemia is a risk during this period. Otherwise, the doe should be left undisturbed. Parturition usually takes place in the morning and lasts less than 30 minutes. When the entire litter has been born, the doe pulls more fur from her body to cover the litter in its nest. Does are particularly susceptible to disturbance in the first few days after parturition and may cannibalize the young. Inexperienced does sometimes mutilate them. The legs or ears may be attacked or the skin stripped over the neck, thorax or abdomen. Cannibalization and mutilation are most likely to take place on the day of parturition and may be an extension of eating the placenta. Sometimes young rabbits are born outside the nest or the doe rejects them. These kits will die from hypothermia unless they are warmed up and returned to the nest. The doe will usually accept them and the chances of survival are far greater if the kit is reared by its natural mother rather than being hand-reared by a human. It is advisable to remove other rabbits from the hutch during late pregnancy. Female companions can cannibalize the young and entire males will mate the doe within hours of her giving birth. Females can lactate and be pregnant at the same time and have a second litter within a few weeks of the first. The doe only feeds the young once or twice daily taking 3–5 minutes (see Section 1.4.). Owners often think the young have been deserted and need reassurance that it is normal for the mother to be out of the nest and that she may be particularly aggressive and protective during this period. Lactation takes place for approximately 5 weeks after parturition.

Baby rabbits are suckled once or occasionally twice daily by a mother and she spends very little time with them. In the wild, although the doe remains in close vicinity of the nest, she does not groom the young or keep them warm. Nests are hidden, well insulated and secure. The babies drink sufficient milk in 2–5 minutes to last 24 h. It is possible for baby rabbits to survive for more than 24-h intervals between feeds, which explains why females can rear litters that exceed their number of nipples (Lang, 1981). Suckling normally takes place in the early morning and, if the doe does return to the nest to feed the young for a second time, then it is usually in the first few days after giving birth. The baby rabbits spend most of the day buried in the warmest part of the nest, tightly grouped together conserving heat and energy. After about 22 h, the whole group becomes active and makes its way to the surface (McBride, 1988). When the mother arrives, she stands over the babies which suckle, changing nipples and position approximately every 30 seconds. After about 3 minutes, the doe leaves the nest and the babies urinate on the surface before digging themselves deep into the bedding to sleep for another 22 h. Young rabbits are totally dependent on milk until day 10. They are usually eating small amounts of solid food by day 15 (Kraus *et al.*, 1984) and start to leave the nest and be weaned at about 3 weeks of age.

The glucose reserve of neonatal rabbits lasts approximately 6 h post partum. Hypoglycaemia results in rapid ketosis and death (Kraus *et al.*, 1984). Passive immunity is obtained through the placenta, although there is some evidence that neonates absorb antibodies from their intestine in the first few hours after birth (Brewer and Cruise, 1994). Rabbit milk has a low lactose content. It is of high nutritive value and the composition changes towards the end of lactation when protein and fat levels increase.

Rabbit owners are usually unaware of the natural lack of maternal behaviour by rabbits and become convinced that a nest of babies has been deserted. Constant interference and 'checking to see if they are alright' increases the likelihood of the mother cannibalizing the young in the first few days. There is also a misconception that all baby animals must be fed every 2–3 h, even during the night. If owners are concerned, the nest can be checked once a day and if the babies are warm, asleep and unwrinkled then they are being fed. Baby rabbits that are not being fed will be restless and crawling around on the surface of the nest. They take on a wrinkled appearance due to dehydration. It is possible to cross-foster orphaned rabbits to another lactating doe. It is not necessary to use any method for destroying the scent of the natural mother or human hand. Females do not make any distinction of young, even if they are of different colours or sizes (Cheeke *et al.*, 1982). Ideally, older rabbits should be introduced to a younger litter. The fostered babies should be placed at the bottom of the nest with the natural kits on top.

3.1.3.1 Rearing orphans

Abandoned or orphaned wild or domestic rabbits can be hand-reared, although the mortality rate is high. Baby rabbits can be fed on powdered cat milk replacers. They will drink 2–30 ml of milk per feed, depending on how old they are. Baby rabbits should be fed when they are restless. Milk replacers are a nutritional compromise and do not match the composition of rabbit milk. Therefore orphan rabbits may need feeding two to three times daily, but care should be taken not to overfeed or force-feed them. Holding newborn rabbits on their backs simulates the natural nursing position. Hypothermic or moribund rabbits can be given fluids or milk replacers by stomach tube to correct hypoglycaemia. The babies should be kept warm and dry in a quiet place with suitable bedding material to burrow into. Shredded tissue paper or kitchen roll is satisfactory for making a nest that can be put in a hay-lined cardboard box and placed in a warm environment such as an airing cupboard.

Most suckling animals are stimulated to urinate and defaecate by the mother licking the perineum and lower abdomen. People that have successfully hand-reared orphans usually advise that baby rabbits should also be stimulated by rubbing the genital region after each feed. Female rabbits do not stay with their young and do not groom them so it may not be necessary to stimulate young rabbits in this way. However, it can do no harm and is therefore advisable.

Mortality can occur from aspiration pneumonia due to inhalation of milk replacer. A syringe with a small amount of tubing cut from a giving set is a satisfactory method of feeding orphans. Healthy babies suck the milk out of the syringe. Squirting milk into the mouth carries a risk of choking the rabbit. Enteritis is a potentially lethal complication of hand-rearing. Rabbits are unusual among young animals in having very few microorganisms in the stomach and small intestine while suckling (Lang, 1981). An antimicrobial fatty acid or 'milk oil' is present in the suckling rabbit. It is produced by an enzymatic reaction in the doe's milk that takes place in the suckling rabbit's stomach (Brooks, 1997). This 'milk oil' controls the gastrointestinal microbial contents of suckling rabbits and protects them from enteric infection. Orphan rabbits that are fed on milk from other species do not develop this antimicrobial factor and are therefore more susceptible to bacterial infections introduced during feeding. It is important that boiled water and sterile syringes and feeding tubes are used to feed orphans and that each feed is made up just prior to being given. Overfeeding can cause digestive upsets. In general, it is preferable to underfeed than overfeed. Small babies can soon make up their weight once they are weaned and able to digest solid food.

Baby rabbits can be offered hay and fresh food from about 18 days of age. Caecotrophs collected from healthy adults may be fed during weaning to colonize the intestinal tract with healthy bacteria and protozoa. It may be necessary to place an Elizabethan collar on an adult rabbit for a day or two to prevent them from eating the caecotrophs so they can be harvested. Weaning is a danger period for any young rabbit, especially orphans. Diarrhoea can result from colonization of the gut by pathogenic bacteria. Probiotics can be useful in this period, especially if no caecotrophs are available.

3.1.4 Pseudopregnancy

Pseudopregnancy mimics true pregnancy. Pseudopregnant does pull fur from their abdomen and chest, make a nest, develop mammary glands and aggressively defend their nesting site. Pseudopregnancy lasts for 16–18 days rather than the 31–32 days of true pregnancy. Because rabbits ovulate in response to sexual stimulation by another rabbit, proximity of a male or mating behaviour between two females housed together can stimulate ovulation and result in pseudopregnancy.

3.1.5 Advice on neutering

Neutering modifies sexual behaviour in rabbits but may not abolish it altogether. Increasing daylength can trigger social, sexual and even aggressive actions in neutered rabbits, although the behaviour is usually mild. In the spring, does may dig out a new burrow and males may have minor skirmishes. Copulatory actions can persist after neutering, as part of dominance or excitement behaviour. It is beneficial for rabbits to be neutered for similar reasons to the dog or cat. Neutering prevents unwanted pregnancies and pseudopregnancies and permits both sexes to be housed together. Male aggression is reduced or abolished so fight and bite wounds are minimized. Neutering also modifies scent marking by spraying urine or depositing faeces. Female reproductive disorders such as uterine or mammary neoplasia and endometritis occur frequently in the middle-aged doe. Spaying is indicated to prevent these diseases. Aggressive behaviour towards owners can be modified by neutering, especially if it is hormone related. Male rabbits make better pets if they are castrated. Entire bucks can attempt to mate their owner's legs or mount toys, mats or other household objects.

Although rabbits can be spayed or castrated at any age, approximately 5 months of age is the best time for both sexes. It is advisable to spay females after puberty but before maturity when large amounts of abdominal fat can complicate the surgery. Pre-pubescent females are difficult to spay because of their tiny uterus and ovaries that can be hard to locate. Males should be left until the testicles have descended. Motile spermatozoa appear in the ejaculate from about 4 months of age. After castration, the male can be considered sterile after a period of 4 weeks.

3.1.6 Leg rings

Pedigree rabbits are identified by an aluminium ring placed over the hock at 8–10 weeks of age. Some breeders use right or left legs according to the gender. Rings are purchased from the British Rabbit Council who keep records of the numbers. Different sizes are needed for different breeds, which are denoted by a letter that prefixes the ring number. The year of birth is also recorded on

Key points 3.2

- Pregnancy can be detected at 10–14 days after mating when fetal units can be palpated as olive-sized masses
- Fetal resorption may take place up to 20 days post mating
- Does should be left alone at the time of parturition
- Mating can take place within a few hours of parturition
- Orphan rabbits can be cross-fostered on to another lactating doe
- Kitten milk replacers can be used as hand-rearing formulas for rabbits
- Baby rabbits do not need feeding every 2–3 h. Two or three feeds a day are sufficient
- Mating behaviour between two females or proximity of a male can induce pseudopregnancy
- Neutering modifies sexual behaviour but may not abolish it altogether
- Neutering is advisable to prevent unwanted pregnancies, reduce aggression and territory marking and remove the risk of uterine adenocarcinoma
- Neutering can be done after 4–5 months of age.

the ring. These rings should be removed as they serve no purpose in the pet rabbit and can trap hair and debris beneath them. Skin necrosis and secondary infection can set in (see Plate 1). In severe cases, the blood supply to the foot is cut off so the leg becomes gangrenous and has to be amputated or the rabbit euthanased. If the rings are not removed, owners must be advised to check them daily.

Ring removal is almost impossible in the conscious animal. Sedation or general anaesthesia is required because leg rings cannot be slipped over the hock and need to be cut. Part of a wooden tongue depressor can be slipped between the ring and the leg to keep the fur our of the way and give some protection to the skin before removing the ring with a hack saw or small saw attachment on a power drill. Care is required to prevent the metal ring from overheating. Cotton wool soaked in water can be used periodically to cool the ring during removal.

3.2 Vaccination

3.2.1 Myxomatosis vaccination

Myxomatosis is a common disease in wild rabbits that can be spread to pet rabbits via insect vectors such as fleas and mosquitoes (see Section 16.6.1.). Those rabbits that are kept in gardens visited by wild rabbits are most at risk. At the present time there is only one type of vaccine available in the UK for the immunization of rabbits against myxomatosis (Nobivac Myxo, Intervet). Live vaccine is prepared from attenuated Shope fibroma virus grown on cell line culture. Shope fibroma virus naturally affects the cottontail rabbit *Sylvilagus floridanus* that is native to North America. It is antigenically related to myxoma virus and cross-immunity occurs. Shope fibroma virus is transmissible to the European rabbit *Oryctolagus cuniculus* in which it produces localized benign fibromas.

In order to stimulate an antigenic reaction and afford immunity, 1 ml of the vaccine is split between two routes; 0.9 ml is administered subcutaneously and the remaining 0.1 ml is given intradermally. Intradermal immunization produces maximum antibody response due to the presence of Langerhans cells within the dermis that act as antigen-presenting cells and increase the activation of T-helper cells. The intradermal route also provides some protection for the antigen by minimizing diffusion into the surrounding tissues and providing a depot effect. The dermis has excellent lymphatic drainage and intradermal injection maximizes exposure of immune cells to the antigen and the subsequent antibody response (Stills, 1994).

The manufacturers recommend using the skin at the base of the ear for the intradermal injection and either administering the remainder of the vaccine subcutaneously at that site or through a separate injection in the scruff. It is also possible to administer both the subcutaneous and intradermal dose through a single injection in the scruff of the neck. The 1 ml dose is drawn into a syringe with a small (23–5 g) needle attached; 0.9 ml is injected into the subcutaneous tissue. The needle, orientated with the bevel up, is then slowly advanced into the overlying dermis and the remaining 0.1 ml injected into the dermis from underneath. A bleb of vaccine can be felt forming in the dermis if the skin over the end of the needle is pinched between the thumb and forefinger as the injection is made.

The vaccine can be given to rabbits over 6 weeks of age. It should not be given during pregnancy. Annual boosters are necessary, although in high-risk situations where pet rabbits are potentially exposed to insects or wild rabbits infected with myxomatosis, the interval between vaccinations can be reduced to 6 months. Myxomatosis tends to be a seasonal disease with outbreaks occurring in the late summer. The optimal time for vaccination is in the late spring to provide good immunity during the summer months. Insect control will also reduce the risk of infection.

3.2.2 Viral haemorrhagic disease

Viral haemorrhagic disease (VHD) is a highly infectious lethal disease of rabbits. It is caused by a host-specific calicivirus (see Section 16.6.2.). VHD virus is spread by oral, nasal and parenteral transmission and is present in urine and faeces from infected rabbits. The virus can survive for long periods outside the host. It is thought that wild birds carried infection across the channel from Europe to wild rabbits in this country. VHD may be transmitted directly from contact with wild rabbits or carried on footwear and clothing. Contaminated foods, such as grass or weeds picked from areas grazed by wild rabbits, can be a source of infection. Hutches and cages that have been occupied by an infected rabbit require thorough disinfection before a new rabbit is introduced. Ideally, only vaccinated animals should be brought in to infected premises. VHD virus can survive outside the host for 10–19 months at room temperature. Exposure to 2% Virkon for 2 h does not inactivate the virus, although 4% Virkon is effective; 1% sodium hydroxide or 10% household bleach are also effective disinfectants (Gorski *et al.*, 1994; Goodly, 2001).

There is a vaccine against viral haemorrhagic disease that is available in the UK (Cylap, Fort Dodge). Rabbits over 10 weeks can be vaccinated with a single dose. It is safe to vaccinate pregnant animals with VHD vaccine. Boosters are given annually.

In contrast with myxomatosis vaccine the whole 1 ml dose should be given subcutaneously. Inadvertent intradermal injection can result in tissue reaction. After subcutaneous administration, it is advisable to massage the vaccination area thoroughly and advise the owner to do the same periodically over the next few hours. In this manner, the vaccine is dispersed in the subcutaneous tissues and is less likely to cause a reaction. Some judges penalize show rabbits that have an area of dermatitis or a scar, so it is important to make sure the owners are aware of the risk. According to the datasheet, accidental self-injection with the vaccine can cause a severe reaction in humans that could result in the loss of a finger.

3.2.3 Simultaneous administration of myxomatosis and VHD vaccine

It is tempting to administer both the myxomatosis and VHD vaccines during a single consultation. There are data to support the efficacy of simultaneous vaccination but no firm conclusions can be drawn because of differences in the type of vaccine. During an outbreak of VHD, 5000 rabbits in Poland were simultaneously vaccinated with myxomatosis vaccine (Myxovac M) and VHD vaccine (Cunivac) without complications. Controlled exposure to infection in the laboratory suggested that rabbits that were simultaneously vaccinated were immune to both diseases (Gorski *et al.*, 1994). However, the manufacturers of the current VHD vaccine in the UK (Cylap, Fort Dodge) have pointed out that their vaccine is different from Cunivac so no conclusions can be drawn from the Polish experience.

At the present time, the manufacturers of both the myxomatosis and the VHD vaccine advise against simultaneous immunization. It is common practice to leave 2 weeks between the two injections.

Key points 3.3

- Pet rabbits in the UK can be vaccinated against both myxomatosis and viral haemorrhagic disease (VHD)
- Myxomatosis vaccine can be given to rabbits over 6 weeks of age. VHD vaccine is given to rabbits over 10 weeks of age
- Myxomatosis vaccine should not be given to pregnant does. VHD vaccine can be given during pregnancy
- Myxomatosis vaccine is given subcutaneously and a small amount (0.1 ml) intradermally
- VHD vaccine must be given entirely subcutaneously and dispersed by massaging the injection area thoroughly
- It is not advisable to administer both myxomatosis and VHD vaccine at the same time. At least 2 weeks should elapse between vaccinations
- Myxomatosis vaccine administered during late spring offers protection over the summer months when the disease is prevalent in wild rabbits.

3.3 Behaviour problems and aggression

Like other species, rabbits respond to handling from an early age. A rabbit that associates humans with pleasurable experiences is less likely to be timid, scared or aggressive than a rabbit that is left to its own devices for most of the time and is chased or handled roughly when it does have human contact. A study into the effect of early handling has suggested that baby rabbits that are picked up and handled between the ages of 26 and 42 days are more willing to approach humans and will remain closer to them (Der Weduwen and McBride, 1999).

Owners frequently seek advice about aggressive tendencies in their rabbits. Sometimes the reason for the aggression is obvious. Two entire males that are kept together are likely to fight and will need to be separated or castrated. Female rabbits are strongly influenced by their hormones and will vigorously defend their 'nesting site', i.e. a hutch or a run, and attack intruders, including other rabbits and humans. These rabbits may be quite docile when they are out of their hutch. For this reason, it is advisable to clean out hutches when they are unoccupied. Spaying usually cures this type of aggression, although it may take some weeks to settle down. Female rabbits can vigorously protect their young and aggressive behaviour can be extended to include the protection of a bonded companion.

Straightforward aggression is not the only reason for rabbits biting their owners. Occasionally fingers are mistaken for food especially if the fingers smell of sweets or biscuits. Overzealous grooming can result in a nibbling response. Young rabbits nibble objects as part of their development and can extend this exploratory behaviour to include their owners. People that smell of other rabbits or animals can be attacked as part of defensive territorial behaviour. In general it is preferable to approach nervous or aggressive rabbits from above. A rabbit that showed periodic aggression following periods of 'stargazing' was found to be seropositive for *Encephalitozoon cuniculi* (Harcourt-Brown, unpublished observation).

As in other species, pain can result in aggressive behaviour. A rabbit that is normally docile but starts to be aggressive should be examined carefully for a source of pain. Dental disease and the formation of sharp hooks on the molars can be extremely painful. Rabbits are also prone to painful musculoskeletal disorders such as arthritis or vertebral spondylitis.

Deafness has been reported as a cause of aggression in rabbits (Rabbit Health News 1991, 1993). Deaf rabbits may be startled by owners coming up on them unexpectedly and sometimes their response is to bite. Deafness can be caused by *Psoroptes cuniculi* infestation occluding the external auditory canal with mites and exudate. Many lop eared rabbits have external ear canals full of wax and debris anyway. In some rabbits, the tympanic bullae are of inspissated pus as a result of ascending *Pasteurella multocida* infection from the nasal cavity. Inspissated pus in the horizontal ear canal is a common *post-mortem* finding in many pet rabbits. Granulomatous encephalitis caused by *Encephalitozoon cuniculi* could cause deafness (see Section 12.4.).

Key points 3.4

- Aggression in rabbits may be hormonal, territorial or a response to pain or alarm
- Obese rabbits have high resting heart rates and can develop hypertension and cardiac hypertrophy. They are prone to developing fatal hepatic lipidosis if they become anorexic
- High fibre diets that would result in weight loss in other species may not be effective in rabbits. Fibre is fermented by the caecal microflora to volatile fatty acids
- Weight reduction can only be achieved in rabbits by providing a diet low in digestible fibre and high in indigestible fibre
- Increased amounts of exercise are an important part of a weight reduction programme
- There are no serious zoonotic diseases that can be spread from rabbits to healthy humans. Immunocompromised AIDS patients may contract *Encephalitozoon cuniculi.* Ringworm and ectoparasites such as fleas or *Cheyletiella parasitovorax* can cause skin lesions in humans
- There are many techniques for handling rabbits. Wrapping them in a towel is an effective method of restraint
- The immobility response (hypnosis) can be used as restraint for minor procedures but is not an alternative to either anaesthesia or analgesia
- The immobility response can be initiated by placing rabbits on their back.

3.4 Obesity

Rabbits are animals that convert food efficiently and are often overfed by indulgent owners. They are used as laboratory models to study the effects of obesity in humans. Obese rabbits have high resting heart rates and can develop hypertension and cardiac hypertrophy (Carroll *et al.*, 1996). Hyperinsulinaemia, hyperglycaemia and elevated serum triglycerides occur in obese rabbits and hepatic lipidosis develops readily after short periods without food, especially if the rabbit is stressed. Obese rabbits are poor surgical candidates.

Fat rabbits are unable to groom inaccessible parts such as the nape of the neck and the base of the tail. They are often unable to reach the perineum to consume caecotrophs. Fly strike and cheyletiellosis can be the result of inadequate grooming and soiled fur. Arthritic conditions are exacerbated by obesity. Sludgy urine and cystitis are also associated with inactive overweight rabbits (see Section 14.4).

Weight reduction can be difficult to achieve in rabbits. It is sometimes difficult to persuade owners that their rabbit has a problem. Many obese rabbits have very little exercise and eating is their main pastime. Owners often feel guilty about not allowing their pet out to exercise and worry about it being bored so they give it lots of food instead. A high fibre, low calorie diet that would result in weight loss in humans and other animals may not have any effect in rabbits. The caecal microorganisms can digest fibre to release volatile fatty acids that can be converted into fat. Only lignocellulose in the form of fibrous, lignified vegetation such as hay, straw or really tough weeds will pass through the digestive tract undigested.

Changing a rabbit's diet can be fraught with difficulty. Many rabbits are finicky, even obese ones, and will steadfastly refuse to eat anything at all if they are not offered their favourite foods. Starvation quickly leads to hepatic lipidosis in obese rabbits. Care should be taken at the outset to ensure that the rabbit is actually eating its new diet and is passing hard faeces. Quantities of cereal mixtures or pellets should be reduced or phased out over a couple of weeks. Eventually a diet of *ad lib* hay or grass with no concentrates can be given until the rabbit has lost weight. Small amounts of vegetables can be given as treat foods. As much exercise as possible is important.

3.5 Health risks from keeping rabbits

For a healthy human, the risk of serious infectious zoonotic disease from pet rabbits is negligible. The main health risks are associated with handling the animal. Rabbits can inflict nasty bites and scratches that can become infected. Owners can develop an allergy to rabbit dander.

Parasites can be transmitted from rabbits to humans. Fleas can be found on pet rabbits, although they are not usually the rabbit flea (*Spilopsyllus cuniculi*) but the cat or dog flea (*Ctenocephalides felis* or *canis*) caught from other pets in the household. *Cheyletiella parasitovorax* is transmissable to humans who handle infested rabbits. The mite causes erythematous pruritic lesions in humans, especially on the arms. Ringworm is occasionally encountered in pet rabbits. Asymptomatic infections have been reported (Vangeel *et al.*, 2000).

Protozoal infections such as giardia (Johnson-Delaney, 1996) can affect both rabbits and humans but transmission between species does not appear to occur. *Toxoplasma gondii* also affects both rabbits and humans but is only transmitted by eating undercooked rabbit meat. It is not transmitted through rabbit faeces. *Encephalitozoon cuniculi* has caused illness in humans but only immunocompromised individuals such as AIDS patients. There are isolated reports of human infections with organisms such as *Salmonella* or *Bordetella bronchiseptica* after contact with infected domestic rabbits (Gueirard *et al.*, 1995). Obscure zoonotic infections occur in wild rabbits such as tularaemia (Gill and Cunha, 1997), plague (*Yersinia pestis*) (Cleri *et al.*, 1997), and listeriosis (Broderson and Gluckstein, 1994).

3.6 Handling rabbits during the consultation

There are many techniques described for handling rabbits (Burgmann, 1991; Quesenberry, 1994; Mader, 1997; Malley, 2000; Richardson 2000). Most pet rabbits are used to human contact and do not object to being picked up and examined. Rough handling and overzealous restraint can be counterproductive and alarm the rabbit and upset the owner. A quiet, gentle but firm approach is preferable, with the option to restrain the animal more firmly should the need arise. Rabbits seldom bite vets in the consulting room even if they bite their owners at home. Instead they can inflict nasty scratches with their powerful hind feet.

It is usually possible to lift pet rabbits out of carriers by placing a hand round either side of the chest and lifting them in the same manner as a cat or small dog. Placing a forefinger around each front leg can be helpful. Fractious or nervous animals can be lifted by the scruff with a supporting hand under the rear end. Very excitable or aggressive rabbits can be caught and removed from the carrier in a towel. Picking rabbits up by their ears is not acceptable and is no longer advocated, although it is recommended in some older texts. After being removed from the carrier, the rabbit can be held on the consulting table and observed while a clinical history is being obtained from the owner. To examine the perineum, the rabbit can be restrained in dorsal recumbency either by holding the scruff and lying the rabbit on its back or by cradling it like a baby in the arms of an assistant or the owner. Dorsal recumbency often evokes an immobility response. An alternative approach is to hold the rabbit upright and rest its rear end on the consulting table. There are many approaches and each clinician will find a method that suits them.

Wrapping a rabbit in a towel is a satisfactory method of restraint for examination of the face and mouth or for venepuncture. A large towel is placed on the table and the rabbit placed on top of it before being wrapped up so the whole body is enclosed with only the head exposed. An assistant, who may be the owner, is needed to hold the rabbit firmly against them or pressed gently on to the table. The front legs can be held. Jackson (1991) found that restraining laboratory rabbits by wrapping them securely in a towel not only reduced the stress of handling but also reduced the incidence of gastrointestinal stasis.

A good method of carrying a rabbit is to hold it with its face tucked in under the handler's arm. The close physical contact and covering the face appears to placate fractious animals.

3.7 Immobility response (freeze response or 'hypnosis')

The immobility response is often described as 'hypnosis', 'the freeze response' or 'trancing'. Hypnosis can be a useful method of restraining rabbits for minor procedures (Bivin, 1994). Although hypnosis has been described for more invasive techniques such as castration (Okerman, 1988), it is not a humane alternative to anaesthesia or analgesia. There is controversy about placing conscious rabbits in dorsal recumbency at all. On one hand, some practitioners lie rabbits on their backs to perform a variety of procedures such as nail clipping, oral administration of medicines and even inserting mouth gags to examine or clip molars. On the other hand, there is a view that the immobility response occurs in stressful situations and that rabbits lying on their backs are terrified and waiting to be eaten. However, it is a useful technique in some situations. For, example, it is possible to immobilize conscious rabbits for long enough to take abdominal radiographs.

The immobility response is exhibited in prey species under conditions that are stressful or threatening. The phenomenon is characterized by lack of spontaneous movement and failure to respond to external stimuli for several minutes. In rabbits, there is hypotonia of flexor and extensor musculature, abolition of the righting reflex, depression of spinal reflexes, miosis, and a drop in blood pressure, heart rate and respiratory rate. An awareness of external stimuli is maintained, although there is a decreased response to noise and painful stimuli (Danneman *et al.*, 1988). This trance-like state is induced in the laboratory by placing the rabbit in dorsal recumbency, covering its eyes with its ears and flexing its chin against the neck. The hind legs are stretched out for a few minutes before releasing the legs and gently stroking the chest and abdomen. As long as the head is flexed, the rabbit remains immobile and restraining devices have been designed to maintain this position (Bivin, 1994). There are similarities between the immobility response and an opiate-induced state. The exact role of endogenous opioid systems is controversial and there are conflicting reports about the effects of naloxone which, theoretically, should prevent or reverse the hypnotic state (Danneman *et al.*, 1988). Sudden noise or painful stimuli can interrupt the trance and there is considerable variation in individual susceptibility to the technique. In a study by Danneman *et al.* (1988), the immobility response could not be evoked in 25% of rabbits. In the consulting room, some pet rabbits can be calmed and restrained by placing them in dorsal or lateral recumbency and gently stroking their stomach while speaking to them quietly. Blowing gently on their face or stroking the bridge of the nose can also be effective.

3.8 Clinical history

It is not always easy to elicit an accurate case history. Owners have preconceived ideas of the correct or incorrect way of keeping rabbits and will often wish to give the 'right' answer rather than a truthful one. For example, owners do not like to admit that the rabbit has not been out of its hutch for months or that it is weeks since they cleaned out its cage. When an owner says they feed 'lots of greens', this can mean half a cabbage leaf once a week or a diet exclusively of hay and vegetables. Misleading information can be given in response to enquiries about the amount of grass a rabbit eats. There seems to be reluctance on the part of owners to pick grass to feed to rabbits although they may be willing to put them out in a run on the lawn to graze. The length of time that a rabbit has access to grass varies considerably, from a couple of hours on two or three occasions during the summer months to several hours a day all year round. Owners often insist that their rabbit will not eat fresh greens, grass and weeds. Because the owner's perception is that the rabbit will not eat such food, they do not offer it. It is interesting how many hospitalized rabbits readily eat grass and dandelions despite their owner's protestations that their pet would not eat such a diet at home.

Recent changes in husbandry can be relevant. For example, a rabbit may not have learnt to use a new automatic drinker. A new batch of food may be unpalatable. Loss of a companion can result in anorexia and depression. Weight loss can result from bullying by a new dominant cage mate that prevents access to food.

Owners may describe symptoms such as tooth grinding or a change in demeanour. Some rabbits exhibit low grade neurological disorders such as head nodding when they are relaxed or appear unaware of loud noises. These behavioural clues are unlikely to take place in the consulting room when the rabbit is apprehensive and have to be elicited from the owner.

3.8.1 Breed incidence

Dwarf breeds appear to be predisposed to developing incisor malocclusion. Giant breeds are more susceptible to cardiomyopathy and arthritic conditions. The giant English and French Lops are prone to superficial pyoderma in the large skin folds that can develop under the chin and around the perineum. Entropion also occurs in these breeds. The thin fur on the hocks of Rex rabbits makes them susceptible to developing sore hocks and the short maxilla and 'squashed in' face of the Netherland Dwarf can alter the anatomy of the nasolacrimal duct so it is prone to blockage. Dwarf breeds appear to have a susceptibility to developing torticollis due to *Encephalitozoon cuniculi* infection (Kunstyr and Naumann, 1983).

3.8.2 Age

Young rabbits that are newly purchased are more likely to be affected by infectious diseases than the adult rabbit kept on its own. Newly weaned rabbits are susceptible to various enteric conditions. Colibacillosis is more prevalent in suckling rabbits and hepatic coccidiosis and mucoid enteropathy are most likely to occur in the post-weaning period. Stress predisposes young rabbits to pasteurellosis. Rhinitis is often seen in young rabbits that have been taken from breeding colonies and exposed for sale in a pet shop. Congenital malocclusion is seen in the young rabbit, whereas the incidence of acquired dental disease, neoplasia and musculoskeletal problems increases with age. Thymomas and a variety of skin tumours are among the other types of neoplasms that have been reported in rabbits. Although tumours are usually encountered in elderly patients, it is possible to discover neoplasms in young animals. Lymphosarcoma has been reported in an 8–10-week-old rabbit (Cloyd and Johnson, 1978).

3.8.3 Husbandry

It is important to find out if the rabbit lives on its own or with a mate. Fur chewing or fights can result in alopecia, wounds or abscesses. Does that are kept with other does or neutered males are more likely to suffer from false pregnancies than those that are housed on their own. Contact with wild rabbits is also a relevant part of the history. It is not unknown for does to dig out of their enclosure, escape and return or be found a few days later. Myxomatosis or pregnancy can be the result. Rabbits kept in enclosures or hutches can be visited by wild rabbits, especially during the night. There is often a pile of droppings as evidence of the visit.

House rabbits are prone to chewing household fixtures. Heavy metal toxicity or electrocution is more likely to occur in a house rabbit than one kept in a hutch outside. They are also at a greater risk of traumatic injuries and fractures. The material that is used in the litter tray is also an important part of the history. For example, pine shavings can cause hepatotoxicity or clay materials can cause caecal impactions.

Hutch rabbits are more likely to suffer from diseases of neglect. It is not uncommon for hutch rabbits with long-standing conditions such as large abscesses, advanced dental disease, and terminal neoplasia to be presented with no clinical history at all. Hutches kept in stuffy sheds predispose to pasteurellosis and upper respiratory tract infections. Hutches exposed to severe weather conditions predispose to heat stroke or stress-related diseases such as gastric stasis following predator attack, a thunderstorm or severe frost.

3.8.4 Eating and drinking

Rabbits normally drink 50–100 ml/kg/24 h (Brewer and Cruise, 1994). The composition and water content of the diet affects this quantity. Rabbits that eat fresh greens may not drink at all (Cheeke, 1987). High protein diets require a high water intake. Fibrous, dry foods absorb water in the intestinal tract and therefore increase thirst. During periods of water deprivation, food intake is reduced, sometimes to the point of anorexia. Conversely, food deprivation results in an increase in thirst with rabbits drinking up to 650% more water (Brewer and Cruise, 1994). Some rabbits never learn to use automatic drinkers and will only drink out of a bowl. Water deprivation eventually leads to dehydration and prerenal azotaemia.

3.8.5 Urination and defaecation

Many owners do not know whether their rabbit is urinating or defaecating normally, especially if it is kept in a hutch or lives with another rabbit. Faecal consistency, size and output are an important part of the clinical history. Sometimes there are some faecal pellets in the carrier that can be examined during the consultation. A healthy rabbit, that is eating well, passes large quantities of hard faeces and eats the soft caecotrophs (see Table 3.1). The number of hard faeces varies with the fibre content of the diet. A healthy 2.5–3 kg rabbit produces about 150 hard faecal pellets a day (Lowe, 1998). Hard pellets can be expelled at any time but are always produced overnight. Absence of hard faeces is indicative of anorexia or reduced intestinal motility. Small faecal pellets are produced following periods of reduced food intake.

Observant owners may see their rabbit ingesting caecotrophs from the anus. Uneaten caecotrophs are sometimes seen as shiny clusters of dark pasty pellets in the bedding of normal animals. Uneaten caecotrophs are often interpreted as diarrhoea. This is not surprising as caecotrophs have a strong smell and a soft consistency in comparison with the hard faecal pellets. Obesity, spinal problems and dental disease are among the many reasons for caecotrophs to be left uneaten (see Figure 10.6). Uneaten caecotrophs can become entangled in the fur under the tail and form an unpleasant, malodorous faecal mass. Changes in the consistency of caecotrophs can follow ingestion of a new food or a succulent

Table 3.1 Significance of faecal output

Clinical condition	*Hard faeces*	*Soft faeces (caecotrophs)*
Normal	Large numbers (~150) of hard pellets produced each day	Usually not seen, although occasional cluster of caecotrophs in the bedding is not abnormal
	Microscopically consist of strands of undigested fibre	Microscopically contain an abundance of bacteria, protozoa and occasional yeast
Anorexia or starvation	Reduced in number and size	Not seen
Gut stasis	Absent	Not seen (absent)
Enteritis	Soft or liquid	Soft or liquid. Cannot be differentiated from hard faeces
Uneaten caecotrophs	Normal, i.e. produced in large quantities	May be seen as clusters in bedding or entangled in fur under tail
Soft uneaten caecotrophs	Normal	Periodic expulsion of soft, faecal paste which easily becomes entangled in fur under the tail

item such as lettuce or fruit. Soft, sticky or liquid caecotrophs may be passed. It is thought that this is due to alterations in the caecal microflora. Rabbits on a high fibre diet have a healthy caecal microflora that can withstand dietary changes. Uneaten caecotrophs are not life threatening although they are unpleasant for the owner and rabbit, and predispose to other conditions such as superficial pyoderma, fly strike and problems with urination due to inflamed painful perineal skin (see Sections 9.7.2, 10.6, and 14.4.3).

Enteritis is signified by excretion of faecal material that cannot be identified as either hard or soft faeces. Microscopic examination of the faecal material can be helpful (see Section 6.8). Caecotrophs consist of a paste that is rich in bacteria that are easily seen on a faecal smear stained with gram's stain. Hard faeces consist of particles of indigestible fibre and little else. Sometimes it is necessary to hospitalize the rabbit to observe faecal output.

Urination should take place with no pain or discomfort. Normal rabbit urine varies considerably in its visual appearance. The colour can vary from the pale yellow colour that is familiar in other species through a range of oranges and brown to a deep red that can be mistaken for blood. The colour depends on the diet and is the result of the excretion of plant pigments. Vegetables such as cabbage, broccoli and dandelions often result in the excretion of red urine. There are clinical conditions such as urolithiasis and uterine disorders that will cause haematuria. Examination of the urine with a dipstick differentiates between blood and plant pigments. Alternatively, a Wood's lamp can be used as urinary pigments fluoresce when exposed to ultraviolet light (Benson and Paul-Murphy, 1999).

Normal rabbit urine can be cloudy due to the presence of calcium carbonate precipitates. The rabbit kidney is adapted for the excretion of large amounts of calcium (see Section 1.6.7). Intestinal absorption is related to the calcium content of the diet and excess amounts are excreted by the kidney. Therefore the amount of calcium carbonate precipitate varies with the calcium content of the diet. The hydration status of the animal and pH of the urine also affect the amount of precipitate. The urine can be clear during periods of high calcium demand such as growth, pregnancy or lactation. A small amount of precipitate is a good sign as it reflects adequate calcium content in the diet. Excessive precipitate can form a thick sludge, especially in the bladder of rabbits that do not urinate frequently (see Section 14.4). High dietary calcium levels exacerbate the problem. Cystitis and urinary incontinence can be the result. It can be difficult to differentiate between normal calcium carbonate deposits and abnormal amounts of sludge. Normal rabbit urine is often radiopaque. Calcium carbonate deposits in the urine of an otherwise healthy animal with no sign of urinary tract disease can be ignored. Similarly, triple phosphate crystals can be a normal finding in rabbit urine.

3.9 Clinical examination

A list of differential diagnoses for some commonly encountered conditions of pet rabbits is given in Table 3.2.

3.9.1 General condition

The general health of a rabbit can be assessed by the state of its coat and its body weight. Obese animals are prone to grooming difficulties, sludgy urine, cystitis, parasitic skin disease, perineal soiling from uneaten caecotrophs, fly strike, cardiovascular disease, arthritis, hepatic lipidosis and death. At the other end of the scale, weight loss is a signi-

Box 3.3 Intestinal obstruction in pet rabbits

Intestinal obstruction in pet rabbits gives a characteristic clinical presentation. The most common cause of obstruction is a felt of hair that is groomed out of the coat, especially the hind feet, during moulting. Dried pulses, foreign objects, tumours, tapeworm cysts are among other causes of obstruction (see Chapter 10). If the condition is recognized early and surgery is performed promptly, there is a reasonable chance of success. If the condition is not recognized and treated, the rabbit will die unless the foreign body happens to pass into the colon.

Presentation

- Sudden onset. The rabbit was well until a few hours before presentation
- Severe mental depression. The rabbit is unresponsive and totally anorexic
- Abdominal distension. The owners may have noticed a bloated appearance although it may be masked by a thick coat
- Palpably distended stomach. A 'strange feeling' or distended abdomen or abdominal pain is a clear indication for abdominal radiography
- Shock, dehydration and collapse. Depending on the site of the obstruction, the rabbit's condition will deteriorate rapidly.

Diagnosis

- Abdominal radiographs are diagnostic. A stomach distended with gas and fluid is clearly visible (See Figure 10.5, Chapter 10). A section of gas-filled intestine can usually be seen radiographically, proximal to the site of obstruction. If the obstruction moves into the colon, gas can be seen in the caecum and proximal colon
- Other causes of gastric dilatation include mucoid enteropathy or dysautonomia, both of which carry a poor prognosis
- Abdominal palpation. An impacted organ, intussusception or foreign body may be palpable, especially if the rabbit is anaesthetized or moribund
- Prompt exploratory laparotomy is indicated.

Treatment

- Motility stimulants are contraindicated prior to surgery. Postoperatively, cisapride or metoclopramide are required to prevent ileus
- Effective analgesia is important. Low dose fentanyl/fluanisone (Hypnorm, Janssen 0.2 ml/kg) provides analgesia, sedation and vasodilation that facilitates intravenous fluid therapy
- Decompress the stomach by passing a stomach tube (a stomach tube should remain in place throughout surgery). This can usually be done after the rabbit has been sedated
- Fluid therapy. Intravenous (or intraosseous) fluid therapy is essential. Subcutaneous fluids will be ineffective in restoring and maintaining blood pressure and correcting dehydration and electrolyte imbalances
- Anaesthesia, gradual mask induction with isoflurane is recommended. Anaesthesia and perioperative care are described in Chapter 5
- Enterotomy. Midline incision. The obstruction is often easy to find. The gas-filled small intestine can usually be identified and followed to the site of the obstruction. (Basic surgical principles in rabbits are described in Chapter 15). Fine suture material (5/0 or 6/0 PDS or Monocryl) is required to repair the intestinal incision. A set of fine instruments is essential (a detailed description of surgical procedure is given in Chapter 10).

Table 3.2 List of differential diagnoses for some common conditions in pet rabbits

Symptoms	*Differential diagnosis*	*Comments*
Abdominal distension	Gastric dilatation	
	Obesity	
	Pregnancy	
	Hepatic coccidiosis	Can cause ascites
	Liver tumour	Can cause ascites
	Uterine adenocarcinoma	
	Cardiac disease	Can cause ascites
Abdominal mass	Pregnancy	
	Neoplasia	Especially uterine adenocarcinoma
	Caecal impaction	
	Extra-uterine pregnancy	
	Abscess	
	Fat necrosis	
	Full bladder, ? urolithiasis	
	Tapeworm cysts	
	Renal enlargement	Neoplasia, hydronephrosis, renal calculi
Abortion	*Listeria monocytogenes*	
	Treponema cuniculi	
Anorexia	Unpalatable diet	
	Stress	Pain, unfamiliar surroundings, predator proximity, loss of companion
	Dental disease	• Spurs on cheek teeth lacerating the tongue • Elongated incisors physically impeding intake of food • Fractured teeth causing pain
	Gastrointestinal hypomotility 'Gut stasis', 'trichobezoars'	Secondary to any stressful situation Predisposed by inadequate dietary fibre
	Intestinal obstruction	Acute onset Associated with severe depression May be caused by ingested felts of hair, foreign bodies such as dried peas and pulses May be due to extramural lesion such as abscesses, tumours or tapeworm cysts
	Mucoid enteropathy	Slow onset Tooth grinding Absence of faeces or mucus ± diarrhoea Associated with stress Juvenile rabbits most commonly affected May have palpably impacted caecum
	Caecal impaction	Idiopathic Excess dietary fibre and inadequate water intake Ingested clay litter material
	Infectious disease	Pasteurellosis, myxomatosis, VHD, enterotoxaemia
	Systemic disease	Renal disease, hepatopathy
	Neoplasia	
	Trauma	Jaw fracture
Ataxia	Spinal cord compression	
	Encephalitozoon cuniculi	
	Ketoacidosis	
	Starvation	
	Trauma	
	Septicaemia	
	Heat stroke	
	Lead poisoning	
Blepharospasm	Keratitis	
	Keratitis in association with dacrocystitis	
	Corneal ulcer	
	Conjunctivitis	May be secondary to poor air quality or dust from hay

continued

Table 3.2 List of differential diagnoses for some common conditions in pet rabbits

Symptoms	*Differential diagnosis*	*Comments*
	Conjunctival foreign body Uveitis Entropion Swollen eyelids	? hay seeds May be congenital or acquired from fight wounds involving eyelids Myxomatosis *Treponema cuniculi* Neoplasia Abscesses
Deafness	Middle ear infection *Encephalitozoon cuniculi* encephalitis Pus, wax and exudate in external ear canal	Pus in tympanic bulla as a result of ascending infection from the eustachian tube
Diarrhoea (see Table 10.2)	Uneaten caecotrophs Uneaten soft caecotrophs Antibiotic-associated diarrhoea Enteritis Enterotoxaemia Coccidiosis	Uneaten caecotrophs are often interpreted by owners as 'diarrhoea' Soft uneaten caecotrophs can be induced by dietary change, especially after introduction of succulent foods such as lettuce Some antibiotics, e.g. oral penicillin, ampicillins, clindamycin and lincomycin can induce diarrhoea by their effects on the gut flora
Exophthalmos: bilateral	Fear Males in breeding season Natural appearance Paraneoplastic disease Bilateral glaucoma Bilateral retrobulbar abscesses	 e.g. short nosed Dwarf breeds Thymoma
Exophthalmos: unilateral	Glaucoma Retrobulbar disease	Congenital Secondary to other diseases such as trauma, tumours or *E. cuniculi* lens rupture Abscess Tumour Haemorrhage Tapeworm cyst Iatrogenic rupture of nasolacrimal duct and infiltration of periorbital space with fluid
Haematuria	Cystitis ('sludgy urine') Urolithiasis Uterine adenocarcinomas Uterine polyps Endometrial venous aneurysms Chronic polypoid cystitis, renal infarcts and disseminated intravascular coagulopathy have also been described as causes of haematuria in laboratory rabbits	 **NB** Blood from the uterus may be voided in urine as the vaginal vestibule fills with urine during micturition. Blood clots may be present
Head tilt	*Encephalitozoon cuniculi* Infection of the vestibular apparatus Other CNS disease (In US) *Baylisascaris* larva	Granulomatous inflammation of central nervous tissue Usually ascending *Pasteurella multocida* from nasal cavity via eustachian tube May be abscesses along vestibular tract Trauma, neoplasia, etc. Raccoons are natural host
Increased respiratory rate	Stress Metabolic acidosis Heat stroke	Due to unfamiliar surroundings or proximity of predators Ketoacidosis Hot stuffy shed Transport by car Hutch situated in sun

continued

Table 3.2 List of differential diagnoses for some common conditions in pet rabbits

Symptoms	*Differential diagnosis*	*Comments*
		Heatpads
	Trauma	? predator attack
		Penetrating injuries of chest wall
		Haemothorax, pneomothorax, etc.
	Rhinitis	Pasteurellosis
		Nasal foreign body, e.g. hay or seed
		Tooth root abscess
	Obstruction of nasopharynx, larynx or trachea	Inflammation caused by pasteurellosis
		Abscess
		Foreign body, hay or seed
		Exudate from lung disease
	Lung disease	Primary bacterial pneumonia, e.g. pasteurellosis
		Secondary pneumonia, e.g. myxomatosis, mucoid enteropathy
		Viral haemorrhagic disease
		Aspiration pneumonia
		Primary or secondary neoplasia
		Pulmonary abscess
	Pulmonary oedema	Congestive heart failure
		Heat stroke
		Electrocution
	Pleural effusion	Neoplasia
		Cardiomyopathy
		Coronavirus
	Congestive heart failure	
Liver disease	Hepatic lipidosis	
	Hepatic coccidiosis	
	Viral haemorrhagic disease	
	Hepatopathy	Has been associated with pine wood shavings as litter material
		Aflatoxin
		Cysticercus pisiformis
	Neoplasia	
	Bile duct obstruction	? Neoplasia
		Adhesions
	Toxoplasma gondii	
Polydypsia	Anorexia	
	Food deprivation	
	Renal disease	*? E. cuniculi*
	? Diabetes mellitus	There is debate about incidence of diabetes mellitus in pet rabbits
Paresis/paralysis	Spinal fracture	Trauma ? predator attack
		Spontaneous due to pre-existing bone disease
	Degenerative disc disease	Disc protrusion may follow trauma
	Spinal deformities	Kyphosis, scoliosis, spondylosis
	Neoplasia	Primary or secondary bone tumours can cause spinal cord compression
	Spinal abscess	Spinal abscess can cause cord compression
	'Floppy rabbit syndrome'	
Pruritus	Flea infestation	Usually dog or cat fleas
	Louse infestation	
	Allergic skin disease	
	Compulsive self-mutilation	
	Ringworm	
Renal disease. *NB* Asymptomatic renal disease can be present due to benign embryonal nephroma,	Nephrolithiasis	
	E. cuniculi	
	Hydronephrosis	
	Renal calcification	

continued

Table 3.2 List of differential diagnoses for some common conditions in pet rabbits

Symptoms	*Differential diagnosis*	*Comments*
congenital renal cysts or encephalitozoonisis		
Reversible azotaemia can occur due to stress, dehydration or water deprivation	Renal abscesses	
	Staphylococcal nephritis	
	Pyelonephritis	
	Lymphoma	
	Neoplasia	
	Amyloidosis	
	Renal agenesis	
	Toxic compounds	
Seizures	Encephalitozoonisis	
	Viral haemorrhagic disease	
	Toxicity, e.g. lead	
	Terminal hepatic lipidosis	
	Arteriosclerosis	
	Toxoplasma	
	Idiopathic epilepsy	
	CNS disease	
Skin lesions: alopecia	Physiological, moulting	Some fluffy haired breeds lose fur in patches
	Fur pulling for nestmaking	Associated with pregnancy or pseudopregnancy
	Treponema cuniculi	
	Barbering	Caused by dominant cage mate
	Fighting	
	Cheyletiellosis	
	Ringworm	
	Nutritional	e.g. essential sulphur amino acid deficiency
Skin lesions: crusty	Ringworm	
	Superficial pyoderma secondary to trauma	
	Ectopic *Psoroptes cuniculi*	
	Allergic dermatitis	
	Atypical myxomatosis	
	Treponema cuniculi	Rabbit syphilis
	Rectoanal papilloma	
Skin lesions : nodules	Primary tumours	e.g. fibromas
	Circumscribed abscesses	
	Atypical myxomatosis	
Skin lesions: swellings	Abscesses	
	Tumours	
	Hernias	
	Subcutaneous *Cysticercus serialis* cysts	Dogs/foxes are intermediate hosts
Sudden death	Enterotoxaemia	
	Viral haemorrhagic disease	
	Intestinal obstruction	
	Choking	Especially rabbits with advanced dental disease that can choke on pieces of hay
	Predator attack	
	Trauma	
	Acute pasteurellosis	
	Electrocution	
	Cardiomyopathy	
	Neoplasia	
	Poisoning e.g. yew	
	Listeriosis	Females in late pregnancy
Weight loss (see also anorexia)	Dental disease	
	Gastrointestinal hypomotility	
	Renal disease	
	Caecal impaction	
	Chronic liver disease	Hepatic coccidiosis in young rabbits
	Neoplasia	
	Change of diet	
	Bullying by cagemate	
	Pseudotuberculosis	

ficant clinical finding as rabbits are seldom given insufficient food unless there is serious neglect taking place. Dental disease, gastrointestinal hypomotility, renal or liver disease or neoplasia can cause weight loss despite the rabbit looking lively and well to its owner.

3.9.2 General demeanour

A healthy rabbit is responsive and alert with its nose constantly twitching. The response to pain is to become quiet, immobile and oblivious of the surroundings. Visceral problems such as gut stasis, or urolithiasis appear to be more distressing to rabbits than the abscesses or fractures. Occasionally, overt signs of pain such as tooth grinding can be evident. This is usually associated with visceral pain especially impactive intestinal problems such as mucoid enteropathy (see Section 10.9). Intestinal obstruction is associated with severe depression and immobility, which gives a characteristic clinical presentation (see Box 3.3). The presence of spurs on the molars that traumatize the sensitive mucosa of the tongue is also very painful for rabbits.

3.9.3 Gait

It is often helpful to allow the rabbit to hop around the consulting room floor, providing the owner and practitioner are confident that the animal can be caught again. Slippery vinyl is a difficult surface for rabbits to move about on. Placing a large towel on a slippery floor aids assessment of the patient's gait. Abnormal gait associated with spinal problems or fractures may be discovered. Neurological deficits can become evident and the rabbit's general demeanour is easier to assess.

3.9.4 Sex, age and sexual maturity

Rabbits can be difficult to sex, especially when they are immature, wriggling and presented individually so no comparison can be made. It is often simpler to sex neonates than animals of 4–6 weeks of age. Adults are usually straightforward because entire males have prominent descended testicles. Bucks tend to be larger and have a broader head than does. Mature, entire males develop a thick skin especially around the scruff and on the dorsum. Females often have a dewlap as a secondary sexual characteristic although some males can develop quite a pronounced dewlap especially if they are castrated or overweight. Pressure on the genital orifice everts either the penis or the vulva. The vulva can look like a small penis to the novice but is shorter, less round and has a slit like opening rather than the circular orifice of the male (see Figure 3.1). Testicles descend at 10–12 weeks, although they can be retracted into the abdomen during periods of ill health or starvation.

There are conflicting reports on the life expectancy of rabbits. Five to 7 years is the life span given by Gillett (1994) with a comment that rabbits can live to be 15. Many pet rabbits live longer than 7 years and can easily attain 11–12 years, although geriatric diseases are common in this age group.

It is difficult to age living rabbits with any degree of accuracy. The epiphyseal line in the tibia closes at approximately 9 months of age. The epiphyses of the lumbar vertebrae close much later. Counting the adhesion lines in the periosteal zone of the mandible by histopathological examination can be used to age mature rabbits accurately (Henderson and Bowen, 1979) but this is not possible during life. The deciduous teeth are shed at birth and so the only criteria to make an assessment of age during clinical examination, are the size and appearance of the rabbit, both of which vary according to breed and state of health. The claws of the rabbit do not project beyond the fur until the rabbit reaches maturity (Sandford, 1996) but this age varies according to breed and size. Fanciers may be able to give an indication of age by feeling the ears that are soft in the young rabbits and become tougher with age (Sandford, 1996). Pedigree rabbits may have rings over their hocks on which the year of birth will be recorded. Smaller breeds mature at 4–5 months of age and the larger breeds mature at 5–8 months (Donnelly, 1997). Bucks reach puberty later than does and so immature females that are housed with their brothers are unlikely to conceive even though he may mount and appear to mate her. Obviously, the two sexes should be separated or

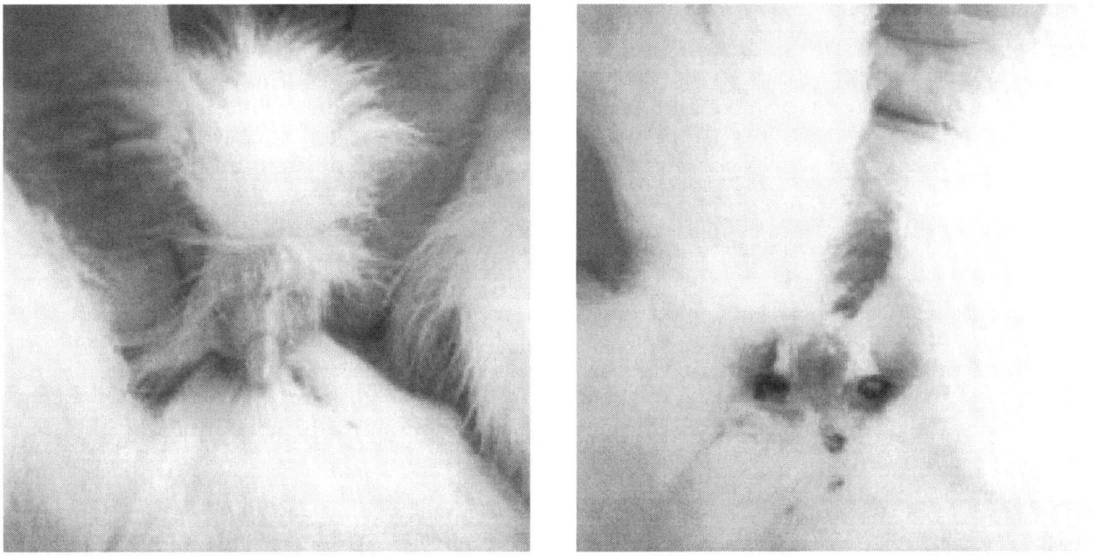

(a) (b)

Figure 3.1. Inguinal skin folds and male and female genitalia. In both sexes, deep skin folds lie on either side of the genital orifice. These folds contain scent glands. It is normal for the folds to contain a waxy, odorous exudate. In (b), a brown exudate can be seen. Rabbits can be sexed by applying gentle pressure on the genital orifice to extrude the genital organ. (a) **Male genitalia**: In the male, the penis is extruded. Testicles can usually be seen in the scrotal sacs of sexually mature rabbits (> 10–12 weeks) although they can be retracted during periods of stress, illness or shortage of food; (b) **Female genitalia**: In the female, the vulva is extruded. The vulva can look similar to a small penis but is shorter, less round and has a slit like opening rather than the circular orifice of the male.

neutered at this stage if pregnancy is to be prevented.

3.9.5 Examination of the skin, fur and mucous membranes

A healthy rabbit will spend a lot of time grooming. Rabbits that are kept together groom each other, especially around the head. There are many clinical conditions that can prevent a rabbit from licking and grooming properly, which are manifested by a dull coat full of dead hair and skin debris. Combing through the fur with a flea comb gives an idea of the amount of dead hair and debris and also reveals the presence of fleas, flea dirt or mites. Mites can just be seen with the naked eye especially under good illumination. A magnifying glass can be used to examine the fur thoroughly. Microscopic examination of skin brushings confirms their presence and gives an idea of numbers. Most rabbits have some degree of infestation, which is not always significant (see Section 9.14.2). The area of skin between the shoulder blades and above the base of the tail are difficult for the rabbit to reach and groom, especially if it obese or has limited flexibility due to spondylosis (see Figure 3.8). Cheyletiellosis often starts to become evident on the back of the neck and along the dorsum. During the summer, soiled fur at the base of the tail or the perineum must be examined closely for the presence of maggots.

The area under the dewlap is prone to superficial pyoderma, predisposed by factors such as poor hygiene, dental disease or obesity. Some rabbits are unable to drink without immersing their dewlap in the water bowl. Excess salivation as a result of dental disease can result in a wet dewlap that is prone to bacterial infection. Fat rabbits with excessive skin folds and large dewlaps experience problems grooming and may lick the cranial surface of the dewlap obsessively as a type of displacement activity because they cannot groom other areas such as the underside of the dewlap or the perineum which is infected, inflamed and sore.

The forelegs are used to clean the face. Examination of the inner aspect of the carpus and metacarpus may show saliva staining indicative of dental disease. Dried mucopurulent material can be found in rabbits with ocular or nasal discharges. Examination of the fore and hind limbs may show evidence of ulcerative pododermatitis. An area of thin, hairless skin over the point of the hock is not unusual. It is protected by thick fur that is directed across it.

Felts of densely matted hair are a cause of intestinal obstruction if the rabbit ingests them during grooming. Large felts can accumulate on the plantar aspect of the hind feet. Owners should be advised to groom these animals daily and ensure that loose felts of hair are removed. Rabbits with dental problems or long-haired breeds such as Angoras are especially at risk.

3.9.6 Examination of the perineum

Examination of the perineum confirms the sex of the rabbit and gives an indication of general state of grooming. Urine scalding, vaginal discharges, adherent caecotrophs, fly strike, perineal fold dermatitis or diarrhoea may be evident on examination of this area (see Figure 3.2)

The two deep folds of skin on either side of the anal orifice are the inguinal glands that are normally filled with a yellow-brown odiferous deposit (see Figure 3.1b).

The perineum is an extremely sensitive area in rabbits. Pain caused by infected, inflamed perineal skin can lead to urine retention, urethritis, cystitis and/or urinary incontinence. Urine scalding can also be due to urogenital disease or indicative of other problems such as vertebral spondylitis, sore hocks or arthritis which prevent the rabbit positioning itself correctly to urinate (see Section 14.4.3). Neurological deficits, abdominal pain or generalized weakness can also lead to urine scalding or perineal soiling. Skin inflammation in the perineal area may be caused by uneaten caecotrophs that have become adherent to the fur and caused superficial pyoderma of the skin beneath. Obesity, dental disease and arthritis prevent grooming around the perineum so the fur becomes matted, soiled and infected. This starts a vicious circle that can be broken by clipping and cleaning the perineal area and treating the painful dermatitis (see Figure 9.1 and Section 9.7.3). Clippers can be used to remove most of the fur. A sharp pair of curved, pointed scissors is useful to tease out and cut matted hair around the genitalia and under the tail. Dead and matted hair can be combed out with a flea comb. It is very easy inadvertently to damage the delicate skin. Patience and the correct equipment are required. Sedation may be needed. The underlying reason for urinary incontinence, cystitis, grooming difficulties or uneaten caecotrophs needs to be addressed to prevent recurrence.

The appearance of the vulva alters according to the state of sexual receptivity. When the doe is non-receptive, the vulva is pale pink and dry. During receptivity, the vulva becomes swollen, moist and red, becoming darker until it is purple at the end of the receptive period. If the doe is mated, the vulva returns to a light pink colour in about 24 h.

Inflamed or crusty skin around the genitalia can be associated with *Treponema cuniculi* or ectopic *Psoroptes cuniculi* infestation. Ear mites can be transferred from the ears to the perineal folds during grooming. Examination of the external ear canal of affected rabbits reveals thick crusty exudate caused by *P. cuniculi*. Rectoanal papillomas can cause crusty lesions that protrude through the anal sphincter.

The hydration status of the rabbit can be assessed during examination of the perineum. Dehydration can occur in the absence of obvious fluid loss due to the redistribution of water and electrolytes associated with alterations of gastrointestinal motility. Although rabbits do not to take on a 'sunken eyed' appearance when dehydrated, the thin skin becomes wrinkled and loses its turgidity. The hairless scrotal skin of males is a useful site to assess hydration status by tenting the skin. The inguinal skin can be used in females.

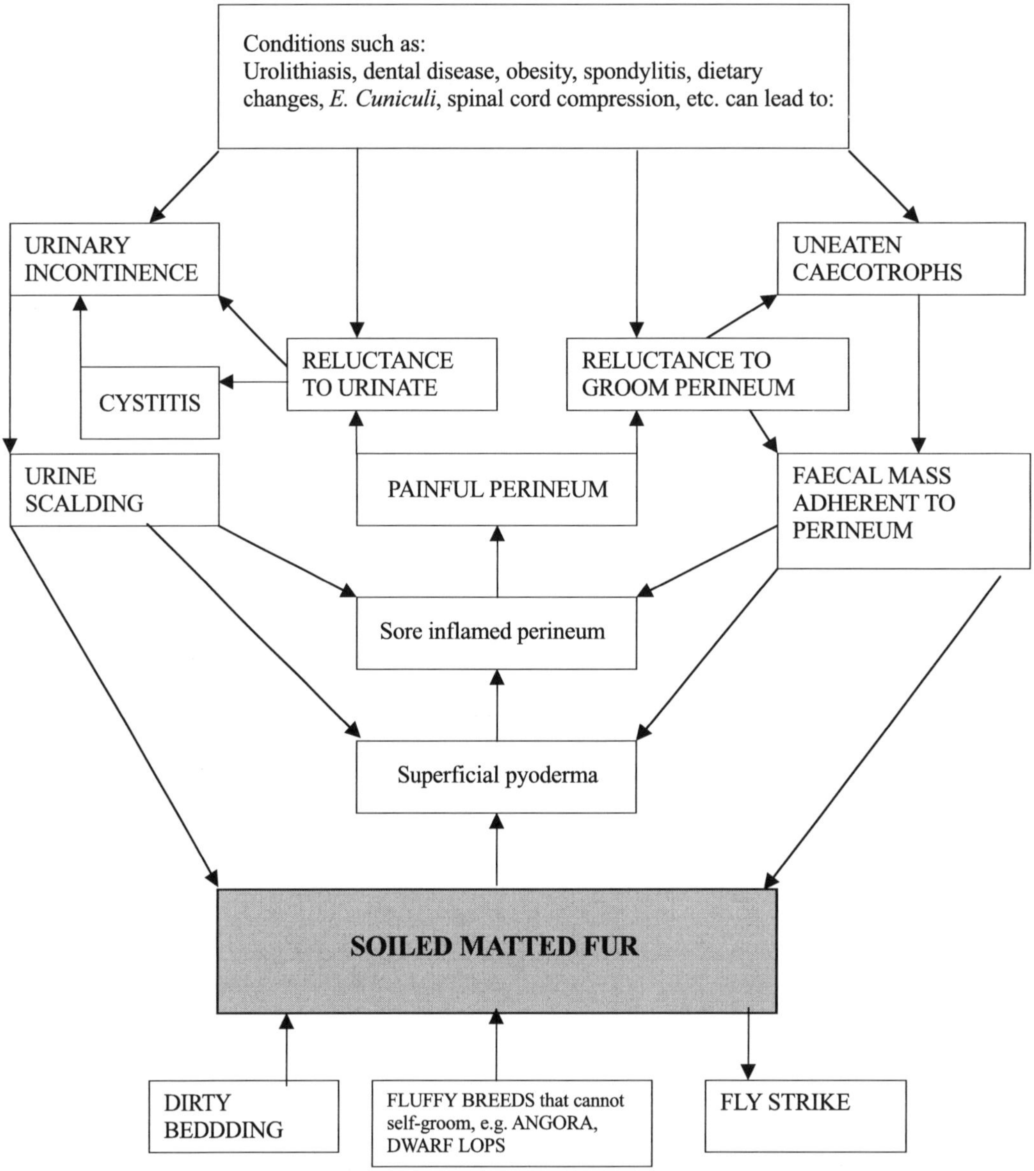

Figure 3.2. Causes of perineal soiling in pet rabbits. A healthy, short-coated rabbit will meticulously groom its perineum and keep it clean. There are many inter-relating factors that can prevent effective grooming of this area and result in matted, soiled fur with or without inflamed underlying skin.

Mucous membranes can be examined by looking at the colour of the nose or by lifting the lip to see the gums and tongue. Cyanosis is evident in advanced cases of cardiovascular or respiratory disease. Mild anaemia is more difficult to elucidate although extreme pallor is obvious.

3.9.7 Rectal temperature

The rectal mucosa is thin and easily damaged. Many practitioners do not routinely take the rectal temperature as part of their clinical examination because of the risk of trauma and the limitations in interpreting its significance.

Key points 3.5

- Rabbits normally drink 50–100 ml/kg/24 h although the amount may vary with diet
- Water deprivation results in anorexia
- Food deprivation can increase thirst
- Normal rabbit urine can be any colour from yellow, to brown orange or red
- Normal rabbit urine is turbid
- Immature rabbits can be sexed by everting the genital orifice. The female has a slit like vulva. The male has a penis. Testicles descend at 10–12 weeks
- Female rabbits have a dewlap
- It is difficult to age live rabbits with any degree of accuracy
- Examination of the perineum is an essential part of clinical examination. Urine scalding or faecal soiling may be indicative of other diseases
- Normal rectal temperature is variable: < 38°C can be considered subnormal. > 40.6°C is significantly high.

Normal rectal temperature of rabbits is 38.5–40°C (103.3–104°F). It is affected by factors such as environmental temperature and restraint. There is a slight seasonal variation with temperatures being higher in the autumn and winter than in spring and summer. Females have a slightly higher rectal temperature than males (Pericin and Grieve, 1984). Temperatures below 38.0°C (100.4°F) can be considered subnormal and temperatures in excess of 40.6°C (105°F) are significant and indicative of pyrogenic infection (Toth and Krueger, 1989) or heat stroke.

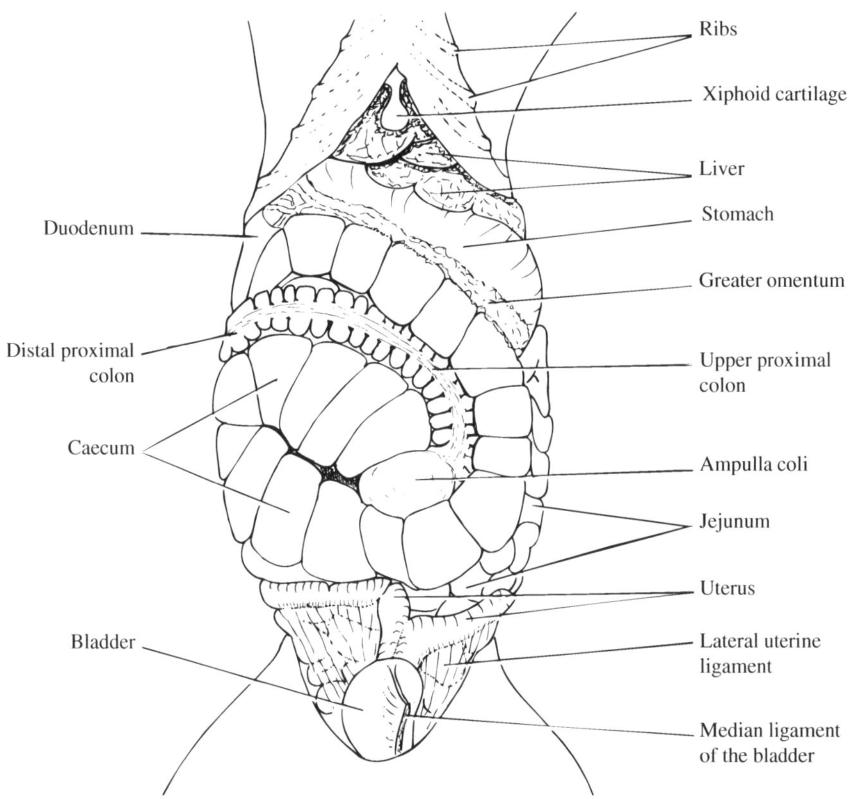

Figure 3.3. Topographic view of the abdomen, ventral view. The ventral abdominal wall has been resected to expose the viscera that are illustrated *in situ*. The diagram was drawn from *post-mortem* specimens using Barone *et al.* (1973) as a reference source.

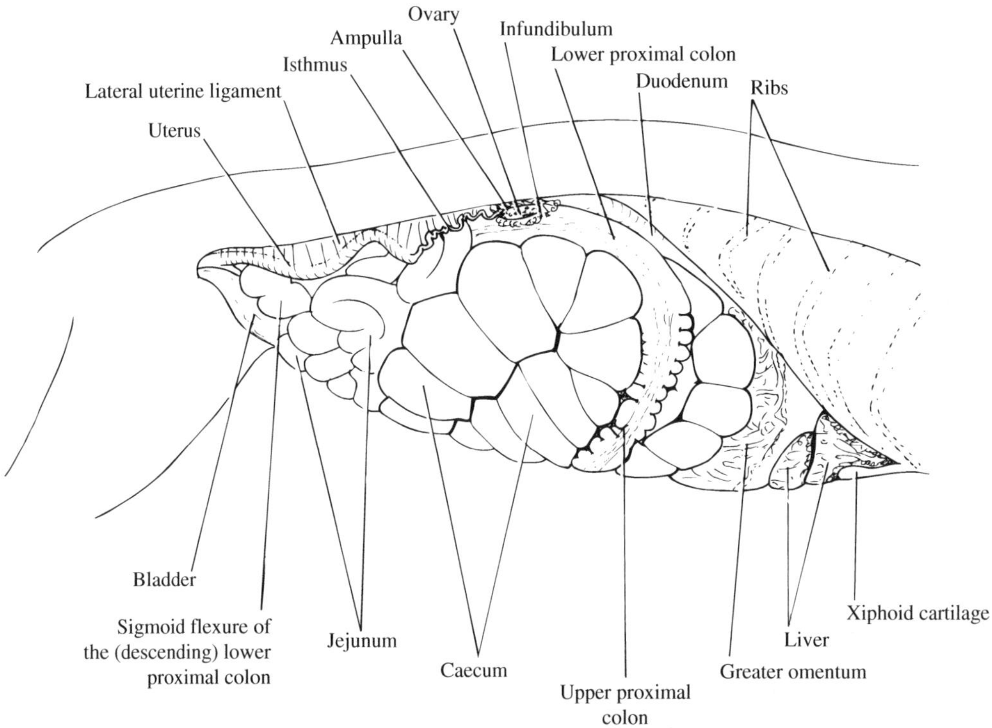

Figure 3.4. Topographic view of the abdomen, right lateral view. The abdominal viscera are illustrated *in situ* after resection of the right abdominal wall. The diagram was drawn from *post-mortem* specimens using Barone *et al.* (1973) as a reference source.

3.9.8 Abdominal palpation and auscultation

The normal topographical anatomy and relative position of the abdominal organs are illustrated in Figures 3.3, 3.4, 3.5. Radiography can be used to differentiate abnormalities detected during abdominal palpation. Ultrasound is also useful. Palpation of the abdomen should be done carefully and gently, as it is easy to traumatize the thin-walled viscera.

The spleen is too small to be palpable and the liver is not felt routinely during abdominal palpation. Both kidneys can usually be identified. They are mobile structures. The left kidney lies caudally to the right kidney, which lies close to the rib cage. The stomach cannot be palpated in the normal rabbit. In some cases of gastric stasis, the stomach may be felt as a hard round mass just behind the ribs on the right hand side. Intestinal obstruction causes gross distension of the stomach with gas and liquid (see Box 3.3). The caecum may be felt as a soft pliable structure in the ventral abdomen. The size and contents vary with diet and time of day. A full caecum may be felt as a doughy mass. Caecal impactions are felt as a hard sausage-like structure. Gas distension of the caecum can result from gastrointestinal hypomotility. In these cases, the caecum may not be differentiated from other organs or can be felt as a gas-filled structure that makes a sloshing sound when palpated. The bladder can be felt in the caudoventral abdomen. It should be palpated with care as it can rupture easily, especially if the urethra is partially obstructed by a urolith. Rabbits suffering from urolithiasis or cystitis often strain in response to bladder palpation and may void small amounts of urine on to the consulting table.

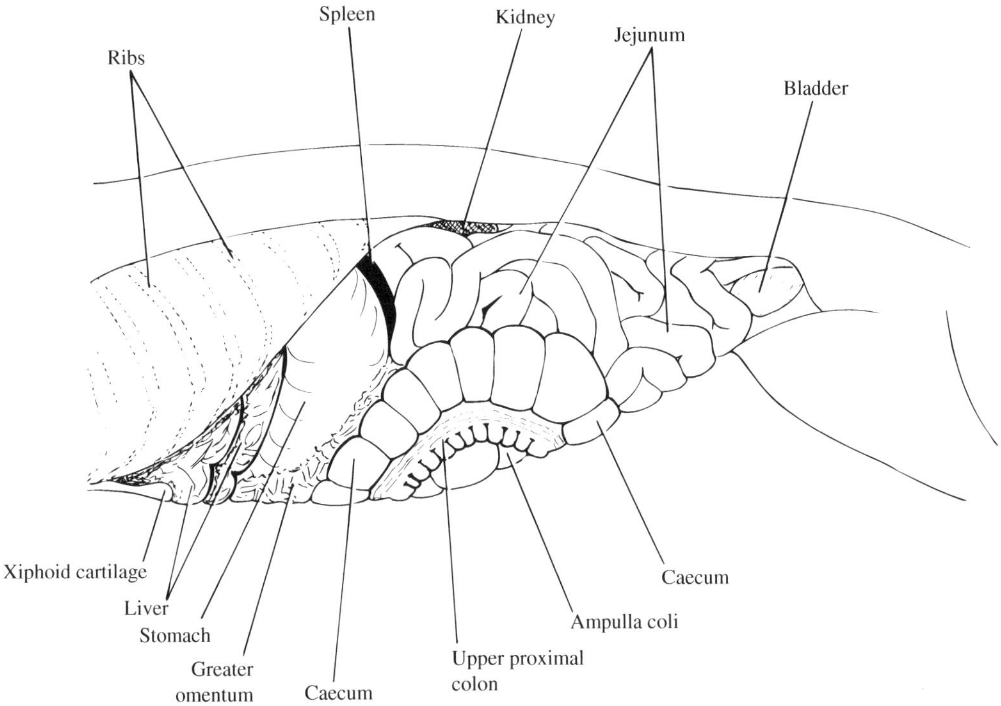

Figure 3.5. Topographic view of the abdomen, left lateral view. The abdominal viscera are illustrated *in situ* after resection of the left abdominal wall. The reproductive tract is not illustrated. The diagram was drawn from *post-mortem* specimens using Barone *et al.* (1973) as a reference source.

Gut sounds are not always evident in the healthy rabbit. Absence of gut sounds does not signify intestinal stasis. Tinkling sounds may be heard in distended gas-filled organs such as the caecum or stomach, indicating a gas/fluid interface.

The uterus lies in the ventral abdomen, caudal to the caecum. The broad ligament may contain large quantities of fat that can be seen radiographically. An enlarged uterus due to pregnancy or neoplasia may be felt. Twelve-to-14-day fetuses can be felt as olive-sized masses in the caudal abdomen. As the uterus enlarges it falls forward into the abdomen.

Abdominal masses may be neoplastic. Common neoplasms include uterine adenocarcinoma, lymphomas, liver and kidney tumours. Abdominal abscesses can occur. Areas of fat necrosis may be felt as hard lumps, especially in the remnants of the broad ligament in spayed females.

The limbs, vertebral column and rib cage can be checked for any obvious fractures or deformities.

3.9.9 Auscultation and assessment of respiration

Rabbits have a small rib cage and thoracic cavity. The diaphragm, rather than the intercostal muscles, brings about respiratory movement. Breathing takes place through the nose. Rabbits do not mouth breathe or pant effectively. Respiratory rate varies between 32 and 60 breaths per minute. Increased respiratory rates are indicative of stress, pain, hyperthermia, infection or respiratory disease. Metabolic acidosis can also be manifested by an increased respiratory rate. Upper respiratory tract disease is common in rabbits (see Section 13.2.3). Occlusion of the nasal passage results in increased respiratory effort and may be accompanied by various snuffles, squeaks and whistles. Some short-nosed breeds always make this type of noise. The differentiation between upper and lower airway disease can be made by observation and auscultation and examination of the nose.

An increase in respiratory rate is brought about by an increase in diaphragmatic rather than intercostal movement and can give the impression of dyspnoea. Dyspnoea is manifested by cyanosis, mouth breathing, depression and distress and may or may not be accompanied by an audible respiratory noise. Abnormal, absent or muffled lung sounds may or may not be heard during thoracic auscultation of rabbits with lower respiratory disease. Chronic lung disease cannot be ruled out by auscultation of the chest. Severe lung changes are a frequent incidental finding during *post-mortem* examination. Abnormal heart sounds can sometimes be detected, although cardiac disease is rare in rabbits in comparison with lung disease. The list of differential diagnoses of dyspnoea is similar to other species.

Normal heart rate varies between 130 and 325 bpm, which is too fast to differentiate heart sounds. Stress increases the heart rate markedly. A pulse can usually be felt in the central artery of the ear (Figure 3.6). A femoral pulse can sometimes be found although it is not as easy to locate in the rabbit as in the dog or cat.

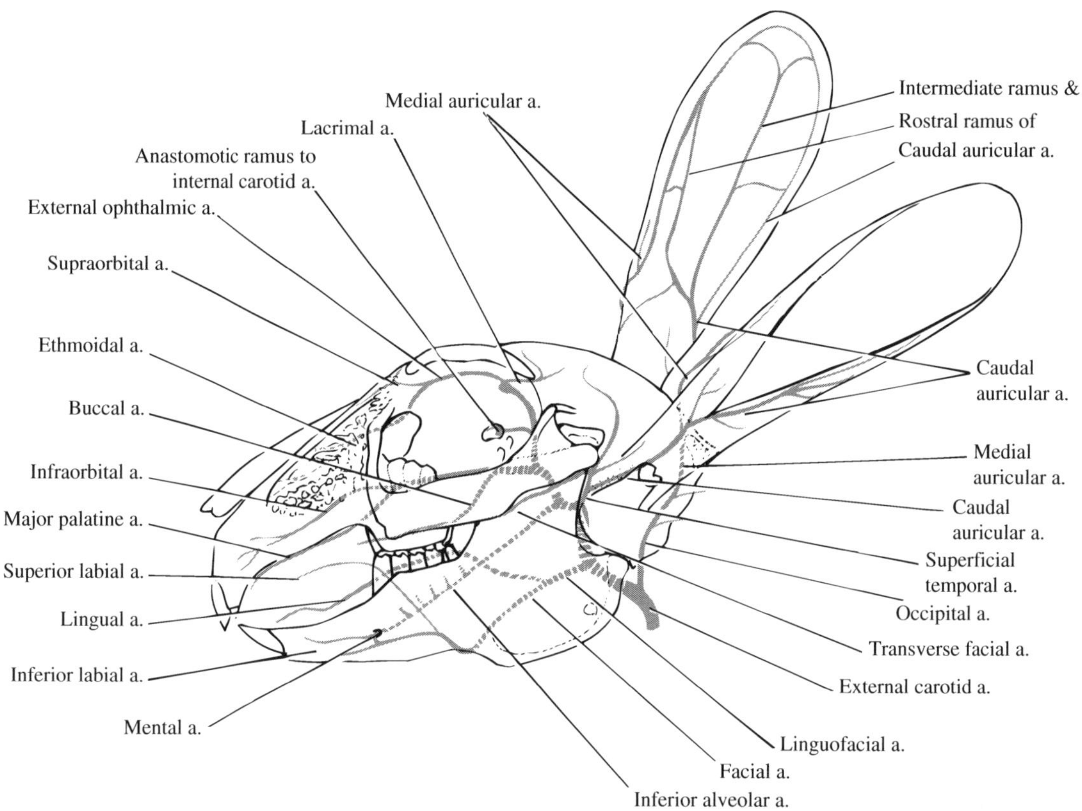

Figure 3.6. Arteries of the head. The arteries of the cheek may be encountered during surgery on facial abscesses in rabbits. The buccal and lingual arteries are in close proximity with the cheek teeth and can be inadvertently punctured during tooth trimming. The arteries of the ear are also illustrated. A pulse can often be detected by placing a finger on the intermediate ramus of caudal auricular (central) artery of the ear.

Key points 3.6

- Care should be taken during abdominal palpation as the thin walled viscera are easily traumatized
- Both kidneys can be felt during routine abdominal palpation
- The spleen is too small to be palpated
- The stomach and liver are not usually palpable
- The caecum may be palpated depending on nature of contents and time of day
- Palpating the bladder can elicit straining and urination in rabbits with cystitis
- The uterus cannot be palpated in the non-gravid, healthy animal. During pregnancy it may be felt in the ventral abdomen
- The thoracic cavity of the rabbit is small
- Breathing takes place through the nose
- Respiration is brought about by movement of the diaphragm rather than the intercostal muscles
- Normal respiratory rate is 32–60 breaths per minute
- Normal heart rate varies between 130 and 325 bpm
- A pulse may be felt in the central artery of the ear.

3.9.10 Examination of the face, head and oral cavity

The rabbit can be wrapped in a towel for this part of the examination and held firmly against the body of the owner or nurse.

Visual inspection of the external ear canal may reveal the typical crusty exudate that is associated with *Psoroptes cuniculi* infestation or the waxy exudate that is often encountered, especially in lop eared breeds. There is a blind ending section of the external ear canal separated by a cartilaginous plate or tragus. Examination of both sides of the tragus can be performed with an auriscope. Auriscopic visualization of the eardrum is difficult due to the length of the auditory canal and the presence of wax and debris.

The skin around the face and head is normally clean and free from debris. Sometimes it is a bonded companion, and not the patient itself, that keeps the head groomed and cleaned. The presence of small scabs in the fur is indicative of a rabbit that is not grooming perhaps due to pain around the face. Saliva staining on the chin or around the mouth is usually indicative of dental disease, although moist dermatitis of deep skin folds under the chin occurs in some loose-skinned breeds. Epiphora causes tear staining and matted fur on the face beneath the medial canthus of the eye, which can lead to superficial pyoderma in that area. Occasionally this is associated with spurs on the upper premolars or molar teeth growing into the mucosa inside the cheek. Grooming the skin over the area becomes painful. The large ears of some lop eared rabbits can sometimes impinge on the eye and surrounding structures causing trauma and irritation.

The head should be palpated and carefully examined for the presence of abscesses on the side of the face, under the masseter muscles or along the bottom of the jaw. One side of the face can be compared with the other. Pain or bony swellings associated with elongated tooth roots can be detected by palpation of the ventral border of the mandible and the zygomatic area (see Section 7.7). The nares should be inspected for signs of a nasal discharge.

The incisors are easily examined by retracting the lips. The molars and premolars can be visualized with the aid of an auriscope or vaginal speculum. With practice, normal and abnormal cheek teeth can be differentiated by this technique, although it is not always possible to determine the cause of an abnormality. Rabbits that resent oral inspection often have problems with their cheek teeth. Excessive saliva, halitosis, presence of food, blood or pus are indicative of dental problems and general anaesthesia is necessary to examine the mouth thoroughly.

3.9.11 Examination of the eyes

Exophthalmos or glaucoma can be seen by comparing the size and shape of the eyes. Fear can cause the eyes to bulge out of the sockets due to engorgement of the orbital vascular sinus (see Figure 3.7) (Eglitis, 1964). Retrobulbar abscesses, tumours or cysts can cause a unilateral exophthalmos. The eyelids should be examined for evidence of wounds, ectropion, entropion, meibomian cysts or myxomatosis. The eyes should be clean and

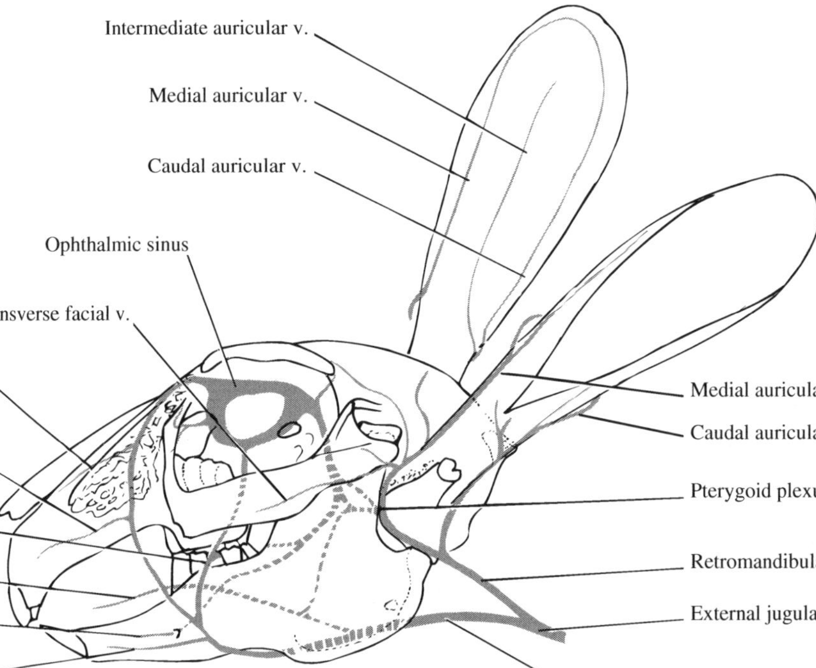

Figure 3.7. Veins of the head. The veins of the head include the marginal ear vein that is a convenient site for venepuncture. The large orbital venous sinus is also illustrated. This sinus may be encountered during enucleation of the eye and can be a source of serious haemorrhage.

free from purulent discharge. The rectus dorsalis muscle can be seen attached to the dorsal sclera when the upper eyelid is retracted. Applying pressure to the area just below the medial canthus of the eye may squeeze pus out of the opening of the nasolacrimal duct in cases with purulent dacrocystitis.

Key points 3.7

- The tragus is a blind-ending section of the external ear canal separated by a cartilaginous plate
- Wax and debris often obscure the ear drum especially in lop eared breeds
- Bilateral exophthalmos can be caused by fear
- Low Schirmer tear tests are of doubtful significance in rabbits
- Rabbits produce atropinesterase that can interfere with topical atropine drops used to induce mydriasis.

Nystagmus may be observed by watching the movement of the eye for a few seconds. Occasionally slow nystagmus can be seen in pet rabbits at rest in association with nodding of the head. Affected individuals are usually seropositive for *Encephalitozoon cuniculi.*

Direct illumination of the eye may reveal pathological conditions of the cornea and uveal tract. Evidence of previous lens rupture and cataract formation is associated with *Encephalitozoon cuniculi.* Local anaesthesia with topical proxymetacaine drops facilitates examination of the cornea and third eyelid. The application of fluorescein will reveal corneal ulceration. The Schirmer tear test has been evaluated in rabbits. The test paper is inserted into the lower conjunctival fold in the lateral third of the eyelid and is held in place for 1 minute. The amount of wetness is measured in millimetres. Topical anaesthesia is not used. Normal values range from 0 to 11.22 mm/min with a mean of 5.30 + 2.96

having been determined. Low values are of doubtful significance (Abrams *et al.*, 1990), although absence of tear production can be a sign of dysautonomia. A low Schirmer tear test result indicates keratoconjunctivitis sicca in other species but this condition has not been reported in rabbits. Impaired tear drainage due to nasolacrimal duct disease can result in high Schirmer tear test results, Excessive tear production can also be associated with corneal irritation due to conjunctivitis, corneal abrasions, ulcerations or foreign bodies. Orbital pain may be due to uveitis, glaucoma or retrobulbar disease.

Ophthalmoscopic examination of the fundus and internal structures of the eye requires mydriasis. Rabbits produce atropinesterase, which can interfere with topical atropine eye drops in some individuals. One drop each of 1% atropine and 10% phenylephrine, three to four times during a 15-minute period has been recommended for rabbits (Kern, 1995) or 0.5% or 1% tropicamide can be used. The optic disc lies above the horizontal midline of the eye and it is necessary to look upward into the eye with an ophthalmoscope to view the optic disc which has a deep natural depression (see Section 11.3). The retina is merangiotic (partially vascularized).

3.10 Hospitalization of rabbits

There are many advantages to hospitalizing rabbits. Conditions such as digestive or respiratory tract disorders require close observation and careful nursing. Medication in the form of intravenous fluids, daily injections or nebulization may be necessary. Regular syringe feeding, clipping and bathing may be required. Observation of behaviour, appetite, faecal and urine output is easier if the rabbit is kept on its own under the careful eye of competent nursing staff. A stress-free environment is required, away from barking dogs and the sight and smell of predators along with a good nursing team who understand the nutritional and physiological requirements of rabbits. Hospitalized rabbits should be provided with a bed of good quality hay to nibble and lie on. The familiar smell of hay gives them security. Some rabbits like a cardboard box to hide in. House rabbits can be very particular in their choice of litter material and may be reluctant to use a tray that does not contain the correct type of litter. Most owners are willing to bring in the correct type of material for their rabbit's litter tray. Fresh water needs to be provided in a drinking container that the rabbit is familiar with. Some rabbits will not use a sipper bottle. It is worth considering hospitalizing a bonded companion of a sick rabbit as they can become stressed if they are separated.

3.11 Euthanasia

Euthanasia is defined as 'an easy or painless death' (Blood and Studdert, 1999). The traditional approach of an intravenous overdose of barbiturate can be difficult to accomplish easily in rabbits. The marginal ear vein is accessible but many rabbits will jump up suddenly in response to venepuncture, which can be distressing for owner, vet and rabbit. Intraperitoneal barbiturate is acceptable but can take some time for the animal to lose consciousness. Sedation prior to intravenous barbiturate injection is preferable if the owner wishes to be present. The owner may wait with their rabbit until the sedative has taken effect. A combination of acepromazine and butorphanol (0.5 mg/kg acepromazine plus 0.1 mg/kg butorphanol) can be given by subcutaneous injection and has the advantage of vasodilation that facilitates venepuncture. Alternatively, fentanyl/fluanisone (0.3–0.5 ml/kg) (Hypnorm, Janssen) can be used but it is given by intramuscular injection, which is more distressing to patient and owner than a subcutaneous injection. Subcutaneous (50 mg/kg) ketamine with or without other agents can be used. Medetomidine, either on its own or in combination with other agents, is an effective sedative but causes peripheral vasoconstriction, which can make the lethal intravenous barbiturate injection difficult.

3.12 Clinical techniques

3.12.1 Chemical restraint

Chemical restraint is useful for the diagnosis and treatment of many conditions in pet rabbits. It is easier to collect a blood sample or take a well-positioned diagnostic radiograph if the patient is immobile and compliant. Soiled, matted fur or maggots can be removed from sedated rabbits and a period of sedation and analgesia allows time for inflamed skin to respond to treatment. Rabbits with gastrointestinal disease that results in gas-filled viscera such as the caecum or stomach can benefit from a period of analgesia. Intravenous fluid therapy is much easier in a sedated animal.

The properties of sedatives and tranquillizers are described in Section 5.4. Fentanyl/fluanisone (0.2–0.3 ml/kg) (Hypnorm) is a particularly useful for rabbits. Fentanyl/fluanisone is vasodilatory which, in conjunction with its sedative properties, makes venepuncture for the blood sampling or intravenous therapy simple. It is satisfactory method of chemical restraint for radiography, dematting or maggot removal. An alternative to fluanisone/fentanyl is a combination of acepromazine and butorphanol (0.5 mg/kg acepromazine plus 0.1 mg/kg butorphanol). This combination is also sedative and vasodilatory. However, it should be used with care in dehydrated animals or those with cardiovascular disturbances (Flecknell, 2000).

There are many other combinations that can be used as chemical restraint in rabbits, especially in the USA where fentanyl/fluanisone is unavailable (Mason, 1997). Anaesthesia and analgesia are discussed in Chapter 5.

3.12.2 Blood sampling

There are several superficial veins that can be used to collect blood from rabbits. Sites for venepuncture and intraosseous fluid therapy are illustrated in Figure 3.8. Although laboratory rabbits are sometimes bled by cardiocentesis, this procedure is not suitable for a pet rabbit. Rabbit blood clots extremely fast and has to be collected quickly but in a manner which does not cause haemolysis. Heparinizing the syringe and needle can be

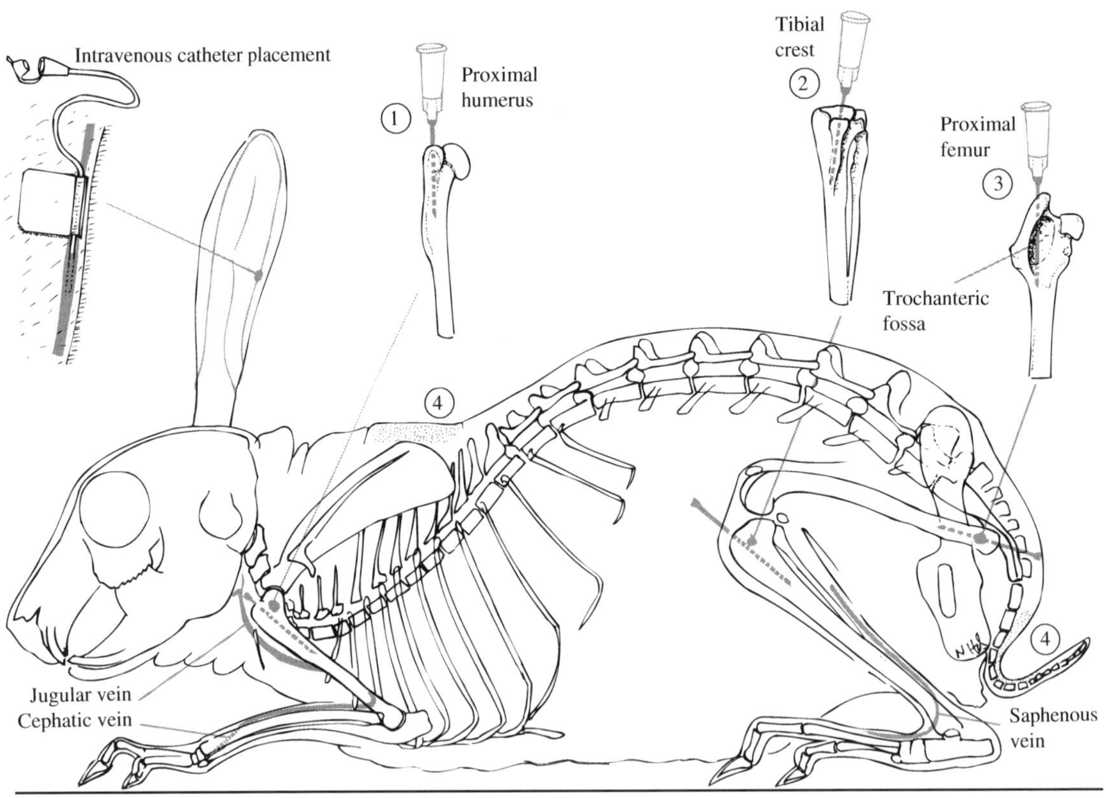

Figure 3.8.

advantageous. As a rough guide it is safe to take up to 1% of the animal's bodyweight of blood (Ramer *et al.*, 1999).

The marginal ear vein is easily visualized and accessible but is too small in some breeds for the blood to flow freely. Blood can be taken quickly from the central ear artery but this procedure carries a small risk of permanent damage to the blood supply to the pinna if the artery is damaged. Part of the pinna may subsequently slough off. Conscious rabbits can jump suddenly and dislodge a needle from an ear vein in response to venepuncture. This response can be avoided

Figure 3.8. Sites for venepuncture and intraosseous fluid therapy plus difficult to groom areas. The jugular, cephalic and saphenous veins are in similar positions to those of other domestic animals such as dogs and cats. All these sites can be used for blood sampling and intravenous injections in rabbits. The jugular vein is the greatest in diameter and is the best site for taking blood samples. The ear vein is also satisfactory in large breeds or for collecting small volumes. The needle and syringe may need to be heparinized as rabbit blood clots very quickly.

Suggested techniques: (Further information is given in Section 3.12, Clinical techniques). Jugular blood sampling: good restraint is required for taking blood from the jugular vein. The rabbit should be wrapped in a towel, placed on the edge of a table and held by an assistant. The head is raised and held back, either by the assistant or by the person collecting the blood. It is important to ensure that the head is held straight. The fur over the jugular furrow is clipped off. Usually, the vein is easily visualized and can be raised by placing a finger at the thoracic inlet. A good quality sample of 5–10 ml of blood can be collected quickly from this site without either haemolysis or clotting.

Intravenous fluid therapy. A simple method of venepuncture for intravenous fluid therapy is to use a 21 gauge or 23 gauge butterfly catheter (see Section 3.12.4.2). One wing is removed before inserting the needle, bevel up, into the marginal ear vein (caudal auricular vein). The remaining wing is 'superglued' to the fur on the ear after the needle has been inserted into the vein. The wing provides a large surface area of contact with the ear. In sedated or moribund rabbits, no bandaging is necessary to keep the needle in place, although a piece of bandage tied around the rabbit's neck can be used to hold the giving set out of the way. An intravenous catheter may be used instead of the butterfly set, but is not as satisfactory because the wing does not have as large a surface area for the bonding agent. Alternative sites for intravenous fluid therapy are the cephalic and saphenous veins.

Intraosseous fluid therapy. In all intraosseous sites, a spinal needle is preferable because the stylet prevents bone clogging the needle. A spinal needle is stronger and more able to penetrate the bone.

Possible sites for intraosseous administration:

1. **Proximal humerus:** this is the easiest site for access to the medullary cavity. An imaginary straight line is made using the greater trochanter of the humerus and the elbow joint as landmarks. The needle is inserted through the greater trochanter and directed along the imaginary line to penetrate into the medullary cavity.
2. **Tibial crest:** an intraosseous catheter can be inserted just caudoproximal to the tibial crest. However, the lateral wall of the tibial cortex curves medially and the needle must be directed towards the medial aspect of the tibia in order to penetrate the medullary cavity. If the needle is mistakenly inserted along an imaginary straight line towards the hock joint, it will go into the cortex of the tibia and miss the medullary cavity.
3. **Proximal femur:** this is the least satisfactory site for intraosseous fluid therapy because of the well-developed trochanteric fossa. This can be seen on the caudal view of the femur. The path of an intraosseous catheter has to pass through this fossa to gain access to the medullary cavity. Therefore, to gain access to the medullary cavity three layers of cortical bone must be penetrated.
4. **Difficult to groom areas.** The areas of skin that are difficult for a rabbit to reach and groom are shown as green shading. Obesity or other flexibility problems hinder grooming in these areas and allow dead hair, skin debris and parasites to accumulate. Signs of skin disease often begin at these sites. The area between the tail and the dorsum can become contaminated by urine, faeces and is often the site that flies choose to lay their eggs. These are the areas that owners should pay particular attention to when grooming their pet.

by the application of a local anaesthetic cream (EMLA, Astra). EMLA is a mixture of lignocaine and prilocaine that produces anaesthesia of full skin thickness. The cream is applied over the marginal ear vein before covering the site with a dressing or clingfilm. After 45–60 minutes a blood sample can be taken (Flecknell, 2000).

The jugular vein is a satisfactory site for the collection of good quality samples in most rabbits. The dewlap of female rabbits does not pose a problem. It may be difficult to visualize the vessels in obese animals. The rabbit should be wrapped in a towel and held securely by an assistant. The head is extended backwards and the hair over the throat clipped off. The jugular vein can usually be visualized in the jugular furrow and is raised by occluding the vessel by a finger at the thoracic inlet. Up to 10 ml of blood can be safely collected from any sized rabbit from this site. Difficulties can arise with short nosed breeds such as the Netherland Dwarf or animals with upper respiratory tract problems that can become distressed or even cyanosed when the head is extended backwards. Alternative sites such as the cephalic or lateral saphenous veins can be used instead. It is a good idea to make a blood film in addition to placing the blood in sample bottles. The film can be quickly stained and examined for a differential white cell count which, in addition to a PCV, will give an immediate assessment of the rabbit's health status in the absence of sophisticated laboratory equipment. As rabbit blood clots so quickly, heparinized syringes may be required. Analysers such as the I-Stat (Heska) requires heparinized blood but is a useful piece of equipment in the assessment of critically ill rabbits as it can measure parameters such as electrolytes, glucose and urea, using only a few drops of blood.

3.12.3 Urine collection

Urinanalysis is covered in Section 6.5. Urine samples can be collected from house rabbits and from many hutch rabbits by providing a clean but empty litter box placed in the site where the rabbit usually urinates. Cystocentesis is an alternative method of urine collection if the bladder can be easily palpated and differentiated from other structures such as a gravid or neoplastic uterus or an abdominal abscess. Ultrasound can be used to identify the bladder. Repetitive puncture of the bladder can cause inflammation and subsequent stone formation. Rabbits are more prone than other species to developing calculi along a cystotomy suture line (Kaminski *et al.*, 1978).

Urine can sometimes be collected by manual expression of the bladder, although this procedure is not without risk. The bladder is thin walled and can rupture during manual expression, especially if there is a urethral obstruction. Chronic cystitis causes thickening of the bladder wall making it less susceptible to rupture. Rabbits with cystitis or urolithiasis often urinate in response to palpation of the bladder and void urine that can be collected, if a suitable container is easily available.

Key points 3.8

- Hospitalization facilitates administration of medication and food and permits observation of demeanour, appetite, thirst, urinary and faecal output
- A stress-free environment is required for hospitalized rabbits
- A bedding of hay provides a familiar smell, a sense of security and a source of indigestible fibre
- Some house rabbits will only use a litter tray containing a familiar substrate
- Peaceful euthanasia can be accomplished by the administration of 0.5 mg/kg acepromazine + 1.0 mg/kg butorphanol given subcutaneously 10–15 minutes prior to intravenous barbiturate injection
- Rabbit blood clots quickly. The marginal ear vein can be used for blood collection in large rabbits. The jugular and cephalic veins may also be used
- Although cystocentesis can be used to collect urine samples, repetitive puncture can cause calculus formation.

3.12.4 Administration of medication

3.12.4.1 Subcutaneous injections

The subcutaneous route is suitable for the administration of most parenteral medications with the exception of some anaesthetic agents. Subcutaneous injections are well tolerated and even owners can inject their rabbit without problems. Occasionally subcutaneous injections of antibiotics or vaccines can result in a skin reaction that may not be noticed until a few days later. These reactions can be minimized by making sure that the needle has penetrated the skin and the medication is injected subdermally rather than intradermally. Massaging the area after giving the injection is also useful. The loose skin over the scruff is the usual subcutaneous injection site. Subcutaneous fluids (10–20 ml/kg) can be administered either into the scruff or the loose skin over the chest.

3.12.4.2 Intramuscular injections

There are a few products that need to be given intramuscularly to rabbits. Large volumes (> 0.5 ml/kg) should be divided and given in two sites. The cranial muscle mass (quadriceps) of the hind leg is the preferred site. The caudal muscle mass can be used, but the sciatic nerve must be avoided by palpating and identifying the semimembranous, semitendinosus and biceps femoris muscles and ensuring that the injection is given into the muscle. Self-mutilation of the foot has been reported in rabbits as a result of nerve damage during intramuscular injection of ketamine and xylazine into the caudal muscle mass (Beyers *et al.*, 1991). Tissue damage and muscle necrosis were found at the injection site.

3.12.4.3 Intravenous injections

The usual site for intravenous injection is the marginal ear vein that is accessible and easily visualized in rabbits (see Figure 3.8). Rabbits can be restrained by wrapping them in a towel. Topical local anaesthesia with EMLA cream (see Blood sampling) or chemical restraint can be used to prevent head shaking and the needle being dislodged. Small gauge needles, adequate light and good eyesight are required especially in dwarf breeds. An alternative site is the cephalic vein similar to the dog or cat. The rabbit's short legs sometimes make raising the vein difficult. Other veins such as the jugular or femoral veins can be used (Malley, 1996) and the choice is largely a matter of individual preference.

The choice of sites is limited for intravenous catheterization and fluid therapy (see Figure 3.8). The femoral or jugular veins are impractical. Usually the marginal ear vein or cephalic vein is used due to the ease of keeping the rabbit in the correct position for intravenous fluids to run once the drip is set up. Intravenous catheters can be held in place with adhesive tape or a few drops of Vetbond or superglue. A simple method is to cut one wing off a 21 g or 23 g butterfly set before placing it in the marginal ear vein. The remaining wing can be superglued to the fur on the pinna to keep the needle in place. No bandaging is required to keep the needle in place in sedated or moribund patients, although a piece of bandage tied around the rabbits neck can be used to hold the giving set out of the way. Most rabbits tolerate the procedure well. Superglue is not as satisfactory for keeping intravenous catheters in place because they have a smaller wing that does not provide a large surface area for the bonding agent.

3.12.4.4 Intraosseous route

This route introduces fluids and drugs into the marrow cavity so they are absorbed into the venous circulation. There are several advantages to this technique which avoids the necessity of cannulating a small collapsed vein in moribund patients. The intraosseous route is often used for small exotic animal patients such as birds, reptiles, guinea pigs and pot-bellied pigs where it is difficult to find a peripheral vein. Most rabbits are large enough and have sufficient accessible veins to use the intravenous route but there are occasions when intraosseous administration of drugs and especially fluids can be life saving. Some practitioners prefer this method of fluid administration and use it routinely. Disadvantages include the risk of introducing infection and causing osteomyelitis. The rate of administration can be slow. These problems can be overcome by using careful aseptic techniques and multiple sites. Immature bones with active growth plates, diseased or fractured bones are not suitable.

A needle is used to bore a hole through a bony prominence into the marrow cavity. Direct penetration of the marrow cavity is easier in the tibia or humerus of the rabbit than the femur. The anatomy of the head of the femur requires penetration of the trochanteric fossa so the cortical bone is penetrated three times instead of once (see Figure 3.8). The humerus is the preferred site. In conscious animals, local anaesthetic is infiltrated around the injection site, which is clipped and sterilized prior to the introduction of the needle. A 20–22 gauge needle that is about half the length of the bone is required, i.e. 4–6 cm (1.5–2.5 inches). Spinal needles with a stylet that prevents a plug of bone clogging up the bore are most suitable but ordinary hypodermic needles can be used with a smaller gauge needle or a length of wire acting as the stylet. The bone is penetrated by using the needle as a drill. The needle should be kept straight when boring the hole in the bone. Moving the needle from side to side results in a larger hole than is required and leakage of fluid around the injection site. Penetration of the cortex can be felt as a sudden lack of resistance. The needle may need to be redirected slightly to push it down the medullary cavity. It is important to be certain that the tip of the needle is in the medullary cavity and not pushed against or penetrating the cortex. At this point the stylet is removed and a syringe attached to the needle to aspirate bone marrow which confirms correct placement of the needle. If there is any doubt, radiography is indicated. If the needle is not placed correctly, it should be withdrawn and a different bone selected to attempt the procedure again. Once the needle is placed it can be glued or sutured in place. Dressings and antiseptics can be used for protection and to reduce the likelihood of infection. Heparin should be introduced into the catheter every 4–6 h. The needle should not be left in place for longer than 72 h. When it is removed a light dressing and some antiseptic can be applied to the site (Anderson, 1995).

3.12.4.5 Intraperitoneal route

This route is seldom required for the treatment of pet animals and is more often used in laboratory rabbits. Ideally the bladder should be empty and care is needed to avoid the thin walled caecum that lies in the right ventral abdomen (see Figure 3.3). The injection should be given caudal to the umbilicus so there is little chance of penetrating the liver, kidneys or spleen. The inguinal quadrant is the site described by Malley (2000). It is important to draw back on the syringe to check for intestinal contents, blood or urine in which case the syringe should be withdrawn and another attempt made.

3.12.4.6 Oral administration

There are therapeutic agents that need to be given by the oral route. Medicating the drinking water is unsatisfactory as many preparations flavour the water and make it unpalatable. Adding sucrose to the water has been advocated as a means of overcoming this problem. It is also difficult to ensure the correct dosage when medication is given in the drinking water and there is experimental evidence to show that antibiotics administered by this route are ineffective (Okerman *et al.*, 1990).

Rabbits can be given tablets, which can be placed in the mouth or administered with a pill giver. Placing tablets in food such as breakfast cereals can be successful and the occasional rabbit will eat tablets voluntarily. Crushing tablets and mixing the powder with honey or baby cereal can also be successful. Powders such as vitamin and mineral supplements can be given with food. Most rabbits will readily accept a piece of bread that has been sprinkled with powder. Liquids can also be given in this way.

Many rabbits are easy to dose with oral liquids. In fact many of them enjoy sweet compounds and will readily accept paediatric syrups or medication mixed with honey or fruit juice such as Ribena. Otherwise the rabbit can be wrapped in a towel and the liquid slowly squirted into the mouth using a syringe inserted in the diastema. Owners can be shown how to do this and most manage well.

3.13 Nutritional support

Nutritional support can be life saving in rabbits. Their metabolism is geared to a constant supply of nutrients from the digestive tract. Anorexia can have dire consequences, especially in fat rabbits as ketoacidosis and hepatic lipidosis can develop rapidly as a result of mobilizing fat reserves. Oral liquids soften and lubricate impacted stomach contents. In the short term, nutritional support is required to provide calories, nutrients, fluids and electrolytes. A readily available source of carbohydrate is required to provide glucose for absorption from the stomach and small intestine and prevent hypoglycaemia and the mobilization of the free fatty acids. In the long term, indigestible fibre and fermentable fibre are required to maintain gut motility and optimal conditions in the caecum for bacterial fermentation. Although fermentable fibre can be administered through a syringe, it is not possible to provide indigestible fibre in this way because it has to be ground down to a fine powder in order to pass through the nozzle. The beneficial effect of long indigestible fibre particles is lost by being ground down to a size smaller than 0.5 mm because particles below this size are moved back into the caecum to undergo bacterial fermentation rather than passing into the colon and stimulating gut motility. Therefore, it is important to encourage sick rabbits to eat as soon as possible. They need a source of palatable indigestible fibre, even if they do not appear to be eating. Hay, grass or dandelions are often the first item to be eaten voluntarily and are often eaten in preference to other foods.

In most instances, nutritional support can be given by syringe feeding three or four times a day. Liquid food (10–20 ml/kg) can be introduced into the mouth through a syringe with or without a small section of tubing attached. Baby foods can be used for this purpose. Cereal based products, pureed fruit or vegetables are palatable and will go through a syringe easily. They are useful in the short term as an immediate source of energy and digestible fibre. Alternatively, extruded rabbit food (SupaRabbit Excel, Burgess) can be moistened and mashed to a paste for syringe feeding, although the fibrous particles tend to block the syringe. The food needs to be ground to a powder to prevent this happening, which detracts from its motility stimulatory properties. Many anorexic rabbits, especially those suffering from dental problems, will eat softened nuggets of extruded food from a dish. Eaten in this way, the food is a source of indigestible fibre.

3.13.1 Nasogastric tubes

Very occasionally a situation can arise where syringe feeding is impossible and it becomes necessary to place a nasogastric tube to provide nutrition. This technique should be used as a last resort because nasogastric tubes stress rabbits and stress reduces gastrointestinal motility and impairs digestive function. An Elizabethan collar is required to prevent a rabbit removing a nasogastric tube and this is not only stress provoking but also prevents caecotrophy. In most cases, syringe feeding is satisfactory and nasogastric tubes can be avoided.

It is easier to place a nasogastric tube in a moribund or anaesthetized rabbit as the nasal mucosa is sensitive and the introduction of a tube can cause sneezing and distress. In the conscious animal, local anaesthetic can be sprayed (Intubeze, Arnolds) or dropped (Opthaine, Ciba) into the nostril. Sufficient time (2–3 minutes) should be allowed to elapse for the anaesthetic to take effect before the tube is introduced. Paediatric tubes (4–8 french) are suitable for this purpose or customized veterinary products are available in varying sizes (Cook Veterinary Products). The tube is measured against the rabbit and marked to give an idea of the position of the tip as the tube is being placed: 3f–4f urinary catheters can be used if a nasogastric tube is not available but holes need to be cut in the side and these can catch on the nasal mucosa as the tube is introduced. To place a nasogastric tube, the rabbit's head is grasped and elevated and the tube introduced into the ventral meatus and directed slightly ventrally (see Figure 3.9) The head is then flexed as the tube passes through the nasopharynx into the oesophagus and down into the stomach. Occasionally resistance is encountered in the nasal passage due to an elongated tooth root. In this instance, the other nostril can be tried.

It is possible to pass a nasogastric tube through the larynx and into the trachea and it is important to ensure that the tube is not placed in the trachea before introducing food. Keeping the head flexed minimizes the risk of tracheal intubation. If the tube has been measured up against the patient prior to placement, the length of the tube that has been passed will indicate whether the end is in the trachea or in the oesophagus. Palpation of the

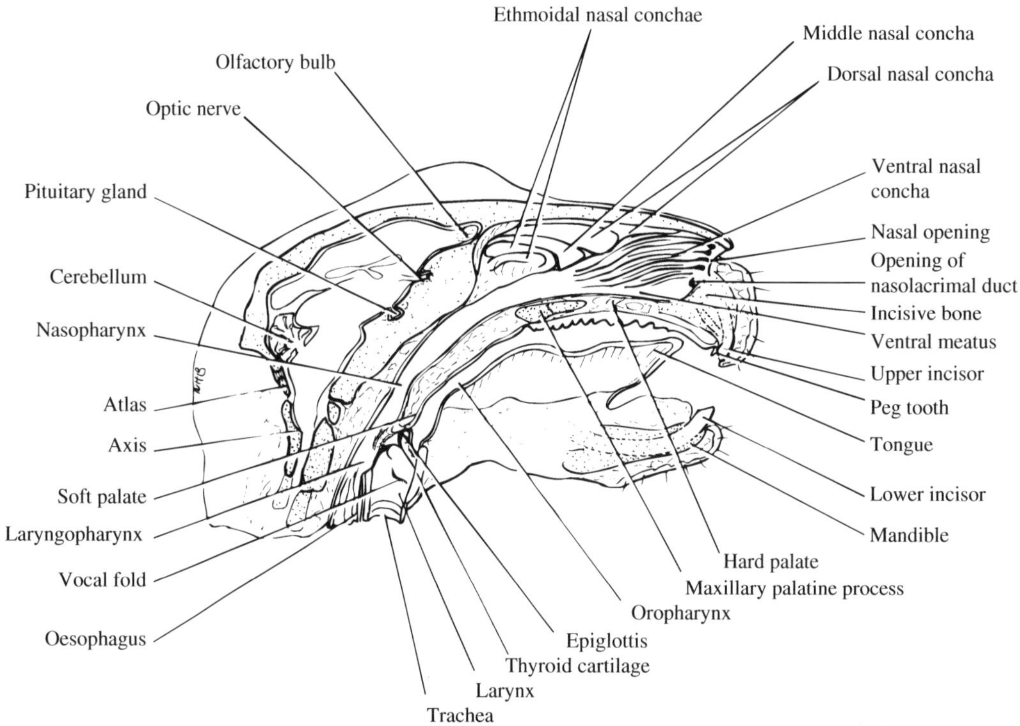

Figure 3.9. Sagittal section through head. This diagram was drawn from a prepared sagittal section of a rabbit's head using Barone *et al.* (1973) as a reference source. The structures of the nasal cavity and the position of the ventral meatus can be seen. The larynx is difficult to visualize through the oral cavity because of the large base of the tongue that occupies most of the nasopharynx and obscures the view.

oesophagus, listening for breath sounds in the tube or instilling a few drops of water or saline can be helpful to confirm the correct placement of the tube in the stomach. If in doubt, a radiograph can be taken to check the tube's position. The nasal end is secured to the skin of the nose and between the ears using tape butterflies and sutures or superglue. Alternatively it can be secured to the Elizabethan collar, which is required to prevent the rabbit removing or damaging the tube. Nasogastric tubes can be left in place for several days. The rabbit is able to eat with the tube in place.

Complications associated with nasogastric tubes include inadvertent introduction of the tube into the trachea and iatrogenic damage to the mucosa. The nasal mucosa is the primary site for *Pasteurella multocida* bacteria to reside and trauma to the tissues can stir up infection. Epistaxis can also result from the passage of a nasogastric tube.

3.13.2 Stomach tubes

There are occasions when it is necessary to pass a stomach tube. The most common indication is to decompress the stomach of rabbits with intestinal obstruction. These patients are usually either moribund or sedated. Some clinicians use stomach tubes for nutritional support or to administer medication. The technique carries a risk of inadvertently traumatizing the larynx or passing the tube into the trachea causing breathing difficulties or aspiration pneumonia. It is also possible for the rabbit to chew through the tube and inhale or swallow a section. A gag can be used to prevent the rabbit from chewing the tubing. A piece of wood with a hole drilled through it can be placed in the diastema.

Despite the difficulty of endotracheal intubation in anaesthetized rabbits it is

COMMON DIFFERENTIAL DIAGNOSES

1) MANAGEMENT FACTORS
- Poor quality food
- Change of diet
- Loss of companion
- Elizabethan collars

2) DENTAL DISEASE:
- Common.
- Usually anorexia is due to spurs on cheek teeth impinging on tongue (see Section 7.6.9)
- Often associated with weight loss, salivation and lack of grooming
- Can be sudden onset
- Requires general anaesthesia and treatment (see Section 7.10.2)

3) GASTROINTESTINAL HYPOMOTILITY
- Usually sequel to pain, stress or fright
- May pick at food. Progresses to total anorexia
- No hard faeces are passed
- Impacted stomach may be palpable
- End point is death from hepatic lipidosis
- Can be treated successfully in early stages (see Section 10.3.4)

4) GASTRIC DILATATION
- Sudden onset, severe depression
- Often associated with intestinal obstruction and treatment is surgical (see Section 10.5)
- Site of obstruction may be identified from gas shadows on abdominal radiographs.

5) CAECAL IMPACTION
- Slow onset
- May be part of to mucoid enteropathy syndrome (see Section 10.9)

6) METABOLIC DISEASE
- Renal failure, may be associated with urolithiasis (see Section 14.5)
- Liver disease

7) NEOPLASIA
- Uterine adenocarcinoma and lymphoma are most common

8) SYSTEMIC DISEASE
- Myxomatosis, enterotoxaemia, VHD, pasteurellosis, coccidiosis are accompanied by other clinical signs
- Toxicity, e.g. lead, plant poisons

EFFECTS OF ANOREXIA
- Reduced intake of indigestible fibre and reduced intestinal motility
- Slow gastric emptying resulting in impaction of stomach contents and trichobezoar formation.
- Reduced supply of nutrients to caecal microflora resulting in changes in caecal pH and balance of microorganisms
- Gas production in bowel, especially the caecum, causing visceral distension and pain.
- Reduced glucose absorption from the gut leading to increased mobilisation of free fatty acids from adipose tissue that can lead to fatal hepatic lipidosis. Obese rabbits are at greater risk as fatty infiltration of the liver is already present.
- Disturbances in electrolyte and water balance
- Gastric ulceration

DIAGNOSTIC APPROACH

STEP 1: HISTORY and CLINICAL EXAMINATION:
- General condition and demeanour
- Duration of anorexia
- Passage of hard faeces. Absent or small hard faeces is a significant finding
- Dental examination (see Section 7.6)
- Abdominal palpation: Look for gastric distension, masses, impacted stomach or caecum
- Look for other signs e.g diarrhoea, dyspnoea, drooling, myxomatous lesions

STEP 2 : HOSPITALIZATION
- Permits observation of appetite and faecal output (see Sections 3.8.4, 3.8.5)
- Nursing is often required (see Section 3.10)
- Intensive medication, injectable analgesics, intravenous fluid therapy and syringe feeding are often needed (see Section 4.11)

STEP 3: DIAGNOSTIC WORKUP
- Low dose Hypnorm [0.2 ml/kg] is useful for radiography and venepuncture).
- Take blood samples: especially for PCV (should be <40%) glucose, urea, electrolytes.Lipaemia or extreme hyperglycaemia carry poor prognosis (see Chapter 6)
- Radiographs show impactions, gas or fluid distensions, uroliths, tumours etc. Painful skeletal conditions may be seen

STEP 4: SURGERY
- Anaesthesia is necessary to trim elongated spurs
- Abdominal surgery is indicated for obstructions, neoplasia, etc. but not indicated for gastric stasis or 'trichobezoars' that can be treated medically
- Surgery needs to be performed promptly

Figure 3.10. Approach to the anorexic rabbit. The anorexic rabbit requires prompt diagnosis and appropriate treatment. Chance medication with antibiotic, vitamin or corticosteroid injections is unlikely to be effective and wastes valuable time.

surprisingly easy to pass a stomach tube into the trachea. Selection of a large tube should prevent this happening. The tube can be measured against the animal and an estimate of the length required to reach the stomach. It is then lubricated with a KY jelly before it is passed over the tongue into the oesophagus. After placing the tube, the animal's respiration should be watched for a moment or two and the colour of the mucous membranes checked. A small amount of water can be introduced before giving any medication or food. If in doubt, a radiograph can be taken to check the placement of the tube. In rabbits with gastric dilation, gas and liquid readily pass up and out of the tube as the stomach decompresses.

3.13.3 Pharyngotomy and gastrotomy tubes

There are clinical situations where syringe feeding is impossible and a nasogastric tube inadvisable. For example, rabbits with skull injuries or a purulent nasal discharge. A technique for placing a pharyngotomy tube has been described for laboratory rabbits. (Rogers *et al.*, 1988). Under general anaesthesia a 1 cm incision is made 5 mm from the midline just anterior to the larynx on the left-hand side. A tube is passed through the oral cavity into the oesophagus and down to the stomach. The tube is grasped with artery forceps through the mouth and pushed against the wall of the pharynx to cause a bulge under the skin incision. The muscle overlying the bulge is carefully incised using the hard tip of the artery forceps in the pharynx as a guide. The pharyngeal wall is incised and the oral end of the stomach tube exteriorized through the incision. The tube is then anchored at the pharyngeal incision before being run through the subcutaneous tissues to emerge at the base of the ear where it is anchored with skin sutures. Pharyngotomy tubes placed in this manner have been left in laboratory rabbits for 6–12 months to ensure accurate doses of the drugs that were being tested. The catheters were well tolerated and the rabbits continued to eat and drink without losing weight. This technique could be applied to pet rabbits. Soft feeding tubes designed for oesophagostomy in cats (Cook Veterinary Products) would be suitable for this purpose.

Percutaneous endoscopical gastrotomy (PEG) tubes have been used to administer enteral nutritional support to rabbits (Smith *et al.*, 1997). This technique does not appear to be as useful in rabbits as it is in dogs and cats. It is difficult to pass an endoscope through the rabbit's mouth and pharynx. In order to have a good endoscopic view, the stomach should be empty which is difficult to achieve in rabbits even if they are prevented from eating caecotrophs. Elizabethan collars or bandages are required to prevent the patient from removing the tube once it is placed and these are not well tolerated.

3.14 Elizabethan collars

Elizabethan collars are used in other species to prevent interference with surgical incisions, wounds, catheters or dressings. There are circumstances when collars need to be fitted to rabbits but there are serious disadvantages. Rabbits fitted with Elizabethan collars can become depressed or even anorexic. The collars are stressful and are most likely to be fitted at a time when it is important to minimize stress levels such as after surgery or during periods of anorexia. Significant elevations in plasma glucose levels have been found in rabbits fitted with collars (Knudtzon, 1988). Elizabethan collars also prevent a rabbit from consuming caecotrophs. Caecotrophs are rich in amino acids and vitamins and necessary for optimum nutrition and wound healing. Good surgical technique, buried subcuticular sutures and the correct choice of suture material reduces the need for Elizabethan collars postoperatively. Alternatively, surgical staples can be used (Dobbins, 2000).

3.15 Nebulization

Nebulization has been described as an adjunct to treatment of upper and lower respiratory tract disease in rabbits (Callaghan and Raftery, 1998). A variety of medications, such as antibiotics, can be mixed with warm saline (38°C) and administered twice a day, via a nebulizer, into the air space of a small

Key points 3.9
- Subcutaneous injections are well tolerated by rabbits
- Intravenous fluids can be given into the marginal ear vein. A butterfly cannula can be superglued to the pinna for easy administration
- The proximal end of the humerus is the preferred site for intraosseous fluid therapy. The trochanteric fossa at the head of the femur precludes direct penetration of the marrow cavity of the proximal femur
- Nutritional support is life saving in rabbits and is preferably given by syringe feeding
- Formulations for nutritional support should include carbohydrate as a source of glucose that can be absorbed from the small intestine to prevent hypoglycaemia and mobilization of free fatty acids
- Powdered formulations given through a syringe cannot provide indigestible fibre to stimulate gastrointestinal motility. It is long particles of indigestible fibre, not small particles of fermentable fibre that stimulate gut motility
- Powdered formulations can be a source of fermentable (digestible) fibre as a substrate for caecal microflora
- A tempting palatable source of indigestible fibre should be available for all sick rabbits. Grass is ideal
- Elizabethan collars can be stressful and prevent caecotrophy. Nasogastric tubes require the placement of Elizabethan collars and are not necessary for the treatment of most anorexic rabbits.

cage containing the rabbit. It is important to use isotonic saline as the vehicle. Experimental nebulization of rabbits with hypertonic saline (3.6%) caused extravasation of water into the subepithelial tissue of the airway wall. The formation of oedema was associated with a decrease in compliance and gas exchange (Hogman *et al.*, 1997).

3.16 Cerebrospinal fluid (CSF) collection and myelography

The increase in status and popularity of rabbits as companion animals has resulted in greater owner expectations of veterinary treatment and there are times when myelography and spinal surgery are required. Cerebrospinal fluid analysis can also be helpful in the differential diagnosis of neurological disease. Cisternal puncture in the rabbit is widely used in laboratory rabbits and the procedure is similar to that for dogs and cats.

References

Abrams, K.L., Brooks, D.E., Funk, R.S., Theran, P. (1990). Evaluation of the Schirmer tear test in clinically normal rabbits. *Am J Vet Res.*, **51**, 1912–1913.

Anderson, N.L. (1995). Intraosseous fluid therapy in small exotic animals. In *Kirk's Veterinary Therapy XII*. pp 1331–1334. W.B Saunders.

Behara, N., Silveira, M., Man, W. *et al.* (1980). Catecholamines and experimental stress ulcer: morphological and biochemical changes in the gastric mucosa (Abstract). *Br J Surg.*, **67**, 624–628.

Benson, K.G., Paul-Murphy, J. (1999). Clinical pathology of the domestic rabbit. *Vet Clin N Am: Exotic Anim Pract.*, **2**, 539–552.

Beyers, T.M., Richardson, J.A., Prince, M.D. (1991). Axonal degeneration and self-mutilation as a complication of the intramuscular use of ketamine and xylazine in rabbits. *Lab Anim Sci.*, **41**, 519–520.

Bivin, W.S. (1994). Basic biomethodology. In *The Biology of the Laboratory Rabbit*, 2nd edn. (P.J. Manning, D.H. Ringler, C.E. Newcomer, eds). pp 72–86. Academic Press.

Blood, D.C., Studdert, V.P. (1999). *Saunders Comprehensive Veterinary Dictionary*. 2nd edn. W.B. Saunders.

Brewer, N.R., Cruise, L.J. (1994). Physiology. In *The Biology of the Laboratory Rabbit*, 2nd edn. (P.J. Manning, D.H. Ringler, C.E. Newcomer, eds). pp 63–70. Academic Press.

Broderson, J.R., Gluckstein, F.P. (1994). Zoonotic and occupational health considerations. In *The Biology of the Laboratory Rabbit*, 2nd edn. (P.J. Manning, D.H. Ringler, C.E. Newcomer, eds). pp 356–366. Academic Press.

Brooks, D. (1997). Nutrition and gastrointestinal physiology. In *Ferrets, Rabbits and Rodents, Clinical Medicine and Surgery*. (E.V. Hillyer, K. Quesenberry, eds). pp 169–175. W.B. Saunders.

Burgmann, P.M. (1991). Restraint techniques and anaesthetic recommendations for rabbits, rodents and ferrets. *J Small Exotic Anim Med.*, **1**, 73–78.

Callaghan, M., Raftery, A. (1998). Rabbit nursing techniques. *Vet Pract Nurse*, **10**, 15–17.

Carroll, J.F., Dwyer, T.M., Grady, A.W. *et al.* (1996). Hypertension, cardiac hypertrophy and neurohumoral activity in a new animal model of obesity (Abstract). *Am J Physiol.*, **271**, H373–H378.

Cheeke, P.R. (1987). *Rabbit Feeding and Nutrition*. Academic Press.

Cheeke, P.R., Patton, N.M., Templeton, G.S. (1982). *Rabbit Production*. Interstate Publishers.

Cleri, D.J., Vernaleo, J.R., Lombardi, L.J. *et al.* (1997). Plague pneumonia disease caused by Yersinia pestis (Abstract). *Semin Respir Infect.*, **12**, 12–23.

Cloyd, G.G., Johnson, G.R. (1978). Lymphosarcoma with lymphoblastic leukemia in a New Zealand white rabbit (Abstract). *Lab Anim Sci.*, **28**, 66–69.

Danneman, P.J., White, W.J., Marshall, W.K., Lang, C.M. (1988). An evaluation of analgesia associated with the immobility response in laboratory rabbits. *Lab Anim Sci.*, **38**, 51–57.

Der Weduwen, S., McBride A. (1999). Behaviour and the effects of early handling. In Refining rabbit housing, husbandry and procedures: report of the 1998 UFAW/RSPCA Rabbit Behaviour and Welfare Group meeting. *Anim Technol.*, **50**, 164.

Dobbins, T.M. (2000). The use of staples for skin closure following elective ovariohysterectomies in pet rabbits. *Clinical Research Abstract*. BSAVA Congress, Birmingham.

Donnelly, T.M. (1997). Basic anatomy, physiology, and husbandry. In *Ferrets, Rabbits and Rodents, Clinical Medicine and Surgery* (E.V. Hillyer, K.E. Quesenberry, eds). pp 147–159. W.B. Saunders.

Eglitis, I. (1964). The glands. In *The Rabbit in Eye Research* (J.H. Prince, ed.) pp 38–56. Charles C. Thomas.

Flecknell, P.A. (2000). Anaesthesia. In *Manual of Rabbit Medicine and Surgery* (P.A. Flecknell, ed.) pp 103–116. British Small Animal Veterinary Association. Gloucester.

Gill, V., Cunha, B.A. (1997). Tularemia pneumonia (Abstract). *Semin Respir Infec.*, **12**, 61–67.

Gillett, C.S. (1994). Selected drug dosages and clinical reference data. In *The Biology of the Laboratory Rabbit*, 2nd edn. (P.J. Manning, D.H Ringler, C.E. Newcomer, eds). pp 468–471. Academic Press.

Goodly, L. (2001). Rabbit hemorrhagic disease. *Compendium on Continuing Education*, **23**, 249–253.

Gorski, J., Mizak, B., Chrobocinska, M. (1994). Control of viral haemorrhagic disease of rabbits in Poland. *Rev Sci Tech.*, **3**, 881–891.

Gueirard, P., Weber, C., le Cousumier, A., Guiso, N. (1995). Human Bordetella bronchiseptica related to contact with infected animals: persistence of bacteria in host (Abstract). *J Clin Microbiol.*, **33**, 2002–2006.

Harcourt-Brown, F.M., Baker, S.J. (2001). Parathyroid hormone, haematological and biochemical parameters in relation to dental disease and husbandry in pet rabbits. *J Small Animal Pract.*, **42**, 130–136.

Henderson, B.A., Bowen, H.M. (1979). A short note: estimating the age of the European rabbit, *Oryctolagus cuniculi*, by counting the adhesion lines in the periosteal zone of the lower mandible. *J Appl Ecol.*, **16**, 393–396.

Hinton, M. (1980). Gastric ulceration in the rabbit. *J Comp Pathol.*, **90**, 475–481.

Hogman, M., Almirall, J., Mork, A.C. *et al.* (1997). Nebulisation of hypertonic saline causes oedema of the airway wall (Abstract). *J Submicros. Cytol Pathol.*, **29**, 59–64.

Jackson, G. (1991). Intestinal stasis and rupture in rabbits. *Vet Rec.*, **129**, 287–289.

Johnson-Delaney, C.A. (1996). Zoonotic parasites of selected exotic animals. *Sem Avian Exotic Pet Med.*, **5**, 115–124.

Kaminski, J.M., Katz, A.R., Woodward, S.C. (1978). Urinary bladder calculus formation on sutures in rabbits, cats and dogs (Abstract). *Surg Gynecol Obstet.*, **146**, 353–357.

Kaplan, B.L., Smith, H.W. (1935). Excretion of inulin, creatinine, xylose and urea in the normal rabbit. *Am J Physiol.*, **113**, 354–360.

Kern, T.J. (1995). Ocular disorders of laboratory animals and pocket pets. *Proc Atlantic Coast Vet Conference.*

Knudtzon, J. (1988). Plasma levels of glucagon, insulin, glucose and free fatty acids in rabbits during laboratory handling procedures. *Z. Versuchstierk*, **26**, 123–133.

Kraus, A., Weisbroth, S.H., Flatt, R.E., Brewer, N. (1984). Biology and diseases of rabbits. In *Laboratory Animal Medicine*. pp 207–237. Academic Press.

Kunstyr, I. and Naumann, S. (1983). Head tilt in rabbits caused by Pasteurella and Encephalitozoonosis. *Lab Anim.*, **19**, 208–213.

Lang, J. (1981). The nutrition of the commercial rabbit. Part 2. *Nutr abstr rev - Series B*, **51**, 287–297.

Lowe, J.A. (1998). Pet rabbit feeding and nutrition. In *The Nutrition of the Rabbit.* (C. de Blas, J. Wiseman, eds). pp 309–332. CABI Publishing.

Mader, D.R. (1997). Basic approach to veterinary care. In *Ferrets, Rabbits and Rodents, Clinical Medicine and Surgery.* (E.V. Hillyer, K.E. Quesenberry, eds). pp 160–168. W.B. Saunders.

Malley, A.D. (1996). The pet rabbit in companion animal practice: 5. The administration of medication. *Irish Vet J.*, **49**, 407–410.

Malley, A.D. (2000). Handling, restraint and clinical techniques. In *Manual of Rabbit Medicine and Surgery.* (P.A. Flecknell, ed.) British Small Animal Veterinary Association.

Mason, D.E. (1997). Anesthesia, analgesia, and sedation for small mammals. In *Ferrets, Rabbits and Rodents. Clinical Medicine and Surgery* (E.V. Hillyer, K.A. Quesenbery, eds). pp 378–391. W.B. Saunders.

McBride, A. (1988). *Rabbits and Hares.* Whittet Books Ltd.

Okerman, L. (1988). *Diseases of Domestic Rabbits.* Blackwell.

Okerman, L., Devriese, L.A., Gevaert, D. *et al.* (1990). *In vivo* activity of orally administered antibiotics and chemotherapeutics against acute septicaemic pasteurellosis in rabbits. *Lab Anim.*, **24**, 341–344.

Pericin, C., Grieve, AP. (1984). Seasonal variations of temperatures in rabbits. *Lab Anim.*, **18**, 230–236.

Quesenberry, K.A. (1994). Disorders of avian and exotic pets. In *Saunders Manual of Small Animal Practice.* (S.J. Birchard, R.G. Sherding. eds). pp 1345–1363. W.B. Saunders.

Rabbit Health News. (1991). *Deaf Rabbits*, **3**, 3. Published by House Rabbit Society, PO Box 3242, Redmond, WA 98073 USA.

Rabbit Health News. (1993) *Aggressive Rabbits*, **8**, 4.

Published by House Rabbit Society, PO Box 3242, Redmond, WA 98073 USA.

Ramer, J.C., Paul-Murphy, J., Benson, K.G. (1999). Evaluating and stabilising critically ill rabbits – Part II. *Compendium of Continuing Education*, **21**, 116–125.

Richardson, V. (2000). *Rabbits. Health, Husbandry and Diseases*. Blackwell Sciences.

Rogers, G., Taylor, C., Austin, J.C., Rosen, C. (1988). A pharyngostomy technique for chronic oral dosing of rabbits. *Lab Anim Sci.*, **38**, 619–620.

Sandford, J.C. (1996). *The Domestic Rabbit*, 5th edn. Blackwell Science.

Smith, D.A., Olson, P.O., Matthews, K.A. (1997). Nutritional support for rabbits using the percutaneously placed gastrotomy tube: a preliminary study. *J Am Hosp Assoc.*, **33**, 48–54.

Stills, H.F. (1994). Polyclonal antibody production. In *The Biology of the Laboratory Rabbit*, 2nd edn. (P.J. Manning, D.H. Ringler, C.E. Newcomer, eds). pp 435–446. Academic Press.

Toft, P., Tonnesen E., Svendsen P., Rasmussen J.W. (1992a). Redistribution of lymphocytes after cortisol administration (Abstract). *APMIS*, **100**, 154–158.

Toft, P., Tonnesen E., Svendsen P. *et al.* (1992b). The redistribution of lymphocytes during adrenaline infusion. An *in vivo* study with radiolabelled cells (Abstract). *APMIS*, **100**, 593–597.

Toth, L.A., Krueger, J.M. (1989). Haematological effects of exposure to three infective agents in rabbits. *J Am Vet Med Assoc.*, **195**, 981–985.

Vangeel, I., Pasmans, F., Vanrobaeys, M. *et al.* (2000). Prevalence of dermatophytes in asymptomatic guinea pigs and rabbits. *Vet Rec.*, **146**, 440–441.

Weber, H.W., Van der Walt, J.J. (1975). Cardiomyopathy in crowded rabbits (Abstract). *Recent Adv Stud Cardiac Struct Metab.*, **6**, 471–477.

4 Therapeutics

4.1 Special considerations when prescribing for rabbits

The use of rabbits in toxicity studies has led to an abundance of information on the actions of drugs on rabbit tissue, both *in vivo* and *in vitro*, but there is a dearth of data on their efficacy in the treatment of clinical disease. In the UK there are only seven products licensed for use in rabbits at the present time (2001). Toxic doses and teratogenic effects may be known, but not actual adverse effects. Young healthy rabbits are used for toxicity studies rather than aged, ill individuals that have not been screened for other diseases. Therefore, the reputation of many preparations in the clinical situation is based on anecdotal evidence from practitioners. The result is a confused picture with conflicting reports of the safety and efficacy of products especially antibiotics and anaesthetic agents. Rabbits differ from other species in many ways and there are some aspects of their physiology that can affect their response to medication.

4.1.1 Digestive physiology

Digestive physiology affects the absorption and metabolism of drugs that are given orally. Substances can be absorbed from the stomach and small intestine into the portal system to be metabolized in the liver before entering the general circulation. This is known as the 'first-pass' effect that can alter the activity of therapeutic agents. The first-pass effect has been demonstrated in rabbits (Huang *et al.*, 1981). Conversely, substances that are absorbed across the buccal mucosa avoid the portal circulation and hepatic metabolism. It is not always possible to extrapolate dosages and effects of an orally administered drug in a rabbit from another species. There are differences between a carnivore, such as a dog, that swallows food without mastication and whose stomach empties completely and a herbivore, such as a rabbit, that chews the food thoroughly and has a stomach that is never empty. The acid pH of the rabbit's stomach can affect ionization and absorption of drugs.

Caecotrophy effectively recycles ingested material and prolongs the length of time that substances are retained in the gut. Fluids and small particles are retained in the caecum, whereas substances that bind with large particles will be excreted rapidly. The absorption of certain drugs may be affected by increased retention time in the caecum (Guillot *et al.*, 1988). The dual production of hard and soft faeces in the rabbit is a complex process controlled by the *fusus coli* that is highly innervated and vascular. The *fusus coli* is affected by hormones, such as aldosterone and prostaglandins, as well as the autonomic nervous system. Pharmacological preparations can affect digestive function through their effect on the *fusus coli*. For example, non-steroidal anti-inflammatory drugs (NSAIDS), such as indomethacin, inhibit endogenous prostaglandin formation and inhibit soft faeces production (Pairet *et al.*, 1986). The ingestion of soft faeces from the anus is triggered by a number of factors including odour, which can be affected by medication. Some drugs, e.g. ampicillin, inhibit normal caecotrophy (Escoula *et al.*, 1981).

4.1.2 Microflora of caecum and digestive tract

The caecum is inhabited by a variety of microorganisms including protozoa and anaerobic bacteria (see Section 1.5.3.2). The balance of microorganisms in the digestive tract, especially in the caecum, is influenced by many factors including antibiotics and other medications. Physiological processes alter caecal pH throughout the day in response to the digestion of food and passage of digesta. Diet affects both the composition of digesta that reaches the caecum and its rate of passage through the gut. Low fibre diets reduce gastrointestinal motility and prolong retention time of digesta in the caecum. Diets high in indigestible fibre promote optimal gastrointestinal motility and a healthy caecal microflora. Therefore rabbits that are fed on high fibre diets may be less susceptible to disruption of the caecal microflora than those that are fed on an exclusively cereal diet. Stress or pain increases circulating catecholamines or cortisol, which can have an effect on the balance of gut bacteria. Increased glucocorticoid levels increase coliform counts and alter the aerobic to anaerobic bacteria ratio in the gut (Straw, 1988).

4.1.3 Antibiotic toxicity in rabbits

In rabbits, antibiotics can alter the gut flora with potentially lethal effects, yet rabbits are prone to bacterial infections that require antibiotics to effect a cure. There are many areas of confusion over the use of antibiotics to treat clinical disease in pet rabbits.

Some antibiotics have the potential to cause enteritis in rabbits by selectively killing certain bacteria and allowing pathogenic species to proliferate. *Clostridia* spp. in particular, can proliferate in the caecum or small intestine and cause rapid death due to the effects of enterotoxins. *Clostridium spiroforme* is the major pathogen in rabbit enterotoxaemia, although *Clostridium difficile* and *Clostridium perfringens* may also be involved on rare occasions (Perkins *et al.*, 1995). A particular strain of *C. spiroforme* is pathogenic to rabbits and produces an iota toxin. *C. perfringens* type E also produces iota toxin. Antibodies against either organism will neutralize the other's iota toxin. This cross-reactivity led people to believe that *C. perfringens* type E was the pathogen in antibiotic-related diarrhoea in rabbits until *C. spiroforme* was identified in 1983 (Carman, 1993). For antibiotic-associated enterotoxaemia to develop in rabbits, both the antibiotic and the clostridium need to be present. *C. spiroforme* is not a normal inhabitant of the rabbit gut flora and normal intestinal ecology of the adult must be disrupted before *C. spiroforme* will colonize (Carman and Borriello, 1984). Glucose is required as a substrate for iota toxin production (Jenkins, 1997) and it is thought that undigested starch in the hindgut of young rabbits fed on cereal diets may increase susceptibility to enterotoxaemia. In young rabbits intestinal absorption of starch is not as efficient as in adults and residual amounts of carbohydrate may reach the caecum to act as a substrate for bacterial fermentation. Adult rabbits appear to digest starch more efficiently, with only small amounts reaching the caeco-colic segment unabsorbed (De Blas and Gidenne, 1998). Therefore high carbohydrate diets are less likely to predispose to enterotoxaemia in adults.

In addition to *Clostridia* spp. there are other pathogenic bacteria that can cause intestinal inflammation, enteritis and diarrhoea. *Escherichia coli* can produce toxins. In a study of the effects of ampicillin and gentamicin on the bacterial flora of the caecum, a strain of *Enterobacter aerogenes* predominated in rabbits treated with ampicillin, 40% of which died (Escoula *et al.*, 1981).

Most of the information about antibiotic-associated diarrhoea in rabbits has been gained from experimental studies rather than from the treatment of clinical cases. Healthy rabbits are used for experimental investigations rather than those that are suffering from some disease. Usually young rabbits are used in experimental studies rather than adults which have a different population of caecal microflora. The effect of diet, particularly indigestible fibre, on experimental results is largely overlooked. In some studies, the effects of antibiotic administration is an incidental finding during the treatment of a disease such as osteomyelitis or lung abscesses, in which rabbits are used as experimental models. For example, ampicillin and clindamycin are considered to be high-risk antibiotics that will readily induce diarrhoea. Yet in one study

Table 4.1 Antibiotic therapy for rabbits

Antibiotic	*Licensed for use in rabbits*	*Effective against Pasteurella Mutocida*	*Risk of antibiotic-associated diarrhoea*	*Suitable for parenteral use*	*Suitable for oral use*	*Suitable for topical use*
Ampicillin			High, especially if given orally	?	No	
Cephalexin		Yes	If given orally	Yes	No	
Clindamycin		No	High	No	No	
Enrofloxacin	Yes	Yes	Negligible	Yes	Yes	
Fusidic Acid	In eye ointment		Low			Yes
Gentamicin	In eye drops	Yes (inactivated by pus	Low	Nephrotoxic		Yes (also can be used in impregnated beads)
Lincomycin		No	High	No	No	
Metronidazole		No	No	If required	Yes (effective against clostridia)	Yes
Penicillin		Yes	If given orally	Yes	No	
Potentiated sulphonamide		Yes (inactivated by pus)	Low	Yes	Yes	
Streptomycin		Variable	Low	Yes		
Tetracycline		Variable	Low	Yes	Yes	
Tilmicosin		Yes	Not known, but there is a risk of fatal adverse reaction			
Tobramycin			Low	Yes		Yes (also can be used in impregnated beads)

(Norden and Budinsky, 1990), rabbits were given high doses of ampicillin (200 mg/kg) three times daily. Half the rabbits died with diarrhoea and inanition but the other half survived. In another study, Mader *et al.* (1989) compared cefazolin (5 or 15 mg/kg) and clindamycin (70 mg/kg) in the treatment of osteomyelitis. The antibiotics were given by subcutaneous injection every 6 h for 28 days. Seven out of 20 rabbits in the clindamycin group died, four with diarrhoea, whereas all the 24 rabbits in the two cefazolin groups survived and none developed diarrhoea.

Experimental investigations of the effects of antibiotics on gut flora in rabbits have given confusing results. For example Milhaud *et al.* (1976) and Escoula *et al.* (1981) reported a high incidence of antibiotic-associated diarrhoea in rabbits given ampicillin, in contrast to Hara-Kudo *et al.* (1996) who reported a low incidence of diarrhoea in rabbits injected with ampicillin in comparison with other antibiotics. Differences in the route of administration and dosages may explain some of these discrepancies but, in many cases, the overall picture is still inconsistent.

4.1.3.1 Prevention of antibiotic-associated diarrhoea and enterotoxaemia

The risk of treating individual pet rabbits with antibiotics is difficult to evaluate, as much information is anecdotal. There are documented reports of high mortality rates in commercial rabbits treated either accidentally, or deliberately with lincomycin at excessive dosages (Thilsted *et al.*, 1981; Maiers *et al.*, 1984).

The choice of antibiotic and route of administration are important factors in the prevention of antibiotic-associated diarrhoea. Clindamycin, lincomycin and oral ampicillin carry a high risk of inducing diarrhoea, whereas enrofloxacin and trimethoprim combinations are apparently safe, even when they are administered orally over a long period of time (Table 4.1). Using high levels of antibiotic increases the risk of enterotoxaemia, especially if they are given orally. Weighing the rabbit and calculating an accurate dose reduces the risk of overdosage.

Oral antibiotics are more likely to induce diarrhoea than those given parenterally. Rabbits are surprisingly easy to inject subcutaneously and most owners can be shown how to give injections themselves. In many cases it easier to inject a rabbit than to medicate it orally. Care should be taken with topical antibiotic preparations as these can be licked off the coat in sufficient quantities to interfere with gut flora. A companion can ingest topical preparation during mutual grooming.

In 'high-risk' situations where enterotoxaemia is likely to develop, cholestyramine can be used prophylactically. Cholestyramine is an ion exchange resin that absorbs enterotoxins. It has been shown to prevent experimental enterotoxaemia associated with clindamycin administration and may also be an effective adjunct to treatment (Lipman *et al.*, 1992; Flecknell, 1998). Probiotics may also be helpful in the prevention and treatment of enteritis (see Table 10.2).

The incidence of enterotoxaemia is greater in intensive situations where the environment is contaminated by clostridial spores. *C. spiroforme* is more commonly encountered in weanling rabbits than in the individual pet animal. Disinfection of buildings by removing organic matter and applying chemical disinfectants can help to reduce the incidence of disease. A sporicidal agent is required.

4.1.4 Legislation

In the UK, there are regulations governing the administration of veterinary medicines. These regulations prohibit the administration of veterinary medicinal products without the authorization of a veterinary surgeon. Veterinary medicinal products are licensed for use for a specific condition in a particular species of animal. There are exemptions to this rule that can permit the use of alternative products. These exemptions are known collectively as the prescribing cascade.

The exemptions are different for food-producing animals and those that are kept as companions. In food-producing animals, to ensure that tissue residue implications have been evaluated, only products that are licensed for other food-producing animals may be used. In companion animals, products authorized for use in any another species or for a different use in the same species may be used. If there is not a suitable veterinary medicine available, then the use of human preparations is acceptable.

In the UK, there are only seven products licensed for use in rabbits at the present time (2000), so most diseases of rabbits require treatment under the prescribing cascade. Rabbits are kept as both food-producing and companion animals so their place in the prescribing cascade is ambiguous. The Veterinary Medicines Directorate takes the view that rabbits should be regarded as food-producing animals '*unless the veterinarian in whose care they have been placed can be satisfied that neither the particular animal(s) being treated nor their produce will enter the food chain. Where the veterinarian is satisfied that the animal(s) concerned are being kept solely as pets and will not be used for food production then those particular animals may be regarded as companion animals for the purposes of the prescribing cascade*' (Veterinary Medicines Directorate, personal communication).

There are people who keep rabbits both as companions and for meat. Exhibition rabbit breeders especially, will kill and eat surplus stock. Rabbit breeders seldom present an animal to a veterinary surgeon for clinical examination. Instead, they treat their rabbits themselves with a variety of home remedies. Magazines and textbooks on rabbit care often describe the use of medicines such as antibiotics, parasiticides and motility stimulants that are only available on prescription. As a result, rabbit breeders may expect veterinary surgeons to supply these medicines on

Table 4.2 Formulary (Products used during anaesthesia are listed separately in Table 5.1)

Disclaimer: There are very few products that are licensed for use in rabbits. The responsibility for the use of unlicensed products lies with the prescribing veterinary surgeon. The following dose rates are based on the current state of knowledge and some dose rates are anecdotal (see end notes). Products that are licensed for use in rabbits appear in **bold** type.

Preparation	*Dosage*	*Route*	*Frequency*	*Type of drug or indication*	*Comments*
Acepromazine	0.5–1 mg/kg	IM, SC		Sedation	Not analgesic
Acepromazine †Butorphanol	0.5 mg/kg + 0.5 mg/kg	SC, IM		Sedation	Can be mixed in same syringe Vasodilatory
Albendazole	20 mg/kg	PO	Daily	Anthelmintic	Used to treat *E. cuniculi* Continue for 3–14 days
Aspirin	100 mg/kg	PO		Analgesic	First aid pain relief
Atropine	0.05 mg/kg (50 μg/kg)	IM		Premedication Organophoshate toxicity	40% rabbits produce atropinesterase that metabolizes atropine
Betamethasone	0.1 mg/kg	IV		Glucocorticoid	
Buserelin (Receptal, Hoechst)	**0.2 ml/rabbit**	**SC**		**FSH/LH**	**Used to induce ovulation and improve conception rate in breeding does**
Carprofen	2–4 mg/kg 1.5 mg/kg	SC PO	sid bid	Analgesic	Care in hypotensive patients Tablets can be mixed with fruit juice, jam or syrup
Cephalexin	15 mg/kg 20 mg/kg	SC SC	bid sid	Antibiotic	
Cholestyramine 'Questran'	0.5 g/kg 2 g/20 ml water	PO	bid or sid	Ion exchange resin	Enterotoxaemia Can be used prophylactically
Chlorphenamine maleate	200–400 μ/kg	PO	bid	Antihistamine	Paediatric syrup available
Cisapride	0.5 mg/kg	PO	bid	Prokinetic	Product withdrawn Contact manufacturers
Cyclizine	8 mg/rabbit	PO	bid	Torticollis	Used to treat labyrinthine disorders in humans
Dexamethasone	1–2 mg/kg	IM, IV		Anti-inflammatory	
Diazepam	1–2 mg/kg	IV, IM		Sedation	Not analgesic
Doxapram	5 mg/kg	IM, IV		Respiratory stimulant	
Enrofloxacin (Baytril, Bayer)	**5 mg/kg** **10 mg/kg** **5–10 mg/kg**	**SC** **SC** **PO**	**bid** **sid** **bid**	**Antibiotic**	**Licensed for use in rabbits**
Fenbendazole	20 mg/kg	PO		Anthelmintic	
Fentanyl/fluanisone (Hypnorm, Janssen)	**0.2–0.3 ml/kg**	**IM, SC**		**Premedication Analgesia Anaesthesia**	**Can be used in combination with midazolam or diazepam (0.5–2 mg/kg)**
Fluid therapy: intravenous subcutaneous	 10–20 ml/kg/hour 10–15 ml/kg				Warm before use
Flunixin	1.1 mg/kg	SC	bid	Analgesia	Care in hypotensive patients
Furosemide	0.3–2 mg/kg	IV, SC, IM		Diuretic	

Fusidic acid: eye drops (Fucithalmic, Leo)	**1 drop/eye**		**sid or bid**	**Conjunctivitis**	
Ointment (Fuciderm, Leo)	Topical		sid or bid	Superficial pyoderma	
Gentamicin (Tiacil, Virbac)	**1–2 drops/eye**		**tid**	**Conjunctivitis**	**Give for 5–7 days**
Glucose 5%	10 ml/kg	IV, SC		Anorexia Perioperatively	Warm before use
Glycopyrrolate	0.01 mg/kg 0.1 mg/kg	IV SC, IM		Premedication OP poisoning	Does not cross blood–brain barrier and cause mydriasis
Griseofulvin	25 mg/kg	PO	sid	Ringworm	Continue for at least 2 weeks
Imidacloprid	10 mg/kg	Topical		Fleas	Active against fleas not mites
Ivermectin	400 μ/kg	SC		Mites	Repeat after 10–14 days
Ketoprofen	1–3 mg/kg	PO	bid	Analgesia	Care in hypotensive patients
Liquid paraffin	1–2 ml/kg	PO	bid	Gastric or impactions	Can be used to soften and lubricate caecal/intestinal contents
Meloxicam	0.1–0.2 mg/kg	PO	sid	Analgesia	Palatable
Metoclopramide	0.5 mg/kg	SC, PO	bid	Motility stimulant	May not be effective in young rabbits
Metronidazole	20 mg/kg	PO	bid	Antibacterial	Treatment of choice for enterotoxaemia
Nandrolone	2 mg/kg	SC, IM		Anabolic steroid	Appetite stimulant Adjunct to treatment for anaemia especially in CRF
Oxytetracycline	15 mg/kg 30 mg/kg (depot) 1 mg/ml 50 mg/kg	SC,IM SC DW PO	sid every 3d	Antibiotic	
Oxytocin	1–2 IU/kg	SC, IM			
Penicillin (Procaine)	40 000 IU/kg (40 mg/kg)	SC	sid	Antibiotic	Contain 1 000 IU/mg
Penicillin Procaine + Benzathine Penicillin	20 mg/kg PP +15 mgBP/kg	SC	wkly	Antibiotic	Treatment of choice for *Treponema cuniculi* Give 3 weekly injections
Penicillamine	30 mg/kg	PO	bid	Chelating agent	Copper and lead toxicity
Praziquantel	6 mg/kg	SC		For treatment of cestodes	Repeat after 10 days
Prednisolone	0.5–2 mg/kg	PO, IM, SC		Anti-inflammatory	
Prochloperazine	0.2–0.5 mg/kg	PO	tid	Torticollis	Doses as high as 30 mg/kg tid are used to treat labyrinthine disorders in humans
Ranitidine	2 mg/kg 2–5 mg/kg	IV PO	sid bid	Gastric ulceration	Gastric ulcers often occur in inappetant rabbits
Selamactin	6–18 mg/kg	Topical	Once only	Mites	Single application appears to be effective
Sodium calciumedetate	27.5 mg/kg or 13 mg/kg	SC SC, IV	qid qid	Lead poisoning	Based on successful treatment of two cases

continued

Table 4.2 *continued*

Disclaimer: There are very few products that are licensed for use in rabbits. The responsibility for the use of unlicensed products lies with the prescribing veterinary surgeon. The following dose rates are based on the current state of knowledge and some dose rates are anecdotal.

Preparation	*Dosage*	*Route*	*Frequency*	*Type of drug or indication*	*Comments*
			for 5 days then every 2–3 days if necessary		General dose rate for cattle, dogs and cats Preparation should be diluted 1:4 in 5% glucose or 0.9% saline prior to use
Sulphadimidene	100–233 mg/l	DW		Coccidiosis	
Trimethoprim/ sulphadiazine	30 mg/kg 48 mg/kg	PO SC	bid	Antibiotic	
Trimethoprim/ sulfamethoxazole	40 mg/kg	PO	bid	Antibiotic Coccidiosis	'Co-trimoxazole' human formulation available as paediatric syrup Continue for 7 days
Toltrazuril	25 ppm 25 mg/kg	DW PO Give daily for 2 days Repeat after 5 days		Coccidiosis	Can be used for treatment of rabbit colonies
Tylosin	10 mg/kg	SC, IM	bid	Antibiotic	
Verapamil	200 μg/kg	SC	tds	To prevent post-surgical adhesions	Start immediately post-op then eight hourly for doses Not used routinely

Rabbits drink approximately 10% of their bodyweight daily and eat approximately 5%.
Abbreviations: sid: once daily; bid: twice daily; tid: three times daily; wkly: once weekly; IV: intravenous injection; SC: subcutaneous injection; IM: intramuscular injection; PO: by mouth; DW: in drinking water.

demand, without consultation, and are unaware of the stringent legislation governing the use of veterinary medicines for rabbits. The prescribing cascade severely limits the choice of medicines that are available for the treatment of rabbits that are destined to be eaten as meat.

4.2 Drugs that are used in rabbits

A formulary of products that are used to treat rabbits is given in Table 4.2.

4.2.1 Antibiotics

There is a temptation to prescribe antibiotics in any situation where there is an ill rabbit and no specific diagnosis. In view of the risk of antibiotic-associated diarrhoea, it is preferable to reserve antibiotic therapy for situations where there is a definite indication for their use. Antibiotics are most successful for the treatment of primary bacterial infections and for preventing secondary bacterial invasion of tissues damaged by viruses, surgery or other disease. Any antibiotic therapy carries a risk of life-threatening diarrhoea and enterotoxaemia in rabbits. This risk is influenced by diet, choice of antibiotic, dose rate, route of administration, presence of pathogenic clostridial species, age, stress, concurrent corticosteroid therapy and fate. The risk of antibiotic therapy needs to be weighed against the risk of not prescribing antibiotics.

Consideration should be given to the causative pathogen and the efficacy of a particular antibiotic against that organism. An effective concentration of the drug at the site of infection for as long as possible is needed to kill bacteria. Concentrations in excess of the mean inhibitory concentration (MIC) are required. MIC depends on the pharmacokinetics of the antibiotic and the microorganism that it is directed at. Ideally, culture and sensitivity identify the causal organism and aid antibiotic selection, but this option is not always available in the clinical setting. Infections may be in inaccessible sites such as the tympanic bulla or anterior chamber of the eye. *Pasteurella multocida* and *Staphylococcus* spp. are frequently isolated from infected sites. *In vitro* rabbit isolates of *P. multocida* are generally sensitive to penicillin, chloramphenicol, tetracycline, erythromycin, novobiocin and nitrofurans with varying susceptibility to streptomycin, kanamycin, neomycin and sulphonamides. They are usually resistant to clindamycin and lincomycin (Manning *et al*., 1989).

It is important to give therapeutic dosages for an antibiotic to be effective. Medicating the drinking water with antibiotics is generally unsatisfactory because it is difficult to ensure correct dosages and the taste of antibiotic can deter the rabbit from drinking the water. Sweetening the water with sucrose or fruit juices can help overcome this problem. In a study by Okerman *et al.* (1990), antibiotics were given to rabbits in the drinking water prior to infecting them with pathogenic *Pasteurella multocida*. *In vitro* sensitivity of the pathogen was confirmed and trimethoprim sulpha, spiramycin, tetracycline, erythromycin, chloramphenicol and enrofloxacin were tested at typical dose rates. Enrofloxacin was given at three different dosages: 25 mg/l, 50 mg/l, and 100 mg/l. Only enrofloxacin at 100 mg/l was effective in preventing infection. Enrofloxacin at 50 mg/l and chloramphenicol prevented rabbits dying but some of the survivors were not in good health. All the rabbits treated with the other antibiotics succumbed to acute pasteurellosis. This study not only highlighted the shortcomings of administering medication in the drinking water but also the importance of giving the correct dose of antibiotic.

It is possible to use potentially toxic antibiotics in a manner that gives high local tissue levels without producing harmful effects. For example, gentamicin, which is known to be nephrotoxic in rabbits, can be injected into abscess capsules or sutured into wounds in the form of antibiotic impregnated beads with no harmful effect on the kidneys.

4.2.1.1 Ampicillin

Ampicillin and amoxycillin have a similar range of antibacterial activity. There is a range of palatable paediatric syrups containing ampicillin that has been used for rabbits due their availability and ease of administration. Unfortunately, ampicillin is a 'high-risk' antibiotic for rabbits and there are numerous reports of diarrhoea and death following its use. In a study by Milhaud *et al.* (1976), rabbits were dosed with oral ampicillin at rates of 50 mg/kg, 15 mg/kg and 5 mg/kg. There was 100% mortality in the 50 mg/kg group and 50% mortality in the other groups. Ampicillin appears to be toxic both parenterally and orally (Escoula *et al*., 1981). Rehg and Yue-Shoung (1981) described a fatal case of diarrhoea in a rabbit that was treated for a respiratory tract infection with 8 mg/kg ampicillin subcutaneously; *C. difficile* was isolated from the caecum. There are numerous other reports in the literature of the toxicity of ampicillin in rabbits. It has been used to induce experimental *C. difficile* infection (Guandalini *et al*., 1988). Ampicillin has no advantages over other antibiotics in the treatment of diseases that affect pet rabbits.

4.2.1.2 Cephalosporins

Cephalosporins are a group of bactericidal, non-toxic antibacterials which contain the beta-lactam ring and are closely related to penicillin. On this basis they have been included in the list of antibiotics that are not suitable for use in rabbits by many authors. Actual reports of antibiotic-associated diarrhoea are scarce if the antibiotic is administered parenterally. In one study, ceftriaxone was administered by daily intramuscular injection for 4 weeks to a group of rabbits without adverse effects (Evans and Nelson, 1993). Cephalosporins are active against a range of gram-positive and gram-negative organisms including *Pasteurella* spp. (Bishop, 1998) and staphylococcal resistance to cephalosporins is less common than to penicillin.

4.2.1.2a Cephalexin

As a cephalosporin, cephalexin has the reputation as an unsafe antibiotic for rabbits

(Laval, 1990; Morris, 2000). Reports of adverse effects can be traced back to a German reference in which oral, not parenteral, cephalexin was administered at high doses (Schröder *et al.*, 1982). At standard dose rates of 15–30 mg/kg daily, parenteral cephalexin is well tolerated by rabbits. Oral preparations are not recommended although during toxicity studies, pregnant rabbits were given oral doses of cephalexin of up to 400 mg/kg daily with no toxic effects (Mallinckrodt, personal communication).

Cephalexin appears promptly in the aqueous humour of the non-inflamed eye of rabbits, in concentrations of 15–20% of serum levels (Gager *et al.*, 1969). Cephalexin is resistant to the action of staphylococcal penicillinase and is therefore active against penicillin-resistant strains of *Staphylococcus aureus* and against *Pasteurella multocida*. It is a useful antibiotic for the treatment of many conditions in pet rabbits including osteomyelitis (Harcourt-Brown, 1997). Parenteral cephalexin can be combined with topical cephalonium eye ointment for the treatment of ocular disease. It is an effective treatment for eye infections especially if there is evidence of uveitis or keratitis. Cephalexin is effective in suppressing signs associated with respiratory infections (Bishop, 1998).

4.2.1.3 Clindamycin

This antibiotic can induce fatal antibiotic-associated diarrhoea if administered orally. There is evidence that it is safer if given parenterally (Lucore *et al.*, 1986), but there is no parenteral preparation available for use in the UK. Many of the strains of *Pasteurella multocida* that affect rabbits are resistant to clindamycin (Manning *et al.*, 1989). Other bacteria such as *Staphylococcus* spp., which can be isolated from abscess cavities, may be sensitive to clindamycin. Local administration of clindamycin into abscess cavities has been described (Chappell, 1994). An antibiotic capsule is punctured and placed in the cavity after surgical drainage and debridement. The skin is sutured to retain the capsule. This simple, cheap technique removes the necessity of administering antibiotic by other routes. However, consideration must be given to the possibility of the antibiotic either being absorbed from a thin walled abscess or reaching the oral cavity through a draining fistula. Antibiotic-associated diarrhoea, which is usually fatal, can result from a clindamycin capsule placed in a site that is groomed or licked by the rabbit or its companion.

4.2.1.4 Enrofloxacin

Enrofloxacin is a fluoroquinolone that is active against a wide range of gram-negative and some gram-positive microorganisms. It is active against *Pseudomonas* spp. and *Mycoplasma* spp. At the present time (2001), enrofloxacin is the only systemic antibiotic that is licensed for use in rabbits. *Pasteurella multocida* is very sensitive to enrofloxacin *in vitro* (Mähler *et al.*, 1995). Enrofloxacin is indicated for the treatment of bacterial infections of the alimentary and respiratory tract. After administration by the oral or subcutaneous route, the drug is rapidly distributed through the tissues before being eliminated. In order to maintain minimum inhibitory concentrations of enrofloxacin for *Pasteurella multocida*, 12 hourly dosing of 5 mg/kg is required either orally or parenterally (Broome *et al.*, 1991). Unfortunately, this regimen may not achieve sufficient tissue concentrations to eliminate infection from the nasal cavity, trachea, middle ear and outer ear where *Pasteurella multocida* frequently resides (Mähler *et al.*, 1995). In a study by Okerman *et al.* (1990), oral administration of enrofloxacin via the drinking water was effective against experimental challenge with highly pathogenic *Pasteurella multocida* infection. A dose rate of 10 mg/kg was found to be more effective than 5 mg/kg. In a study by Suckow *et al.* (1996), experimental *Pasteurella multocida* intranasal infections of pregnant does were not eliminated with enrofloxacin given either in the drinking water (200 mg/l) or intramuscularly (5 mg/ kg bid), although the antibiotic prevented transmission of the organism to the kits. There is no documentary evidence that enrofloxacin disrupts intestinal flora or predisposes to enteric problems even when administered orally. It is a very safe antibiotic in rabbits and can be given over long periods. There is evidence that quinolones can cause arthropathy in juvenile rabbits. (Sharpnack *et al.*, 1994).

4.2.1.5 Fusidic acid

Fusidic acid is a steroidal antibiotic isolated from the fermentation products of the fungus

Fusidium coccineum. It is chemically related to cephalosporin P1 (Taylor *et al*., 1987) and has bacteriostatic or bactericidal activity mainly against gram-positive bacteria by selectively inhibiting bacterial protein synthesis (Bishop, 1998). The antibiotic is available for veterinary use as topical preparations. It is particularly effective against pathogenic staphylococci (Saijonmaa-Koulumies *et al*., 1998). Fusidic acid can penetrate avascular tissue even in large collections of pus (Taylor *et al*., 1987). Topical application penetrates the cornea and aqueous humour of rabbits giving levels of fusidic acid well above minimum inhibitory concentrations for most gram-negative organisms for at least an hour after application. Minimum inhibitory concentrations persist for up to 24 h in the cornea against gram-positive infections (Taylor *et al*., 1987). Fusidic acid viscous eye drops (Fucithalmic Vet, Leo Laboratories Ltd) give significantly higher tear fluid concentrations than chloramphenicol viscous eye drops (van Bijsterveld *et al*., 1987) and the preparation has sustained release properties. The carbomer base increases the concentration of fusidic acid in the tear film so this preparation is useful for the treatment of conjunctivitis and keratitis in rabbits, especially as it only needs to be applied once or twice daily. The gel preparation of fusidic acid in combination with betamethasone (Fuciderm, Leo Laboratories Ltd) can be used to treat inflamed perineal skin folds. The ointment is applied once daily for 2–3 days after the area has been clipped and cleansed and the underlying problem addressed. Fusidic acid does not appear to cause antibiotic-associated diarrhoea.

4.2.1.6 Gentamicin

Gentamicin is an aminoglycoside that is bactericidal and active against gram-negative organisms and some gram-positive ones, but not streptococci. Antibiotic resistance by enteric organisms can occur rapidly, especially if subtherapeutic doses are given (Bishop, 1998). Absorption does not occur from the digestive tract so oral administration is ineffective unless enteric infections are being treated. The antibiotic is ineffective against anaerobes and is not indicated for enteric infections in rabbits. Gentamicin does not appear to cause disturbances in caecal microflora (Escoula *et al*., 1981). It is poorly distributed into the eye, brain or cerebrospinal fluid. Excretion is solely by the kidney and the drug is potentially nephrotoxic. Purulent material binds and inactivates aminoglycosides (Elliott, 1998) so gentamicin is only effective for the topical treatment of abscesses if all the necrotic material has been removed by thorough debridement.

Parenteral gentamicin was not found to be as effective as penicillin in the treatment of rhinitis in a group of laboratory rabbits infected with *Pasteurella multocida* (Gaertner, 1991). As gentamicin is potentially nephrotoxic, its systemic use is not recommended.

The main indications for gentamicin in rabbits are for topical treatment of conjunctivitis and for local treatment of abscesses. Gentamicin ophthalmic solution (Tiacil, Virbac) is one of the few licensed preparations available for rabbits. Gentamicin is poorly absorbed into the inflamed eye and not at all in the normal eye of rabbits (Behrens-Baumann, 1996).

Gentamicin is also used in rabbits for the treatment of abcesses. It can be packed into abscess cavities incorporated into beads of polymethylmethacrylate (bone cement). The technique of implanting antibiotic impregnated substances into infected wounds or compound fractures has increased in human medicine in recent years and gentamicin is often used. It has been routinely incorporated in the bone cement used in human hip replacements. Gentamicin withstands the exothermic process that takes place during curing of the cement. In veterinary medicine, septic arthritis in both horses and cattle has been successfully treated using gentamicin impregnated polymethylmethacrylate beads (Butson *et al*., 1996). The beads can be purchased ready made as 7 mm spheres (Septopal, Merck) or made in a variety of sizes from gentamicin impregnated bone cement (see Section 8.3.4). Gentamicin can also be injected into the wall of abscesses (Brown, 1998).

4.2.1.7 Metronidazole

Metronidazole is a nitroimidazole that is bactericidal to most gram-negative and many anaerobic gram-positive bacteria. It has negligible activity against aerobic gram-positive infections and is not effective in the treatment of pasteurellosis. Nitroimidazoles have antiprotozoal properties, although *in vitro* testing suggests that metronidazole is ineffective against *Encephalitozoon cuniculi* (Franssen *et al.*, 1995). Metronidazole has been cited as a treatment of choice for enterotoxaemia caused by *Clostridium spiroforme* (Carman, 1994) and has been found to be effective in preventing abscess formation after experimental septic peritonitis in rabbits (Simopoulos *et al.*, 1994). The antibiotic is safe and easy to administer. Paediatric suspensions are available for oral dosing in addition to veterinary preparations suitable for parenteral administration.

4.2.1.8 Penicillin

Procaine penicillin can be used on its own or combined with benzathine penicillin as a depot injection. Penicillin is generally active against staphylococci, β-haemolytic streptococci and *Pasteurella* spp., although many staphylococci are now becoming resistant to the antibiotic. It is inactive against *Bordetella bronchiseptica*. In rabbits, penicillin is the treatment of choice for venereal spirochaetosis caused by *Treponema cuniculi.*

Penicillin is an example of conflicting information about the safety of a particular antibiotic in rabbits. Penicillin is often cited as a high-risk antibiotic for causing enterotoxaemia (Laval, 1990) but it has been used extensively to treat both venereal spirochaetosis (Cunliffe-Beamer and Fox, 1981) and pasteurellosis (Jaslow *et al.*, 1981; Gaertner, 1991) without complications. Benzylpenicillin is particularly active against gram-positive aerobes and anaerobes including *Clostridium* and *Bacteroides* species (Bishop, 1998). Clinically, it seems that penicillin is a safe antibiotic to use parenterally but not orally. There are no indications for its oral use.

Penicillin is useful for the treatment of pasteurellosis. In order to achieve blood levels that reach minimum inhibitory concentrations against *Pasteurella multocida*, penicillin needs to be given 8 hourly by intramuscular injection (Welch *et al.*, 1987), although daily injections of long-acting preparations have been used to overcome the practical problems associated with 8-hourly injections (Gaertner, 1991).

Many reference sources give dosages of penicillin in international units (IU). There are 1000 IU per milligram.

Long-acting depot injections are useful for rabbits. A combination of short-acting procaine penicillin is combined with benzathine penicillin that is slowly absorbed and maintains therapeutics blood levels over 3–4 days. Toxic effects from the procaine component have been described if high doses are used (Harkness and Wagner, 1995). There are reports of the death of kits when nursing does have received procaine penicillin. The deaths have been attributed to the toxic effects of procaine (Collins, 1995)

4.2.1.9 Potentiated sulphonamides

Sulphonamides are an antibacterial group of compounds that act by competing with tissue factors such as p-aminobenzoic acid. They have a wide range of activity. They are effective against some protozoa, including toxoplasma and coccidia (Bishop, 1998). Sulphonamides diffuse well into body tissues. They are partly inactivated in the liver. The acetylated derivatives are relatively insoluble in acid urine and can precipitate in renal tubules leading to crystalluria and renal failure. Rabbits excrete alkaline urine and are therefore less likely to develop crystalluria and subsequent renal damage as a result of sulphonamide therapy. However, kidney function is a consideration when selecting any therapeutic agent, including sulphonamides.

Sulphonamides can be combined with folate reductase inhibitors such as baquiloprim, ormetoprim or trimethoprim to form a preparation that is bactericidal and has a wide antibacterial spectrum including anaerobic bacteria. The half-life of some sulphonamides that are combined with trimethoprim is shorter in rabbits than in other species. For example, sulphadiazine, which is the sulphonamide component of most veterinary preparations, only has a half-life of about an hour in rabbits in comparison with 5–10 h in other species (Morris, 2000).

Potentiated sulphonamides diffuse well into body tissues and are good choice of antibiotic for rabbits due to their low toxicity, availability and ease of administration. However, potentiated sulphonamides are inactivated by exudate and debris (Whittem and Gaon, 1998) and are not as effective in the treatment of established purulent infection. There are no reports of antibiotic-associated diarrhoea with potentiated sulphonamides and so trimethoprim combinations can be used safely as a prophylactic antibiotic during surgery where wound contamination could occur.

Sulphonamides are used to treat coccidiosis in a number of species including rabbits. They have activity against the spectrum of life cycle stages. In most cases, they are only available in large quantities suitable for medicating large numbers of farmed rabbits. For the individual rabbit, co-trimoxazole is a trimethoprim/sulpamethazole combination that is available for human use. A paediatric oral suspension is available that be can used to treat coccidiosis. Alternatively, sulphadimethoxine is available for treatment of coccidiosis in pigeons and may be purchased in small quantities.

Oral dosing is straightforward using either paediatric syrups or preparations suitable for piglets. Prolonged administration of certain sulphonamides can cause keratoconjunctivitis sicca in dogs and antagonize vitamin K in poultry.

4.2.1.10 Tetracyclines

Tetracyclines are broad-spectrum antibiotics that are effective against *Mycoplasma* and *Chlamydia* spp. and some protozoa as well as a range of gram-positive and gram-negative bacteria. Tetracyclines are bacteriostatic and many organisms, especially *Staphylococcus aureus*, are now resistant to their effects. Tetracyclines have a synergistic effect with tylosin against *Pasteurella*. Many rabbit isolates of *P. multocida* are susceptible to tetracyclines *in vitro*. In the past, tetracyclines have been used extensively in commercial rabbit units both as growth promoters and prophylactically. They were administered either in the feed or in drinking water. However, it has been demonstrated that the administration of tetracycline in the drinking water does not produce detectable levels of the antibiotic in the serum, even at a high dosage (1600 mg/l). Medication of the water is also associated with a significant drop in water intake (Percy and Black, 1988). Therefore, this method of administration is unlikely to be effective. High parenteral dosages (30 mg/kg every 8 h) resulted in anorexia and diarrhoea in a study by McElroy *et al.* (1987), so this antibiotic does have toxic potential in rabbits, although the risk is small. It is safer than many other antibiotics. The main indication for tetracyclines is in the treatment of Tyzzer's disease caused by *Clostridium piliforme* (Harkness and Wagner, 1995). Depot injections of oxytetracycline or doxycycline have been used for the prolonged treatment of pasteurellosis or abscesses in pet rabbits (Laval, 1990; Malley, 1995).

4.2.1.11 Tilmicosin

Tilmicosin is a bacteriostatic macrolide that is used to treat pasteurella pneumonia in cattle and sheep. It is designed as a single dose therapy. It has been used successfully in the treatment of *P. multocida* in rabbits (Harvey, 1997). Experimentally, tilmicosin has proved 93% effective in eliminating the organism from the body (McKay *et al.*, 1996) at a dose of 25 mg/kg. However, the drug can cause a fatal adverse reaction in rabbits and a test dose of 5 mg/kg is advised prior to administration of 10 mg/kg daily for 3 days or once weekly (Harvey, 1997). There are many

Key points 4.1

- Although rabbits are used extensively as laboratory models of human disease and in pharmacological, physiological and toxicity studies, there is a dearth of information relating to the use of therapeutic agents in the clinical diseases that affect rabbits
- Physiological differences between rabbits and other species affect the pharmacokinetics of therapeutic agents
- Parenterally administered antibiotics carry a lower risk of inducing antibiotic-associated diarrhoea than those given orally
- Clindamycin, lincomycin and ampicillin carry a high risk of inducing antibiotic-associated diarrhoea
- Enrofloxacin and trimethoprim/sulpha combinations are unlikely to cause diarrhoea even if given orally
- Penicillin and cephalosporins are safe if given parenterally but should not be administered orally
- Antibiotics administered in the drinking water are unlikely to reach therapeutic levels in the body. The taste can deter rabbits from drinking medicated water.

warnings on the datasheet about adverse effects that can occur in humans. This antibiotic should only be used with the owner's understanding that adverse reactions have been reported and can be fatal.

4.2.1.12 Tylosin

Tylosin is a macrolide antibiotic with good activity against mycoplasma and gram-positive organisms (Bishop, 1998). There are reports of its use in rabbits, although its efficacy or potential for inducing enterotoxaemia are unclear.

4.2.1.13 Vancomycin

Vancomycin is a glycopeptide antibiotic that is active against gram-positive bacteria. The antibiotic is listed as one of three drugs effective against *Clostridium spiroforme* based on *in vitro* testing (Carman and Wilkins, 1991) and is cited as a treatment of choice for enterotoxaemia (Carman, 1994). A parenteral human preparation is currently available in the UK. Intravenous doses of 75 mg/kg resulted in 100% mortality in a study in rabbits by Nicolau *et al.* (1993). An acute adverse reaction took place that was prevented by reducing the dose to 50 mg/kg and giving the injection more slowly.

4.3 Probiotics

Probiotics are products that contain microorganisms in vegetative or arrested states that are capable of colonizing the gut. The microorganisms are non-pathogenic and reduce the adverse effects of potential pathogens. Their effects are thought to be due to competition for space and nutrients or to the production of substances that inhibit bacterial growth. Most probiotic preparations contain *Lactobacillus, Enterococcus* spp. and yeasts.

In rabbits, *Bacteroides* spp. predominate in the caecal flora that has a wide variety of gram-positive and gram-negative rods, cocci, filaments, coccobacilli and spirochaetes. In a review of the literature by Straw (1988), *Escherichia coli* and *Lactobacillus* were absent from the caecal microflora of healthy rabbits in most studies. However, *Lactobaccillus* was isolated from a group of rabbits that were fed on green foods and another group fed pellets containing antibiotics. The significance of these findings is unclear.

In recent years, there has been considerable interest in the use of probiotics in the prevention and treatment of enteric disease in rabbits. As *Lactobacillus* is generally absent from the normal gut flora of rabbits, its efficacy in questionable in this species. Penny *et al.* (1986) found no changes in the gut flora of rabbits fed on a diet supplemented with a commercial *Lactobacillus* preparation. The low pH of the stomach is likely to kill bacteria before they reach the small intestine, although an increase in pH during digestion of caecotrophs may permit bacteria to pass into the small intestine. Straw (1988) cites a study by Jilge and Meyer (1975) into the effect of caecotrophy on the populations of anaerobic bacteria in the stomach and small intestine. They found that soon after caecotroph consumption the populations were high but that after 5 h no bacteria could be isolated from the stomach and after 6 h, no viable cells were recovered from any part of the small intestine. In most probiotic preparations, organisms are encapsulated to prevent digestion in the stomach.

Despite theoretical doubts about the efficacy of probiotics in rabbits, there are many anecdotal reports that they are effective. There is also some experimental evidence to support this view. Hollister *et al.* (1989, 1990) concluded that probiotics were effective in reducing the incidence of enteritis and improving weight gain in newly weaned rabbits. The bacterial components of the probiotics appeared to be of greater importance than yeasts. However, the gastrointestinal flora of adult rabbits is different from newly weaned ones and the benefit of probiotics in adult animals remains controversial. As probiotics are not harmful, they can only be either beneficial or ineffective. Many authorities recommend their routine use in rabbits that are unwell especially those that have been treated with antibiotics or have compromised digestive function due to inadequate diet or intercurrent stress. Concurrent antibiotic administration can kill the beneficial microorganisms that are present in probiotics.

An alternative to probiotics is caecotrophs from a healthy rabbit which contain organisms that normally colonize the rabbit's gastrointestinal tract. Caecotrophs are coated in mucus that protects the contents from stomach acid and enzymes. The caecotrophs are eventually digested in the stomach and small intestine. Collection of caecotrophs can be difficult. Some pet rabbits on a plentiful diet may occasionally leave uneaten caecotrophs in the bedding which are usually found in the morning. Alternatively, a collar may be fitted to a healthy, donor rabbit for a day or two in order to prevent caecotrophy. Caecotrophs can be blended with pureed vegetables for syringe feeding. Feeding faeces from one animal to another is not only distasteful but there is a risk of transmitting disease, although the risk is small. Caecotrophs should only be collected from rabbits that are known to be healthy. Endoparasites are not a problem in pet rabbits. Coccidiosis cannot be transmitted by fresh caecotrophs, as the maturation process requires 48 h before oocysts are infective.

4.4 Corticosteroids

Corticosteroids are used in human and veterinary medicine for their anti-inflammatory and immunosuppressive properties. The main indications for their use are in the treatment of allergic and autoimmune diseases and the management of some neoplastic conditions such as lymphomas or mast cell tumours. Corticosteroids are also used to suppress inflammation in arthritic conditions and to treat metabolic disorders such as ketosis in cattle and sheep. Sometimes they are used indiscriminately, but effectively, as 'symptom suppressors' where no accurate diagnosis can be made.

There is little information about either the efficacy or the adverse effects of corticosteroids in the treatment of rabbits. Veterinary treatment of pet rabbits is still in its infancy in comparison with other domestic species and protocols for the treatment of allergies, autoimmune disease or neoplasia are yet to be developed. There are anecdotal reports of successful treatment with corticosteroids of 'shock' in rabbits associated with trauma or blood loss. Prednisolone has proven to be life saving in experimental rabbit models of toxic shock syndrome (Parsonnet *et al.*, 1987) when the corticosteroid and toxin were administered concurrently.

Inflammatory conditions such as granulomatous encephalitis caused by *Encephalitozoon cuniculi* have been treated with high doses of prednisolone with apparent success (Feaga, 1997).

There are potential hazards associated with the use of corticosteroids in rabbits. Chronic administration can affect wound healing (Kim *et al.*, 1993). The immunosuppressive properties of corticosteroids may allow latent infections such as *Pasteurella multocida*, *Encephalitozoon cuniculi* or *Clostridium piliforme* (Tyzzer's disease) to flare up. Some pet rabbits, especially those suffering from dental disease, have very low lymphocyte counts and may already be immunosuppressed (Harcourt-Brown and Baker, 2001) (see Figure 6.1).

In ruminants, glucocorticoids are used in the treatment of ketosis and pregnancy toxaemia. Glucocorticoids are used to stimulate gluconeogenesis and increase blood glucose levels and could be considered a suitable treatment for anorexic rabbits. However, glucocorticoids also stimulate mobilization of free fatty acids from adipose tissue and could also contribute to the development of hepatic lipidosis, which is a potentially fatal sequel to anorexia in rabbits. As a general rule, non-steroidal anti-inflammatory drugs (NSAIDs) are preferable to corticosteroids in rabbits for the non-specific treatment of pain and inflammation. NSAIDs are safe, effective and well tolerated.

4.5 Anabolic steroids

Anabolic steroids are synthetic derivatives of testosterone with some androgenic activity but less virilizing effects. They are used to promote nitrogen retention in animals with catabolic disease and cause retention of sodium, calcium, potassium, chloride, sulphate and phosphate (Bishop, 1998). Anabolic steroids stimulate appetite, increase muscle mass, retain intracellular water, increase skin thickness, increase skeletal mass, close growth plates prematurely and increase production of erythrocytes. In small animal practice, their main indications are the treatment of anaemia, especially uraemic anaemia, and the treatment of debilitating disease such as neoplasia. They are usually used in conjunction with other drugs. Anabolic steroids are contraindicated in animals with impaired hepatic function.

In rabbits, there are anecdotal reports of the successful use of anabolic steroids to stimulate appetite. Experimentally, daily doses of 2 mg/kg nandrolone decanoate were found to ameliorate the adverse effects of chronic corticosteroid administration on intestinal healing in rabbits and doses as high as 20 mg/kg had no apparent adverse effect (Kim *et al.*, 1993).

4.6 Non-steroidal anti-inflammatory drugs (NSAIDs)

Non-steroidal anti-inflammatory drugs are nearly all weak carboxylic or enolic acids (Bishop, 1998) that act by inhibiting cyclo-oxygenase and reducing the synthesis of prostaglandins and related compounds. Cyclo-oxygenase is an enzyme that promotes the formation of prostaglandin from cell membrane arachidonic acid. There are two cyclo-oxygenase isoforms COX1 and COX2. All NSAIDs are analgesic, antipyretic and have anti-inflammatory properties. Their potential for causing toxic effects is related to the cyclo-oxygenase isoforms. COX1 has a range of physiological roles and inhibition of COX1 accounts for the major toxic effects of NSAIDs. COX2 is produced at inflammatory sites to generate inflammatory mediators. Potency ratios for the inhibition of COX1:COX2 vary between NSAIDs and are high for products such as aspirin and phenylbutazone and low for newer NSAIDs such as meloxicam and carprofen, which should therefore have less toxic side effects. Carprofen, however, is a weak cyclo-oxygenase inhibitor and has fewer toxic effects because of this. It appears to have another mechanism of action.

The isomeric structure of the molecule also influences its pharmacological effects, especially in the group of NSAIDs that belong to the 2-arylproprionic acid subgroup (carprofen, ketoprofen and vedaprofen). Formulations are usually a mixture of the two structural mirror images (enantiomers). Metabolism within the body can alter the ratio of the two enantiomers and therefore modify the pharmacokinetics of the drug. Marked species differences occur in the way these drugs are metabolized (Bishop, 1998).

In general, the dose interval of NSAIDS should be increased in neonates and aged animals to avoid toxicity (Bishop, 1998). Inhibition of normal prostaglandin regulation of renal blood flow can result in poor perfusion of the kidney in hypotensive patients and could result in acute renal failure. This situation can occur during anaesthesia, especially if there is excessive blood loss, but can be avoided by maintaining blood pressure with appropriate fluid therapy. It is advisable to leave 24 h between the administration of different types of NSAID.

In rabbits, the anti-inflammatory and analgesic properties of NSAIDs are used to treat many clinical conditions, although no products are currently licensed for use in this species. NSAIDs can be used to reduce inflammatory oedema in acute inflammatory conditions such as pneumonia or enteritis. They are invaluable for postoperative analgesia and for the treatment of chronic osteoarthritic conditions. The effect of NSAIDs on prostaglandin synthesis is significant in rabbits. Prostaglandins stimulate elimination of soft faeces by inhibiting motility of the proximal colon and stimulating motility in the distal colon. Experimentally, the infusion of prostaglandin is followed by elimination of soft faeces. NSAIDs inhibit the synthesis of prostaglandins and inhibit the elimination of soft faeces (Pairet *et al.*, 1986). NSAIDs can be used to treat conditions in which a temporary reduction in soft faeces production is advantageous, e.g. in rabbits that have perineal dermatitis exacerbated by uneaten caecotrophs.

4.6.1 Aspirin

Aspirin combines irreversibly with cyclo-oxygenase (COX1) and therefore has more potential toxic effects than some newer preparations. Aspirin is an effective analgesic for rabbits (Deeb, 1992). It is useful as a first aid measure because most households have some aspirin available for human use. The drug reaches its maximum concentration in the serum after 1–2 h in rabbits. Aspirin can cause a reduction in platelet numbers and bleeding tendencies have been noted in laboratory rabbits treated with aspirin (Marangos *et al.*,1995). The analgesic properties are weak in comparison with some of the newer NSAIDS such as carprofen or flunixin.

4.6.2 Carprofen

Carprofen is a weak cyclo-oxygenase inhibitor with a low COX1:COX2 ratio that has minimal toxic effects. It is a useful product for rabbits although it is not licensed for use in this species. Dose rates are empirical. Carprofen can be routinely administered postoperatively to all surgical patients. Although it may be given orally, once daily subcutaneous or intravenous injection is satisfactory. Injection reactions can occur in the skin following subcutaneous injections of carprofen. The incidence of injection reactions is reduced by ensuring that the product is given subcutaneously rather than intradermally and by massaging the area thoroughly after the injection is made. Carprofen is indicated as an analgesic for acute painful conditions such as fractures or trauma. It can also be used as part of the treatment protocol for painful gastrointestinal diseases.

4.6.3 Flunixin

Flunixin is a potent cyclo-oxygenase inhibitor that is used effectively as an anti-inflammatory drug in large herbivores such as cattle and horses. The manufacturers recommend that the drug should not be administered until the patient is fully recovered from general anaesthesia as this NSAID can compromise renal blood flow. It should not be given with other potential nephrotoxic drugs such as gentamicin.

Flunixin can be used as an analgesic and for its anti-inflammatory properties in rabbits (More *et al.*, 1989; Brown, 1998). The cyclo-oxygenase inhibitory properties of flunixin could be useful in the treatment of enterotoxaemia.

4.6.4 Ketoprofen

The use of ketoprofen has been described in small mammals including rabbits (Flecknell, 1998). It is an alternative to carprofen or meloxicam.

Key points 4.2

- Probiotics contain *Lactobacillus* that is not a normal inhabitant of the gut flora in rabbits
- There are many reports that probiotics are useful in the prevention and treatment of enteric disease in rabbits
- An alternative to probiotics are caecotrophs collected from a healthy rabbit
- Although corticosteroids may be beneficial in the treatment of shock, autoimmune disease, allergies and inflammatory conditions such as *Encephalitozoon cuniculi*, they may also allow latent infections such as pasteurellosis to flare up
- Anabolic steroids can be used to stimulate appetite or as part of the treatment of uraemia and debilitating disease
- Non-steroidal anti-inflammatory drugs are useful for many conditions in rabbits. Carprofen can be given perioperatively as a routine analgesic and meloxicam is available as a honey-flavoured oral preparation that is palatable to rabbits and is useful for long-term treatment.

4.6.5 Meloxicam

Meloxicam is a NSAID with a low COX1: COX2 ratio (Bishop, 1998). It has potent anti-arthritic effects and a reduced potential to cause gastric irritation in animals in comparison with other NSAIDS. Toxicity studies showed good tolerance and excellent tissue tolerability (Stei *et al.*, 1996). The rate of gastric emptying or intestinal transport in the rat is not influenced by therapeutic doses of meloxicam, which has only mild effects on gastric acidity. In doses well above those required for anti-inflammatory action, meloxicam had no influence on water, electrolyte or creatinine excretion during pharmacological studies of the drug (Engelhardt *et al.*, 1996).

In rabbits, the oral preparation, which is a honey flavoured syrup, is very palatable making it a useful preparation for long-term analgesia for painful, chronic conditions such as arthritis or spondylosis.

4.7 Motility agents

4.7.1 Cisapride

Cisapride is a prokinetic, which is a class of drugs that enhance the passage of intraluminal contents through the gastrointestinal tract (Blood and Studdert, 1999). Cisapride belongs to the group of serotonergic or 5-hydroxytrytamine (5-HT) drugs that bind 5-HT receptors and have antagonistic effects on enteric cholinergic neurons and consequently stimulate contractions of gastrointestinal smooth muscle (Washabau and Hall, 1997). In humans, cisapride is indicated for the treatment of gastro-oesophageal reflux, delayed gastric emptying, ileus, intestinal pseudo-obstruction and constipation. Fatal adverse drug interactions in humans have resulted in the withdrawal of cisapride in many countries including the UK. For more information about the current situation, the manufacturers of cisapride (Janssen) should be contacted.

In rabbits, cisapride promotes gastric emptying, increases gastrointestinal and colonic motility and is used in the treatment of gastrointestinal hypomotility or gut stasis. Following administration cisapride is rapidly and almost completely absorbed from the gastrointestinal tract (Michiels *et al.*, 1987). The effects last for 4–10 h. Stimulation of gastric contractility not only facilitates gastric emptying but also stimulates appetite, especially for fibrous foods such as grass or hay. Many rabbits will start to eat soon after administration.

Cisapride is contraindicated in patients with mechanical gastrointestinal obstruction, haemorrhage or perforation. In other species, cisapride can cause GI disturbances such as stomach cramps, borborygmi and diarrhoea and has some potential adverse drug interactions. For rabbits, the most notable interaction is with anti-fungal drugs such as ketoconazole, itraconazole or miconazole, which can result in fatal cardiac arrhythmias. Cisapride has caused embryotoxic and fetotoxic effects in rabbits when administered at high dose (FitzSimons, 1999).

4.7.2 Metoclopramide

Metoclopramide is a dopaminergic antagonist with gastrointestinal prokinetic and antiemetic properties (Hall and Washabau, 1997). It exerts its effects via antagonism of dopaminergic D_2 receptors and agonism of serotonergic 5-HT receptors. In rabbits metoclopramide promotes gastric emptying and increases gastrointestinal motility. There is *in vitro* evidence that metoclopramide is only effective in adult rabbits (Langer and Bramlett, 1997). Atropine and opioid analgesics can antagonize the effects of metoclopramide (Washabau and Hall, 1997). Like cisapride, metaclopramide is contraindicated in cases of gastrointestinal obstruction.

4.7.3 Buscopan compositum

Buscopan compositum (Boehringer Ingelheim) is an analgesic/spasmolytic preparation that is indicated for the relief of pain associated with spasm in the gastrointestinal and urinary tracts. It is a combination of metamizole (a NSAID) and hyoscine. Buscopan compositum has been used either prophylactically to prevent gastroenteric problems or in the treatment of diarrhoea. In a study by Morisse (1978), ampicillin was given used to induce diarrhoea in rabbits. The mortality rate was apparently reduced by the concurrent administration of Buscopan, although it is not clear whether it was the spasmolytic or analgesic effects of the preparation that were effective in reducing the incidence of enterotoxaemia.

Hyoscine is contraindicated in cases of gastrointestinal hypomotility, although it may be beneficial in cases of enteritis where gut motility is increased, e.g. due to infectious agents or plant toxins.

4.8 Parasiticides

4.8.1 Albendazole

Albendazole is a member of the benzimidazole group of parasiticidal agents that disrupt parasite energy metabolism by binding to tubulin, a constituent cell protein required for the uptake of nutrients (Bishop, 1998). The anthelmintic activity of the benzimidazoles is related to the duration of therapeutic blood concentrations. Doses may need to be repeated in pigs, dogs and cats while single doses are sufficient in ruminants because the rumen or large intestine acts as a reservoir. Albendazole is available as a modified release oral anthelmintic for use in cattle and sheep. Although the product is not licensed for use in rabbits, the pharmacokinetics have been investigated in this species using a dose of 20 mg/kg (Li *et al.*,1995). *In vitro* studies show that albendazole is an effective antimicrosporidial agent. Spores of *Encephalitozoon cuniculi* are killed in rabbit kidney cell tissue culture by albendazole without evidence of cytopathic change. It appears that the drug is effective against the early stages of microsporidia development, as mature spores are not produced during drug treatment (Weiss *et al.*, 1994). Albendazole can be used to treat encephalitozoonosis in rabbits (see Section 16.4.2.5). The duration of treatment has not been determined. In humans, immunocompromised AIDS patients require lifelong treatment. In rabbits, an empirical approach is required. Anecdotally, albendazole therapy is continued for 3–14 days. The agent appears to be safe, although it should be used with caution in breeding does as albendazole has been demonstrated to have teratogenic effects (Bishop, 1998).

4.8.2 Fenbendazole

Fenbendazole is a benzimidazole that is used widely in domestic animals as an anthelmintic. In rabbits, fenbendazole is used to treat nematode infections such as *Passalurus ambiguus*. The compound is metabolized to oxfendazole after oral dosing (Short *et al.*, 1988). The compound is well tolerated and no teratogenic effects have been recorded. Fenbendazole has been demonstrated to be effective against *Encephalitozoon cuniculi* infection. In a controlled study by Suter *et al.* (2001), fenbendazole was administered for 7 days prior to inoculation of *E. cuniculi* to laboratory rabbits and continued for 21 days after inoculation. No serological response was found in the treated rabbits and no parasite was detected in brain tissue. Fenbendazole was given at a dose rate of 0.1 mls/kg twice daily (Panacur, 10%, Hoechst Roussel).

4.8.3 Avermectins

4.8.3.1 Ivermectin

Ivermectin is a member of the avermectins group of drugs that are effective against a wide range of mature or immature nematodes and arthropods but have no activity against cestodes or trematodes. Ivermectin does not readily cross the blood–brain barrier and has a wide margin of safety. There are a variety of preparations available for use in farm animals that can be given orally, parenterally or as a pour-on. Although the manufacturers state that ivermectin should not be used in species other than cattle, sheep or pigs, it has been used extensively in rabbits without adverse effect. There is no ectoparasiticide that is licensed for use in this species.

In rabbits, ivermectin is an effective treatment for mite infestations. A subcutaneous dose of 400 μg/kg produces high and sustained tissue concentrations of ivermectin for at least 13 days. The drug is carried throughout the body in the bloodstream and is effective against blood sucking lice and mange mites. After injection, high concentrations of ivermectin are achieved in the skin and therefore the drug is likely to be effective against mites that are active in the keratin layer (McKellar *et al.*, 1992). The propylene glycol can cause local irritation when injected subcutaneously.

The rabbit ear mite, *Psoroptes cuniculi* is particularly sensitive to ivermectin (Curtis *et al.*, 1990). Ivermectin does not kill *Psoroptes cuniculi* eggs, but the persistence of the drug in the tissues is sufficiently long to kill new generations of mites as they hatch. The eggs hatch after 4 days. Dosages of 400 μg/kg are required, 200 μg/kg were found to be inadequate in the elimination of ear mites in a study by Wright and Riner (1985). There is a report of the use of ivermectin to treat experimental *Eimeria infections* in rabbits (Arafa and Wanas, 1996). Ivermectin is ineffective against *Passalurus ambiguus* (Morrisey, 1996).

In a study by Ali (1990), high doses of ivermectin (2.5 mg/kg) in rabbits altered haematological parameters causing anaemia, whereas dose rates of 0.2 mg/kg or 1 mg/kg had no effect on blood parameters.

4.8.3.2 Selamectin

Selamectin is a topical avermectin that is licensed for use in dogs and cats (Stronghold, Pfizer). It is effective against fleas and a range of mites. The product is available in prepacked pipettes containing varying amounts of either 60 mg/ml or 120 mg/ml spot-on solution. In rabbits, selamectin can be used as a topical treatment for mite infestations at the dose rate of 12 mg/kg. In a study by Hack *et al.* (2001), selamectin was effective against *Psoroptes cuniculi* at dose rates of 6 mg/kg and 18 mg/kg. No adverse effects were seen.

4.8.4 Fipronil

Fipronil (Frontline, Merial) is a phenylpyrazole insecticide that acts by blocking the action of the neurotransmitter γ-aminobutyric acid. It is effective against fleas, ticks and mites in dogs and cats and has been used to treat canine cheyletiellosis effectively (Chadwick, 1997). Fipronil spray is effective against mite infestations of rabbits (Cutler, 1998) but carries a manufacturers' warning against its use in species other than cats and dogs (Cooper and Penaliggon, 1997). The warning followed a number of reports of adverse reactions in young or small rabbits treated with fipronil spray. Affected rabbits were presented within a week of treatment with a history of depression and reduced appetite. The reaction is potentially fatal and has been observed following treatment with both the spray and the spot-on preparation (Merial, personal communication) and is therefore not solely attributable to the alcohol vehicle or chilling of small rabbits. If fipronil is to be used then it is wise to obtain written consent from the owner and to disclaim responsibility for any adverse effects.

4.8.5 Imidacloprid

Imidacloprid (Advantage 40, Bayer) is a chloronicotinyl nitroguanide that acts by binding nicotinic acetylcholine receptors in the insect CNS leading to inhibition of cholinergic transmission resulting in paralysis and death.

The product is used to control fleas in dogs and cats. Imidacloprid is well tolerated by rabbits and can be used to control fleas that are caught from dogs or cats in the household (Hutchinson *et al.*, 2001). Imidacloprid is not effective against mites in rabbits.

4.9 Miscellaneous preparations

4.9.1 Buserelin

Buserelin (Receptal, Hoechst Roussel Vet Ltd) is a synthetic releasing analogue that is equivalent to the natural luteinizing hormone (LH) and follicle stimulating hormone (FSH) produced in the hypothalamus. It causes simultaneous release of LH and FSH from the pituitary. Buserelin is one of the few licensed products available for use in rabbits. It is used to improve conception rate and induce ovulation in commercial does.

4.9.2 Cholestyramine

Cholestyramine is an ion exchange resin. It is used in humans to reduce elevated serum cholesterol levels in patients who do not respond to dietary modification. Cholestyramine is not absorbed but binds to bile acids in the intestine, which are then excreted from the gut rather than being reabsorbed. Bile acids are derived from cholesterol so bile acid loss requires increased cholesterol metabolism to produce bile acids for fat digestion.

Cholestyramine also binds fat soluble and bacterial toxins and is effective in the treatment of enterotoxaemia if it is given in the early stages of the disease. In a study by Rateau *et al.* (1986), cholestyramine reduced the loss of water and electrolytes from the ileum of rabbits treated with cholera toxin. It was also effective in preventing death from enterotoxaemia in rabbits treated with clindamycin (Lipman *et al.*, 1992) even if treatment was delayed until 48 h after the administration of the antibiotic.

Chlolestyramine is widely available from pharmacies in sachets of 'Questran', which is a palatable powder that can be sprinkled on food or dissolved in water for syringe feeding. It can be administered to rabbits that are considered to be at risk of developing enterotoxaemia. Besides binding with bile acids and toxins, cholestyramine binds to numerous drugs such as digoxin (Cady *et al.*, 1979), iboprofen (El Sayad *et al.*, 1994), phenylbutazone and phenobarbitone. It has been used to delay absorption of toxic substances from the gut in cases of toxic overdose in the dog, although activated charcoal is now considered the treatment of choice (Gfeller and Messonier, 1997). Cholestyramine also binds to the fat-soluble vitamins A, D, E and K. In humans large doses can cause severe constipation (CRC Desk Reference of Clinical Pharmacology, 1998).

4.9.3 Anti-ulcer drugs

4.9.3.1 H_2 antagonists

H_2 antagonists inhibit the secretion of gastric acid and reduce pepsin output. H_2 antagonists include cimetidine and ranitidine, which are products that are available as human preparations for the treatment of gastric and duodenal ulceration. This group of drugs is used in veterinary medicine for the treatment of ulcers in horses, dogs and cats but their use has not been described in rabbits. Gastric ulceration is frequently seen during *post-mortem* examination of rabbits (Hinton, 1980). The condition is associated with stress and reduced gut motility. The use of anti-ulcer drugs can be a useful adjunct to treatment of rabbits with hypomotility disorders (see Section 10.4). Rabbits are included in many laboratory investigations into the effects and toxicity of these drugs so their effects on rabbits are known. Ranitidine (Zantac, Glaxo Wellcome) is available as tablets or as an injectable preparation. It has a stimulatory effect on intestinal motility in the rat and guinea pig and on isolated strips of rabbit fundus and colon (Bertaccini *et al.*, 1983; Kounensis *et al.*, 1992). In rabbits, ranitidene is effective in decreasing gastric acid and pepsin secretion (Redfern *et al.*, 1991), although it is ineffective in resolving indomethacin-induced gastric ulceration (Wallace and McKnight, 1993).

4.9.3.2 Omeprazole

Omeprazole (Losec, Astra) is a human anti-ulcer drug that acts by inhibiting the hydrogen-potassium adenosine triphosphatase system that is responsible for gastric acid production by the parietal cells.

Experimentally, omeprazole significantly reduces gastric ulcer formation in rabbits treated with indomethacin (Lee *et al.* 1996) and elevates postprandial intragastric pH above 5 (Redfern *et al.*, 1991). At the present time, omeprazole is only available in capsules, which are difficult to divide.

4.9.4 Chelating agents

4.9.4.1 Sodium calciumedetate

Sodium calciumedetate mobilizes lead from bone and is widely used for the treatment of lead poisoning in all species. It enhances removal of lead from the body by forming a stable water-soluble lead complex that is readily excreted by the kidneys. It is not suitable for oral administration as it can enhance absorption of lead from the gastrointestinal tract (Gfeller and Messonier, 1997). Excessive lead mobilization from bone can enhance intoxication and result in renal tubule damages (Bishop, 1998). The preparation can be given subcutaneously or intravenously up to four times a day. Dilution of 1:4 in 0.9% sodium chloride 5% glucose is recommended prior to administration in cattle and dogs (Sodium calciumedetate (strong) datasheet, Animalcare, 1999).

4.9.4.2 Penicillamine

Penicillamine is a chelating agent that is used to treat copper and lead poisoning. It is the principal agent used to treat copper hepatotoxicity in dogs. Penicillamine is administered orally and may have the side effect of enhancing lead absorption from the gastrointestinal tract. Side effects at higher doses are reported in dogs in which it causes vomiting. D-penicillamine has been used to treat copper poisoning in rabbits that had chewed and ingested electric cables.

4.9.5 Verapamil

Verapamil is a calcium channel blocker whose main indication in veterinary medicine is in the treatment of supraventricular arrhythmias in dogs. It can also be used to prevent adhesions. In humans, surgical adhesions cause postoperative complications after gynaecological procedures and rabbits have been used as experimental models to investigate the problem. Rabbits readily develop surgical adhesions and under experimental conditions verapamil inhibits this process. Doses of 200 μg/kg subcutaneously every 8 h for nine doses significantly reduced adhesion formation in rabbits which had one uterine horn traumatized by ligation followed by burns induced with thermocautery. The animals tolerated surgery and recovery without overt evidence of cardiopulmonary compromise (Steinleitner *et al.*, 1990). Verapamil reduces the response of colonic smooth muscle to motilin *in vitro* (Depoortere *et al.*, 1991). It is worth considering the use of verapamil in surgical situations where adhesions are likely to occur, such as surgery on the caecum or colon. Treatment is started immediately postoperatively.

4.9.6 Vitamin C (ascorbic acid)

Rabbits are able to synthesize vitamin C and do not have a dietary requirement. However, in a study by Verde and Piquer (1986), plasma ascorbic acid concentrations decreased while cortisol levels increased during periods of stress induced either by heat or noise. The authors postulated that the fall in ascorbic acid values was due to increased utilization of vitamin C by the adrenal gland during stressful periods and that depletion of ascorbic acid reserves may play a part in reducing immune function.

Most vegetables provide vitamin C, especially green peppers and blackcurrants. Vitamin C-containing cranberry tablets have been advocated as part of the regimen for the treatment of urolithiasis (Brown, 1998).

4.10 Topical preparations

Although there are no licensed topical preparations for treating skin conditions in rabbits, there are products for use in dogs and cats that are useful. Many skin complaints in rabbits result from the animal's inability to groom and so it is unlikely that topical creams and ointments will be licked off. However, it is important to consider potential systemic effects if the patient or its companion licks the product off the skin and ingests it. This is a potential complication of antibiotic and corticosteroid preparations.

Corticosteroids can be absorbed across the skin and cause significant adrenocortical suppression in healthy animals (Zenoble and Kemppainen, 1987). There are a number of factors that influence the extent of absorption of topical corticosteroids and its effects. In general, the anti-inflammatory effect of a topical corticosteroid bears a close correlation with its potential to produce adverse effects. Hydrocortisone and prednisolone are the weakest of the corticosteroids that are used in veterinary topical preparations, followed by betamethasone and triamcinolone, which are classified as 'potent' (Sneddon, 1976). The vehicle and the concentration of the steroid in the cream or ointment also affects absorption, which is greater from an ointment than from a cream. Application of occlusal dressings can increase steroid penetration by as much as a factor of one hundred in humans (Monk, 1995). In animals, skin folds can exert a similar effect. There is greater absorption of steroids by inflamed skin. The thin skin of rabbits absorbs corticosteroids well. Topical skin preparations are useful but should be used with caution in rabbits. The main indication for their use is in the treatment of the inflamed ano-genital region that results from urine scalding or uneaten caecotrophs. Clipping, cleaning and bathing the area are necessary and the application of topical ointments speeds recovery (see Section 9.7.3).

4.10.1 'EMLA' cream

EMLA cream (Astra) is a topical preparation containing 2.5% lidocaine and 2.5% prilocaine that provides local anaesthesia of full thickness skin. The product is supplied with an occlusive dressing to place over the cream while the local anaesthetic takes effect. EMLA cream takes 45–60 minutes to become effective. It can be used to anaesthetize skin over superficial abscesses that require lancing or it can be used for taking skin biopsies. Additional sedation is usually required. EMLA cream also prevents head shaking in response to venepuncture of the marginal ear vein.

4.11 Fluid therapy

The principles of fluid therapy for rabbits are the same as in other species. The objective of fluid therapy is to restore blood volume and correct aberrations in plasma pH, glucose and electrolytes. Fluid replacement is required in conditions that cause loss of intracellular fluid and dehydration. Assessment of the degree of dehydration is a recognized procedure in dogs and cats (Schaer, 1989) and can be used in rabbits. Although there may be no obvious fluid loss in vomit or diarrhoea, rabbits with digestive disorders such as intestinal obstruction or gut stasis can rapidly become dehydrated. Saliva is constantly secreted and normal gastrointestinal motility is required to maintain water absorption and excretion along the digestive tract (see Figure 1.2). Mild gastrointestinal hypomotility can be compared with the dog with gastroenteritis and the degree of dehydration estimated at approximately 5%. Dry mucous membranes and decreased skin turgor suggest a 5–8% degree of dehydration. Marked degree of decreased skin turgor, dry mucous membranes, a fast, weak pulse, slow capillary refill time and mental depression indicate a 10–12% degree of dehydration. Mental depression associated with dehydration and electrolyte imbalance is marked in rabbits and often exacerbated by abdominal pain caused by a distended viscus such as a gas-filled stomach, caecum or loop of intestine. Packed cell volume (PCV) measurement is a useful assessment of hydration status. The haematocrit of a hydrated pet rabbit is approximately 32–40% (Harcourt-Brown and Baker, 2001). Values of 45–50% are indicative of dehydration. Obviously there are many other diseases and physiological factors that can affect the haematocrit and so the PCV should be considered in conjunction with other parameters.

4.11.1 Choice of fluid therapy for rabbits

The complex secretion and absorption of water and electrolytes along the digestive tract results in rapid dehydration and electrolyte imbalance if digestive function is altered. In rabbits, there are many digestive disorders that are life threatening due to their effect on electrolyte and water balance. For example, a feature of intestinal obstruction in rabbits is gastric dilatation and the presence of excessive fluid in the stomach and small intestine. This situation is analogous to gastric dilatation/volvulus in dogs and the effects on electrolyte balances and blood pH are profound. In the ideal world, blood pH and electrolytes would be monitored but, in reality, immediate facilities for measuring these parameters are often unavailable and the electrolyte and acid–base status of the patient remains speculative. Analysers such as the I-Stat (Heska) are extremely useful to measure electrolytes and other critical parameters and assist the selection of fluid therapy.

Rabbits cannot vomit and metabolic alkalosis is unlikely. Acidosis is a major problem due to the limited ability of the rabbit kidney to excrete excess hydrogen ions (see Section 1.6.5). Ketoacidosis develops during periods of anorexia. Hepatic lipidosis is a significant and serious complication of anorexia especially in obese animals. Although parenteral glucose can be useful to restore blood glucose levels in the early stages of anorexia, in the later stages, glucose can stimulate synthesis of triglycerides in the liver and may further compromise hepatic lipid metabolism. The safest choice of fluid for most situations is lactated Ringer's or Hartmann's solution.

4.11.2 Blood transfusion

Blood transfusion is feasible in the rabbit. The circulating blood volume of a rabbit is 55–65 ml/kg (Gillett, 1994) and up to 10% of this amount can be lost without untoward effect. Above 20–25% loss results in shock. Ideally whole blood is required to replace the loss. Blood can be obtained from a donor and cross-matching is not required in the first instance (Flecknell, 1996). The jugular vein is the most satisfactory site for collection as rabbit blood clots quickly and problems can be encountered collecting blood from smaller peripheral veins. Fentanyl/fluanisone is a good sedative for this procedure. Other agents such as medetomidine are peripheral vasoconstrictors that can make blood collection difficult. Citrate anticoagulant can be collected from a human blood collection pack and diluted 1:3.5 with donor blood. It is preferable to use the blood within 4–6 h, as platelet function and red cell viability are likely to be well maintained for this period (Flecknell, 1996). One percent of the donor's weight in blood can be safely collected (10 ml/kg). Blood should be replaced at a rate of 6–12 ml/kg/h. Colloidal plasma volume expanders (Haemaccell, Hoechst, or Gelofusine, Arnolds) can be used to prevent hypovolaemic shock if donor blood is unavailable.

4.11.3 Route of delivery

The route of fluid delivery depends on the patient's physical condition, state of dehydration and temperament. Oral fluid therapy is useful in rabbits. Oral rehydration fluids can be given instead of water and are useful to maintain a supply of electrolytes in rabbits that are suffering from diarrhoea. Products formulated for dogs or cats can be used (e.g. Lectade, Pfizer). They can be administered by syringe feeding, stomach or nasogastric tube (see Section 3.13).

Subcutaneous fluids can be used for animals that are mildly dehydrated. This route is not suitable for ill, dehydrated or hypotensive patients as absorption of fluids from under the skin is poor when peripheral tissue perfusion is reduced in shocked or hypovolaemic patients. Many veterinary surgeons routinely give a prophylactic subcutaneous bolus of fluids perioperatively. Isotonic fluids should be used and warmed prior to use. A reservoir of cold fluid beneath the skin increases the risk of hypothermia in the anaesthetized patient.

Some practitioners favour intraperitoneal injections. The technique is described in Section 3.12.4.5. Again, it is important to warm the fluids. Hypertonic solutions should not be used, as they will add to any dehydration that the animal is suffering. Intraperitoneal injections are contraindicated in cases of abdominal sepsis, ascites or peritonitis and are not advisable for animals that are about to undergo abdominal surgery.

Ideally, fluid therapy should be given intravenously. Blood volume and blood pressure are restored in addition to a rapid supply of electrolytes. The intraosseous route can also be used in small individuals or rabbits that are moribund with collapsed veins that are hard to find. The sites and techniques for intravenous and intraosseous therapy are described in Section 3.12.4 and illustrated in Figure 3.8. The rate of administration and amount of fluids depends on the degree of dehydration and the physical state of the patient. In most instances a rate of 10–20 ml/kg/h for the first 2 h followed by 100 ml/kg/day will satisfactorily rehydrate the animal. Subcutaneous and intravenous fluids can be given simultaneously. Fluids should be warmed prior to administration. Care should be taken to calculate the amount of fluid required and avoid overloading the circulation. A syringe driver or similar device that administers a measured quantity of fluid is useful. It is important to keep the patient free from pain and stress as far as possible. The catecholamine release that results from

Key points 4.3

- Due the constant absorption and excretion of fluid and electrolytes along the gastrointestinal tract, rabbits can become dehydrated without obvious fluid loss. Fluid replacement therapy is an important part of treatment for most digestive disorders
- A haematocrit of 45–50% is indicative of dehydration
- The safest choice of fluid for most situations is lactated Ringer's or Hartmann's solution
- Although oral and subcutaneous fluids can be given as a source of water and electrolytes, intravenous or intraosseous fluid therapy is often necessary to restore blood volume and blood pressure
- Blood transfusion is feasible in rabbits. Cross-matching is not required for the first transfusion. Citrate collected from a human blood collection pack can be diluted 1:3.5 with donor blood. It is safe to collect 10 ml/kg of blood from a donor
- As a general rule, intravenous fluid therapy can be given at 25 ml/kg/h for first 2 h followed by 100 ml/kg/day
- Stress can cause oliguria, so it is important to keep rabbits stress free and not overload the circulation during fluid therapy.

stress or pain can result in a marked and prolonged reduction in renal plasma flow and filtration and cause oliguria and death (Brod and Sirota, 1949).

References

Ali, B.H. (1990). The effect of ivermectin on some haematological indices in rabbits: influence of vitamin K treatment (Abstract). *Clin Exp Pharmac Physiol.*, **17**, 735–738.

Arafa, M.A., Wanas, M.Q. (1996). The efficacy of ivermectin in treating rabbits experimentally infected with *Eimeria* as indicated parasitologically and histologically (Abstract). *J Egypt Soc Parasitol.*, **26**, 773–780.

Behrens-Baumann, W. (1996). Absorption of topically administered ciprofloxacin, ofloxacin, and gentamicin in the inflamed rabbit eye (Abstract). *Ophthalmologica*, **210**, 119–122.

Bertaccini, G., Poli, E., Adami, M., Coruzzi G. (1983). Effect of some new H_2-receptor antagonists on gastrointestinal motility (Abstract). *Agents Actions*, **13**, 157–162.

Bishop, Y.M. (1998). *The Veterinary Formulary*, 4th edn. Royal Pharmaceutical Society of Great Britain and British Veterinary Association.

Blood, D.C., Studdert, V.P. (1999). *Saunders Comprehensive Veterinary Dictionary*, 2nd edn. W.B. Saunders.

Brewer, N.R. and Cruise, L.J. (1994). Physiology. In *The Biology of the Laboratory Rabbit*, 2nd edn. (P.J. Manning, D.H. Ringler, C.E. Newcomer, eds). pp 63–70. Academic Press.

Brod, J., Sirota, J.H. (1949). Effects of emotional disturbance on water diuresis and renal blood flow in the rabbit. *Am J Physiol.*, **157**, 31–39.

Broome R.L., Brooks D.L., Babish J.G. *et al.* (1991). Pharmacokinetic properties of enrofloxacin in rabbits. *Am J Vet Res.*, **52**, 1835–1841.

Brown, S.A. (1998). *BSAVA Specialist Session Course notes.* British Small Animal Veterinary Association.

Butson, R.J., Schramme, M.C., Garlick, M.H., Davies, J.V. (1996). Treatment of intrasynovial infection with gentamicin-impregnated polymethylmethacrylate beads. *Vet Rec.*, **138**, 460–464.

Cady, W.J., Rehder, T.L., Campbell, J. (1979). Use of cholestyramine in the treatment of digitoxin toxicity (Abstract). *Am J Hosp Pharm.*, **36**, 92–94.

Carman, R.J. (1993). Antibiotic associated diarrhea of rabbits. *J Small Exotic Anim Med.*, **2**, 69–71.

Carman, R.J. (1994). Clostridial enteropathies of rabbits. *J Small Exotic Anim Med.*, **2**, 179–181.

Carman, R.J., Borriello, S.P. (1984). Infectious nature of *Clostridium spiroforme*-mediated rabbit enterotoxaemia. *Vet Microbiol.*, **9**, 497–502.

Carman, R.J., Wilkins, T.D. (1991). *In vitro* susceptibility of rabbit strains of *Clostridium spiroforme* to antimicrobial agents. *Vet Microbiol.*, **28**, 391–397.

Chadwick, A.J. (1997). Use of a 0.25% fipronil pump spray formulation to treat canine cheyletiellosis. *J Small Anim Pract.*, **38**, 261–262.

Chappell, S. (1994). The rabbit abscess and antirobe. *Antirobe In-Focus. Magazine* produced by Upjohn Ltd, Animal Health Division, Crawley, West Sussex, RH10 2LZ.

Collins, B.R. (1995). Antimicrobial drug use in rabbits, rodents and other small mammals. *Proceedings of symposium on Antimicrobial Therapy and The North American Veterinary Conference, Orlando.*

Cooper, P.E., Penaliggon, J. (1997). Use of frontline spray on rabbits. *Vet Rec.*, **140**, 535–536.

CRC Desk Reference of Clinical Pharmacology. (1998). CRC Press.

Cunliffe-Beamer, T.L., Fox, R.R. (1981). Venereal spirochaetosis of rabbits: Epizootology. *Lab Anim Sci.*, **31**, 366–382.

Curtis, S.K., Housley, R., Brooks, D.L. (1990). Use of ivermectin for treatment of ear mite infestation in rabbits. *J Am Vet Med Assoc.*, **196**, 1139–1140.

Cutler, S.L. (1998). Ectopic *Psoroptes cuniculi* infestation in a pet rabbit. *J Small Anim Pract.*, **39**, 86–87.

De Blas, E., Gidenne, T. (1998) Digestion of starch and sugars. In *The Nutrition of the Rabbit.* (C. de Blas and J.Wiseman, eds). pp 17–38. CABI Publishing.

Deeb, B. (1992). Pain and analgesia in rabbits. *Rabbit Health News*, **5**, 1–2.

Depoortere, I., Peeters, T.L., Vantrappen, G. (1991). Motilin receptors of the rabbit colon (Abstract). *Peptides*, **12**, 89–94.

El-Sayad, Y.M., al-Meshai, M.A., al-Angary, A.A. *et al.* (1994). The effect of colestipol and cholestyramine on the systemic clearance of intravenous ibuprofen in rabbits (Abstract). *J Pharm Pharmacol.*, **46**, 73–75.

Elliott, J. (1998). Logical antibacterial drug prescribing – the theory behind the practice. *CPD Vet Med.*, **1**, 55–60.

Engelhardt, G., Homma, D., Schlegel, K. *et al.* (1996). General pharmacology of meloxicam – Part 1: Effects on CNS, gastric emptying, intestinal transport, water, electrolyte and creatinine excretion (Abstract). *Gen Pharmacol.*, **27**, 673–677.

Escoula, L., Camguilhem, R., Larrieu, G., More, J. (1981). Sensibility of rabbits to treatment with ampicillin and gentamycin (English Abstract, article in French). *Ann Rech Vet.*, **12**, 1–17.

Evans, R.P., Nelson, C.L. (1993). Gentamicin impregnated polymethyl methacrylate beads compared with systemic antibiotic therapy in the treatment of chronic osteomyelitis. *Clin Orthopaed Rel Res.*, **295**, 37–42.

Feaga, W.P. (1997). Wry neck in rabbits. *J Am Vet Med Assoc.*, **210**, 480.

FitzSimons, H. (1999). Cisapride. *Compendium of Continuing Education*, **21**, 324–326.

Flecknell, P.A. (1996). Anaesthetic management. In *Laboratory Animal Anaesthesia.* pp 75–101. Academic Press.

Flecknell, P.A. (1998). Developments in the veterinary care of rabbits and rodents. *In Practice*, **20**, 286–295.

Franssen, F.F.J., Lumiej, J.T., Van Knapen, F. (1995).

Susceptibilty of *Encephalitozoon cuniculi* to several drugs *in vitro*. *Antimicrob Agents Chemother.*, **39**, 1265–1268.

Gaertner, D.J. (1991). Comparison of penicillin and gentamycin for treatment of pasteurellosis in rabbits. *Lab Anim Sci.*, **41**, 78–79.

Gager, W.E., Elsasa, F.J., Smith, J.L. (1969). Ocular penetration of cephalexin in the rabbit. *Br J Ophthalmol.*, **53**, 403–406.

Gfeller, R.W., Messonnier, S.P. (1997). *Handbook of Small Animal Toxicology and Poisonings*. Mosby.

Gillett, C.S. (1994). Selected drug dosages and clinical reference data. In *The Biology of the Laboratory Rabbit*, 2nd edn. (P.J. Manning, D.H. Ringler, C.E. Newcomer, eds). pp 468–472. Academic Press.

Guandalini, S., Fasano, A., Migliavacca, M. *et al.* (1988). Pathogenesis of postantibiotic diarrhoea caused by *Clostridium difficile*: an *in vitro* study in the rabbit intestine (Abstract). *Gut*, **29**, 598–602.

Guillot, P., Sanders, P., Mourot D. (1988). Pharmacokinetic study of chloramphenicol in the rabbit (Article in French, English abstract). *Ann Rech Vet.*, **19**, 27–33.

Hack, R.J., Walstrom, D.J., Hair, J.A. (2001). Efficacy and safety of two different dose rates of selamectin against naturally acquired infestations of *Psoroptes cuniculi* in rabbits. *Scientific Proceedings of British Small Animal Association Congress 2001*, p. 552.

Hall, J.A., Washabau, R.J. (1997). Gastrointestinal prokinetic therapy: dopaminergic antagonistic drugs. *Compendium of Continuing Education*, **19**, 214–220.

Hara-Kudo, Y., Mirshita, Y., Nagaoka, Y. *et al.* (1996). Incidence of diarrhoea with antibiotics and increase of Clostridia in rabbits. *J Vet Med Sci.*, **12**, 1181–1185.

Harcourt-Brown, F.M. (1997). Diagnosis, treatment and prognosis of dental disease in pet rabbits. *In Practice*, **19**, 407–421.

Harcourt-Brown, F.M., Baker, S.J. (2001). Parathyroid hormone, haematological and biochemical parameters in relation to dental disease and husbandry in pet rabbits. *J Small Anim Pract.*, **42**, 130–136.

Harkness, J.E., Wagner, J.E. (1995). *The Biology and Medicine of Rabbits and Rodents*, 4th edn. Williams and Wilkins.

Harvey, C. (1997). Abscesses in rabbits. In *Rabbit Medicine and Procedures for Practitioners Program and Abstracts*, House Rabbit Society Veterinary Conference.

Hinton, M. (1980). Gastric ulceration in the rabbit. *J Comp Path.*, **90**, 475–481.

Hollister, A.G., Cheeke, P.R., Robinson, K.L., Patton. N.M. (1989). Effects of water-administered and acidifiers on growth, feed conversion and enteritis mortality of weanling rabbits. *J Appl Rabbit Res.*, **12**, 143–147.

Hollister, A.G., Cheeke, P.R., Robinson, K.L., Patton, N.M. (1990). Effects of dietary probiotics and acidifiers on performance of weanling rabbits. *J Appl Rabbit Res.*, **13**, 6–9.

Huang, S.M., Huang, Y.C., Chiou, W.L. (1981). Oral absorption and presystemic first-pass effect of chlorpheniramine in rabbits (Abstract). *J Pharmacokinet Biopharm.*, **9**, 725–738.

Hutchinson, M.J., Jacobs, D.E., Bell, G.D., Mencke, N. (2001). Evaluation of imidacloprid for the prevention of cat flea (*Ctenocephalides felis felis*) infestations on rabbits. *Veterinary Record*, **148**, 695–696.

Jaslow, B.W., Ringler, D.H., Rush, H.G., Glorioso, J.C. (1981). Pasteurella associated rhinitis of rabbits: Efficacy of penicillin therapy. *Lab Anim Sci.*, **31**, 382–385.

Jenkins, J.R. (1997). Gastrointestinal diseases. In *Ferrets, Rabbits and Rodents, Clinical Medicine and Surgery*. (E.V. Hillyer, K.E. Quesenberry, eds). pp 176–188. W.B. Saunders.

Jilge, B., Meyer, H. (1975). Coprophagy dependent changes of the anaerobic bacterial flora in the stomach and small intestine of the rabbit (cited by Straw, 1988). *Z versuchstierkd*, **17**, 308–314.

Kim, C.S., Buchmiller, T.L., Fonkalsrud, E.W., Phillips, J.D. (1993). The effect of anabolic steroids on ameliorating the adverse effects of chronic corticosteroids on intestinal anastomotic healing in rabbits (Abstract). *Surg Gynecol Obstet.*, **176**, 373–379.

Kounensis, G., Koutsoviti-Papadopoulou, M., Elezoglou, A., Voutsas. A. (1992). Comparative study of the H_2 antagonists cimetidene, ranitidine, famotidine, and nazatidine on the rabbit stomach fundus and sigmoid colon (Abstract). *J Pharmacobiodyn.* **15**, 561–565.

Langer, J.C., Bramlett, G. (1997). Effects of prokinetic agents on ileal contractility in a rabbit model of gastroschisis (Abstract). *J Paediatr Surg.*, **32**, 605–608.

Laval, A. (1990). Choix de l'anti-infectieux chez le lapin d'agrement (Article in French). *Rec Med Vet.*, **167**, 375–379.

Lee, M., Kallal, S.M., Feldman, M. (1996). Omeprazole prevents indomethacin-induced gastric ulcers in rabbits (Abstract). *Aliment Pharmacol Ther.*, **10**, 571–576.

Li, T., Qiao G.L., Hu G.Z. *et al.* (1995). Comparative plasma and tissue pharmacokinetics and drug residue profiles of different chemotherapeutants in fowls and rabbits (Abstract). *J Vet Pharmacol Ther.*, **18**, 260–273.

Lipman, N.S., Weischedel, A.K., Connors, M.J. *et al.* (1992). Utilization of cholestyramine resin as a preventive treatment for antibiotic (Clindamycin) induced enterotoxaemia in the rabbit. *Lab Anim.*, **26**, 1–8.

Lucore, C.L., McDonald, M.I., Wharton, M., Durack, D.T. (1986). Experimental anaerobic liver abscess: observations on treatment (Abstract). *Liver*, **6**, 125–132.

Mader, J.T., Adams, K., Morrison, L. (1989). Comparative evaluation of cefazolin and clindamycin in the treatment of experimental *Staphylococcal aureus* osteomyelitis in rabbits. *Antimicrob Agents Chemother.*, **33**, 1760–1764.

Mähler, M., Stunkel, S., Ziegowski, C., Kunstyr, I. (1995). Inefficacy of enrofloxacin in the elimination of Pasteurella multocida in rabbits. *Lab Anim.*, **29**, 192–199.

Maiers, J.D., Mason, S.J., Griffin H.C. (1984). Lincomycin-associated enterocolitis in rabbits. *J Am Vet Med Assoc.*, **185**, 670–671.

Malley, A.D. (1995). Rabbits. *Lecture notes for BSAVA Continuing Education Course* 24.11.95.

Manning, P.J., Digiacomo, R.F., Delong, D. (1989). Pasteurellosis in laboratory animals. In *Pasteurella and Pasteurellosis.* (C. Adlam, J.M. Rutter, eds). pp 264–289. Academic Press.

Marangos, M.N., Onyeji, C.O., Nicolau, D.P., Nightingale, C.H. (1995). Disposition kinetics of aspirin in female New Zealand White rabbits. *Lab Anim Sci.*, **45**, 67–69.

McElroy, D.E., Ravis, W.R., Clark, C.H. (1987). Pharmacokinetics of oxytetracycline in rabbits (Abstract) *Am J Res.*, **48**, 1261–1263.

McKay, S.G., Morck, D.W., Merrill, J.K. *et al.* (1996). Use of tilmicosin for pasteurellosis in rabbits. *Am J Vet Res.*, **57**, 1180–1184.

McKellar, Q.A., Midgley. D.M., Galbraith, E.A. *et al.* (1992). Clinical and pharmacological properties of ivermectin in rabbits and guinea pigs. *Vet Rec.*, **130**, 71–73.

Michiels, M, Monbaliu, J, Hendriks, R. *et al.* (1987). Pharmacokinetics and tissue distribution of the new gastrokinetic agent cisapride in rat, rabbit and dog (Abstract). *Arzneimittelforschung*, **37**, 1159–1167.

Milhaud, G., Renault, L., Vaissaire, J., Maire, C. (1976). Sensibilite du Lapin a l'ampicilline (Article in French). *Rec Med Vet.*, **152**, 843–847.

Monk, B. (1995). Safe prescription and use of topical steroids. *Dermatology in Practice.* March/April 1995 14–17.

More, R.C., Kody, M.H., Kabo, J.M. *et al.* (1989). The effects of two nonsteroidal anti-inflammatory drugs on limb swelling, joint stiffness and bone torsional strength following fracture in a rabbit model (Abstract). *Clin Orthop.*, **247**, 306–312.

Morisse, J.P. (1978). Induction d'une enterite de type colibacillaire chez le lapin. *Revue Med Vet.*, **129**, 625–632.

Morris, T.H. (2000) Therapeutics. In *Manual of Rabbit Medicine and Surgery.* (P.A. Flecknell, ed.). British Small Animal Veterinary Association pp. 89–101.

Morrisey, J.K. (1996). Parasites of ferrets, rabbits and rodents. *Sem Avian Exotic Pet Med.*, **5**, 106–114.

Nicolau, D.P., Freeman, C.D., Nightingale, C.H., Quintiliani, R. (1993). Pharmacokinetics of minocycline and vancomycin in rabbits. *Lab Anim Sci.*, **43**, 222–225.

Norden, C.W., Budinsky, A. (1990). Treatment of experimental chronic osteomyelitis due to staphylococcus aureus with ampicillin/sulbactam. *J Infect Dis.*, **161**, 52–53.

Okerman, L., Devriese, L.A., Gevaert, D. *et al.* (1990). *In vivo* activity of orally administered antibiotics and chemotherapeutics against acute septicaemic pasteurellosis in rabbits. *Lab Anim.*, **24**, 341–344.

Parsonnet, J., Gillis, Z.A., Richter, A.G., Pier, G.B. (1987). A rabbit model of toxic shock syndrome that uses a constant, subcutaneous infusion of toxic shock syndrome toxin 1 (Abstract). *Infect Immun.*, **55**, 1070–1076.

Pairet, M., Bouyssou, T., Ruckesbuch, Y. (1986). Colonic formation of soft feces in rabbits: a role for endogenous prostaglandins. *Am J Physiol.*, **250**, G302–G308.

Penney, R.L., Folk, G.E., Galask, R.P., Petzold, C.R. (1986). The microflora of the alimentary tract of rabbits in relation to pH, diet and cold. *J Appl Rabbit Res.*, **9**, 152–156.

Percy, D.H., Black, W.D. (1988). Pharmacokinetics of tetracycline in the domestic rabbit following intravenous or oral administration. *Can J Vet Res.*, **52**, 5–11.

Perkins, S.E., Fox, J.G., Taylor, N.S. *et al.* (1995). Detection of *Clostridium difficile* toxins from the small intestine and cecum of rabbits with naturally acquired enterotoxaemia. *Lab Ani. Sci.*, **45**, 379–447.

Rateau, J.G., Brouillard, M., Morgant, G., Aymard, P. (1986). Experimental study in the rabbit of the effect of cholestyramine in the treatment of infectious diarrhoea caused by cholera. (English Abstract, Article in French). *Ann Gastroenterol Hepatol. (Paris)*, **22**, 289–296.

Redfern, J.S., Lin, H.J., McArthur, K.E. *et al.* (1991). Gastric acid and pepsin secretion in conscious rabbits. *Am J Physiol.*, **261**, G295–G304.

Rehg, J.E., You-Shoung, L. (1981). *Clostridium difficile* colitis in a rabbit following antibiotic therapy for pasteurellosis. *J Am Vet Med Assoc.*, **179**, 1296–1297.

Saijonmaa-Koulumies, L., Parson, E., Lloyd, D.H. (1998). Elimination of *Staphylococcus intermedius* in healthy dogs by topical treatment with fusidic acid. *J Small Anim Pract.*, **39**, 341–347.

Schaer, M. (1989). General priciples of fluid therapy. *Vet Clin N Am; Small Anim Pract.*, **19**, 203–213.

Schröder, C., Matthes, S., Löliger, H. (1982). Untersuchungen über die verträglichkiet oraler antibiotikamedikation beim kaninchen. *Kleintierpraxis*, **27**, 221–268.

Sharpnack, D.D., Mastin, J.P., Childress, C.P., Henningsen, G.M. (1994). Quinolone arthropathy in juvenile New Zealand White rabbits (Abstract). *Lab Anim Sci.*, **44**, 436–442.

Short, C.R., Barker, S.A., Hsieh, L.C. *et al.* (1988). Disposition of fenbendazole in the rabbit. *Res Vet Sci.*, **44**, 215–219.

Simopoulos, C., Kouskoukis, C., Polychronides, A., Bezirtzoglou, E. (1994). Effect of different combinations of antibiotics on experimental septic peritonitis in rabbits (Abstract). *Int J Clin Lab Res.*, **24**, 167–170.

Sneddon, I.B. (1976). Clinical use of topical corticosteroids. *Drugs*, **11**, 193–199.

Stei, P., Kruss, B., Weiglab, J., Trach, V. (1996). Local tissue tolerability of meloxicam, a new NSAID; indications for parenteral, dermal and mucosal administration. (Abstract). *Br J Rheumatol.*, **35**, 44–50.

Steinleitner, A., Lambert, H., Kazensky, C. *et al.* (1990). Reduction of primary postoperative adhesion formation under calcium channel blockade in the rabbit. *J Surg Res.*, **48**, 42–45.

Straw, T.E. (1988). Bacteria of the rabbit gut and their role in the health of the rabbit. *J Appl Rabbit Res.*, **11**, 142–146.

Suckow, M.A., Martin, B.J., Bowersock, T.L., Douglas, F.A. (1996). Derivation of *Pasteurella multocida*-free rabbit litters by enrofloxacin treatment (Abstract). *Vet Microbiol.*, **51**, 161–168.

Suter, C., Müller-Doblies, U.U., Hatt, J.-M., Deplazes, P. (2001). Prevention and treatment of *Encephalitozoon cuniculi* in rabbits with fenbendazole. *Veterinary Record*, **148**, 478–480.

Taylor, P.B., Burd, E.M., Tabbara, K.F. (1987). Corneal and intraocular penetration of topical and subconjunctival fusidic acid (Abstract). *Br J Ophthalmol.*, **71**, 598–601.

Thilsted, J.P., Newton, W.P., Crandell, R.A., Bevill, R.F. (1981). Fatal diarrhoea in rabbits resulting from the feeding of antibiotic contaminated feed. *J Am Vet Hosp Assoc.*, **179**, 360–361.

Van Bijsterveld, O.P., Andriesse, H., Neilsen, B.H. (1987). Fusidic acid in tear fluid: pharmacokinetic study with fusidic acid viscous eye drops (Abstract). *Eur J Drug Met Pharmacokinet.*, **12**, 215–218.

Verde, M.T., Piquer, J.G. (1986). Effect of stress on the cortisone and ascorbic acid content of the blood plasma of rabbits. *J Appl Rabbit Res.*, **9**, 181–182.

Wallace, J.L., McKnight, G.W. (1993). Characterisation of a simple animal model for nonsteroidal anti-inflammatory drug induced antral ulcer (Abstract). *Can J Physiol Pharmacol.*, **71**, 447–452.

Washabau, R.J., Hall, J.A. (1997). Gastrointestinal prokinetic therapy: Serotonergic drugs. *Compendium of Continuing Education*, **19**, 473– 479.

Weiss, L.M., Michalakakis, E., Coyle, C.M. *et al.* (1994). The *in vitro* activity of albendazole against *Encephalitozoon cuniculi. J Eukaryotic Microbiol.*, **41**, 65S.

Welch, W.D., Lu, Y.S., Bawdon, R.E. (1987). Pharmacokinetics of penicillin-G in serum and nasal washings of *Pasteurella multocida* free and infected rabbits. *Lab Anim Sci.*, **37**, 65–68.

Whittem, T., Gaon, D. (1998). Principles of microbial therapy. *Vet Clin N Am: Small anim pract.*, **28**, 197–211.

Wright, F.C., Riner, J.C. (1985). Comparative efficacy of injection routes and doses of ivermectin against Psoroptes in rabbits (Abstract). *Am J Vet Res.*, **46**, 752–754.

Zenoble, R.D, Kemppainen, R.J. (1987). Adrenocortical suppression by topically applied corticosteroids in healthy dogs. *J Am Vet Med Assoc.*, **191**, 685–688.

Anaesthesia and analgesia

5

5.1 Problems associated with anaesthetizing rabbits

Anaesthetizing rabbits is perceived by many vets and owners as a high-risk procedure and it is usually the anaesthetic agent that is blamed for any problems that occur, despite the inherent safety of most of the present day drugs. There are other factors that can affect anaesthetic risk, especially in rabbits. Stress, hypoxia and pre-existing disease are the biggest threats, especially if more than one of these factors is present in the same animal (see Box 5.1).

Box 5.1 Problems associated with rabbit anaesthesia

There are three main problems associated with rabbit anaesthesia. Anaesthetic safety can be improved by considering the following risk factors and taking steps to minimize them.

Stress that can be caused by:

- Unfamiliar surroundings
- Transport to surgery
- Loud noises
- Proximity of predators
- Rough handling
- Restraint
- Pain due to dental disease, gastrointestinal disease, surgery
- Surgical intervention

Hypoxia that can be caused by:

- Anaesthetic agents causing a drop in oxygen tension
- Respiratory depression
- Breath holding
- Poor positioning causing occlusion of the airway or increased weight of viscera on diaphragm
- Pre-existing lung disease
- Firm restraint around chest

NB Rabbits are prone to hypoxia due to their small lung capacity and restricted nasopharynx, especially in short nosed breeds. Their tidal volume is 4–6 ml/kg

Pre-existing disease such as:

- Dental disease that can cause pain, malnutrition and salivation
- Lung disease caused by pasteurellosis
- Dehydration or electrolyte imbalances caused by gastrointestinal disease or excessive salivation

These factors predispose to cardiac arrest during surgery and gut stasis leading to the development of fatal hepatic lipidosis in the days following surgery.

Anaesthetic safety can be improved by:

- Providing food until a few of hours before anaesthesia. Rabbits do not need to be fasted. They cannot vomit
- Providing a quiet secluded environment with familiar bedding material (hay) for rabbits awaiting or recovering from surgery
- Quiet, gentle handling
- Induction of anaesthesia with injectable agents to avoid breath holding in response to the smell of anaesthetic vapours
- Gradual introduction of volatile agents to prevent breath holding
- Careful positioning to ensure an unobstructed airway and taking the weight of the viscera away from the diaphragm
- The administration of oxygen throughout anaesthesia. Endotracheal intubation if possible
- Routine use of effective analgesia for *all* rabbits undergoing surgery
- Careful anaesthetic monitoring
- Providing tempting food in the postoperative period to restore appetite and stimulate gut motility. Fresh grass and vegetables will tempt most rabbits to eat and provide a source of indigestible fibre.

It is vital that owners are advised to make certain that their rabbit is eating and passing hard faeces in the 24–48 h following surgery. If not, it should be brought back for treatment.

Loud noises, unfamiliar surroundings and the sight, smell or sound of predators is stressful to rabbits that are awaiting or recovering from surgery. Restraint causes endogenous catecholamine release that can cause cardiac arrhythmias. Pain is especially stressful. It reduces appetite, slows gut motility and can lead to gut stasis and the ultimate development of fatal hepatic lipidosis. Rabbits appear to be particularly susceptible to the effects of pain after surgical intervention, especially after abdominal surgery and incisor removal.

Hypoxia can easily develop in rabbits. Their lung capacity is small (see Figures 10.9 and 13.3). Endotracheal intubation is difficult. The anatomy of the mouth, nasopharynx and trachea does not lend itself to visualization of the mucous membranes, nasopharynx or larynx (see Figure 3.9). The conformation of the short nosed breeds, such as the Netherland Dwarf, can impair respiratory function and gas exchange. The tidal volume of rabbits is only 4–6 ml/kg (Gillett, 1994) and the lungs occupy a small volume in comparison with the abdominal contents. Inspiratory and expiratory movement is primarily due to movement of the diaphragm rather than the actions of the intercostal muscles. Positioning anaesthetized rabbits with the weight of the abdominal viscera against the diaphragm can interfere with respiratory movement. Pre-existing lung disease, e.g. from *Pasteurella multocida* infection, can compromise alveolar gas exchange. In addition to these problems, the response of a lightly anaesthetized rabbit to the smell of an anaesthetic vapour is to hold its breath. Apnoea is associated with bradycardia and hypercapnia. In a study by Flecknell *et al.* (1996), a period of apnoea lasting between 30 seconds and 2 minutes was the response to both isoflurane and halothane delivered either by mask or in an induction chamber. Some anaesthetic agents (e.g. medetomidine/ketamine) induce a fall in arterial oxygen tension (Hellebrekers *et al.*, 1997) and add to the risk of hypoxia.

Many rabbits that are undergoing general anaesthesia are not healthy. Dental problems or gastrointestinal disturbances can result in malnourishment and debility. Some rabbits with dental problems salivate profusely, which results in dehydration and electrolyte loss. Obese rabbits have high resting heart rates and can develop hypertension and cardiac hypertrophy (Carroll *et al.*, 1996). Hyperinsulinaemia, hyperglycaemia and elevated serum triglycerides occur in obese rabbits and hepatic lipidosis develops readily after short periods without food, especially if the rabbit is stressed. Obese rabbits are poor surgical candidates.

Even apparently healthy rabbits can be suffering from latent infections such as pasteurellosis or encephalitozoonosis. Congenital heart defects, such as ventricular septal defects, occur and cardiomyopathy is sometimes present, especially in giant breeds such as the French lop (see colour plate 30). Repeated anaesthesia with ketamine/xylazine infusion has been linked with heart disease and death. Marini *et al.* (1999) postulated that repeated episodes of hypoxaemia lead to cell death and necrosis resulting in myocardial fibrosis. The rabbit has limited collateral myocardial circulation and is therefore predisposed to ischaemia by vasoconstriction

5.2 Reducing anaesthetic risk in rabbits

Clinical examination prior to anaesthesia gives an idea of the general health status of the rabbit. Some debilitated patients need nutritional support prior to anaesthesia. Dehydrated, shocked or hypotensive patients require intravenous or intraosseous fluid therapy. Rabbits cannot vomit so pre-anaesthetic fasting is not required, although a short starvation period of 1–2 h is required to ensure the mouth is empty and the stomach is not overfull.

An accurate weight is required to calculate the dosages of drugs that are to be used. The amount of digesta in the gastrointestinal tract fluctuates throughout the day and influences bodyweight. Rabbits can have large amounts of food in their digestive tract, especially in the caecum. Fasting reduces bodyweight but does not necessarily reduce the amount of medication that is required. Fat animals require lower dose rates than thin ones. Because of these considerations, some authors advocate calculating dosages on metabolic body size i.e. $W_{kg}^{0.75}$ (Aeschbacher, 1995).

Stress levels can be reduced by the provision of a quiet, secluded kennel both before and after anaesthesia. Long periods without food and water, confined in a carrier can be stressful. If facilities are available, a cage with familiar bedding (i.e. hay) is beneficial postoperatively and may be necessary preoperatively if there is a long delay between admission and surgery. Ideally, rabbits awaiting or recovering from anaesthesia should be kept away from predators such as dogs, cats, ferrets or raptors. Quiet, gentle handling reduces stress levels in rabbits. A tight grip around the chest or throat can compromise respiratory function.

Good anaesthetic equipment, the correct range of drugs and an observant anaesthetist improve anaesthetic safety. Although anaesthetic monitoring equipment is advantageous, it cannot replace a human being who is closely observing the patient. During anaesthesia, the risk of hypoxia is reduced by positioning the patient so the airway is unimpeded and the weight of the abdominal viscera is not against the diaphragm. Extending the neck and pulling the tongue out of the mouth not only allows the anaesthetist to observe the colour of the mucous membranes but also moves the base of the tongue away from the epiglottis and opens the airway. Careful observation by the anaesthetist ensures an unimpeded airway during surgical procedures. Respiratory effort is largely diaphragmatic and observation of shallow respiratory movements can be difficult. Drapes and surgeons can obscure the anaesthetist's view of the patient. If respiration monitors are not available, it can be difficult for the anaesthetist to be certain that the animal is breathing and cooperation between the surgeon and anaesthetist is required. Clear plastic drapes facilitate observation of respiratory movements during surgery.

Anaesthetized rabbits require the administration of oxygen throughout the anaesthetic period. A period of preoxygenation before masking down decreases the risk of hypoxia should breath holding occur. Oxygen can be delivered through a facemask, endotracheal tube, nasal tube or even a tube placed in the pharynx through the mouth.

As in other species, a balanced anaesthetic is required to permit surgery but can be difficult to achieve in rabbits. A light plane of anaesthesia not only causes breath holding in response to the volatile agent, but also results in movement or even 'screaming' in response to surgical stimuli. Screaming is an alarm response of rabbits to unpleasant stimuli and can occur during light anaesthesia. The patient maintains expiration for an alarming length of time and can become hypoxic or even cyanosed. The actual scream may not be audible, especially if the rabbit is intubated. The anaesthetist's reaction to the prolonged period of respiratory arrest is often to turn down the concentration of anaesthetic agent. The result is a lightening of anaesthesia and increased response to surgical stimuli. An increased concentration of the volatile agent is then required to deepen anaesthesia. If the rabbit is not intubated, the smell of the anaesthetic agent stimulates breath holding and failure to inhale the anaesthetic vapour and surgical anaesthesia is then difficult to achieve. The administration of additional quantities of injectable agents is possible, but undesirable because of the length of time for it to take effect and uncertainty about the required dose. This type of unsatisfactory anaesthetic can be overcome by using an injectable induction agent and maintaining anaesthesia with a volatile agent. The slow introduction of volatile gases prevents breath holding if a facemask is used. If anaesthesia is induced with a facemask, an effective premedicant is required. Endotracheal intubation overcomes the problem of breath holding. It also permits the continuous administration of oxygen and gives greater control of the depth of anaesthesia. Endotracheal intubation allows intermittent positive pressure ventilation if it is needed.

Good postoperative care and routine analgesia are important to reduce pain and stress, restore appetite and prevent the development of hepatic lipidosis.

5.3 Anaesthetic equipment

Specialized but simple anaesthetic equipment is required for rabbit anaesthesia. Clear facemasks permit observation of the colour of the nose and mucous membranes. A range of small, uncuffed endotracheal tubes (2.0–5.0 mm) are required for endotracheal intubation. Soft 3–4 f nasogastric catheters can be used for nasal intubation. Rabbits have a small tidal volume (4–6 ml/kg) and anaesthetic circuits with low dead space are

Table 5.1 Formulary for products used during anaesthesia

Disclaimer: There are very few products that are licensed for use in rabbits. The responsibility for the use of unlicensed products lies with the prescribing veterinary surgeon. The dose rates are based on the current state of knowledge, some dose rates are anecdotal. Products that hold a product licence in the UK for use in rabbits appear in **bold** type.

Preparation	*Dosage*	*Route/ frequency*	*Indication*	*Comment*
Acepromazine	0.5–1 mg/kg	IM, SC	Premedication	Not analgesic
Acepromazine + Butorphanol	0.5 mg/kg + 0.5 mg/kg	SC, IM	Sedation	Can be mixed in same syringe Vasodilatory
Adrenaline	20 μg/kg	SC, IV	Cardiac arrest	Some products need diluting from 1:1000 (1 mg/ml) to 1:10 000 (100 μg/ml) Can be given into the trachea
Atipamezole	1 mg/kg	SC, IM, IV		Reversal of medetomidene
Atropine	0.05 mg/kg (50 μg/kg)	IM	Premedication	40% rabbits produce atropinesterase that metabolises atropine so glycopyrrolate is preferable
Buprenorphine	0.01–0.05 mg/kg	IV, SC	Analgesia	Can be used to reverse the effects of fentanyl/fluanisone Analgesic effects last 6–12 h
Butorphanol	0.1–0.5 mg/kg	SC, IM, IV	Analgesic	Can be used in combination with acepromazine for sedation Can be used for pre-emptive analgesia medetomidine/ketamine Can be used to reverse effects of fentanyl/fluanisone Effects last 2–4 h
Carprofen	4 mg/kg 1.5 mg/kg	SC sid PO bid	Analgesia	Care in hypotensive patients Can be mixed with jam, fruit juice or syrup for oral administration Effects last 24 h
Diazepam	1–2 mg/kg	IV, IM	Sedation	Not analgesic
Doxapram	5 mg/kg	IM, IV	Respiratory stimulant	Effects last 15 minutes
Fentanyl/ fluanisone (Hypnorm, Janssen)	**0.2–0.3 ml/kg**	**IM**	**Premedication Sedation Anaesthesia Analgesia**	**Contains 0.315 mg/ml fentanyl citrate equivalent to 0.20 mg/ml fentanyl+10 mg/ml fluanisone Can be used in combination with midazolam or diazepam (0.5–2 mg/kg) Anaesthetic time: 20–40 mins Sleep time: 1–4 h**
Fluid therapy: intravenous subcutaneous	 10–20 ml/kg/h 10–15 ml/kg			 Warm before use
Glucose 5%	10 ml/kg	IV, SC	Anorexia Perioperatively	Warm before use
Glycopyrrolate	0.01 mg/kg 0.1 mg/kg	IV SC, IM	Premedication	Does not cross blood–brain barrier and cause mydriasis
Ketamine	25–50 mg/kg	IM	Sedation	Can be used in combination with other agents for anaesthesia
Ketamine + xylazine	35 mg/kg + 5 mg/kg	IM	Anaesthesia	Anaesthetic time: 20–30 min Sleep time: 1–2 h
Ketoprofen	1–3 mg/kg	SC bid	Analgesia	Care in hypotensive patients Lasts 12–24 h
Medetomidine	0.1–0.5 mg/kg	IM	Premedication or sedation	Not analgesic

Suggested combination:				
Medetomidine + Ketamine + Butorpanol	0.2 mg/kg + 10 mg/kg + 0.05 mg/kg	SC	Induction of anaesthesia	Can be mixed together and given in same syringe Doses can be increased to 0.25 mg/kg medetomidine + 0.15 mg/kg ketamine Anaesthetic time: 30–40 min Sleep time: 1–4 h
Midazolam	0.5–2 mg/kg	IV	Tranquillizer	Can be given IV to effect after premedication with fentanyl/fluanisone to induce anaesthesia Can be used as sole agent for sedation for minor procedures Precipitates in Hartmann's solution
Naloxone	10–100 μ/kg	IM, IV, IP	Opioid antagonist	Reverses the effects (including analgesia) of narcotic analgesics
Pethidine	5–10 mg/kg	SC or IM	Analgesic	Lasts 2–3 h

Abbreviations: sid: once daily; bid: twice daily; IM: intramuscular injection; IV: intravenous injection; SC: subcutaneous injection.

required. Paediatric connectors can be used to make up a Bain circuit or T-piece (Portex, Arnolds). Although a gag is not necessary for intubation, purpose-made rodent gag and cheek dilators are useful to visualize the oral cavity and pharynx. A laryngoscope with a small blade (0 or 1) can be used to visualize the larynx and aid intubation.

Pulse oximetry can be used as an adjunct to anaesthetic monitoring. The tongue is the best site for the sensor but is not always accessible, e.g. if the rabbit is undergoing dentistry or anaesthesia is maintained with a facemask. A satisfactory signal is sometimes found in either the pinna or the base of the tail if the hair is clipped off and a suitable sensor is available. A rectal probe may also be used. Poor peripheral perfusion in rabbits anaesthetized with medetomidine or ketamine may prevent a satisfactory signal. Respiration monitors can be used in larger rabbits but can prove unreliable in small breeds. Electrocardiography can be used for cardiac monitoring.

Rectal temperature is monitored with a standard thermometer or a digital thermometer with a remote sensor. A maximum/minimum digital thermometer with a remote sensor designed for measuring household indoor and outdoor environmental temperatures can be used. The sensor is lubricated and carefully inserted into the rectum permitting remote monitoring of body temperature throughout the anaesthetic period.

5.4 Drugs, analgesics and anaesthetic agents used in rabbit anaesthesia

A formulary of drugs used during rabbit anaesthesia is given in Table 5.1.

5.4.1 Controlled drugs

Many of the narcotic analgesics that are used in rabbits are drugs that are capable of being abused by humans and are classed as controlled drugs that are scheduled under UK law. Schedule 1 includes drugs such as cannabis and LSD that are not used therapeutically in either veterinary or human medicine. Schedule 2 drugs include fentanyl, pethidine, and morphine and require a written requisition signed by a veterinary surgeon to obtain the preparation from the wholesalers. A register must be maintained recording the purchase and supply of these drugs that are kept in a locked, immovable cabinet. Schedule 3 drugs include buprenorphine and barbiturates and also require a written requisition but transactions do not need to be recorded in a register. Buprenorphine needs to be kept in a locked cupboard. Some benzodiazepines, such as temazepam or diazepam, require a written requisition. It is advisable to keep all such preparations in a locked cupboard including butorphanol and ketamine, which are not included on the controlled drugs list.

5.4.2 Atropine and glycopyrrolate

Atropine and glycopyrrolate are anticholinergic agents that are used to reduce bronchial and salivary secretions and protect the heart from vagal inhibition. In rabbits, anticholinergics are not required as a routine premedicant, although they can be used to counteract the cardiovascular effects of xylazine during anaesthesia with a combination of xylazine and ketamine. About 40% of rabbits produce atropinesterase that rapidly breaks down atropine, so if an anticholinergic drug is required, glycopyrrolate is preferable. A potentially undesirable effect of anticholinergic agents is the reduction of gastrointestinal motility

5.4.3 'EMLA' cream

EMLA cream (Astra) is a topical preparation containing 2.5% lidocaine and 2.5% prilocaine that is supplied with an occlusive dressing to place over the cream while the local anaesthetic takes effect. The cream can be applied to the marginal ear vein to provide local anaesthesia of full thickness skin and prevents the rabbit shaking its head and dislodging the needle in response to venepuncture (Flecknell, 1998a). EMLA cream takes 45–60 minutes to become effective.

5.4.4 Acepromazine

Acepromazine is a phenothiazine derivative that has a depressant action on the central nervous system. It is a dopamine inhibitory, alpha-adrenergic blocking agent with weak antimuscarinic activity (Bishop, 1998). Acepromazine is a sedative that potentiates the effects of other anaesthetic agents and facilitates a smooth recovery. It is used routinely as a premedicant in dogs and other species. Acepromazine is hypotensive and does not have analgesic properties. In rabbits, acepromazine can be used for premedication prior to induction with volatile agents. It can also be combined with butorphanol to provide sedation.

5.4.5 Benzodiazepines: diazepam and midazolam

Diazepam and midazolam are effective sedatives in rabbits. They produce good muscle relaxation and potentiate the effect of anaesthetics and narcotic analgesics. Cardiovascular and autonomic side effects are negligible (Green, 1975). Midazolam and diazepam have a similar spectrum of effects except that midazolam has a shorter duration of action (Flecknell, 1984). Diazepam is poorly soluble in water and is therefore prepared in an oily solvent (Valium, Roche) that is locally irritant and can cause tissue damage and skin sloughing if administered perivascularly. A water-soluble diazepam preparation is available that requires dilution before use (Diazemuls, Roche). Midazolam is water soluble (Hypnovel, Roche) and does not cause a tissue reaction if it is administered perivascularly. Intramuscular or intravenous midazolam has been recommended as a routine short-acting sedative for diagnostic procedures (Ramer *et al.*, 1999). It is absorbed across mucous membranes and can be given intranasally if required.

Midazolam can be given after premedication with fentanyl/fluanisone (Hypnorm, Janssen) to induce anaesthesia (see Box 5.4).

5.4.6 Alpha-2-adrenergic agonists

5.4.6.1 Xylazine

Xylazine (Rompun, Bayer) produces moderate sedation and minimal analgesia in rabbits. It is seldom used as a sole agent but is given in combination with ketamine. The combination causes cardiovascular and respiratory depression and cardiac arrhythmias are produced at high doses. Xylazine and ketamine have been associated with a high mortality rate (Flecknell *et al.*, 1983). Atipamezole, an alpha-adrenergic blocking drug that is used to reverse the effects of medetomidine, can be used to reverse the effects of xylazine.

5.4.6.2 Medetomidine

Medetomidine (Domitor, Pfizer) is a more specific alpha-2 agonist than xylazine and has a lower incidence of side effects. It is relatively expensive and rabbits require comparatively larger doses than other species. Medetomidine can be used on its own as a premedicant or it can be combined with ketamine to provide surgical anaesthesia. Medetomidine causes peripheral vasoconstriction, which gives mucous membranes a slight mauve appearance that may be mistaken for cyanosis. The vasoconstriction is not dangerous but the poor colour of the mucous membranes could mask a true cyanosis should it occur. Hypoxia occurs during anaesthesia with medetomidine and oxygen should be administered throughout the anaesthetic period (Flecknell, 2000). Vasoconstriction can prevent satisfactory pulse oximetry and venepuncture for blood collection or intravenous fluid therapy. Medetomidine can cause hypothermia and diuresis.

Medetomidine has some advantages. It can be given by subcutaneous rather than intramuscular injection. It provides good laryngeal relaxation for endotracheal intubation. It is not respiratory depressant and recovery is usually complete within 3 h. Recovery can be hastened by reversal with atipamezole. The use of medetomidine in combination with ketamine is described in Box 5.4

5.4.7 Analgesics

Analgesia is the 'absence of sensibility to pain, particularly the relief of pain without loss of consciousness' (Blood and Studdert, 1999). Endogenous opioids are released in response to pain and other stressful stimuli and reduce pain perception and recognition. Inflammation or tissue hypoxia at the site of injury stimulate the release of nociceptive substances such as kinins which, in turn, stimulate prostaglandin release. Nonsteroidal analgesics (NSAIDs) interfere with this process (see Section 4.6). Narcotic analgesics reduce pain perception and recognition by interacting with opioid receptors.

5.4.7.1 Narcotic analgesics

A variety of opioid receptors are found in the brain, spinal cord and other opioid responsive tissues such as the gastrointestinal tract. Opioids produce a variety of effects depending on the type of receptor that is stimulated and there are species differences in the responses that are elicited. μ (mu) receptors are mainly responsible for supraspinal analgesia, euphoria, respiratory depression and, in humans, physical dependence. κ (kappa) receptors are mainly responsible for spinal analgesia, miosis and sedation. σ (sigma) receptors are responsible for dysphoria, hallucinations, respiratory stimulation and various vasomotor effects. Other receptors such as δ (delta) receptors exist in a variety of tissues (Jenkins, 1987). It is the effect on the μ and κ receptors that is most important for pain relief. Other effects such as respiratory depression, sedation or interference with gastrointestinal motility may or may not be desirable, depending on the situation in which the drugs are used. Morphine is a μ agonist, i.e. it activates μ receptors to produce analgesia, euphoria and respiratory depression. Its effects can be reversed by the administration of a μ antagonist, such as naloxone, that binds to the receptors but does not activate them thereby blocking the effects of morphine. Some opioids are μ antagonists but κ agonists so they inactivate μ receptors and activate κ receptors resulting in spinal analgesia, miosis and sedation. Such products are known as mixed agonists/antagonists and can be used to reverse the effects of μ agonists while still providing some analgesia by their effect on the κ receptors. They can also be used as analgesics in their own right. Butorphanol is an example of a mixed agonist/antagonist. The situation is further complicated by the mixed effects of some drugs. Buprenorphine is a partial agonist due to its agonist effects on the μ receptors but will also antagonize pure μ agonists such as morphine. Therefore a wide range of opioid effects and side effects can be produced and reversed using the variety of opioid agonists and antagonists that is available. The dose rate is an important factor in producing the desired effect without side effects such as respiratory depression. Combinations of small quantities of different compounds can be used for this purpose.

In rabbits, narcotic analgesics are used extensively to provide analgesia and, in some cases, anaesthesia. They can also be used to reverse anaesthesia while retaining analgesic effects. Side effects of narcotic analgesics that can cause concern in rabbits are respiratory and mental depression, hypothermia and bradycardia.

5.4.7.2 Buprenorphine (Schedule 3)

Buprenorphine is a potent long-acting analgesic with mixed agonist/antagonist properties. In man, it does not appear addictive and so the drug is not under the same stringent controls as fentanyl/fluanisone. In rabbits, buprenorphine is used for long-term analgesia as its effects persist for 7 h after administration. It can be used postoperatively or for the treatment of painful conditions. Buprenorphine is also used to reverse the respiratory depressant effects of fentanyl postoperatively in rabbits that have been anaesthetized with fentanyl/fluanisone and benzodiazepine combinations (Flecknell *et al.*, 1989). Analgesia is maintained for several hours, although the rabbits may remain sedated due to the residual effects of fluanisone and the benzodiazepine. Buprenorphine can be administered at the outset of anaesthesia to provide pre-emptive analgesia for potentially painful procedures. There is evidence that preoperative buprenorphine administration reduces the amount of isoflurane required to maintain anaesthesia (Flecknell, 1998b).

5.4.7.3 Butorphanol

Butorphanol is a synthetic opioid with mixed agonist/antagonist properties. It is analgesic with a potency three to five times greater than morphine in humans and up to 30 times greater than morphine in rats (Wixson, 1994). Butorphanol provides analgesia and mild sedation but does not cause respiratory depression unless high dose rates are used. In some tests, the dose response curve of butorphanol is bell-shaped suggesting that higher doses can have less analgesic effect than lower ones (Flecknell, 1984). The half-life of butorphanol in rabbits, at a dose rate of 0.5 mg/kg, has been calculated to be 1.64 h after intravenous administration in comparison with 3.16 h if the drug is given subcutaneously (Portnoy and Hustead, 1992). Butorphanol can be used to reverse the respiratory depressant effects of μ agonists such as fentanyl, morphine or pethidine and still retain some analgesic properties. The analgesic effects of butorphanol last for 2.5 h (Flecknell *et al.*, 1989).

Butorphanol is used in combination with medetomidine and ketamine to produce surgical anaesthesia (see Box 5.4). It can also be used in combination with acepromazine for sedation. The combination is vasodilatory, which facilitates blood collection and intravenous injections.

5.4.7.4 Fentanyl/fluanisone (Hypnorm, Janssen) (Schedule 2)

Fentanyl is a potent opioid agonist acting primarily on μ receptors and therefore induces analgesia, respiratory depression and, in man, euphoria. It is a potent analgesic and is 20–100 times more effective than morphine (Green, 1975). Its analgesic effect is potentiated by a butyrophenone sedative, fluanisone, that also partially antagonizes respiratory depression. It has the advantage of holding a product licence for use in rabbits in which it is used for sedation and anaes-

Key points 5.1

- Approximately 40% of rabbits produce atropinesterase that rapidly breaks down atropine. If an anticholinergic agent is required for premedication, glycopyrrolate can be used
- Acepromazine, midazolam, medetomidine, fentanyl/fluanisone (Hypnorm, Janssen) or a combination of acepromazine and butorphanol can be used as sedatives for rabbits
- Fentanyl/fluanisone (Hypnorm, Janssen) is vasodilatory and facilitates venepuncture for intravenous therapy and blood collection. Acepromazine/butorphanol is also vasodilatory but should be used with care in dehydrated patients. Medetomidine causes peripheral vasoconstriction
- Fentanyl/fluanisone is a Schedule 2 controlled drug and needs to be kept in a locked immovable cabinet with a register recording purchase and supply
- Buprenorphine is a Schedule 3 drug that needs to be kept in a locked immovable cabinet but does not require a record of transactions.

thesia. Profound analgesia lasts for 3 h after administration (Flecknell *et al.*, 1989). Fentanyl/fluanisone is classified as a Schedule 2 dangerous drug. A written requisition is required to obtain the drug and it has to be stored in a locked immovable cabinet. Records must be kept of the purchase and supply.

The combination of fentanyl/fluanisone is one the most useful preparations available for rabbits. It can be used as a premedicant, sedative, potent analgesic or, in combination with midazolam, as an anaesthetic agent (see Boxes 5.3, 5.4).

5.4.7.5 Pethidine

Pethidine is an opioid agonist acting primarily on μ receptors with some activity on κ and δ receptors (Bishop, 1998). It is less potent than morphine and relatively short acting. It is only effective for 2–3 h. Pethidine has some antimuscarinic activity and affects gastrointestinal motility. In horses, it is used as a spasmolytic (Bishop, 1998). In rabbits, pethidine is not used routinely although it may be useful as an analgesic if alternative products are unavailable.

5.4.8 Drugs that are used to counteract effects of narcotic analgesics

5.4.8.1 Doxapram

Doxapram (Dopram-V, Willows Francis) is a respiratory stimulant that is sometimes used to counteract the respiratory depression that accompanies premedication with fentanyl/fluanisone (Hypnorm, Janssen). There is evidence that doxapram not only reverses the respiratory depressant effects of fentanyl but also reduces its analgesic effect (Flecknell *et al.*, 1989). The respiratory stimulant effect lasts for 15 minutes (Cooper, 1989) so a temporary loss of analgesia at the outset of anaesthesia may not be important. Doxapram can be used to treat respiratory arrest during anaesthesia.

Doxapram has been recommended in conscious rabbits to overcome the breath holding response during induction with volatile agents such as halothane or isoflurane. Exposure to volatile agents appears to be distressing to rabbits, so forcing the animal to inhale the vapour by stimulating respiration may be equally distressing. It is unnecessary if an injectable induction agent is used and the volatile agent introduced slowly.

5.4.8.2 Naloxone

Naloxone is a pure opioid antagonist that is chemically related to the opioid analgesics and is able to reverse all their actions including respiratory depression and analgesia. There is a possibility of relapse as the effects wear off.

5.4.9 Injectable induction agents

5.4.9.1 Alphaxalone-alphadolone

Alphaxalone-alphadolone (Saffan, Schering Plough) is licensed as a dissociative anaesthetic agent in cats and has been used in rabbits. The cremophor vehicle causes anaphylaxis in dogs but this effect has not been reported in rabbits (Wixson, 1994). The agent can be given incrementally to maintain a light plane of anaesthesia with good muscle relaxation but poor analgesia. Higher doses cause respiratory depression and can cause apnoea and cardiac arrest. The agent is not recommended for use in rabbits (Flecknell, 2000).

5.4.9.2 Barbiturates

Thiopentone can be used as an induction agent in rabbits. Pentobarbitone has been used as an anaesthetic agent for laboratory rabbits, although the safety margin is small (Greene, 1975). Respiratory depression or arrest may occur before surgical anaesthesia is achieved. There is a narrow difference between the doses required for anaesthesia and euthanasia (Wixson, 1994). Hypoxia, hypercapnia and acidosis can occur in rabbits under barbiturate anaesthesia (Flecknell *et al.* 1983). Pentobarbitone sodium 6% w/v (Sagatal, Meriel) carries a product licence as a sedative and general anaesthetic in rabbits, although it is not recommended and should not be used in animals intended for human consumption.

5.4.9.3 Propofol

Propofol (Rapinovet, Mallinckrodt), a substituted phenol derivative, has been approved for general use in human patients since 1986 and is licensed for use in dogs and cats. As an induction agent, it has many advantages, including a moderate to high hypnotic potency and therapeutic ratio, rapid onset and rapid smooth recovery. In other species, repeated doses do not accumulate and propofol can be used to maintain anaesthesia by continuous infusion.

In rabbits, propofol can be used as an induction agent. A dose of 5–14 mg/kg gives sufficient time for the experienced anaesthetist to intubate (Aeschbacher and Webb, 1993a). Transient apnoea occurs after intravenous administration and high doses can cause respiratory arrest. Propofol is not recommended for long-term anaesthesia in rabbits (Aeschbacher and Webb, 1993b).

5.4.9.4 Ketamine

Ketamine is a dissociative agent that can be used as a sole agent for induction of anaesthesia or in combination with other agents for induction and maintenance. As a sole agent, ketamine has a sympathomimetic effect leading to an increase in heart rate, cardiac output and blood pressure. Ketamine does not abolish ocular, laryngeal and swallowing reflexes and is characterized by muscular rigidity. Poor muscular relaxation makes ketamine an unsatisfactory sole agent for surgical procedures. However, in combination with another agents, such as xylazine or medetomidine, xylazine provides surgical anaesthesia.

5.4.10 Inhalational anaesthetic agents

5.4.10.1 Nitrous oxide

Nitrous oxide is used as an adjunct to anaesthesia with volatile agents. It is analgesic, has minimal effect on cardiovascular and respiratory function and reduces the amount of the volatile agent required to maintain anaesthesia.

In rabbits, nitrous oxide has half the anaesthetic potency of that in humans (Wixson, 1994) and is primarily used to facilitate the uptake of a volatile agent. Nitrous oxide also appears to interact with the opiate receptor system to provide analgesia (Wixson, 1994). There are disadvantages associated with the use of nitrous oxide. It can contribute to hypoxia and diffuse into closed gas spaces. Long periods of nitrous oxide administration have been shown to cause gastric dilation in rabbits (Kumar *et al.*, 1993).

A 50/50% mixture of nitrous oxide and oxygen aids smooth induction and helps to achieve balanced anaesthesia if it is administered during the introduction of volatile agents. Once a satisfactory plane of anaesthesia is reached, the nitrous oxide should be switched off because of the risk of diffusion into gas-filled organs such as the caecum. The risk of diffusion into gas-filled organs is greater in rabbits suffering from gastrointestinal hypomotility.

5.4.10.2 Halothane

For many years, halothane was the volatile agent of choice for rabbits although it has now been superseded by isoflurane. Halothane is non-flammable, produces rapid induction and recovery and good muscle relaxation. It is vasodilatory and hypotensive. Halothane can sensitize the myocardium to catecholamines that can be released during rabbit anaesthesia. In common with isoflurane, masking down with halothane evokes breath holding and hypoxia.

5.4.10.3 Isoflurane

Isoflurane is a volatile halogenated ether that is administered by inhalation and quickly distributed throughout the body. In rabbits, it is rapidly excreted via the respiratory system with only a small fraction (0.2%) metabolized by the liver (Marano *et al.*, 1997). It is a safe anaesthetic for animals with compromised hepatic or renal function and has several advantages over halothane and is recommended for maintenance of anaesthesia in rabbits (see Box 5.5). The depth of anaesthesia can be adjusted rapidly and isoflurane does not depress myocardial contractility as much as halothane (Marano *et al.*, 1997). The minimum alveolar concentration (MAC) % of rabbits is believed to be 2.05% (Meriel, personal communication) in comparison with 1.34% in birds or 1.68% in cats. MAC is the concentration of an anaesthetic in the alveoli that prevents a muscular response to a painful stimulus in 50% of the subjects (Blood and Studdert, 1993). Induction is rapidly induced at concentrations of 2–3% and anaesthesia can be maintained at concentrations of 0.25–2%. Isoflurane does not provide analgesia. The main problem with its use in rabbits is the breath holding response to the odour that can occur during induction or in lightly anaesthetized patients.

5.5 Maintenance of anaesthesia

5.5.1 Endotracheal intubation

Endotracheal intubation is not easy in rabbits due to the difficulty of visualizing the larynx. The rabbit's mouth does not open widely and the large base of the tongue that occupies most of the nasopharynx obscures the view of the larynx (see Figure 3.9). It is impossible to see the larynx without a laryngoscope, auriscope or endoscope. Even with this type of equipment, it can still be difficult to see the larynx in small breeds. The *rima glottidis* or

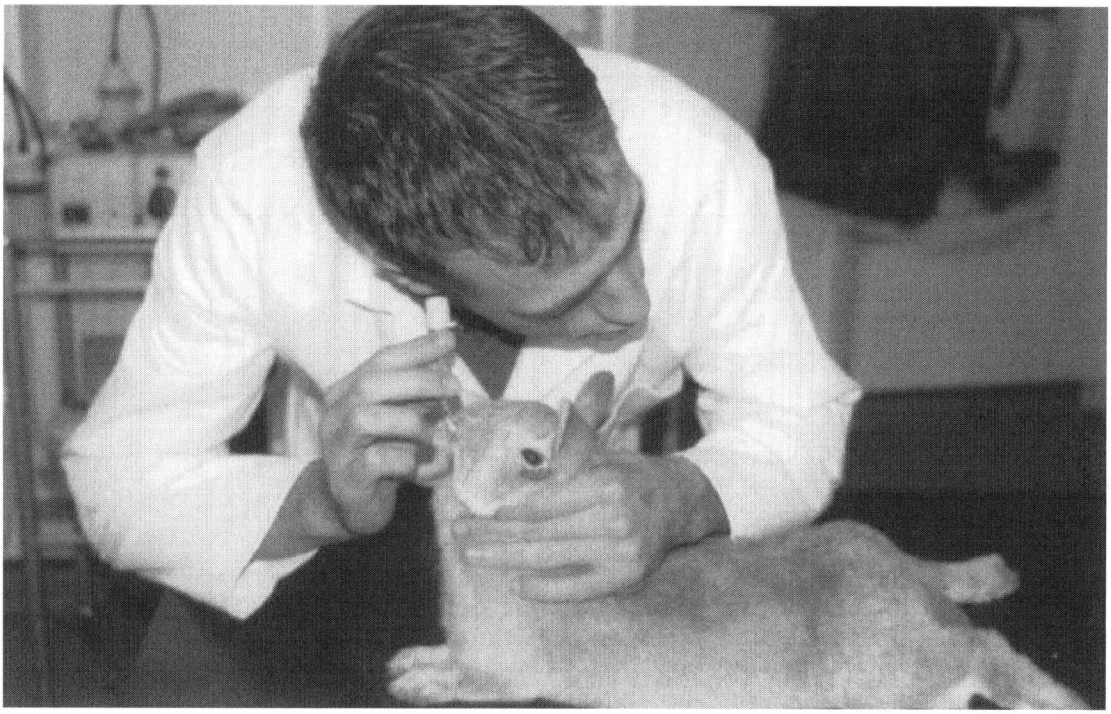

Figure 5.1. Positioning the rabbit for blind endotracheal intubation. For blind endotracheal intubation, the anaesthetized rabbit is placed in sternal recumbency with its head extended. Some local anaesthetic solution (Lidocaine: Intubeaze, Arnolds Veterinary Products) is sprayed into the pharynx and the tip of the tube lubricated. The larynx is palpated and the endotracheal tube measured against the rabbit to estimate the length between the lips and the entrance to the larynx. The estimated length of tube is inserted over the tongue and into the pharynx. At this stage, if necessary, additional local anaesthetic can be sprayed into the tube to trickle down into the larynx. An accurate idea of the position of the end of the tube can be gained by putting an ear to the end of the tube, watching the respiratory movements and listening to the breath sounds. Once breath sounds are heard, the tube is slowly advanced during each inspiration. The rabbit usually coughs as the tube passes into the trachea. A description of blind endotracheal intubation in rabbits is given in Section 5.5.1.1.

entrance to the larynx is relatively small and will only admit a small endotracheal tube. Uncuffed tubes are required to maximize internal diameter. As a general rule, a 2.5 kg rabbit can be intubated with a 2.5 mm uncuffed tube. There are several techniques that can be used to intubate rabbits. Care is required to prevent iatrogenic damage to the larynx and pharynx or cause laryngospasm and respiratory distress. Endotracheal intubation is easier in large breeds.

5.5.1.1 Blind intubation

It is possible to intubate rabbits without visualizing the larynx. After induction of anaesthesia, the rabbit is placed in sternal recumbency and neck extended so there is a straight line from the mouth to the larynx. A gag is not required and can be counterproductive as it stimulates jaw movement unless the patient is deeply anaesthetized. Lignocaine hydrochloride (Intubeze, Arnolds) is sprayed as far back into the mouth as possible with the head held up so the liquid can trickle over the tongue on to the larynx. An uncuffed endotracheal tube is measured against the rabbit to estimate the length required to reach the larynx, which can be palpated. A water-soluble lubricant such as KY Jelly can be used to lubricate the end of the tube. After a minute or two, when the local anaesthetic spray has taken effect, the tube is inserted through the diastema and advanced to the entrance to the larynx. An accurate idea of the position of the end of the tube is gained by putting an ear to the end of the tube and listening to the breath sounds (see Figure 5.1). Once breath sounds are heard, the tube is slowly advanced during each inspiration. It is helpful to watch the rabbit's respiratory movements at the same time as advancing the tube. The breath sounds become louder until the tip is situated at the entrance of the larynx. At this point the breath sounds are at their loudest. If breath sounds are lost when the tube is advanced further, then it has almost certainly passed into the oesophagus. Resistance is felt if this is the case. If the tube goes through the rima glottidis into the larynx, the rabbit will usually cough and breath sounds can still be heard through the tube. Condensation from the end of the tube on the surface of the operating table confirms correct positioning. If the tube has been inadvertently placed in the oesophagus, it can be palpated alongside the trachea. If the first attempt is unsuccessful, then the procedure can be repeated using a smaller tube.

5.5.1.2 Intubation by visualizing the larynx

In large rabbits, the larynx can be seen through an auriscope, laryngoscope or endoscope. Auriscopes or Wisconsin laryngoscopes (Size 0–1) designed for paediatric use are suitable. It can be difficult to see the larynx in Dwarf breeds by this method because of their small pharynx.

To intubate the rabbit, it is placed either in dorsal or sternal recumbency with the neck extended. The soft palate may need to be pushed away from the epiglottis with the end of the endotracheal tube before the characteristic triangular entrance to the larynx can be seen. Introducers can be used to facilitate intubation. A small gauge urinary catheter (3–5 f) threaded through the endotracheal tube prior to insertion into the larynx can be used to guide the tube after it (Gilroy, 1981). Alternatively, a small 1.9 mm semi-rigid endoscope (Needlescope, Storz) used as an introducer, permits simultaneous visualization and guidance of the endotracheal tube into the larynx.

5.5.2 Nasal intubation

An alternative to the endotracheal tube is a nasal tube that is positioned to lie in the nasal passages. Small soft nasogastric tubes or 1.0–1.5 mm endotracheal tubes (Cook Veterinary Products) are suitable. The technique requires high flow rates to create positive pressure and force the anaesthetic mixture into the nasopharynx to be successful. Nasal intubation is useful in small rabbits that are difficult to intubate through the larynx. Occasionally it is not possible to pass a nasal tube in rabbits if incisor tooth roots have penetrated the nasal passages.

An alternative technique is to advance the endotracheal tube through the nasal passages and pharynx and into the trachea (Mason, 1997).

Box 5.2 Anaesthetic emergencies

If respiratory arrest occurs:
- Check the plane of anaesthesia. Breath holding can be a response to the smell of anaesthetic vapours in lightly anaesthetized patients
- Check the airway is clear
- Check the heart and pulse (the pulse can often be felt by applying gentle digital pressure to the central auricular artery)
- Gently compress the chest between finger and thumb to move air in and out of the lungs and stimulate respiration. The chest can be compressed at a rate of once per second
- Administer oxygen. Use a face-mask if the patient is not intubated
- Attempt intubation if the patient is deeply anaesthetized
- Start intermittent positive pressure ventilation if the patient is intubated
- Administer doxapram at 5 mg/kg (0.25 ml/kg, Dopram-V, Fort Dodge). Dopram-V injection may be given intravenously or intramuscularly. Dopram-V drops may be applied topically to the oral or nasal mucous membranes
- Consider tracheotomy if there is respiratory obstruction or to introduce oxygen into the lungs if the rabbit is not intubated. A large hypodermic needle can be used to penetrate the trachea.

If cardiac arrest occurs:
- Check the airway is clear
- Administer oxygen
- If possible, place an endotracheal tube
- Start intermittent positive pressure ventilation
- Use external cardiac massage over the heart at rate of approximately 70–90 times per minute
- Administer atipamezole if appropriate. Atipamezole can be given intravenously, intramuscularly or subcutaneously. If possible, the intravenous route should be used
- Administer adrenaline, it can be given i.v., s.c. or squirted into the trachea. Solutions come as 1mg/ml, i.e. 1:1000 that need to be diluted in sterile water. (0.2 ml/kg of 1:10 000 solution)

Nasal intubation carries a risk of introducing pathogens, such as *Pasteurella multocida*, from the nasal cavity into the trachea and subsequently the lung.

5.6 Monitoring anaesthesia

The colour of the mucous membranes is assessed by looking at the nose, lips or tongue. Rectal temperature can be monitored. The heart beat can be felt by placing a finger on either side of the chest. In most rabbits a pulse can be detected by gentle palpation of the central auricular artery (see Figure 3.6). Alternatively the pulse can be monitored by pulse oximetry, electrocardiography or direct auscultation of the chest. Typical heart rates are 240–280 bpm, although rates of 120–160 bpm can occur in rabbits that have received medetomidine (Flecknell, 2000). An oesophageal stethoscope can be used in large rabbits in which it is possible to place the tube without compromising respiratory function. In some small breeds the nasopharynx is not large enough to accommodate the stethoscope without occluding the airway.

There are several parameters that are used to assess the depth of anaesthesia in rabbits. These parameters differ with each anaesthetic protocol and do not compare with the responses of dogs or cats. For example, absence of a corneal reflex denotes a dangerous depth of anaesthesia in rabbits unless they have been anaesthetized with medetomidine combinations (Hellebrekers *et al.*, 1997). In general, the palpebral reflex cannot be relied upon to give a correct assessment of the depth of anaesthesia. The toe pinch, leg withdrawal reflex is more reliable using the hind rather than the fore feet. Rate, depth and pattern of respiration are the most useful indicators of anaesthetic depth. The absence of an ear pinch reflex and loss of jaw tone are reliable indicators of surgical anaesthesia. Respiratory depression can be considered to be severe at less than 4 breaths per minute (Flecknell *et al.*, 1983). Emergency procedures during respiratory or cardiac arrest are summarized in Box 5.2.

Box 5.3 Recommended technique for sedation for minor procedures (e.g. dematting, radiography etc.)

Fentanyl/fluanisone (Hypnorm, Janssen)

- Fentanyl/fluanisone provides sedation and profound analgesia
- Fentanyl/fluanisone induces a state of narcosis that enables the rabbit to be placed in almost any position. It can be used for radiography, dematting, removal of maggots, cleaning wounds etc.
- Rabbits that are sedated with fentanyl/fluanisone are indifferent to their surroundings. They tolerate minor procedures, including venepuncture, without movement
- The vasodilatory effects of fentanyl/fluanisone facilitate blood collection and administration of intravenous fluids. The sedative effects of fentanyl/ fluanisone last for approximately 3 h
- The usual dose rate is 0.3 ml/kg but this can be reduced to 0.2 ml/kg for poor risk patients
- If radiological or other findings indicate that surgery is required, general anaesthesia can be induced by subsequent intravenous administration of midazolam (0.5–2 mg/kg) to effect. Alternatively, the rabbit can be masked down with isoflurane
- Recovery can be hastened by the administration of a mixed agonist/antagonist. Either buprenorphine (0.01–0.05 mg/kg) or butorphanol (0.1–0.5 mg/kg) can be given either subcutaneously or intravenously to reverse the effects of fentanyl and maintain analgesia. Butorphanol is more effective than buprenorphine in reversing the effects of fentanyl but the subsequent period of analgesia is longer with buprenorphine (Flecknell, 2000).

Box 5.4 Recommended anaesthetic techniques

Option 1: Combination of medetomidine, ketamine and butorphanol

A combination of medetomidine, ketamine and butorphanol can be used on its own for short procedures such as tooth trimming or radiography. It can also be used to induce anaesthesia prior to maintenance with an inhalational agent for routine surgical procedures such as neutering or prolonged dental procedures such as burring cheek teeth or incisor extraction. Intubation is required for prolonged dental procedures, as anaesthesia cannot be maintained with a facemask. Inhalational anaesthesia is also recommended for flushing tear ducts because it can be an extremely stimulatory procedure.

- An induction dose of 0.2 mg/kg medetomidine combined with 10 mg/kg ketamine and 0.5 mg/kg butorphanol is given subcutaneously. This dose translates as 0.2 ml/kg Domitor (Pfizer), 0.1 ml/kg ketamine and 0.05 ml/kg Torbugesic (Fort Dodge). Occasionally the injection appears to sting. The combination takes 5–10 minutes to become effective
- Anaesthesia with this combination lasts for approximately 20 minutes. Full recovery takes place over a period of 2–4 h. The introduction of an inhalational agent is required for most surgical procedures
- After the rabbit has lost consciousness, it can be intubated. Alternatively, anaesthesia can be maintained with a facemask. A tightly fitting mask is needed in order to permit satisfactory scavenging of anaesthetic gases. Breath holding often occurs in lightly anaesthetized rabbits exposed to anaesthetic gases delivered via a facemask. The breath holding response to the smell of isoflurane (or halothane) is proportional to the concentration of the anaesthetic vapour. This response can be overcome by gradual introduction of the volatile agent that is introduced after a period of preoxygenation (2–3 minutes). Introducing isoflurane at a concentration of 0.5% for a few minutes before increasing it to 1% then 1.5% overcomes problems with breath holding. The rabbit can be prepared for surgery during this period
- Nitrous oxide facilitates smooth induction of anaesthesia with inhalation agents. It can be used during induction in a 50:50

Box 5.4 *continued*

mixture with oxygen. Once surgical anaesthesia is attained the nitrous oxide is switched off. It is not advisable to administer nitrous oxide for prolonged periods in rabbits because of the risk of diffusion into gas-filled spaces such as the caecum

- During surgery, anaesthesia is usually maintained with concentrations of 1.5–2.5% isoflurane delivered in 100% oxygen
- At the end of surgery, a period of breathing pure oxygen is required if nitrous oxide has been used in the previous 10 minutes
- If necessary, at the end of surgery, medetomidine can be reversed with atipamezole (1 mg/kg or 0.1 ml/kg) (Antisedan (Pfizer). A period of 15–40 minutes should elapse between administration of medetomidine and atipamezole as resedation can take place because the effects of atipamezole do not last as long as medetomidine. The analgesic effects of medetomidine can also be reversed by the atipamezole
- Without reversal, recovery from anaesthesia is complete in 1–2 h and allows a period of relaxation during which the effects of surgery can wear off and postoperative NSAIDs can become effective
- Routine analgesia with NSAIDs is essential.

Option 2: Induction using isoflurane after premedication with fentanyl/fluanisone (Hypnorm, Janssen)

Induction of anaesthesia using a facemask allows rapid recovery. Premedication is essential. Fentanyl/fluanisone is recommended as a premedicant because it provides effective sedation and postoperative analgesia. Hypnorm also carries a product licence for use in rabbits.

- Fentanyl/fluanisone (0.3 ml/kg) is given by intramuscular injection 10–20 minutes before induction of anaesthesia. Fentanyl/fluanisone can be given subcutaneously but may be less sedative by this route.
- A period of preoxygenation is required before introducing isoflurane at a low concentration via a facemask
- Nitrous oxide can be included in the anaesthetic mixture for induction. It is switched off at the start of surgery
- During induction, the rabbit is gently restrained and observed closely. Wrapping in a towel is not recommended as it masks respiratory movement
- A slow induction, increasing the concentration of isoflurane to 1.5–2.5%, over a period of approximately 5 minutes reduces the risk of breath holding.

Option 3: Combination of fentanyl/fluanisone (Hypnorm, Janssen) and midazolam

Fentanyl/fluanisone and benzodiazepine combinations can be used as sole agents for short procedures such as minor dentistry. An advantage of this technique is the absence of anaesthetic equipment, such as masks or endotracheal tubes that impede the view of the oral cavity. Respiratory depression and prolonged recovery time are potential problems, so respiration must be observed closely during the anaesthetic period. Oxygen can be administered via a facemask when dentistry is not taking place.

- Fentanyl/fluanisone in combination with midazolam provides surgical anaesthesia for 30–45 minutes
- Fentanyl/fluanisone is given by intramuscular injection 10–20 minutes before induction of anaesthesia with intravenous midazolam (0.5–2 mg/kg) into the marginal ear vein. A dose of 2 mg/kg of midazolam is drawn up and a quarter to half the dose given initially and the rest to effect
- The sedative and vasodilatory effects of fentanyl/fluanisone facilitate the intravenous injection that takes place without resistance from the rabbit
- At the end of surgery, the effects of fentanyl/fluanisone can be reversed with subcutaneous or intravenous buprenorphine (0.01–0.05 mg/kg) or butorphanol (0.1–0.5 mg/kg), although the rabbit will remain slightly sedated
- Without reversal, the effects of fentanyl/fluanisone and midazolam wear off after approximately 4–6 h during which time analgesia is provided and the rabbit remains relaxed and quiet. Food and water can be offered as soon as the rabbit adopts sternal recumbency and many rabbits will eat and drink despite residual sedation.

Box 5.5 Recommended technique for anaesthesia of critically ill patients (e.g. for abdominal surgery such as acute intestinal obstruction)

Gradual induction with a volatile agent, especially isoflurane, is recommended for critically ill, poor risk patients. Isoflurane is safe and recovery is rapid. Ill rabbits are unlikely to struggle during induction and do not seem to breath hold in response to the smell of anaesthetic agents as much as their healthy counterparts.

- Many rabbits will have already received a premedicant, a first aid analgesic or sedative for radiography and diagnostic work. Fentanyl/fluanisone at a reduced dose of 0.2 ml/kg is an efficient analgesic and prolonged recovery is not a problem at this dose rate. Residual postoperative sedation prevents patient interference with surgical wounds and intravenous fluid apparatus so Elizabethan collars and other stressful devices are not required
- Buprenorphine can be used as an alternative premedicant if a period of postoperative sedation is undesirable
- It is important to preoxygenate for a few minutes before the introduction of nitrous oxide (50%). Nitrous oxide appears to calm rabbits and aid a smooth induction
- A slow gradual introduction of isoflurane starting with low concentrations minimizes struggling and breath holding
- The rabbit can be intubated as soon as surgical anaesthesia is achieved. Endotracheal intubation gives greater control over the anaesthetic and permits intermittent positive pressure ventilation if required. If endotracheal intubation is not possible, anaesthesia can be maintained with a tightly fitting facemask or nasal tube
- The nitrous oxide is switched off as soon as surgical anaesthesia is attained
- Fluid therapy and analgesia are essential parts of the treatment of critically ill rabbits, especially those that are undergoing surgery on the gastrointestinal tract. Blood loss or dehydration can result in hypotension and electrolyte imbalances and increase the risk of cardiac failure.

Recommended anaesthetic protocols are summarized in Boxes 5.3–5.5.

5.7 Postoperative care

5.7.1 Recovery from anaesthesia

Hypothermia can occur during prolonged recovery from anaesthesia. Clipping off large amounts of fur or using copious quantities of spirit during skin preparation potentiate heat loss and the development of hypothermia, especially in small rabbits with no fat reserves. Towels or other bedding can be used as insulation against cold or wet surfaces, or the rabbit can be placed on a heat pad or in a heated kennel for recovery. Heating devices should be switched off as soon as body temperature is within normal range as rabbits cannot pant effectively and are susceptible to hyperthermia. They also chew through electric cables.

Pain or stress stimulate the sympathetic nervous system and reduce gastrointestinal motility. Reduced gut motility can trigger a sequence of events that, left unchecked, culminate in the development of hepatic lipidosis and death. To reduce stress, rabbits should recover in a quiet, comfortable environment with a warm ambient temperature. Ideally, they should be kept away from barking dogs and the smell of predators. Food and water needs to be available as soon as the rabbit has recovered enough to eat and drink. Some rabbits appear thirsty and drink a substantial amount of water as soon as they come round from an anaesthetic. Grass, hay and other fibrous foods are often eaten in preference to cereal mixtures or pellets. Fresh grass, dandelions, cabbage, carrots or other vegetables should be offered to tempt rabbits to eat as soon as they recover from anaesthesia. Good quality hay placed in the cage acts as a source of fibre and as a familiar bedding material once the rabbit adopts sternal recumbency.

5.7.2 Pain assessment

The assessment of pain in rabbits can be difficult. Rabbits do not exhibit many of the pain responses that are encountered in other species. They do not howl or whimper. Instead, their response to pain is to sit very still in the back of the cage and appear oblivious to their surroundings. Physiological parameters such as body temperature, respiratory and heart rate are affected by pain, but it is difficult to evaluate these changes without handling the rabbit which, in itself, alters these parameters. An assessment of pain can be made by observing the animal, but familiarity with normal behaviour patterns is required to make a comparison. Rabbits in pain do not come to front of the cage to investigate a bowl of food or a human hand. They do not groom and can become aggressive to cagemates or resent being picked up and nip or bite. Abdominal pain is manifested by the adoption of a crouched position and tooth grinding. Sometimes, the rabbit is restless and will jump up and circle the cage periodically. Rabbits with urinary tract problems may strain and appear uncomfortable in association with urination. Complete anorexia is a feature of pain.

Analgesia in laboratory animals, including rabbits, has been extensively investigated. In order to assess the effectiveness of analgesic agents, pain scoring systems have been devised. However, individual variation in both the animals and in the observers make such a system of evaluation difficult, especially for the assessment of mild pain (Flecknell, 1996a). The dose rates required to provide analgesia vary according to the stimulus (Flecknell, 1984). Therefore an empirical approach is required to analgesia in rabbits that can be based on an anthropomorphic perception of pain. As analgesia is so safe and effective, it must be given to all rabbits that may need it as, apart from the humane aspect, pain is a life-threatening condition to rabbits.

5.7.3 Choice of postoperative analgesic

The duration of action is a consideration when choosing an analgesic regimen. Although exact information about the duration of action of NSAIDs in rabbits is not available, most injectable preparations are estimated to last for 12–24 h (Flecknell, 2000). In comparison, the effects of opioid drugs only last for a few hours. Buprenorphine is effective for 6–12 h, whereas pethidine and butorphanol are effective for 2–4 h (Flecknell, 2000). Narcotic analgesics are required for up to 72 h postoperatively.

NSAIDs are used for their analgesic and anti-inflammatory properties. Drugs such as flunixin and carprofen provide effective pain control that is comparable to opioid analgesics. Non-steroidal analgesics are considered to be more beneficial in the treatment of somatic or integumentary pain rather than visceral pain (Jenkins, 1987). Therefore, abdominal surgery may require opioid analgesia, whereas NSAIDs are more effective following dental extractions or fracture repair. To ensure adequate analgesia, both opioid and non-steroidal analgesics can be administered together without adverse effect.

Key points 5.2

- The larynx of a rabbit is impossible to visualize without equipment such as a laryngoscope, auriscope or endoscope
- A blind technique for endotracheal intubation can be used that is very satisfactory once the technique is mastered
- It is possible to maintain anaesthesia using a facemask or nasal tube to deliver the anaesthetic gases although these techniques are not as satisfactory as endotracheal intubation
- Nitrous oxide can diffuse into gas-filled viscera and cause caecal or gastric dilatation. Although it may be useful for induction, it should not be used for long periods in rabbits
- The pulse of a rabbit can often be felt by gentle digital pressure on the central auricular artery
- Eye reflexes and withdrawal reflexes are not reliable indicators of the depth of anaesthesia in rabbits
- Pulse oximetry is useful, especially if the sensor is placed on the tongue. Medetomidine causes peripheral vasoconstriction that can prevent a satisfactory signal in other accessible sites such as the pinna.

Table 5.2 Comparison of fentanyl/fluanisone/midazolam with medetomidine/ketamine. (Advantages are in bold type)

Fentanyl/fluanisone (Hypnorm) + midazolam	*Medetomidine + ketamine + butorphanol*
Intramuscular and intravenous injection is required	**Can be given subcutaneously**
Fentanyl/fluanisone is licensed for use in rabbits	Products are not licensed for use in rabbits
Under the Dangerous Drugs Act, Fentanyl/fluanisone is a Schedule 2 drug that has to be kept in a locked cupboard and records kept of its use	**No records need to be maintained**
Fentanyl/fluanisone needs to become effective before administration of midazolam. Period for induction can be 20–30 minutes	**Onset of anaesthesia within 10 minutes of injection**
Fentanyl/fluanisone is an effective analgesic	Butophanol is not as effective an analgesic as fentanyl/fluanisone
Fentanyl/fluanisone causes peripheral vasodilation that facilitates venepuncture for blood sampling or administration of intravenous therapy	Medetomidine/ketamine causes peripheral vasoconstriction
The colour of the mucous membranes remains a reassuring pink colour Can cause respiratory depression Full recovery can take several hours. Hypothermia can develop during the recovery period Administration of buprenorphine (or butorphanol) reverses respiratory depression but full recovery can still be prolonged	Mucous membranes become pale mauve, which could mask shock or cyanosis **Recovery usually complete within 3 hours even without reversal of medetomidine** **Option to effectively reverse anaesthesia by administering atipamizole**
Cheaper than medetomidine and ketamine	Relatively expensive

5.7.4 Other postoperative pain relieving factors

Practical considerations such as the type of diet for a rabbit recovering from dental extractions or immobilization of a fractured or injured limb can reduce postoperative pain. Soft, mashed or grated food should be offered to rabbits following incisor extraction. Good surgical technique and the placement of sutures that are not too tight minimize discomfort from a surgical wound. A warm quiet environment with dry, familiar, comfortable bedding (hay) with food and water within easy reach also adds to the comfort of the patient postoperatively.

Key points 5.3

- Hypothermia can occur during prolonged recovery from anaesthesia. Heatpads can be used but need to be switched off once body temperature has returned to normal. Rabbits are susceptible to hyperthermia and can chew through electric cables
- Routine postoperative analgesia is essential to reduce pain and stress, and to restore appetite and gut motility
- Fresh grass, dandelions, vegetables and favourite foods should be offered as soon as rabbits have recovered from anaesthesia
- A bed of hay provides familiarity, a sense of security and a source of indigestible fibre to rabbits recovering from anaesthesia
- Careful observation is required to see signs of pain in rabbits. They do not vocalize but remain quiet and immobile in the back of the cage
- Practical considerations such as a soft diet and comfortable sutures minimize postoperative pain
- It is vital that owners are advised to make certain that their rabbit is eating and passing hard faeces within 24–48 h of surgery and to bring it back for treatment promptly if required.

5.7.5 Instructions to owners

When the rabbit is discharged, it is vital that owners are instructed to observe their rabbit carefully and make certain that it is eating and passing hard faeces. The rabbit should be brought back for re-examination if it does not eat for more than 24 h. If the owners cannot be relied upon, or the rabbit's appetite is in doubt, then hospitalization overnight is necessary. Rabbits that do not eat postoperatively require treatment to prevent gastrointestinal stasis (see Table 10.3) and re-appraisal of the primary diagnosis.

References

Aeschbacher, G. (1995). Rabbit anesthesia. *Compendium on Continuing Education*, **17**, 1003–1011.

Aeschbacher, G., Webb, A.I. (1993a). Propofol in rabbits. 1 Determination of an induction dose. *Lab Anim Sci.*, **43**, 324–326.

Aeschbacher, G., Webb, A.I. (1993b). Propofol in rabbits. 2. Long term anaesthesia. *Lab Anim Sci.*, **43**, 328–335.

Blood, D.C., Studdert, V.P. (1999). *Saunders Comprehensive Veterinary Dictionary*, 2nd edn. W.B. Saunders.

Bishop, Y.M. (1998). *The Veterinary Formulary*. 4th edn. (Y.M. Bishop, ed.). Royal Pharmaceutical Society of Great Britain and British Veterinary Association.

Carroll, J.F., Dwyer, T.M., Grady, A.W. *et al.* (1996). Hypertension, cardiac hypertrophy and neurohumoral activity in a new animal model of obesity (Abstract). *Am J Physiol.*, **271**, H373–H378.

Cooper, J.E. (1989). Anaesthesia of exotic species. In *Manual of Aneasthesia for Small Animal Practice*. (A.D.R. Hilbery, ed.) p. 144. British Small Animal Veterinary Association.

Flecknell, P.A. (1984). The relief of pain in laboratory animals. *Lab Anim.*, **18**, 147–160.

Flecknell, P.A. (1996a). *Laboratory Animal Anaesthesia*. Academic Press.

Flecknell, P.A. (1998a). Developments in the veterinary care of rabbits and rodents. *In Practice*, **20**, 286–295.

Flecknell, P.A. (1998b). Analgesia in small mammals. *Sem Avian Exotic Pet Med.*, **7**, 41–47.

Flecknell, P.A. (2000). Anaesthesia. In *Manual of Rabbit Medicine and Surgery*. (P.A. Flecknell, ed.) pp 103–116. British Small Animal Veterinary Association.

Flecknell, P.A., John, M., Mitchell, M. *et al.* (1983). Neuroleptanalgesia in the rabbit. *Lab Anim.*, **17**, 104–109.

Flecknell, P.A., Liles, J.H., Wootton, R. (1989). Reversal of fentanyl/fluanisone neuroleptanalgesia in the rabbit using mixed agonist/antagonist opioids. *Lab Anim.*, **23**, 147–155.

Flecknell, P.A., Cruz, I.J., Liles, J.H., Whelan, G. (1996). Induction of anaesthesia with halothane and isoflurane in the rabbit: a comparison of the use of a face-mask or an anaesthetic chamber. *Lab Anim.*, **30**, 67–74.

Gillett, C.S. (1994). Selected drug dosages and clinical reference data. In *The Biology of the Laboratory Rabbit*, 2nd edn. (P.J. Manning, D.H. Ringler, C.E. Newcomer, eds). pp 468–472, Academic Press.

Gilroy, A. (1981). Endotracheal intubation of rabbits and rodents. *J Am Vet Med Assoc.*, **183**, 1295.

Green, C.J. (1975). Neuroleptanalgesic drug combinations in the anaesthetic management of small laboratory animals. *Lab Anim.*, **9**, 161–178.

Harcourt-Brown, F.M., Baker, S.J. (2001). Parathyroid hormone, haematological and biochemical parameters in relation to dental disease and husbandry in pet rabbits. *J Small Anim Pract.*, **42**, 130–136.

Hellebrekers, L.J., de Boer, E.J., van Zuylen, M.A., Vosmeer H. (1997). A comparison between medetomidine-ketamine and medetomidine-propofol anaesthesia in rabbits. *Lab Anim.*, **31**, 58–69.

Jenkins, W.L. (1987). Pharmacologic aspects of analgesic drugs in animals: an overview. *J Am Vet Med Assoc.*, **191**, 1231–1240.

Kumar, R.A., Boyer, M.I., Bowen, C.V.A. (1993). A reliable method of anesthesia for extensive surgery in rabbits. *Lab Anim Sci.*, **43**, 265–266.

Marano, G., Formigari, R., Grigioni, M., Vergari, A. (1997). Effects of isoflurane versus halothane on myocardial contractility in rabbits: assessment with transthoracic two-dimensional echocardiography. *Lab Anim.*, **31**, 144–150.

Marini, R.P., Xiantung, L., Harpster, N.K., Dangler, C. (1999). Cardiovascular pathology possibly associated with ketamine/xylazine anesthesia in Dutch Belted rabbits. *Lab Anim Sci.*, **49**, 153–160.

Mason D.E. (1997). Anesthesia, analgesia, and sedation for small mammals. In *Ferrets, Rabbits and Rodents, Clinical Medicine and Surgery*. (E.V. Hillyer, K.E. Quesenberry, eds). pp 378–391. W.B. Saunders.

Portnoy, L.G., Hustead, D.R. (1992). Pharmacokinetics of butorphanol tartrate in rabbits. *Am J Vet Res.*, **53**, 541.

Ramer, J.C., Paul-Murphy, J., Benson, K.G. (1999). Evaluating and stabilizing critically ill rabbits. Part II. *Compendium on Continuing Education*, **21**, 116–125.

Wixson, S.K. (1994). Anesthesia and analgesia. In *The Biology of the Laboratory Rabbit*, 2nd edn. (P.J. Manning and D.H. Ringler, eds). pp 87–109. Academic Press.

Clinical pathology

6

6.1 Haematology and biochemistry

As rabbits are used extensively for toxicological and physiological studies, there are many scientific papers about the effects of experimental infections, drugs and toxic substances on haematological and biochemical parameters. There is also information about diseases of commercial rabbits, which are mainly investigated by *post-mortem* examination. In contrast, there is a dearth of literature about the effects of clinical diseases on the blood picture of rabbits or the use of blood tests as diagnostic or prognostic indicators. It is not always possible to extrapolate from other species, especially carnivores such as dogs and cats to the herbivorous rabbit with its specialized physiology. At the present time, much of the information that is available on the haematology and biochemistry of pet rabbits is anecdotal, although it can be helpful and is better than no information at all.

6.1.1 Sample collection

The collection of blood and urine samples is covered in Section 3.12. Parameters such as glucose, creatine kinase and aspartate aminotransferase (AST) can be altered by stress associated with handling and restraint, or tissue damage that has occurred during sample collection. For example, potassium results appear less reliable in samples taken with a plastic cannula as opposed to a hypodermic needle (Robson *et al.*, 1981).

Rabbit blood haemolyses easily and clots quickly (Perry-Clark and Meunier, 1991). Small clots affect haematology results and haemolysis affects certain biochemistry results, especially potassium and serum inorganic phosphorus that are released from erythrocytes. Rapid clotting can affect the performance of some analysers and heparinized syringes and needles are required.

6.1.2 Fasting and other physiological considerations

It is not possible to take a guaranteed fasting sample from a rabbit because they ingest caecotrophs. Parameters such as blood glucose are affected by digestion. Some parameters such as bile acids, cholesterol and urea follow a diurnal rhythm that also affects the total and differential white cell count (Fox and Laird, 1970; Fekete, 1989; Loeb and Quimby, 1989). Stress associated with car journeys or a period in unfamiliar surroundings will increase blood glucose and alter haematological parameters such as the distribution of neutrophils and lymphocytes. Pregnancy affects parameters such as protein, haematocrit, cholesterol, alkaline phosphatase, triglycerides (Viard-Drouet *et al.*, 1984), glucose, sodium, calcium, phosphate and red cell indices (Palm, 1997). Serum cholesterol is the parameter that is most affected and can be up to 30% lower in pregnant than in non-pregnant animals (Palm, 1997).

Anaesthesia affects some blood parameters such as potassium (Robson *et al.*, 1981). The effect of anaesthesia on biochemical parameters is minimized by taking samples within 5 minutes of induction. Intravenous or intraosseous fluids will also affect haema-

Table 6.1 Conversion factors for units

To convert	From Units used in this book	To Units used by other authors	Multiply by
Albumin	g/l	g/dl	0.1
Bilirubin	µmol/l	mg/dl	0.059
Calcium	mmol/l	mg/dl mEq/l	4 2
Cholesterol	mmol/l	mg/dl	38.7
Creatinine	mg/dl	µmol/l	88.4
Globulin	g/l	g/dl	0.1
Glucose	mmol/l	mg/dl	18
Haemoglobin	g/dl	g/l mmol/l	10 0.62
Lead	µg/dl	µmol/l	0.0483
Packed cell volume	l/l	% or ml/dl	100
Phosphate (inorganic)	mmol/l	mg/dl mEq/l	3.1 1.8
Potassium	mmol/l	mEq/l mg/dl	1 3.9
Sodium	mmol/l	mEq/l mg/dl	1 2.3
Total protein	g/l	g/dl	0.1
Urea	mmol/l	mg/dl	6

tological findings (Ros *et al.*, 1991) and blood samples should be taken prior to treatment.

6.1.3 Reference ranges

There are a number of published reference ranges for haematological and biochemical parameters in rabbits. Conversion factors for the variety of units that are used in reference ranges are given in Table 6.1. Differences in analytical techniques between laboratories can lead to disparity in results. Laboratory data are often derived from populations of rabbits of the same breed, sex and age that are not genetically diverse. In contrast, the pet rabbit population is made up of a variety of breeds, cross breeds and is composed of rabbits of all ages. Significant breed and sex differences have been noted for some parameters in laboratory rabbits (Kozma *et al.*, 1974).

Published reference ranges for pet rabbits are either derived from sets of data from laboratory rabbits or from data collected by the author. Some reference ranges are an amalgamation of other references ranges and result in a range so wide that almost any result will fall within it. For example, the reference range for serum albumin concentrations of pet rabbits is given as 27–46 g/l (Malley, 1996) based on four published sets of data. Gillett (1994) gives an even wider range of 27–50 g/l for laboratory rabbits based on five sets of data. For some parameters there are big differences between published reference ranges. An example is blood calcium. Gillett (1994) gives a range of 1.5–3.4 mmol/l in comparison with 3.4–4.0 mmol/l by Harkness and Wagner (1995). Differences in calcium content of the diet between the groups of rabbits or differences in analytical technique could explain these discrepancies. Different laboratory methods can result in large differences between reference ranges. An example is alkaline phosphatase. Collins (1988) gives a reference range of 4.1–16.2 IU/l in comparison with 10–70 IU/l (Gillett, 1994) or 112–350 IU/l (Harkness and Wagner, 1995).

Automated flow cytometers are designed to measure numbers of human blood cells. Rabbit erythrocytes are smaller in diameter than human erythrocytes and also vary in diameter. These differences cause problems with some automated analysers. Automated differential white cells counts cannot be relied upon for rabbit blood and accurate results can only be obtained using manual counting methods (Kabata *et al.*, 1991).

Key points 6.1

- Rabbit blood clots quickly and haemolyses easily
- Food deprivation does not guarantee a fasting blood sample as rabbits ingest caecotrophs
- Stress associated with transport or handling can affect parameters such as blood glucose and the distribution of neutrophils and lymphocytes
- Pregnancy, anaesthesia, blood collection techniques and intravenous fluid therapy will influence some blood results
- Time of day can influence blood results as many parameters follow a duirnal rhythm in common with many physiological processes in rabbits
- Laboratory reference ranges are often derived from animals of the same breed and strain. Pet rabbits come from a more genetically diverse population
- Reference ranges for pet rabbits are often an amalgamation of laboratory reference ranges that can be so wide that almost any result will fall within them
- Different analytical techniques can result in disparity between laboratory reference ranges
- Automated flow cytometry is not suitable for differential white cell counts in rabbits. Accurate results can only be obtained by manual counting methods.

6.2 Haematology

6.2.1 Morphological characteristics of blood cells

Some morphological characteristics of rabbit blood cells are different from other species. The red blood cells vary in diameter within a range of 5.0–7.8 μm (Sanderson and Philips, 1981). This variation in diameter (anisocytosis) is a feature of blood smears from rabbits and is not a significant finding (see Plate 2). The red cell distribution width (RDW) is a measurement of the variation in size of erythrocytes and is higher in rabbits (11–15, Idexx reference range) than in dogs and cats (8–10; Bush, 1981). In dogs and cats, anisocytosis is indicative of the presence of reticulocytes and a regenerative anaemia. In rabbits, 1–4% of circulating erythrocytes may be reticulotytes. Polychromasia and reticulocytes in rabbit blood smears have been attributed to the short life span and high turnover of erythrocytes (Kraus *et al.*, 1984). Nucleated red cells and Howell-Jolly bodies can also be found occasionally (McLaughlin and Fish, 1994).

Rabbit neutrophils have an almost colourless cytoplasm and contain two types of granules. The smaller granules stain pink giving a pinkish colour to the cytoplasm. Larger granules stain a deeper pinkish-red. The overall colour of the neutrophils varies according to the proportion of large and small granules. The granular appearance of the cytoplasm has led to different nomenclature. Rabbit neutrophils may be called heterophils, pseudoeosinophils, acidophils or amphophils depending on the text (Sanderson and Philips, 1981; Benson and Paul-Murphy, 1999). Neutrophils measure 10–15 μm in comparison with eosinophils that measure 12–16 μm (Sanderson and Phillips, 1981).

Small lymphocytes are seen more commonly than large lymphocytes. The average cell diameter for small lymphocytes is 7–10 μm (Cooke, 2000). The lymphocytes are round cells with the typical morphology described for other species. An occasional large lymphocyte may have a few azurophilic granules in the cytoplasm (Jain, 1986).

Monocytes are large nucleated cells measuring 15–18 μm (Cooke, 2000). The nucleus has a diffuse lacey chromatin pattern that lightly stains a purple blue. The vacuolar cytoplasm stains light blue.

Eosinophils can be distinguished from neutrophils by their greater size and large acidophilic granules.

In contrast to other laboratory species, basophils are frequently found in the circulation of rabbits in small to modest numbers (Jain, 1986).

6.2.2 Interpretation of haematology results

A reference range for haematological parameters is given in Table 6.2. The haematological picture gives an indication of the general health status of a rabbit. Stress and a range of diseases will alter haematological parameters. Hinton *et al.* (1982) analysed the haematolog-

Table 6.2 Haematological reference range

	Laboratory reference range (Gillett, 1994)	Comment
Erythrocytes	4–7 × 10^{-12}/l	Anisocytosis, polychromasia, small numbers of nucleated red blood cells and Howell-Jolly bodies can be normal findings in rabbit blood films
Haemoglobin	10–15 g/dl	
PCV	33–48% (0.33–0.48 l/l)	31–40% usual range for pet rabbits
MCV	60–75 μm^3(fl)	
MCH	19–23 pg	
MCHC	34.5 g/dl	
Reticulocytes	2–4%	
Platelets	250–600 ×10^{-3}/l (10^{-9}/l)	
White cells	5–12 × 10^{-3}/l (10^{-9}/l)	
Neutrophils	30–50%	Neutrophil:lymphocyte ratio is approximately 1:1 in a healthy adult
Lymphocytes	30–60%	
Eosinophils	0–5%	
Basophils	0–8%	
Monocytes	2–10%	

From: Gillett, C.S. (1994). Selected drug dosages and clinical reference data. In *The Biology of the Laboratory Rabbit.* 2nd edn. (P.J. Manning, D.H. Ringler, C.E. Newcomer, eds). pp 467–472. Academic Press.
Sanderson, J.H., Philips, C.E. (1981). Rabbits: In *An Atlas of Laboratory Animal Haematology.* p. 6. Oxford University Press.

ical findings in 117 healthy and diseased rabbits and found that blood cellularity was a good indicator of disease especially with regard to erythrocyte and lymphocyte counts. These findings are in agreement with studies of experimental infections in rabbits (Toth and Krueger, 1988, 1989) and in a clinical study by Harcourt-Brown and Baker (2001). In this study, significantly higher red cell counts, haemoglobin values, haematocrits and lymphocyte counts were found in rabbits kept outside with unlimited access to grazing and exercise. A comparison was made with rabbits kept in hutches and those suffering from dental disease (see Figure 6.1).

6.2.3 Red cell parameters

Reference ranges for packed cell volumes (PCV) vary between sources with values between 30% and 50% (Malley, 1996). Pet rabbits tend to have PCV values at the lower end of the range, typically between 30 and 40% (Harcourt-Brown and Baker, 2001). Values greater than 45% are indicative of dehydration, especially in rabbits suffering from gut motility problems. Values of less than 30% indicate anaemia that can be classified into non-regenerative and regenerative in a similar manner to other species.

A regenerative anaemia is associated with chronic blood loss, e.g. due to heavy flea infestation or from a site that intermittently bleeds such as a uterine endometrial aneurysm. Uterine adenocarcinomas are a common finding in middle-aged does. Lead poisoning can result in a regenerative anaemia with the presence of nucleated erythrocytes, hypochromasia, poikilocytosis and cytoplasmic basophilic stippling (Fudge, 2000). A non-regenerative anaemia is caused by diseases such as lymphoma or chronic renal failure. Autoimmune haemolytic disease has not been described as a clinical phenomenon in pet rabbits although there are reports that it occurs. Autoimmune haemolytic anaemia has been reported in laboratory rabbits in association with lymphosarcoma (Weisbroth, 1994). Chronic debilitating disease such as dental disorders or abscesses often cause a mild anaemia in pet rabbits (Harcourt-Brown and Baker, 2001) (see Figure 6.1).

Nucleated red blood cells can be associated with acute infectious processes although a few may be present in normal blood films. Experimentally, infections with *Escherichia coli* and *Staphylococcus aureus* cause an increase in

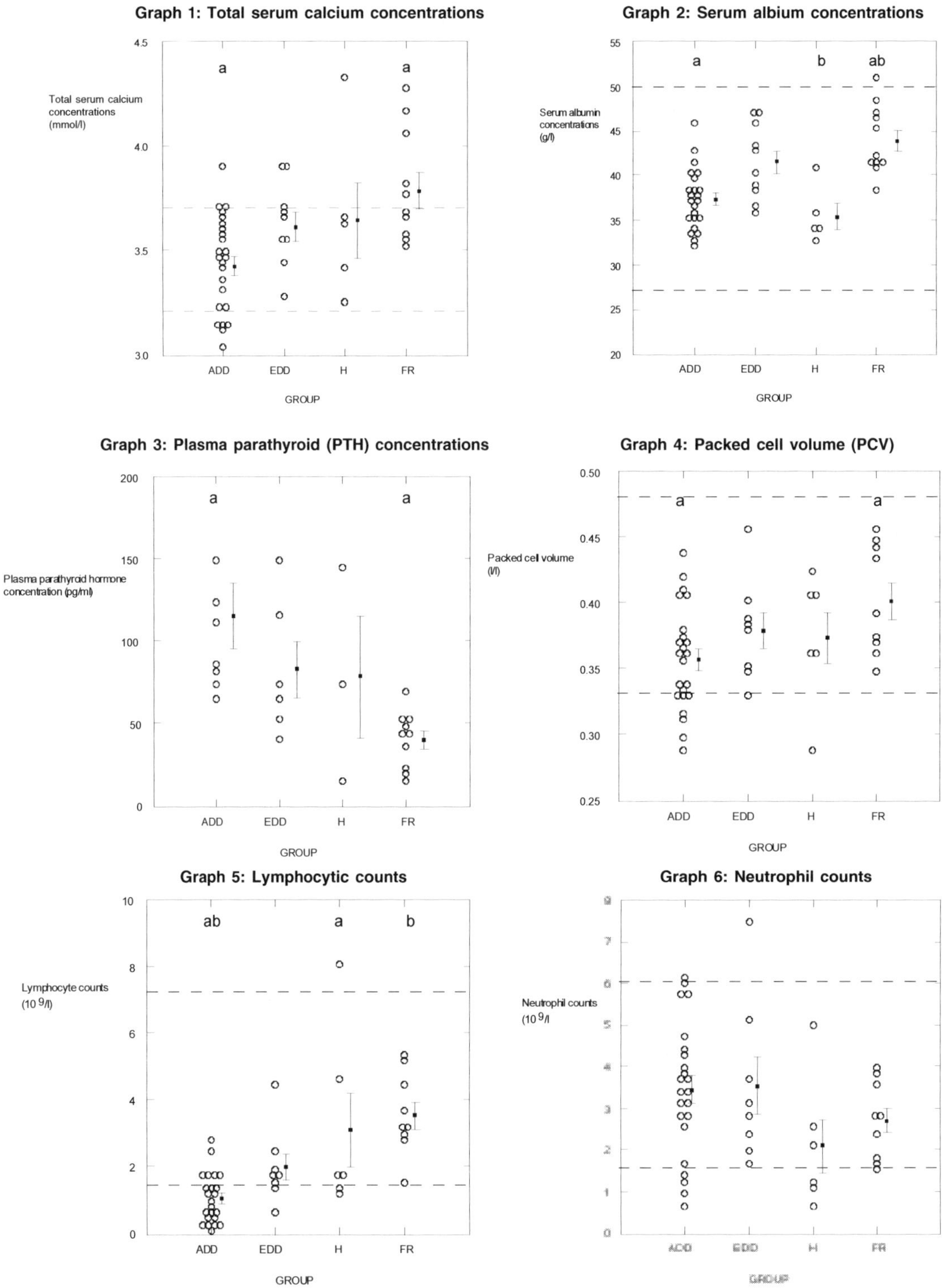

Dashed line indicates upper and lower limits of reference range for laboratory rabbits (Gillett, 1994)

Figure 6.1.

number of circulating nucleated red blood cells during the septicaemic phase of the disease (Toth and Krueger, 1988, 1989).

6.2.4 White blood cells

6.2.4.1 Total white blood cell count

There is a natural diurnal variation in total white cell count with lowest counts occurring during the late afternoon and evening (Fox and Laird, 1970). The white cell count also varies with age (Jain, 1986). It is higher in young rabbits of approximately 3 months of age and in adults over 1 year old. The first peak in leucocyte count is due to an increase in the number of lymphocytes. The second peak is due to an increase in the number of neutrophils.

In other species, an increased white blood cell count is seen in response to bacterial infection or in response to endogenous or exogenous corticosteroids. Rabbits do not develop marked leucocytosis after either acute infectious challenge or the intramuscular injection of cortisone acetate (Toth and January, 1990). In two studies by Toth and Krueger (1988, 1989) controlled experimental infections with *Staphylococcus aureus, Streptococcus pyogenes, Escherichia coli* and *Candida albicans* resulted in fever, increased plasma cortisol concentrations, neutrophilia and lymphopaenia but no significant increase in total white blood cell count. High white cell counts can be found in rabbits with suffering from lymphosarcoma (McLaughlin and Fish, 1994). Low white blood cell counts can be found in association with chronic disease (Hinton *et al.*, 1982).

Figure 6.1. Comparison of some blood parameters of pet rabbits. As part of an investigation into the relationship of metabolic bone disease with dental disease, blood samples were taken from pet rabbits presented for veterinary treatment or for health checks. At the time of sampling the rabbits were assigned to one of four groups: ADD (advanced dental disease), EDD (early dental disease), H (healthy rabbits kept in hutches), FR (rabbits kept in free-range conditions in a large enclosure with unlimited access to exercise and natural daylight all year round). No rabbits in the free-range group (FR) showed signs of dental disease; all the rabbits in the ADD, EDD and H groups were kept in hutches. Blood results from rabbits that were found to be suffering from other conditions, such as renal disease or neoplasia, were not included in the statistical analysis.

The ADD group consisted of rabbits that were presented for veterinary treatment for dental disorders such as acquired malocclusion or abscesses. All the other rabbits in the EDD, H and FR groups were presented for neutering, health checks, vaccination or euthanasia. Rabbits in the EDD group had signs of early dental disease, such as horizontal ribs on the incisors, swellings along the ventral border or the mandible or epiphora related to elongation of the roots of the upper primary incisors.

The investigation was conducted to compare blood parameters related to calcium metabolism in rabbits with or without dental disease. The healthy free-range group was used as a control. During the course of the study, differences in haematological pictures and albumin values emerged among rabbits kept under the different husbandry regimens. Complete blood counts from free-range rabbits were comparable with laboratory reference ranges whereas there were significantly lower red cell and lymphocyte counts in rabbits suffering from advanced dental disease. The low lymphocyte counts of rabbits with dental disease suggest they suffered from chronic stress.

Serum albumin values were significantly higher in rabbits kept in free-range conditions than in those suffering from advanced dental disease or those unaffected by dental disease but kept in hutches. Total serum calcium concentrations were highly correlated with serum albumin levels. Rabbits kept in hutches showed trends towards anaemia and lymphopaenia. Plasma parathyroid hormone (PTH) concentrations were higher and total serum calcium concentrations were lower in hutch-kept rabbits with advanced dental disease in comparison with rabbits kept in free-range conditions. These results indicated that acquired dental disease of pet rabbits is related to husbandry and is associated with alterations in calcium metabolism. Reprinted from Harcourt-Brown and Baker (2001) with kind permission from the *Journal of Small Animal Practice.*

6.2.4.2 Differential white cell counts

Although the total white cell count of rabbits seldom alters in diseased rabbits, the differential white cell count may show a number of changes due to the redistribution of white blood cells. A feature of many diseases in rabbits is an alteration in the ratio of neutrophils to lymphocytes and a reduction in blood cellularity (Hinton *et al.*, 1982). The neutrophil: lymphocyte ratio has been suggested as a method of predicting whether a rabbit is normal or abnormal (McLaughlin and Fish, 1994). Jain (1986) described a physiological variation in the neutrophil: lymphocyte ratio according to the age of the rabbit. The ratio changes from 33:60 in the second month of life to 45:45 in rabbits over 1 year of age. Stress and increased cortisol levels can affect this ratio as well as disease.

6.2.4.3 Effect of stress on the differential white cell count

Stress alters the differential white cell count in any species. Rabbits are particularly susceptible to the effects of stress. A car journey to the surgery, a period in the waiting room next to a barking dog or the excitement of handling can be reflected in the blood picture. Adrenaline and cortisol affect the distribution of lymphocytes throughout the body. Administration of exogenous adrenaline to rabbits results in redistribution of lymphocytes from spleen and bone marrow to peripheral blood, lungs and liver (Toft *et al.*, 1992a). Conversely, exogenous corticosteroid administration results in a redistribution of lymphocytes from the peripheral blood, bone marrow and spleen to the lymphatic tissue in rabbits (Toft *et al.*, 1992b). Prolonged periods of stress cause neutrophilia and lymphopaenia. Marked changes in white cell distribution with a relative neutrophilia and lymphopaenia were found in a study of the cortisol levels and haemograms of rabbits after transport, either by air or by lorry. The changes in white cell distribution lasted for 24–48 h and were correlated with increased cortisol levels (Toth and January, 1990).

Disease is stressful as well as having a direct effect on the production and distribution of white cells.

Rabbits with experimental infections exhibit a neutrophilia and lymphopaenia in comparison with control rabbits handled and sampled in exactly the same manner but inoculated with heat killed cultures (Toth and Krueger, 1989). Rabbits inoculated with a heat-killed culture do not experience the same rise in plasma cortisol concentrations as those inoculated with a live culture, indicating that the stress response is initiated by disease rather than by handling. Therefore the stressful effects of a long car journey to the surgery or a morning spent in a kennel next to a barking dog is more likely to affect the neutrophil:lymphocyte ratio than the excitement response of taking blood.

6.2.4.4 Neutrophils

Neutrophils function primarily as phagocytes and are important in infectious conditions and in inflammation. In other species, a neutrophilia occurs in response to inflammation, especially bacterial infection. An increase in the number of circulating neutrophils causes a rise in total white blood cell count. This response is not marked in rabbits. However, a change in the distribution of white cells can occur in response to infection with a relative neutrophilia and lymphopaenia but no alteration in total white cell count (Toth and Krueger, 1989). A mature neutrophilia accompanied by an increase in plasma cortisol can also be associated with stress (Toth and January, 1990).

6.2.4.5 Lymphocytes

Lymphocytes are involved in immunological responses and are distributed throughout the body in various tissues including blood, bone marrow, lymph nodes, spleen and gut-associated lymphoid tissue. The number of lymphocytes in the blood reflects a balance between cells leaving and entering the circulation and does not necessarily reflect a change in lymphopoiesis. Increased cortisol levels cause a lymphopaenia and increased adrenaline levels cause lymphocytosis (Toft *et al.*, 1992a, b).

In rabbits, lymphopaenia is a feature of a variety of clinical diseases (Hinton *et al*, 1982). Marked lymphopaenia has been reported as a feature of differential white cell counts of pet rabbits especially those suffering from dental disease (see Figure 6.1) (Harcourt-Brown and Baker, 2001).

Lymphoma is a relatively common tumour of rabbits and atypical lymphocytes can be found in the peripheral blood of these patients.

6.2.4.6 Eosinophils

The main function of eosinophils is detoxification either by inactivation of histamine, or histamine-like toxic materials. Eosinophils are important in the allergic response and are capable of phagocytosis (Kerr, 1989). Chronic eosinophilia can be seen in diseases of tissues that contain large numbers of mast cells such as the skin, lungs, gastrointestinal tract and uterus. Eosinophilia can be associated with parasitism, especially when parasites are migrating through tissue. Mild eosinophilia has been associated with experimentally induced chronic ascarid parasitism in rabbits (Gupta and Trivedi, 1981). However, heavy worm burdens are rare in pet rabbits. Encephalitozoonosis does not appear to cause an eosinophilia. Slight to moderate elevations in eosinophil counts can be observed after traumatic wound repair in rabbits (Fudge, 2000).

Although eosinopaenia can be a significant finding in other species, low eosinophil counts or a zero count are not unusual in rabbits.

6.2.4.7 Basophils

Basophils are similar to neutrophils but have dark blue cytoplasmic granules. Although basophils are rare in blood films from species such as the dog, they may be seen commonly in rabbit blood (Kerr, 1989). Basophil counts as high as 30% have been reported in clinically normal animals (Benson and Paul-Murphy, 1999).

6.2.4.8 Monocytes

In other species, monocytosis is associated with chronic disease, particularly chronic inflammatory conditions. In rabbits, increased monocyte counts can be associated with chronic bacterial infection. Hinton *et al.* (1982) noted increased monocyte counts in rabbits with subcutaneous abscesses, mastitis and 'labyrinthitis'. However, monocyte counts within the laboratory reference do not signify the absence of chronic infection. Rabbits with chronic osteomyelitis due to dental disease can have monocyte counts within the laboratory reference range (Harcourt-Brown, unpublished data).

Key points 6.2

- Rabbit erythrocytes vary in diameter and anisocytosis can be a normal finding in rabbit blood films
- Polychromasia and small numbers of reticulocytes and nucleated red cells may be seen on normal blood films
- Rabbit neutrophils have a granular cytoplasm and may be mistaken for eosinophils
- There are several different terms for the rabbit neutrophil. Some authors use terms such as heterophil, pseudo-eosinophil, acidophil or amphophil instead of neutrophil
- Basophils are frequently found on blood films from rabbits
- Low blood cellularity, i.e. anaemia and lymphopaenia, is a non-specific feature of disease in rabbits
- High numbers of nucleated red blood cells may be associated with infectious disease
- The neutrophil:lymphocyte ratio should be approximately 1:1 in adult rabbits. Alterations in the ratio can be associated with stress or disease
- Adrenaline causes a shift of lymphocytes from the spleen and bone marrow to blood. Cortisol causes a shift of lymphocytes away from the bloodstream to the spleen and lymphatic tissue
- An increase in total white cell count is unusual in rabbits even in the presence of infection
- A neutrophilia with a left shift occurs in response to infection
- Monocytosis can be seen in association with chronic infection.

6.3 Biochemistry

A reference range for biochemical parameters is given in Table 6.3.

Table 6.3 Biochemistry. (NB: A fasting sample cannot be guaranteed by withholding food from rabbits as they ingest caecotrophs)

Ref source	*Parameter*	*Reference range*
b	Albumin	27–50 g/l
b	Alkaline phosphatase	10–70 IU/l
b	ALT	25–65 IU/l
b	AST	10–98 IU/l
b	Amylase	200–500 U/l
b	Bilirubin	3.4–8.5 µmol/l
g	Bile acids	> 40 µmol/l
a f	Blood lead	3.7-5.3 µg/100 ml(dl) 2-27 µg/dl (0.002-0.027 mg/dl)
c	Calcium (total)	3.2–3.7 mmol/l (anecdotal range of 3–4.2 mmol/l for pet rabbits on a varied diet)
h	Calcium (ionized)	1.71 (+ 0.11) mmol/l
b	Cholesterol	0.3–3.00 mmol/l
b	Creatinine	44.2–229 µmol/l
b	Triglycerides	1.4–1.76 mmol/l
d	Gamma GT	0–7.0 IU/l
b	Globulin	15–27 g/l
b	Glucose	4.2–7.8 mmol/l
b	Inorganic phosphate	1.28–1.92 mmol/l
b j	Potassium	3.5–7 mmol/l 3.2 + 0.1 mmol/l (**NB**. Values can be affected by anaesthesia)
b	Sodium	138–150 mmol/l
a	T_4	6.4–8.3 µg/100 ml (dl) or 82.37–106.82 nmol/l
b	Total protein	54–75 g/l
e	Urea	6.14–8.38 mmol/l
b	Vitamin A (plasma)	30–80 µg/ml ± < 10 µg/ml indicates deficiency (Liver levels of < 10 µg/g liver denote deficiency)
b	Vitamin E (plasma κ-tocopherol)	> 1 µg/ml (< 0.5 µg/ml indicates deficiency)

Reference sources: a: Jones, R.T. (1975); b: Gillett, C.S. (1994); c: Goad, D.L. *et al.* (1989); d: Okerman, L. (1994); e: Collins, B.R. (1988); f: Swartout, M.S., Gerken, D.F. (1987); g: Kerr, M. (1989); h: Warren, H.B. *et al.* (1989); j: Robson, W.L. *et al.* (1981).

6.3.1 Glucose

Herbivores, such as rabbits, differ from carnivores in their carbohydrate metabolism. Carnivores eat periodically and have sudden large intakes of nutrients that must be stored for utilization during the fast between meals. Herbivores graze for long periods of the day and are continually absorbing nutrients from the digestive tract. In rabbits, volatile fatty acids are produced from bacterial fermentation in the caecum and are continually absorbed as an energy source. A fasting sample is difficult to obtain from a rabbit. Withholding food does not prevent caecotrophy and the digestion of caecotrophs provides a source of glucose. Blood samples taken after 96 h of food deprivation may show no alteration in blood glucose levels (Kozma *et al.*, 1974).

Hyperglycaemia is a relatively common finding in rabbits and can be accompanied by glycosuria. Handling alone can cause an increase in blood glucose to the order of 8.5 mmol/l experimentally (Knudtzon, 1988) and 15 mmol/l or more anecdotally. Diabetes mellitus has not been described in pet rabbits and there is some difference of opinion about its importance as a clinical disease (Hoefer, 2000; Jenkins, 2000; Rosenthal, 2000). Herbivorous animals withstand the absence of insulin more readily than carnivorous ones (Bentley, 1998) and are therefore not so susceptible to diabetes mellitus. Diabetes mellitus has been induced in laboratory rabbits by the administration of alloxan. It has also been described as a hereditary disease in rabbits. A laboratory strain was selectively bred as an animal model of human diabetes mellitus. (Roth and Conaway, 1982). Affected animals were polydipsic, polyuric and polyphagic with severely impaired insulin release. Elevated glycosylated haemoglobin values of 12.2% were observed in the overtly diabetic animals in comparison with 3.9% in normal animals. Increased glycosylated haemoglobin levels did not correlate with plasma glucose concentrations (Cannon and Conaway, 1981). Histologically there was hypergranulation of β-cells of the islets of Langerhans. Obesity and ketoacidosis were not features of diabetes mellitus in the laboratory rabbits. The hyperglycaemia was in the region of 540–590 mg/dl (30–33.4 mmol/l) and there was marked glycosuria. Roth and Conaway (1982) described the maintenance of one diabetic individual on insulin at a dose of up to 8 units per day for 3 years. Ketonuria was not observed.

In pet rabbits, a diagnosis of diabetes mellitus cannot be made on a single blood sample and requires serial blood and urine sampling to confirm the diagnosis. In view of the physiological factors that can increase blood glucose levels it is advisable to take repeat blood samples from hyperglycaemic rabbits with time of day, phase of digestion, anaesthesia, influence of handling or car journeys in mind. Mild glycosuria is not a significant finding.

Hyperglycaemia can be seen in the terminal stages of gut stasis and is a poor prognostic sign (Harcourt-Brown, personal observation). It is associated with fatty degeneration of the liver at *post-mortem* examination. Marked hyperglycaemia is also seen in association with painful conditions such as acute intestinal obstruction. Blood glucose levels can rise to 20–25 mmol/l and return to normal once the condition is resolved (Harcourt-Brown, unpublished observation). Experimental haemorrhagic or traumatic shock results in hyperglycaemia proportional to the severity of the condition. Hyperthermia also results in hyperglycaemia (McLaughlin and Fish, 1994). Diseases that elevate serum glucose levels in other species, such as hyperadrenocorticism or acute pancreatititis have not been reported in pet rabbits, although they could occur.

Hypoglycaemia is a significant finding in rabbits and is associated with anorexia, starvation or disturbances in the digestion and absorption of carbohydrates. It can be a sign of hepatic dysfunction. A drop in blood glucose leads to mobilization of free fatty acids from adipose tissue and contributes to the development of ketoacidosis and fatty degeneration of the liver. Measurement of serum glucose is of value in moribund rabbits as a basis for the selection of appropriate fluid therapy. Other causes of hypoglycaemia such as Addison's disease or insulinomas have not been reported in pet rabbits although such conditions could occur.

6.3.2 Total protein

Interpretation of total protein concentrations is similar to other mammals. Artefactual increases in protein concentrations can result from excessive venous stasis during blood collection. Fluid and small molecules leave the plasma, resulting in a relative increase in proteins. This situation can occur in rabbits, especially in miniature breeds with small veins.

An increase in total protein indicates dehydration, chronic and immune-mediated disease. In rabbits dehydration due to water deprivation or gastrointestinal disturbances commonly occurs. Examination of the haematocrit and albumin and globulin fractions can assist differential diagnosis.

Liver disease, chronic enteropathy, starvation or malnutrition may result in reduced protein levels. Glomerulonephropathy or protein-losing enteropathy are uncommon conditions that could cause low total protein levels in rabbits. A decrease in both albumin and globulin may be associated with haemorrhage or exudative skin lesions such as fly strike.

6.3.3 Albumin

The liver is the sole site of albumin synthesis and hypoalbuminaemia is feature of advanced liver disease in all species. In rabbits, heavy parasitism is a cause of liver disease. *Eimeria steidae* causes hepatic coccidiosis (see Section 10.10.1.2). *Cysticercus pisiformis,* the larval stage of *Taenia pisiformis,* migrates through the liver and results in the development of fibrous tracks and necrotic foci (see Section 16.3.2). Severe infestations can result in low albumin levels. Non-hepatic causes of low serum albumin include glomerulonephropathy, protein-losing enteropathy, malabsorption and cardiogenic ascites.

Laboratory reference ranges for serum albumin levels in rabbits can be wide and vary between sources. Sex differences have been reported in laboratory rabbits. One study showed that female New Zealand White rabbits had higher serum albumin levels than males, although other studies have found no sex differences (Kozma *et al.*, 1974).

In rabbits, hypoalbuminaemia is most likely to be associated with nutritional factors such as abnormal caecotrophy, incorrect diet, starvation or malnutrition associated with dental disease. Primary or secondary hepatic neoplasia occasionally occurs in pet rabbits. Hepatic coccidiosis is a cause of low serum albumin levels, especially in young rabbits that have been kept in colonies.

A high serum albumin concentration is not a feature of any specific disease, although an increased albumin level in conjunction with a raised PCV is indicative of dehydration. In a study by Harcourt-Brown and Baker (2001), pet rabbits kept in free-range conditions had significantly higher serum albumin concentrations than rabbits that were suffering from advanced dental disease. They were also significantly higher than rabbits kept in hutches that were not suffering from dental problems (see Figure 6.1). The difference in albumin levels was attributed to differences in diet and husbandry. Caecotrophs are a source of amino acids for rabbits and normal caecotrophy is an important element of their protein metabolism. Low fibre diets, obesity, dental disease or skeletal abnormalities can prevent rabbits ingesting caecotrophs from the anus and reduce the available amino acids for protein synthesis. Rabbits that are kept in hutches are more likely to be eating a low fibre diet and to suffer from obesity and skeletal problems than rabbits living outside with unrestricted access to natural vegetation and exercise.

6.3.4 Globulin

Plasma globulins are made up of a range of proteins including carrier proteins and immunoglobulins or antibodies. The types of globulin can be separated into five fractions by electrophoresis. The γ-globulin fraction is almost entirely composed of immunoglobulins. Some globulins can be synthesized in the liver but immunoglobulins are synthesized exclusively in lymphoid tissue. Acute inflammation, chronic disease or immune-mediated disease can cause an increase in globulin levels. Myeloproliferative disease results in abnormal levels of immunoglobulin production.

There are few published data on the significance of globulin concentrations in rabbits. Lipaemia can artefactually elevate protein levels with some analytical methods. Experimental infections with rabbit coronavirus result in hypergammaglobulinaemia. Analogies have been made between coronavirus infection in rabbits and feline infectious peritonitis in cats (DiGiacomo and Mare, 1994). Coronavirus occurs in laboratory rabbits but is an unlikely diagnosis in the pet rabbit.

6.3.5 Cholesterol and triglycerides

Cholesterol is synthesized in the liver or absorbed from the diet. It is a metabolic precursor of steroid hormones. Cholesterol is broken down in the liver and excreted in bile. In other species, elevated cholesterol levels are indicative of a variety of metabolic disorders such as hypothyroidism, hepatopathy, diabetes mellitus, and hyperadrenocorticism. Low levels can occur in association with impaired hepatic function. Changes in serum triglyceride levels reflect a similar range of diseases. Blood levels of triglycerides increase after a meal, especially if it is a fatty meal.

In rabbits, there are some physiological factors that affect cholesterol levels. Male rabbits have lower cholesterol levels than females and there is a diurnal variation with higher levels occurring during the late afternoon (Loeb and Quimby, 1989). Large variations in blood cholesterol and triglyceride values can occur between individual rabbits (Yu *et al.*, 1979). A fasting blood sample is required for cholesterol and triglyceride assay. In rabbits, it is difficult to obtain a fasting sample because of caecotrophy. Abnormal cholesterol or triglyceride levels are most likely to be associated with dietary factors or hepatic impairment. In anorexic rabbits, especially obese ones, a lipaemic sample is a poor prognostic indicator as it signifies impaired fat metabolism and the presence of hepatic lipidosis (see Section 10.3). A rise in triglyceride levels has been found in association with experimentally induced chronic renal failure in rabbits (Tvedegaard, 1987).

6.3.6 Amylase

In other species, amylase is found in the pancreas and to a lesser extent in the salivary glands, liver and small intestinal mucosa. Amylase has a short half-life and is rapidly removed from the circulation. It is excreted by the kidney. Elevated levels indicate pancreatic disease or renal insufficiency.

In rabbits, amylase is present in pancreatic tissue in high concentrations. Low concentrations are found in the salivary glands and none is produced by the liver (Jenkins, 2000). Amylase is also produced by caecal microorganisms and is present in caecotrophs aiding conversion of glucose to lactic acid during digestion in the stomach and small intestine. Serum amylase levels are lower in rabbits than other species (McLaughlin and Fish, 1994). Pancreatic duct obstruction or pancreatic disease can result in a rise in blood amylase values. Rabbits can survive experimental ligation of the pancreatic duct (Brewer and Cruise, 1994).

6.3.7 Bilirubin

The rabbit secretes a large amount of bile, approximately seven times as much as a dog on a weight basis (Brewer and Cruise, 1994). The rabbit also differs from other species in the excretion of breakdown products of haemoglobin. The rabbit has low biliverdin reductase activity (Fekete, 1989) and only 30% of biliverdin is converted to bilirubin. Bilirubin values can be affected by fasting. Glucose administration to rabbits lowers serum bilirubin concentrations by modifying hepatic conjugation and increasing biliary secretion (McLaughlin and Fish, 1994).

In rabbits, biliary obstruction results in jaundice and raised serum bilirubin values. In young rabbits, hepatic coccidiosis is the most usual cause of jaundice. In older rabbits, bile duct obstruction from neoplasia is more likely. Aflatoxicosis from the ingestion of mouldy feed can result in hepatic fibrosis and jaundice (Krishna *et al.*, 1991). Viral haemorrhagic disease (VHD) causes acute hepatic necrosis with elevated bilirubin concentrations in association with dramatic increases in AST and ALT concentrations. VHD is invariably fatal, although some rabbits may survive long enough to develop jaundice before they die.

There is little on information on haemolytic disease as a cause of jaundice in pet rabbits. Haemolytic anaemia has been reported in association with lymphosarcoma in laboratory rabbits (Weisbroth, 1994).

6.3.8 Alanine aminotransferase (ALT)

In other species, ALT is used as an indicator of hepatocellular damage, especially in dogs and cats. ALT is also in found in other tissues such as muscle and red blood cells. An increase in ALT signifies cell damage, although the degree of the increase does not correlate with the severity of hepatic disease and is not a prognostic indicator (Willard *et al.*, 1999).

In rabbits, liver ALT activity is lower than in other species and there is less organ specificity (Rosenthal, 1997). ALT is also present in cardiac muscle. The half-life of ALT in the rabbit is approximately 5 h. In the dog the half-life is 45–60 hours (Jenkins, 2000).

Hepatic coccidiosis due to *Eimeria steidae* is a cause of increased blood ALT concentrations especially in conjunction with an increase in alkaline phosphatase, bilirubin and gamma GT. Elevated ALT values have been found in asymptomatic house rabbits and have been attributed to the effects of organic solvents in wood shavings used as litter material. Other liver diseases such as neoplasia can cause a rise in ALT but sometimes not until the condition is advanced (McLaughlin and Fish, 1994). Low doses of aflatoxin caused a significant rise in ALT concentrations in a group of laboratory rabbits (Fekete and Huszenicza, 1993). Hepatic lipidosis will elevate ALT levels.

6.3.9 Aspartate aminotransferase (AST)

In other species AST is widely distributed throughout the body. In particular, it is found in skeletal muscle, cardiac muscle, liver and erythrocytes. Like ALT, AST is an indicator of tissue damage. It is sometimes used as an indicator of liver disease, especially in horses in which ALT is not liver specific.

In rabbits, AST is found in liver, heart, skeletal muscle, kidney and pancreas with the highest activity in the liver and skeletal muscle (Benson and Paul-Murphy, 1999). Physical exertion or tissue damage during blood collection can elevate results. Raised AST levels can be found in association with liver disease.

6.3.10 α-Glutaryltransferase (GGT)

GGT is found in liver and kidney tissue. In other species, GGT is used as an indicator of hepatobiliary disease especially in horses and ruminants where it is associated with long-term liver damage. Although GGT is found in high concentrations in renal tubular cells, kidney disease does not lead to elevated blood levels, probably because the enzyme is excreted in the urine (Bush, 1991).

In the rabbit GGT is located predominantly in the renal epithelium with low activity in the liver. Liver GGT is present primarily in bile duct epithelial cells and is therefore an indicator of hepatobiliary disease rather than hepatocellular damage (McLaughlin and Fish, 1994). In cases where there is renal tissue damage, urine GGT may be increased in addition to plasma concentrations.

6.3.11 Alkaline phosphatase (AP)

Alkaline phosphatase consists of a group of several isoenzymes that hydrolyse phosphates at an alkaline pH (Kerr, 1989). It is one of the most widely distributed enzymes in the body. Alkaline phosphatase is found particularly in bone, liver and intestinal wall. Different isoenzymes are produced from each site. Increases in plasma activity are usually due to the isoenzymes derived from liver and bone. Higher concentrations are found in young animals with high osteoblastic activity.

In rabbits, alkaline phosphatase is present in nearly all tissues. It is found in association with cell membranes and especially in intestinal epithelium, renal tubules, osteoblasts, liver and placenta. The rabbit has three AP isoenzymes – the intestinal form as well as two isoenzymes present in both liver and kidney (McLaughlin and Fish, 1994). There is a wide variation between laboratory reference ranges for AP values for rabbits. Examples include: 4.1–16.2 IU/l (Collins, 1988); 10–70 IU/l (Gillett, 1994); 112–350 IU/l (Harkness and Wagner, 1995). Different analytical techniques could account for these variations.

In a survey of blood parameters relating to calcium metabolism in pet rabbits, serum alkaline phosphatase values varied widely even in apparently healthy individuals (Harcourt-Brown and Baker, 2001). Increased levels of alkaline phosphatase are seen in biliary obstruction, e.g. neoplasia or hepatic coccidiosis. Experimental ligation of the common bile duct results in increased levels of alkaline phosphatase up to 600 IU/l (McLaughlin and Fish, 1994). Enteric disease can also elevate alkaline phosphatase values (Jenkins, 2000).

6.3.12 Bile acids

Bile acids are derived from cholesterol and are secreted into the intestine to aid fat digestion. From the gut, they are reabsorbed into the circulation and transported to the liver to be resecreted in the bile. Impaired hepatic function results in increased concentrations of bile acids in peripheral blood. There are physiological variations in circulatory bile acid concentrations in association with the digestion of food and stimulation of the gall bladder to release bile into the small intestine. In most species, a fasting sample should have a low concentration of bile acids of less than 15 μmol/l (Kerr, 1989). Impaired hepatic function can result in marked rises in fasting serum bile acid concentrations.

In rabbits, the production of bile acids shows a circadian rhythm (Fekete, 1989). There is a problem in obtaining a fasting sample from rabbits due to the ingestion of caecotrophs. Bile acids are not included in published reference ranges for rabbits at the present time. Bile acid levels in excess of 100 µmol/l have been found in association with hepatic coccidiosis in comparison with levels that are generally less than 40 µmol/l (Harcourt-Brown, unpublished data).

6.3.13 Urea

Urea is a nitrogenous waste product that is formed in the liver as the end product of deamination of amino acids. It is transported in the blood to the kidney where it is excreted in the urine. In other species, high blood urea concentrations are indicative of impaired renal function that may be due to renal disease or poor perfusion due to circulatory disorders or cardiac disease. Low blood urea levels can reflect hepatic dysfunction.

In rabbits, many physiological factors influence the concentration of urea in the blood. Dietary protein concentrations and quality, withholding food and natural diurnal rhythms can all affect blood urea concentrations. Higher levels occur in the late evening (Loeb and Quimby, 1989). The rabbit's urea metabolism is further complicated by urea utilization by caecal microflora during catabolism or during periods of dietary excess. Therefore small fluctuations in serum urea concentrations are difficult to interpret. Laboratory reference ranges apply to animals that are fed a standard diet and have usually been bled at a specific time of day. Pet rabbits are subject to greater fluctuations in blood urea values due to the variation in diet and other factors, and can have values slightly higher than laboratory reference ranges. Prerenal azotaemia associated with poor renal perfusion occurs during periods of dehydration. The rabbit has a limited capacity to concentrate urea and a greater volume of urine is required when urea load increases (Brewer and Cruise, 1994). Increased blood urea values were recorded in a study by Licois *et al.* (1978) of young rabbits with diarrhoea experimentally induced with coccidiosis. The authors suggested that the blood urea values rose as a result of intense nitrogen catabolism during weight loss associated with the disease. Water deprivation can lead to high blood urea values as high as 40 mmol/l in association with creatinine values in excess of 200 µmol/l (Harcourt-Brown, unpublished data). Water deprivation can be due to a lack of available drinking water, caused either by an oversight by the owner or by a faulty mechanism on the drinking bottle.

In rabbits, dehydration can cause urea and creatinine values that would signify renal disease in the dog and cat. High levels usually return to normal once the animal is rehydrated. Therefore, urea and creatinine values should be checked before making an absolute diagnosis of renal failure. As in other species, elevated blood urea values in rabbits are associated with renal insufficiency. Nephrolithiasis is a cause of kidney disease in the rabbit (see Section 14.5). Abdominal radiography is indicated in rabbits with raised urea and creatinine levels. *Encephalitozoon cuniculi* can cause low-grade kidney disease in rabbits with mild elevations in blood urea. Most cases are subclinical. *E. cuniculi* infection causes granulomatous lesions in the kidneys that become pitted and scarred with fibrotic areas. The parasite has been associated with chronic renal failure with blood urea values in the region of 152.7 mg/dl (25.45 mmol/l) and creatinine of 5.8 mg/dl (512.72 µmol/l) in a study by Ewringmann and Göbel (1999). Affected rabbits were anaemic with low haemoglobin and red cell counts and had elevated serum potassium concentrations. Neoplasia, interstitial nephritis, nephrotoxicity also occur in rabbits and cause renal disease.

Low blood urea values in association with impaired hepatic function and the use of anabolic steroids have been described (Benson and Paul-Murphy, 1999).

6.3.14 Creatinine

Creatinine is a nitrogenous waste product that, like urea, is transported in the blood to the kidney where it is excreted in the urine. Creatinine is not the product of amino acid breakdown but of creatine which is a substance present in the muscle and is involved in high energy metabolism (Kerr, 1989). The slow catabolism of creatine results in a slow inflow of creatinine to the plasma at a rate which is directly proportional to the individual's muscle mass but is unaffected by any change in muscular activity or muscle damage. Any changes in blood creatinine concentrations are due to changes in excretion and are a reflection of renal function. Concentrations rise quickly at the outset of renal disease and decrease when an improvement of renal function takes place. Creatinine deteriorates in plasma and readings from old samples (>24 h) cannot be relied upon. There is interference from a variety of other substances such as bilirubin (which decreases creatinine) or cephalosporins (which increase creatinine).

Key points 6.3

- Stress of handling can cause a marked elevation of blood glucose levels in rabbits. Levels as high as 15 mmol/l can occur in association with handling. Higher levels (> 20 mmol/l) may be seen in association with stressful or painful diseases such as intestinal obstruction
- There is debate about the occurrence of diabetes mellitus in domestic rabbits. It has been induced in laboratory rabbits and a genetically susceptible laboratory strain has been bred
- Large individual variations in blood cholesterol and triglyceride values can occur in rabbits
- Jaundice is unusual in rabbits but may be seen in association with cholestasis in diseases such as hepatic coccidiosis or neoplasia
- There is a wide variation between laboratory reference ranges for alkaline phosphatase values
- Blood urea and creatinine values can be high in cases of prerenal azotaemia in rabbits and do not always signify renal failure. Causes include dehydration or water deprivation.

6.3.15 Electrolytes

The rabbit's complex digestive physiology and the compromised renal capability of correcting acid–base disorders make the rabbit a prime candidate for electrolyte imbalances (see Section 1.6). Dietary deficiency of electrolytes such as sodium and potassium is unlikely in the herbivorous diet of rabbits. Instead, electrolyte problems are more likely to be associated with abnormal losses. Although rabbits do not vomit, water and electrolyte absorption and secretion are affected by gastrointestinal disease. If facilities are available, electrolyte assays, especially potassium, can be a valuable part of the diagnostic workup for critically ill rabbits.

6.3.15.1 Sodium

In general, changes in sodium concentrations reflect the osmolality of extracellular fluid rather than the total body sodium content. Increased blood sodium concentrations (hypernatraemia) can be the result of water deprivation or the loss of low sodium fluids. Decreased sodium concentrations (hyponatraemia) may occur as a result of chronic renal failure when the kidney cannot concentrate urine and fast urine flow through the renal tubules prevents effective sodium/potassium exchange. Lipaemia or hyperproteinaemia can artefactually reduce affect sodium concentrations if certain laboratory methods are used.

At the present time, there are few data available on clinical conditions that affect sodium concentrations in rabbits.

6.3.15.2 Potassium

About 95% of the total body potassium is intracellular, so measurement of extracellular potassium in blood samples does not give a true reflection of the potassium status of the patient. The balance between intracellular and extracellular potassium is regulated by aldosterone, insulin and catecholamines and is affected by blood pH. Aldosterone stimulates renal excretion of potassium. Insulin promotes the movement of potassium into cells. The effects of these hormones prevent large diet-induced changes in plasma potassium concentrations. Potassium is an important ion in the maintenance of membrane potential. Abnormally high or low potassium concentrations can have life-threatening consequences due to impaired electrical activity of cells. High blood potassium concentrations can result in cardiac arrest.

Alterations in blood potassium levels can be due to alterations in dietary intake and excretion, or redistribution across cell membranes. To maintain electroneutrality, potassium ions shift from intracellular to extracellular fluid in exchange for hydrogen ions. In other species, hypoadrenocorticism (Addison's disease) reduces the exchange of sodium and potassium ions across the cell membrane and results in increased serum potassium and decreased serum sodium concentrations. Hyperkalaemia can be the result of impaired renal excretion of potassium due to kidney disease or from tissue trauma such as crushing injuries that release large amounts of potassium into the circulation. Acidosis causes a redistribution of potassium across the cell membrane. Artefactually high levels of potassium can result from leakage from red cells in haemolysed samples or those that have not been separated until several hours after the blood was taken.

Low blood potassium can cause muscular weakness and depression. Hypokalaemia can be the result of dietary potassium deficiency or as a result of potassium loss from the gastrointestinal tract. Diuresis or the use of potassium-free intravenous fluids also cause hypokalaemia. Alkalosis can cause redistribution of potassium and sodium across the cell membrane and result in hypokalaemia. Artefactually low potassium concentrations are uncommon although they can occur secondarily to hyperlipidaemia or hyperproteinaemia (Willard *et al.*, 1999). Blood collection through a catheter that contains residual potassium-free fluids can lead to erroneously low results.

In rabbits, the effect of blood collection methods on plasma potassium levels has been investigated. Discrepancies in results were found between blood collected from the ear and from the carotid artery when the blood was collected with a plastic catheter but not with a 21 g needle (Robson *et al.*, 1981). General anaesthesia with pentobarbitone depressed plasma potassium values but sedation with chlorpromazine did not affect results. Serum potassium concentrations were found to be higher than plasma and in venous rather than arterial blood (Robson *et al.*, 1981).

Low serum potassium values have been found in unanaesthetized rabbits in conjunction with signs of muscular weakness (Harcourt-Brown, unpublished data). Affected animals can still eat and drink but are unable to move. It is not known whether hypokalaemia is the cause of the muscular weakness. Possible causes of hypokalaemia are discussed in Section 12.6.1.1. Further investigations of serum potassium concentrations of rabbits are required to know the clinical significance of measured values and the influence of various physiological states. In horses, blood potassium concentrations can fall to 2.0 mmol/l after prolonged exercise due to potassium loss in sweat and to 2.5 mmol/l while eating hay due to potassium loss in saliva. During moderate exercise concentrations can rise to 4.0 mmol/l due to potassium release from muscle cells (Kerr, 1989). Similar physiological variations could occur in the rabbit.

6.3.15.3 Calcium

Calcium is an essential element that is involved in many body systems. Most of the body's calcium is stored in bone in conjunction with phosphate. Calcium is an essential part of the structure of bones and teeth. It is an important cation in intracellular and extracellular fluid where it is required for muscle metabolism, enzyme activation, blood coagulation and osmoregulation. Calcium is found in the blood in three forms: ionized, bound to other anions (especially phosphate) and bound to protein (especially albumin). Because of the protein binding capacity of calcium, total serum calcium concentrations are proportional to albumin concentrations. Ionized calcium is the physiologically active component of blood and is involved in the permeability of cell membranes. Hypocalcaemia is a life-threatening condition. In many species, a high demand for calcium during late pregnancy and lactation can result in hypocalcaemic tetany. There are also some metabolic disorders that can result in alterations in serum calcium concentrations in other species. Examples include renal, pancreatic and neoplastic diseases.

The rabbit has a different calcium metabolism from other domestic species (see Section 1.6.7). Dietary calcium is readily absorbed from the intestine and total plasma values reflect dietary intake. Total blood calcium levels are higher and can vary over a wider range than other species. An erroneous diagnosis of hypercalcaemia is often made because of the rabbit's high total serum calcium levels in comparison with other animals. Parathyroid hormone (PTH) regulates calcium metabolism in a similar manner to other animals, but a reduction in plasma PTH level occurs at a higher plasma calcium concentration than in other species (Warren *et al.*, 1989). The kidney plays an important role in calcium regulation and has a high fractional excretion for calcium when blood levels are high. Calcium is excreted in the urine in which it forms calcium carbonate precipitate. Some authors have suggested monitoring blood calcium concentrations as part of the protocol for treating 'sludgy urine'. However, high blood calcium levels are not the sole cause of urinary tract disease in rabbits (see Section 14.4.1).

There are differences between published reference ranges for total serum calcium values in rabbits. Variations in dietary calcium intake could account for some of the discrepancies. The peak blood level that was obtained by increasing dietary calcium intake in laboratory rabbits was 5.42 mmol/l (21.7 mg/dl) in a study by Chapin and Smith (1967a). Experimental calcium restriction resulted in minimum serum concentrations of 3.22–3.5 mmol/l (13–15 mg/dl) before a rapid decline just before death in a separate study by Chapin and Smith (1967b).

A reference range of 3.2–3.7 mmol/l taken from eight laboratory reference sources has been made by Goad *et al.* (1989). Values outside this range are encountered in otherwise healthy individuals and a range of 3.0–4.2 mmol/l is acceptable for pet rabbits on a varied diet.

Total blood calcium levels in rabbits are also affected by age and reproductive status. Kamphues *et al.* (1986) found that increased calcium intake only resulted in higher total plasma calcium concentrations in adult rabbits and not young ones of 5–19 weeks. Serum calcium concentrations in growing rabbits are fixed at a value of approximately 3.5 mmol/l (14 mg/dl) (Kamphues *et al.*, 1986, Gilsanz *et al.*, 1991). Blood calcium levels decrease during pregnancy (Assane *et al.*, 1993).

Due to the protein binding properties of calcium, albumin levels can also affect total calcium concentrations. Albumin concentrations in pet rabbits are variable and appear to be affected by the manner in which they are kept (Harcourt-Brown and Baker, 2001). In dogs and man, total serum calcium values can be adjusted by using a mathematical formula that takes albumin concentration into account. (Adjusted calcium concentration = measured serum total calcium concentration – serum albumin (g/dl) + 3.5). This formula is unreliable in cats (Flanders *et al.*, 1989) and has not been investigated in rabbits.

At present, most published reference ranges for pet rabbits refer to total serum calcium concentrations. Ideally, ionized calcium should be measured for an accurate assessment of calcium status but special sample handling and equipment is required that precludes its measurement in most practice situations. However, affordable equipment is now becoming available that can be used in the practice laboratory. Measurements of ionized calcium have been made during experimental investigations using rabbits. Warren *et al.* (1989) found a linear relationship between total serum calcium and ionized calcium values. A group of 29 non-pregnant female and male rabbits were found to have ionized serum calcium levels of 1.71 + 0.11 mmol/l. Kamphues *et al.* (1986) reported ionized calcium values of 6.94 + 0.21 mg/dl (1.73 + 0.05 mmol/l) in adult rabbits on an average dietary calcium intake (0.85%).

Hypocalcaemic tetany has been reported in lactating does (Barlet, 1980). Hypercalcaemia is seen in rabbits with chronic renal failure and impaired calcium excretion (see Section 14.5.3.1). In a study by Tvedegaard (1987), experimentally induced chronic renal failure resulted in total serum calcium concentrations of 4.82 + 0.77 mmol/l. Levels in excess of 4.25 mmol/l have been recorded in association with neoplasia (Voelkel *et al.*, 1978).

6.3.15.4 Phosphate

Inorganic phosphate is involved in many enzyme systems and is important in carbohydrate and muscle metabolism as well as forming a major component of bone. Phosphate is obtained from the diet. Vitamin D and PTH influence intestinal absorption of phosphorus in a similar manner to calcium. PTH stimulates renal excretion of phosphate and renal conservation of calcium. The pH of intestinal contents and the presence of cations such as calcium and magnesium can affect the availability of dietary phosphate.

Abnormalities of phosphate metabolism are complex and interdependent with many other factors. Blood phosphate values can be difficult to interpret and need to be examined alongside other parameters. In other species, physiological activities such as feeding and exercise reduce serum phosphorus concentrations (Aitken and Allen, 1994). There are drug interactions that alter serum phosphorus values. Examples include phosphate binders, anaesthetic agents, bicarbonate, parenteral glucose, anabolic steroids, diuretics and tetracyclines (Willard *et al.*, 1999). Phosphorus can shift between the intracellular and extracellular space in response to alterations in acid–base metabolism. In addition to these problems of interpretation, phosphate values are subject to artefactual error caused by poor sample handling. Haemolysis releases phosphate from erythrocytes, which results in elevated values.

In rabbits, there is little information about the clinical relevance of serum phosphate concentrations. Rabbit blood clots easily and good quality non-haemolysed samples can be difficult to obtain. Hyperphosphataemia can be due to impaired renal phosphorus excretion due to kidney disease. Hypophosphataemia may result from dietary deficiency, impaired intestinal absorption or metabolic disorders.

6.4 Miscellaneous assays

6.4.1 Lead estimation

Blood lead concentrations are given in different units depending on the source. The conversion factor for μg/dl to μmol/l is 0.0483.

A study by Roscoe *et al.* (1975) evaluated three diagnostic tests for lead toxicity in rabbits. Whole blood lead concentrations of greater than 0.03 mg/dl (1.45 μmol/l) were considered a reliable indicator of lead ingestion. Measurement of urinary delta-aminolevulinic acid (δALA) was considered unreliable. Erythrocytes from rabbits that were given lead fluoresced red when exposed to light rays of 320–400 nm. The fluorescent erythrocyte test (FET) was considered a convenient and reliable test for lead ingestion.

Swartout and Gerken (1987) described two clinical cases of lead poisoning that had blood levels of 70 μg/dl (0.07 mg/dl) and 40 μg/dl (0.04 mg/dl). They gave a range of 2–27 μg/dl (0.002–0.027 mg/dl) as a normal range for laboratory rabbits.

6.4.2 Parathyroid hormone (PTH)

PTH is released by the parathyroid gland in response to both a fall in blood calcium and low serum 1,25-$(OH)_2D_3$ levels. It is responsible for the minute to minute regulation of calcium, due to its quick, short duration response. PTH stimulates conversion of (25-OH-D) to the active from of vitamin D (1,25-$(OH)_2D_3$) that, in turn, stimulates intestinal absorption of calcium. PTH also stimulates osteoclastic resorption of bone to release calcium, phosphorous and magnesium into the circulation. PTH stimulates renal conservation of calcium but not phosphorous, which results in an increase in blood calcium without an increase in phosphorous concentrations.

In animals with disturbances in calcium metabolism that result in bone demineralization, PTH levels are high, and PTH can be used to investigate metabolic bone disease that is often nutritional in origin. Dietary calcium deficiency, or a failure to absorb calcium are reasons for metabolic bone disease. Failure to absorb calcium can be due to vitamin D deficiency or unavailability of calcium due to binding with substances such as oxalates, fats or phosphates in the gut.

PTH assays are available in commercial laboratories that specialize in endocrinological investigations. PTH assays have been performed on pet rabbits as part of an investigation of the possibility of metabolic bone disease as a cause of poor tooth and bone quality and the development of dental disease in rabbits (Harcourt-Brown and Baker, 2001). Sample handling is of paramount importance as the hormone is labile and haemolysis interferes with the assay. Samples require separating and freezing immediately after collection and must be shipped in the frozen state to a laboratory. Sufficient, non-haemolysed blood to harvest 1–2 ml of serum or plasma needs to be collected. As PTH is responsible for the minute to minute regulation of blood calcium, values can vary over a wide range making interpretation of a single result difficult. Diet, age, pregnancy, lactation, diurnal rhythms cause physiological variations in results. Warren *et al.* (1989) reported PTH values of 59.6 + 41.2 pg/ml in a group of 29 non-pregnant farm and laboratory rabbits and Harcourt-Brown and Baker (2001) reported values of 40.3 + 10.7 pg/ml in a group of 12 pet rabbits kept outside under free-range conditions all year round (see Figure 6.1). Values as high as 100–200 pg/ml have been recorded in baseline samples from laboratory rabbits (Warren *et al.*, 1989). Values in excess of 230 pg/ml have been found in pet rabbits, one of which was found to have a liver tumour on subsequent *post-mortem* examination (Harcourt-Brown, unpublished data).

6.4.3 Serology

In the UK, serological tests are available for *Encephalitozoon cuniculi*, *Toxoplasma gondii*, myxomatosis, viral haemorrhagic disease and *Treponema cuniculi* as part of the commercial health screening of laboratory rabbits. Commercial laboratories may accept individual samples from pet rabbits for serological screening. It is advisable to consult a veterinary laboratory in the first instance. In the USA, serology and a PCR test are also available to detect *Pasteurella multocida* infection (Sanchez *et al.*, 2000) but these tests are not available in the UK at the present time (September, 2000).

Serological testing for *Encephalitozoon cuniculi* antibodies can be useful in the differential diagnosis of neurological diseases such as vestibular syndrome or paraplegia (Section 12.4) or uveitis (Section 11.7.3.1). It is also indicated in animals with mild renal insufficiency (Section 14.5.1). Serological and histological tests from naturally infected rabbits have demonstrated the presence of antibodies before the organism can be seen in the kidney. Lesions were not seen in the brain until at least 8 weeks after the first detectable antibodies, suggesting that serology is a sensitive procedure for early diagnosis (Cox and Gallichio, 1978). Therefore animals with clinical signs that are seronegative are unlikely to be suffering from encephalitozoonosis, although experimental infections with *Encephalitozoon cuniculi* have shown the presence of granulomas in the brain of animals that had become seronegative (Kunstyr *et al.*, 1986). Conversely, asymptomatic rabbits can be seropositive. Therefore serology can only be used as a guide in the diagnosis of *Encephalitozoon cuniculi* infection. Antibody titres can be helpful in distinguishing between recent and chronic infection. Simultaneous detection of IgM and IgG suggest recent infection.

Key points 6.4

- Serum potassium values in rabbits can be depressed by anaesthesia. In unanaesthetized rabbits, low potassium values have been associated with generalized muscular weakness
- Blood calcium levels in rabbits vary over a wide range and are higher than other domestic species
- Total blood calcium values are correlated with serum albumin levels and are affected by diet, age and reproductive status
- Parathyroid hormone (PTH) can be measured, but requires careful sample handling. Interpretation of a single result is difficult
- In the UK, serological tests are available for *Encephalitozoon cuniculi, Toxoplasma gondii,* myxomatosis, viral haemorrhagic disease and *Treponema cuniculi.*

6.5 Urine examination

Urinanalysis is summarized in Table 6.4. Urine collection is described in Section 3.12.3. In common with other herbivorous species, rabbits excrete alkaline urine. Urinary pH is approximately 8–8.2. Rabbit urine is normally turbid due to the presence of calcium carbonate that can be seen as sediment in collected samples. The urine from anorexic, pregnant, lactating or young rabbits is often clear. The colour of normal urine can vary from pale yellow, to orange, brown or red, mimicking haematuria. Plant porphyrin pigments are the cause of red coloured urine and can be distinguished from haematuria with urinanalysis dipstick tests. Alternatively, a Wood's lamp can be used, as urinary pigments fluoresce when exposed to ultraviolet light (Benson and Paul-Murphy, 1999). In addition to the presence of calcium carbonate crystals, oxalate or ammonium magnesium phosphate crystals can also be found in normal rabbit urine. The specific gravity of rabbit urine is difficult to evaluate accurately due to the presence of mineral deposits (Goad *et al.*, 1989) but is approximately 1.003–1.036. Traces of glucose and protein can be present in normal rabbit urine. As in other species, rabbit urine can be spun and the sediment examined microscopically for the presence of crystals, red cells, inflammatory cells and bacteria. Cultures can be taken to confirm bacterial infection and aid antibiotic selection. Examination of urine sediment stained with gram stain can reveal *Encephalitozoon cuniculi* spores that are oval, strongly gram-positive with a coiled filament inside (Pye and Cox, 1977; Patton, 2000). Ketones may be detected in the urine of anorexic rabbits and is a poor prognostic sign as it is associated with the development of hepatic lipidosis.

Table 6.4 Urinanalysis

Specific gravity	1.003–1.036 **NB** Difficult to measure accurately due to mineral deposits
pH	7.6–8.8
Protein	Small quantities of albumin may be a normal finding especially in young rabbits
Cells	A small number of leucocytes and erythrocytes are a normal finding in rabbit urine
Crystals	Ammonium magnesium phosphate (struvite) and calcium carbonate deposits are a normal finding in rabbit urine. Oxalate crystals can also be seen

6.6 Faeces examination

Rabbits produce two types of faeces: hard dry pellets that are composed of compressed indigestible fibre and soft caecotrophs that are composed of a smooth paste rich in bacteria and other microorganisms. The first step in faeces examination is to determine which type of faeces has been collected. It is often samples of soft faeces or caecotrophs that are collected for examination because their consistency is abnormally loose or the owner has mistaken uningested caecotrophs for diarrhoea. Microscopically the two types of faeces are completely different. Hard faeces contain indigestible fragments of plant debris and little else. Caecotrophic material contains a wide range of microorganisms including large gram-negative bacilli, *Bacteroides*, large metachromic staining bacilli and many other bacteria including oval and fusiform rods. In some types of diarrhoea, a mixture of indigestible fragments of plant material can be seen alongside a range of typical caecal microorganisms. This signifies a failure of the proximal colon to separate the indigestible and digestible fractions of the diet. Coccidial oocysts or eggs of the non-pathogenic oxyurid *Passalurus ambiguus* can be found in both hard and soft faeces of infected rabbits. Coccidial oocysts can be confused with a non-pathogenic *Saccharomyces*, a budding sporogenous yeast that can be present in large numbers in rabbit faeces (see Figure 6.2).

Clostridium spiroforme is a large gram-positive, semicircular or spiral-shaped bacterium that may be seen in faecal smears from diarrhoeic rabbits or those that have died from enterotoxaemia. Centrifuging faecal material at 20 000 rpm for 15 minutes and gram staining the residue after the supernatant has been removed improves the chance of diagnosis (Langan and O'Rourke Schaeffer, 2000). Although the presence of semicircular bacteria in the faeces or caecal material is suggestive of clostridial enterotoxaemia, it is not a reliable diagnostic criterion. *Clostridia* species can be present in the normal caecal flora and proliferate after death. The demonstration of the toxin and anaerobic culture of the organism is required for positive diagnosis (Carman and Borriello, 1983).

Clostridium piliforme, the causative organism of Tyzzer's disease, is not detected in faeces. A PCR test is available in the USA for detection of this organism. *Escherichia coli* is not a normal inhabitant of the rabbit gut flora

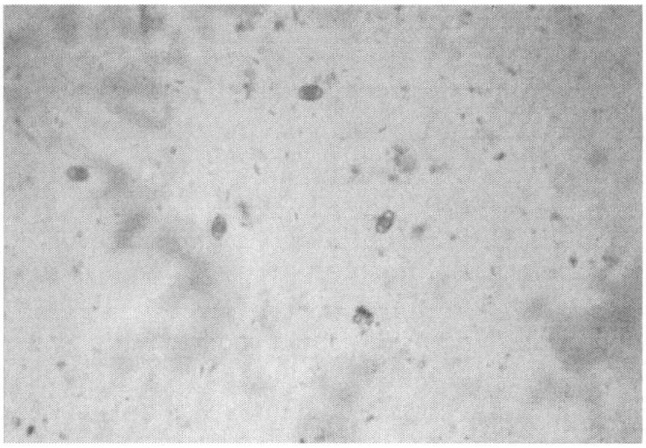

(a)

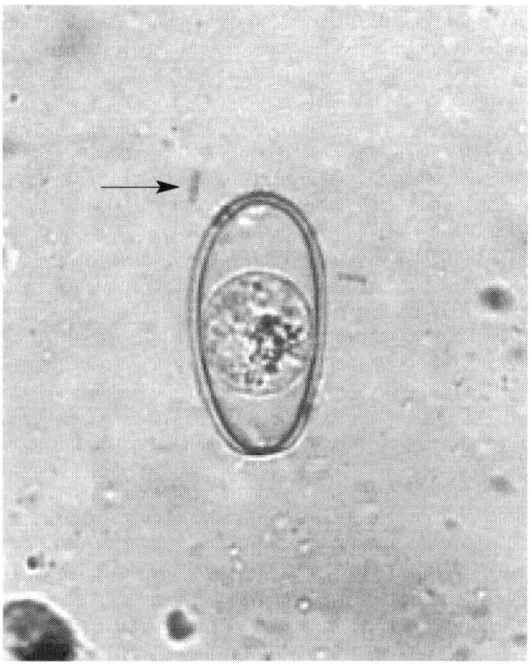

(b)

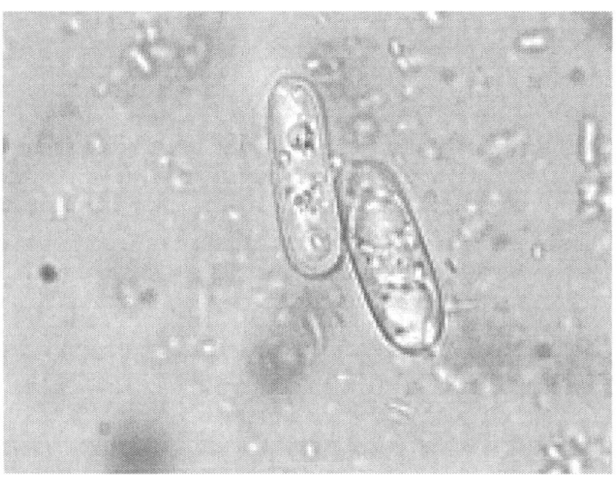

(c)

Figure 6.2. Coccidial oocysts in faeces samples from rabbits. Coccidial oocysts can be confused with non-pathogenic *Saccharomyces guttulatus*, a budding sporogenous yeast that can be present in large numbers in rabbit faeces.

(a) **Coccidial oocysts and saccharomyces** (× 100). Shows large numbers of coccidial oocysts interspersed with *Saccharomyces guttulatus.* The faecal sample was from a 14-week-old, thin rabbit that was suffering from diarrhoea. Faecal material was emulsified with water before being passed through a fine sieve to remove the coarse debris. The homogenate was then centrifuged and the supernatent discarded. The residue was mixed with saturated salt solution and centrifuged again. After the sample had been spun, more saturated salt solution was added to the test tube until a meniscus formed. A cover slip was placed over the meniscus and the sample left for approximately 30 minutes for the oocysts or worm eggs to float to the top of the tube. At the end of this period, the cover slip and surface film was removed from the test tube, placed on a microscope slide and examined under low power.

(b) **Eimeria steidae** (high power) (Image kindly supplied by Dr Sheelagh Lloyd, Division of Animal Pathology, University of Cambridge). Several *Eimeria* spp. affect rabbits and mixed infections occur. The species can be differentiated by the morphological characteristics of the oocysts. The most pathogenic species is *Eimeria steidae,* which causes hepatic coccidiosis (see Section 16.4.1). *E. steidae* invades the epithelial cells of the bile ducts and can cause severe liver damage. Oocysts may be seen in faeces from infected rabbits or in smears of bile collected from rabbits during *post mortem* examination. The relative sizes of coccidial oocysts and *Saccharomyces guttulatus* can be seen in (a,b). Worm eggs are larger than coccidial oocysts. The most common helminth infestation of pet rabbits is *Passalurus ambiguus.* Adult worms or ova from *P. ambiguus* may be seen in rabbit faeces. The ova are ovoid, slightly flattened and asymmetrical with a cap at one end.

(c) **Saccharomyces guttulatus** (high power) (Image kindly supplied by Idexx Laboratories, Wetherby). *Saccharomyces guttulatus* is a budding yeast that is commonly found in the faeces of rabbits, chinchillas and guinea pigs. It is not believed to be pathogenic. Some texts call the yeast *Cyniclomyces guttulatus.*

although small numbers may be present in some animals. Enteropathogenic strains can be found in association with diarrhoea in weanling rabbits. Pathogenic *Salmonella* spp. may be isolated although *post-mortem* material is usually available in these cases. Infectious enteritis is rare in the individual pet rabbit.

Key points 6.5

- Rabbit urine may be coloured red due to the presence of plant pigments. Dipsticks can be used to differentiate haematuria from red urine
- Normal rabbit urine contains calcium carbonate sediment. Small quantities of triple phosphate and oxalate crystals may be present
- Traces of glucose and protein can be present in normal rabbit urine
- Rabbits produce two types of faeces that differ in composition. The first step in faeces' examination is to determine which type of faeces has been collected
- Hard faeces are composed of compressed strands of indigestible fibre
- Soft faeces or caecotrophs are composed of a strong smelling paste rich in bacteria
- Some rabbits with diarrhoea excrete a mixture of hard and soft faeces signifying a failure of the proximal colon to separate the indigestible and digestible fractions of the diet
- Coccidial oocysts and ova from *Passalurus ambiguus* may be seen in both types of faeces
- A non-pathogenic yeast *Saccharomyces guttulatus* may be seen in large numbers and can be mistaken for coccidial oocysts (see Figure 6.2)
- *Clostridium spiroforme* can sometimes be seen in large numbers on a gram-stained smear of faeces collected from a rabbit suffering from enterotoxaemia.

6.7 Laboratory examination of hair

Plucked hair samples may be examined visually for the presence of mites that are just visible with the naked eye. Under good illumination, *Cheyletiella* mites can be seen in scale and skin debris that has been brushed out of the coat. After a few minutes, individual mites can be seen moving into the warmth of the illuminating light. Egg cases and cuticles from developmental stages of the fur mite *Leporacus gibbus* (formerly known as *Listrophorus gibbus*) may also be seen on visual examination of hair brushings. They remain attached to hair shafts after hatching or moulting and give the fur a characteristic 'salt and pepper appearance' in heavy infestations. Visual evidence of *L. gibbus* is seen more easily on white or light coloured areas of fur, especially if it is wet. Occasionally lice may be found.

Microscopic examination of acetate strips applied to the skin of alopecic areas can be used to detect *Cheyletiella parasitovorax*. All stages of the life cycle of *C. parasitovorax* can be seen by this method. Skin brushings can also be examined microscopically. Fleas, flea dirt, *Cheyletiella parasitovorax* and *Leporacus gibbus* can be seen in skin brushings examined under low magnification.

A trichogram is useful in differentiating between conditions that cause alopecia. For this technique a sample of hair is plucked from as close to skin as possible using forceps. The hair is placed on a microscope slide, taking care to ensure the hairs remain orientated in the same direction. A drop of mineral oil and a cover slip are applied before examining the shafts of hair under the microscope. Abrupt, fragmented, distal ends of the hair shaft suggest barbering by a companion. Egg cases, cuticles or adult mites, usually *Leporacus gibbus*, may be seen attached to hair shafts. The presence of fungal spores in broken hair shafts plucked from a lesion is diagnostic of dermatophytosis.

Dermatophyte infection can be demonstrated by the presence of mycelia or ectothrix arthospores in potassium hydroxide preparations of macerated scale. Asymptomatic infections can be detected by brushing the entire body with a sterile toothbrush and incubating the brushings at 25°C on dermasel agar (Oxoid). Plates that do not show fungal growth within 3 weeks can be considered negative (Vangeel *et al.*, 2000). Dermatophyte infections are usually due to *Trichophyton mentagrophytes* that does not fluoresce under ultraviolet light. *Microsporum canis* infections can also occur that are evident from the characteristic apple green spores that fluoresce under a Wood's lamp.

Exudate from crusty lesions may be examined for the presence of mites. Although *Psoroptes cuniculi* normally inhabits the ear canal, the mite can be found in other areas of the body such as the perineal skin folds and can be seen on microscopic examination of the exudate from affected areas. Skin scrapings may be required to demonstrate sarcoptic mange mites in scabies cases that are characterized by intense pruritus and crusty lesions. Dark field microscopy can be used to look for *Treponema cuniculi* organisms in crusty lesions suggestive of rabbit syphilis (Section 16.5.9). The organism is a motile corkscrew-shaped spirochaete. Lesions are found on the mucocutaneous junctions of the anus and genitalia or on the nose, lips and eyelids (see plate 10). The lesion is abraded with a sterile saline-soaked swab. Serum from the lesion is then expressed on to a slide and covered with a cover slip before being examined immediately (DiGiacomo *et al.*, 1984). The slide can be placed in a moisturized chamber. The differential diagnosis of exudative skin lesions in rabbits can be difficult and histopathological examination of biopsy specimens may be required.

Key points 6.6

- *Cheyletiella parasitovorax*, fur mites (*Leporacus gibbus*), lice (*Haemodipsus ventricosus*), fleas or flea dirt can be seen in skin brushings from affected animals
- Acetate tape strips can be used to detect all stages of the life cycle of *Cheyletiella parasitovorax*
- A trichogram can differentiate between dermatophytosis and barbering. Mites, cuticles and egg cases may be seen attached to the hair shafts
- *Psoroptes cuniculi*, the rabbit ear mite, can sometimes be seen on microscopic examination of smears from skin lesions in other parts of the body such as the perineum
- Dark field microscopy may be used to detect *Treponema pallidum* organisms.

6.8 Cerebrospinal fluid

Cerebrospinal fluid can be collected from the cisterna magna of rabbits in a similar manner to other animals. Some normal parameters are summarized in Table 6.5. Depressed glucose concentrations (< 56 mg/dl) may be indicative of purulent inflammation (Kusumi and Plouffe, 1980).

Table 6.5 Cerebrospinal fluid

Ref	Parameter	
b	Glucose	56–135 mg/dl
a	WBC	0–7 cells/mm^3 (Up to 20 cells/mm^3 have been found in healthy rabbits)
a	Lymphocytes	40–79%
a	Monocytes	21–60%
b	Total protein	16–66 mg/dl

Reference sources: a: Curiel T.J. *et al.* (1982); b: Kusumi, R.K., Plouffe, J.F. (1980).

References

Aitken, M., Allen M. (1994). Minerals and electrolytes Part 1. *In Practice*, **16**, 78–83.

Assane, M., Gongnet, G.P., Coulibaly, A., Sere, A. (1993). Influence of dietary calcium/phosphorous ratio on blood calcium, phosphate and magnesium during gestation in the rabbit. (Article in French, English Abstract). *Reprod Nutr Dev.*, **33**, 223–228.

Barlet, J.P. (1980). Plasma calcium, inorganic phosphorus and magnesium levels in pregnant and lactating rabbits. *Reprod Nutr Develop.*, **20**, 647–651.

Benson, K.G., Paul-Murphy, J. (1999). Clinical pathology of the domestic rabbit. *Vet Clin N Am: Exotic Anim Pract.*, **2**, 539–552.

Bentley, P.J. (1998). *Comparative Vertebrate Endocrinology*, 3rd edn. Cambridge University Press.

Brewer, N.R., Cruise, L.J. (1994). Physiology. In *The Biology of the Laboratory Rabbit*, 2nd edn. (P.J. Manning, D.H. Ringler, C.E. Newcomer, eds). pp 63–70. Academic Press.

Bush, B.M. (1981). *Interpretation of Laboratory Results for Small Animal Clinicians*. Blackwell.

Carman, R.J., Borriello, S.P. (1983). Laboratory diagnosis of *Clostridium spiroforme*-mediated diarrhoea (iota enterotoxaemia) of rabbits. *Vet Rec.*, **113**, 184–185.

Cannon, D.J., Conaway, H.H. (1981). Glycosylated haemoglobin levels in a colony of spontaneously diabetic rabbits (Abstract). *Diabetologia*, **20**, 242–243.

Chapin, R.E. Smith, S.E. (1967a). The calcium tolerance of growing rabbits. *Cornell Vet.*, **57**, 482–491.

Chapin, R.E. Smith, S.E. (1967b). Calcium requirement of growing rabbits. *J Anim Sci.*, **26**, 67–71.

Collins, B.R. (1988). Common diseases and medical management of rodents and lagomorphs. In *Contemporary Issues in Small Animal Practice: Exotic Animals* (E.R. Jacobson, G.V Kollias, eds). pp 261–306. Churchill Livingstone.

Cooke, S. (2000). Clinical chemistry. In *Manual of Rabbit Medicine and Surgery.* (P.A. Flecknell, ed.) pp 103–116. British Small Animal Veterinary Association.

Cox, J.C., Gallichio, H.A. (1978). Serological and histological studies on adult rabbits with recent naturally acquired encephalitozoonosis. *Res Vet Sci.*, **24**, 260–261.

Curiel, T.J., Perfect, J.R., Durack, D.T. (1982). Leucocyte subpopulations in cerebrospinal fluid of normal rabbits (Abstract). *Lab Anim Sci.*, **32**, 622–624.

DiGiacomo, R.F., Lukehart, S.A., Talburt, C.D. *et al.* (1984). Clinical course and treatment of venereal spirochaetosis in New Zealand White rabbits. *Br J VenerDis.*, **60**, 214–218.

DiGiacomo, R.F., Mare J. (1994). Viral diseases. In *The Biology of the Laboratory Rabbit*, 2nd edn. (P.J. Manning, D.H. Ringler, C.E. Newcomer, eds). pp 171–197. Academic Press.

Ewringmann, A., Göbel, T. (1999). Untersuchungen zur Klinik und Therapie der Encephalitozoonose beim Heimtierkaninchen (Article in German, English Abstract). *Kleintierpraxis*, **44**, 357–372.

Fekete, S. (1989). Recent findings and future perspectives of digestive physiology in rabbits: a review. *Acta Vet Hungar*, **37**, 265–279.

Fekete, S., Huszenicza, G. (1993). Effects of T-2 toxin on ovarian activity and some metabolic variables of rabbits. *Lab Anim Sci.*, **43**, 646–649.

Flanders, J.A., Scarlett, J.M., Blue, J.T., Neth, S. (1989). Adjustment of total serum calcium concentration for binding to albumin and protein in cats: 291 cases (1986–1987). *J Am Vet Med Assoc.*, **194**, 1609–1611.

Fox, R.R., Laird, C.W. (1970). Biochemical parameters of clinical significance in rabbits. II. Diurnal variations. *J Hered.*, **61**, 261–265.

Fudge, A.M. (2000). Rabbit hematology. In *Laboratory Medicine. Avian and Exotic Pets* (A.M. Fudge, ed.) pp 273–275. W.B. Saunders.

Gillett, C.S. (1994). Selected drug dosages and clinical reference data. In *The Biology of the Laboratory Rabbit*, 2nd edn. (P.J. Manning, D.H. Ringler, C.E. Newcomer, eds). pp 467–472. Academic Press.

Gilsanz, V., Roe, T.F., Antunes, J., Carlson, M. *et al.* (1991). Effect of dietary calcium on bone density in growing rabbits. *Am J Physiol.*, **260**, E471–E476.

Goad, D.L., Pecquet, M.E., Warren, H.B. (1989). Total serum calcium concentrations in rabbits. *J Am Vet Med Assoc.*, **194**, 1520–1521.

Gupta, S.P., Trivedi, K.K. (1981). Effect of *Ascaris suum* infection on blood picture of rabbits in relation to the production of immunity (Abstract), *Zool Anz Jena.*, **206**, S246–S251.

Guyton, A.C. (1991). *Textbook of Medical Physiology.* W.B. Saunders.

Harcourt-Brown, F.M., Baker, S.J. (2001). Parathyroid hormone, haematological and biochemical parameters in relation to dental disease and husbandry in pet rabbits. *J Small Anim Pract.*, **42**, 130–136.

Harkness, J.E., Wagner, J.E. (1995). *The Biology and Medicine of Rabbits and Rodents*, 4th edn. Williams and Wilkins.

Hinton, M., Jones D.R.E., Festing M.F.W. (1982). Haematological findings in healthy and diseased rabbits, a multivariate analysis. *Lab Anim.*, **16**, 123–129.

Hoefer, H.L. (2000). Rabbit and ferret renal diagnosis. In *Laboratory Medicine. Avian and Exotic Pets* (A.M. Fudge, ed.) pp 311–318. W.B. Saunders.

Jain, N.C. (1986). Hematology of laboratory and miscellaneous animals. In *Schalm's Veterinary Hematology*, 4th edn. pp 276–282. Lea and Febiger.

Jenkins, J.R. (2000). Rabbit and ferret liver and gastrointestinal testing. In *Laboratory Medicine. Avian and Exotic Pets* (A.M. Fudge, ed.) pp 291–304. W.B. Saunders.

Jones, R.T. (1975). Normal values for some biochemical constituents in rabbits. *Lab Anim.*, **9**, 143–147.

Kabata, J., Gratwohl, A., Tichelli, A. *et al.* (1991). Hematological values of New Zealand White rabbits determined by automated flow cytometry. *Lab Anim Sci.*, **41**, 613–619.

Kamphues, V.J., Carstensen, P. Schroeder, D. *et al.* (1986). Effect of increasing calcium and vitamin D supply on calcium metabolism in rabbits (Article in German, English Summary). *J Anim Physiol Nutr.*, **50**, 191–208.

Kerr, M. (1989). *Veterinary Laboratory Medicine. Clinical Biochemistry and Haematology.* Blackwell Scientific Publications.

Knudtzon, J. (1988). Plasma levels of glucagon, insulin, glucose and free fatty acids in rabbits during laboratory handling procedures. *Z Versuchstierk*, **26**, 123–133.

Kozma, C., Macklin, W., Cummins, L.M., Mauer, R. (1974). The anatomy, physiology and the biochemistry of the rabbit. In *The Biology of the Laboratory Rabbit.* (S.H. Weisbroth, R.E. Flatt, A.L. Kraus, eds). pp 50–69. Academic Press.

Kraus A., Weisbroth S.H., Flatt R.E., Brewer N. (1984). Biology and diseases of rabbits. In *Laboratory Animal Medicine.* pp 207–237. Academic Press.

Krishna L., Dawra R.K., Vaid J., Gupta V.K. (1991). An outbreak of aflatoxicosis in Angora rabbits (Abstract). *Vet Hum Toxicol.*, **33**, 159–161.

Kunstyr, I., Lev, L., Naumann, S. (1986). Humoral antibody response to rabbits to experimental infection with *Encephalitozoon cuniculi. Vet Parasitol.*, **21**, 223–232.

Kusumi, R.K., Plouffe, J.F. (1980). Cerebrospinal fluid glucose and protein values in normal rabbits. *Lab Anim.*, **14**, 41–42.

Langan, G.P., O'Rourke Schaeffer, D. (2000). Rabbit microbiology and virology. In *Laboratory Medicine* (A.M. Fudge, ed.) pp 325–333. W.B. Saunders.

Licois, D., Coudert, P., Mongin, P. (1978). Changes in hydromineral metabolism in diarrhoeic rabbits 2. Study of the modifications of electrolyte metabolism. *Ann Rech Vet.*, **9**, 453–464.

Loeb, W.F., Quimby, F.W. (1989). *The Clinical Chemistry of Laboratory Animals.* Pergamon.

Malley, A.D. (1996). The pet rabbit in companion animal practice 4: Haematological and biochemical reference values. *Irish Vet J.*, **49**, 354–355.

McLaughlin, R.M., Fish, R.E. (1994). Clinical biochemistry and haematology. In *The Biology of the Laboratory Rabbit*, 2nd edn. (P.J. Manning, D.H. Ringler, C.E. Newcomer, eds). pp 111–124. Academic Press.

Okerman, L. (1994). *Diseases of Domestic Rabbits*, 2nd edn. Blackwell.

Palm, M. (1997). Clinical pathology values in pregnant and non-pregnant rabbits. *Scand J Lab Anim Sci.*, **24**, 177–182.

Patton, S. (2000). Rabbit and ferret parasite testing. In *Laboratory Medicine. Avian and Exotic Pets.* (A. Fudge, ed.) pp 358–365. W.B. Saunders.

Perry-Clark, L.M., Meunier, L.D. (1991). Vascular access ports for chronic serial infusion and blood sampling in New Zealand White rabbits. *Lab Anim Sci.*, **41**, 495–497.

Pye, D., Cox, J.C. (1977). Isolation of *Encephalitozoon cuniculi* from urine samples. *Lab Anim.*, **11**, 223–224.

Robson, W.L., Bayliss. C.E., Feldman, R. *et al.* (1981). Evaluation of the effect of pentobarbitone anaesthesia on the plasma potassium concentration of the rabbit and the dog. *Can Anaesth Soc J.*, **28**, 210–216.

Ros, S.P., McMannis, S.I., Kowal-Vern, A. *et al.* (1991). Effect of intraosseous saline infusion on hematological parameters. *Ann Emergency Med.*, **20**, 243–245.

Roscoe, D.E., Nielsen, S.W., Eaton, H.D., Rousseau, J.E. (1975). Chronic plumbism in rabbits: a comparison of three diagnostic tests (Abstract). *Am J Vet Res.*, **36**, 1225–1229.

Rosenthal, K. (1997) Interpretation of selected clinical pathology values in ferrets and rabbits. *Proceedings of Atlantic Coast Veterinary Conference*, pp. 1–3.

Rosenthal, K. (2000). Ferret and rabbit endocrine disease. In *Laboratory Medicine. Avian and Exotic Pets* (A.M. Fudge, ed.) pp 319–324. W.B. Saunders.

Roth, S., Conaway, H.H. (1982). Spontaneous diabetes mellitus in the New Zealand White rabbit. *Am J Pathol.*, **109**, 359–363.

Sanderson, J.H., Philips, C.E. (1981). Rabbits. In *An Atlas of Laboratory Animal Haematology*. p. 6. Oxford University Press.

Sanchez, S., Mizan, S., Ritchie, B.W., Lee, M.D. (2000). Pasteurellosis in rabbits. *Compendium on Continuing Education*, **22**, 344–360.

Swartout, M.S., Gerken, D.F. (1987). Lead induced toxicosis in two domestic rabbits. *J Am Vet Med Assoc.*, **191**, 717–719.

Toft, P., Tonnesen E., Svendsen P., Rasmussen J.W. (1992a). Redistribution of lymphocytes after cortisol administration (Abstract). *APMIS*, **100**, 154–158.

Toft, P., Tonnesen E., Svendsen P. *et al.* (1992b). The redistribution of lymphocytes during adrenaline infusion. An *in vivo* study with radiolabelled cells (Abstract). *APMIS*, **100**, 593–597.

Toth, L.A., Krueger, J.M. (1988). Alteration of sleep in rabbits by staphylococcus aureus infection. *Infect Immun.*, **56**, 1785–1791.

Toth, L.A., Krueger, J.M. (1989). Haematological effects of exposure to three infective agents in rabbits. *J Am Vet Med Assoc.*, **195**, 981–985.

Toth, L.A., January, B. (1990). Physiological stabilization of rabbits after shipping. *Lab Anim Sci.*, **40**, 384–387.

Tvedegaard, E. (1987). Arterial disease in chronic renal failure. An experimental study in the rabbit. *Acta Pathol Microbiol Immunol Scand Section A. Suppl.*, **290**, 95, 3–28.

Vangeel, I., Pasmans, F., Vanrobaeys, M. *et al.* (2000). Prevalence of dermatophytes in asymptomatic guinea pigs and rabbits. *Vet Rec.*, **146**, 440–441.

Viard-Drouet, F., Provot, F., Coudert, P. (1984). Changes in plasma parameters in rabbit does as a function of their physiological state and feed rationing (Abstract). *Ann Rech Vet.*, **15**, 417–424.

Voelkel, E.F., Levine, L., Alper, C.A. *et al.* (1978). Acute phase reactants ceruloplasmin and haptaglobin and their relationship to plasma prostaglandins in rabbits bearing the VX2 carcinoma (Abstract). *J Exp Med.*, **147**, 417–424.

Warren, H.B., Lausen, N.C., Segre, G.V. *et al.* (1989). Regulation of calciotropic hormones *in vivo* in the New Zealand White rabbit. *Endocrinology*, **125**, 2683–2689.

Weisbroth, S.H. (1994). Neoplastic diseases. In *The Biology of the Laboratory Rabbit*, 2nd edn. (P.J. Manning, D.H. Ringler, C.E. Newcomer, eds). pp 259–292. Academic Press.

Willard, M.D., Tvedten, H., Turnwald, G.H. (1999). *Small Animal Clinical Diagnosis by Laboratory Methods*, 3rd edn. W.B. Saunders.

Yu L., Pragay D.A., Chang, D., Whicher L. (1979). Biochemical values of normal rabbit serum. *Clin Biochem.*, **12**, 83–87.

Dental disease

7

7.1 Dental anatomy of the domestic rabbit *Oryctolagus cuniculus*

The domestic rabbit *Oryctolagus cuniculus* belongs to the order of lagomorphs. A characteristic of lagomorphs is the presence of four upper incisors. There is a second set of small incisors or 'peg teeth' situated just behind the large upper primary incisors. All lagomorph teeth are open rooted and, in healthy animals, grow continually throughout life. In rodents, such as rats, mice and hamsters, it is only the incisors that continually grow; the premolars and molars do not. All the teeth of histricomorphs (e.g. guinea pigs and chinchillas) grow throughout life but histricomorphs and rodents do not have peg teeth.

Rabbits have two sets of teeth. A deciduous set is present in fetal rabbits and is shed just before or just after birth (Wiggs and Lobprise, 1995). The deciduous set comprises:

$$I: \frac{2}{1} \quad C: \frac{0}{0} \quad P: \frac{3}{2} \quad M: \frac{0}{0} \quad = 16$$

The permanent set of teeth erupts during the first 5 weeks of life and comprises:

$$I: \frac{2}{1} \quad C: \frac{0}{0} \quad P: \frac{3}{2} \quad M: \frac{3}{3} \quad = 28$$

Rabbits' teeth have the same structural components as other animals, i.e. dentine, enamel, cementum and pulp. The main body of the tooth is made up of dentine composed of hydroxyapatite crystals similar to those in bone, but much denser. The crystals are embedded in a collagen matrix that is also similar to bone but without the osteocytes, osteoclasts, osteoblasts or blood vessels. Dentine is nourished by a layer of odontoblasts that line its inner surface along the pulp cavity. The odontoblastic layer contains free sensory nerve endings, some of which extend into the dentine through tubules. Species with continually erupting teeth, such as rabbits, have smaller and fewer axons in the dentine than animals with permanent dentition (Byers,1984). In the rabbit, tubular dentine is formed at the apex of the tooth and becomes thicker as it migrates occlusally. Enamel is formed at the apex by a layer of ameloblasts (Bishop, 1995).

The upper incisor teeth have a single deep groove on the labial aspect that runs longitudinally along the length of the tooth. The amount of enamel covering the crowns of the incisors varies with each type of incisor tooth (Hirschfield *et al.*, 1973). The large upper primary incisors have a thick layer of enamel on the labial aspect but none on the lingual side. The other incisors have enamel on both the labial and lingual aspects. This distribution of enamel permits the formation of sharp cutting edges to the tips of the teeth (see Figure 7.1). The incisors are primarily used for slicing through vegetation, although they can be used for gnawing and biting. Canine teeth are absent. There is a large diastema between the incisors and premolars. The premolars and molars are indistinguishable from each other and form a row of grinding cheek teeth.

The mandibular cheek teeth are arranged in a straight line. The maxillary cheek teeth are similarly arranged, except that the intermediate premolars and molars are wider than the first premolar and the last molar giving the buccal side of the alignment a convex shape. The circumference of the cheek teeth exhibit deep grooves or embrasures, which are deep on the buccal aspect and fit into a corresponding groove in the alveolar wall (see Figures 7.2 and 7.3).

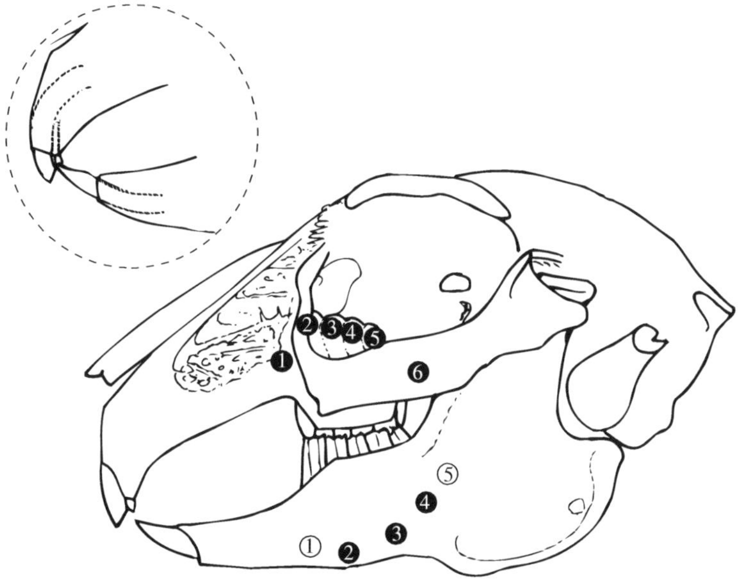

Figure 7.1. Normal incisor occlusion and sites of bone penetration by elongated roots of the cheek teeth. The incisors are used to slice through vegetation like scissors. The lower incisors can also be moved in a rostrocaudal direction to gnaw through bark or wood. The large upper primary incisors have a thick layer of enamel on the labial aspect but none on the lingual side. This distribution of enamel permits the formation of sharp cutting edges to the tips of the upper primary incisors as the lingual aspect is worn against the lower incisor. During grinding of food between the cheek teeth, chewing movements in rabbits are made in a lateral direction (see Figure 7.4), rather than the rostrocaudal action that takes place in rodents. During mastication, the jaw is moved through an arc that also brings the mandibular incisors into contact with the peg teeth. This action wears the tips of the mandibular incisors to a cutting edge.

Root elongation occurs as part of the syndrome of acquired dental disease that affects pet rabbits. Alterations in the shape and curvature of the teeth tend to follow a characteristic pattern. Elongated roots penetrate the bone and emerge through the periosteum in predictable sites. Periapical abscesses occur at the site of root penetration. The site of the abscess can be helpful in predicting which tooth root is infected. In the figure the penetration sites of elongated roots of the cheek teeth (molariform teeth) are shown. The solid circles (●) are roots that curve and penetrate the bone laterally. The empty circles (○) are roots that curve penetrate the bone medially. The circle contains the number of the tooth so, the fourth molariform tooth, deviating laterally, is ❹.

Figure 7.2. Structure of the cheek teeth.

(a) **Lateral aspect of the second lower right molar (molariform tooth number 4).** Shows the lateral aspect of the second lower right molar that illustrates some morphological characteristics of the cheek teeth of rabbits. The premolars and molars are very similar. Some texts use the term 'molariform teeth'. Longitudinally, the root and the crown of the cheek teeth are not morphologically distinct. Wild rabbits and those pet rabbits that eat grass and natural vegetation may have brown staining on the supragingival crowns of the teeth (see Plate 11).

(b) **Longitudinal section through the second lower right molar.** A longitudinal section through the tooth as illustrated in (a). It show the two laminar extensions of the pulp cavity. These extensions converge at the apex of the tooth to form a single pulp chamber that contains a range of differentiated and undifferentiated cells and a nerve supply. Towards the occlusal end, the two pulp chambers taper and close, and the dentine transforms from tubular to thicker atubular tissue in which there are no blood vessels. There is a deep longitudinal

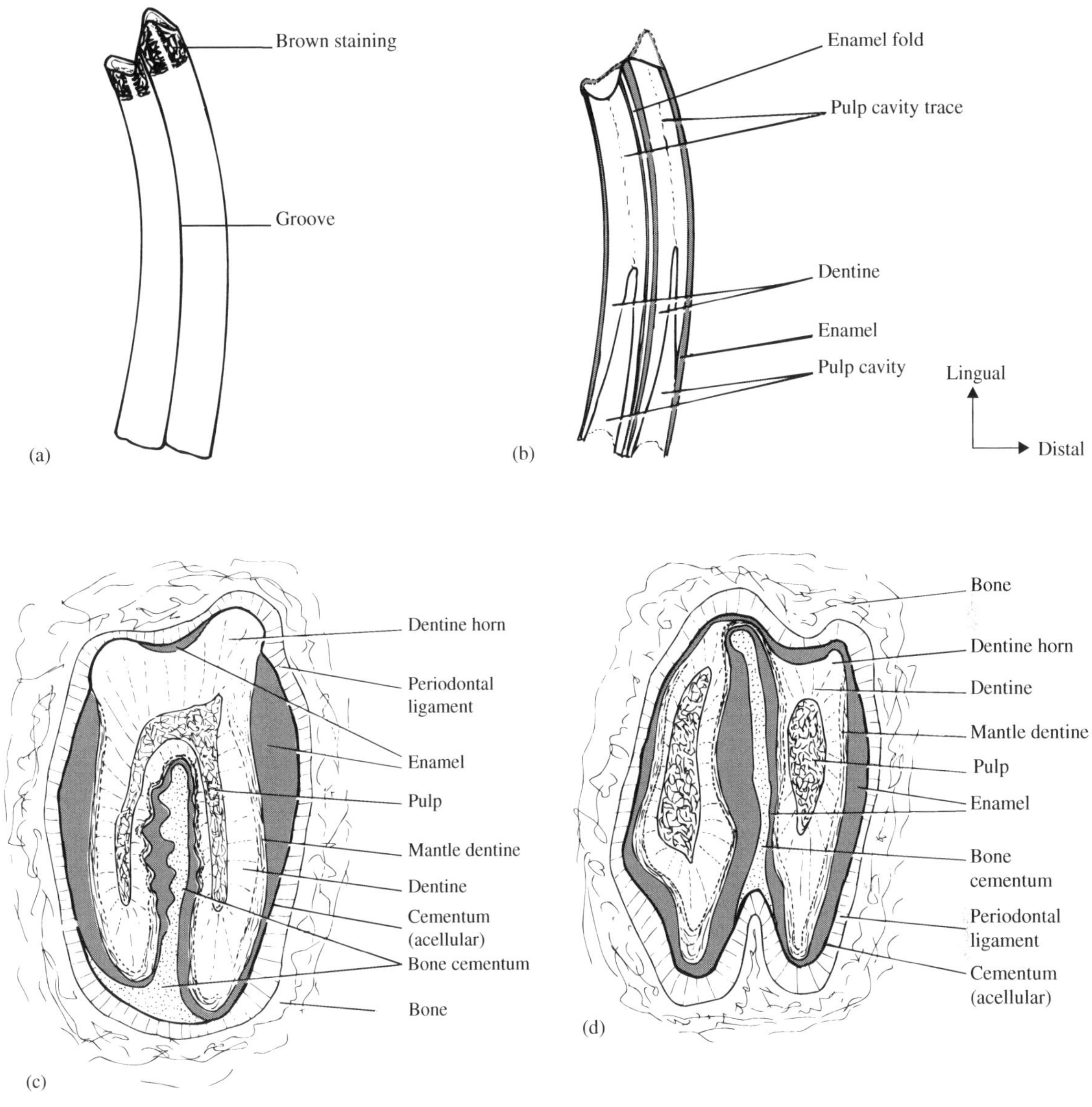

fold of enamel in the centre of the tooth, which can be seen as a radiodense line in the cheek teeth on lateral radiographs of the skull.

(c) **Transverse section through a maxillary (upper) cheek tooth and (d) transverse section through a maxillary (lower) cheek tooth:** (c) and (d) are transverse sections of the cheek teeth. The external surface of the cheek teeth is made of enamel that is covered by a layer of acellular cementum into which the fibres of the periodontal ligament are embedded. The opposing ends of the fibres are embedded into alveolar bone anchoring the tooth into the alveolar socket. The circumference of the mandibular cheek teeth exhibits deep grooves that fit into a corresponding groove in the alveolar wall. All the cheek teeth, except the first and last of the upper jaw, possess an enamel fold which runs across the tooth from the vestibular to lingual surface. The fissure in the enamel fold is filled with a type of vascular bone cementum that is contiguous with the avascular cementum surrounding the tooth. On the lower cheek teeth, this enamel fold almost divides the tooth in two.

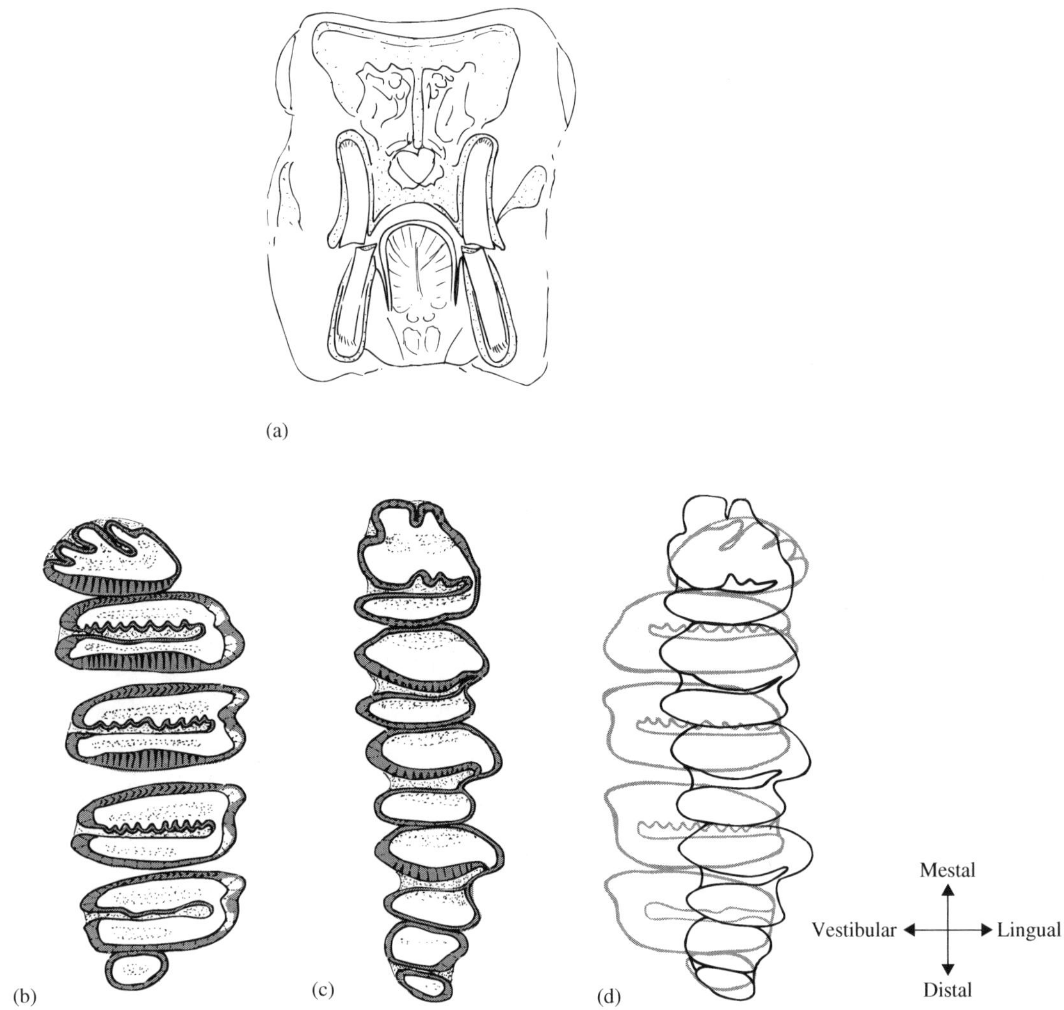

Figure 7.3.

Longitudinally, the root and the crown of the cheek teeth are morphologically indistinct (see Figure 7.2). Wild rabbits and those pet rabbits that eat grass and natural vegetation sometimes have brown staining on the supragingival crowns of the teeth, especially the cheek teeth (see Plates 12 and 13).

Examination of transverse sections across the long axis of the cheek teeth shows the pulp cavity in the two laminar extensions that converge at the apex of the tooth to form a single pulp chamber containing a range of differentiated and undifferentiated cells and a nerve supply. At the occlusal end, the two pulp chambers taper and close, and the dentine transforms from tubular to thicker atubular tissue in which there are no blood vessels (Bishop, 1995). There is a deep longitudinal fold of enamel in the centre of the molars and premolars (see Figures 7.2 and 7.3). This fold can be seen as a radiodense line running longitudinally in the cheek teeth on lateral radiographs of the skull (see Figure 7.7). The circumference of the tooth is made up of enamel covered by a layer of acellular cementum in which the fibres of the periodontal ligament are embedded. The opposing ends of the fibres are embedded into alveolar

Figure 7.3. Occlusion of the cheek teeth.
(a) **The transverse section through the head of a wild rabbit shows the anatomical relationship of the upper and lower cheek teeth.** This was drawn from a decalcified head sectioned at the level of the interdental space between the first second and second lower premolars. The upper second premolar has been sectioned across the tooth. The head was taken from a mature adult wild rabbit with no evidence of dental disease. It can be seen that the jaws are isognathic, i.e. the rows of teeth in the lower jaw are closer together than those in the upper jaw. This only allows the cheek teeth one side of the mouth to be in occlusion at any time.
(b) **The occlusal surfaces of the (left) maxillary cheek teeth;** (c) **The occlusal surfaces of the (left) mandibular cheek teeth;** and (d) **Superimposition of the outline of the maxillary cheek teeth onto the mandibular cheek teeth to show their occlusal relationship.** In (b) and (c) the illustrations were drawn from the teeth of a wild rabbit. In *Nomina Anatomica Veterinarium*, the five surfaces of the teeth are named occlusal, mesial and distal, lingual and vestibular. Vestibular replaces buccal and labial. The vestibular surface is so named because this surface faces *vestibulum oris*.
There are six molariform cheek teeth in the upper jaw and five in the lower jaw. The mandibular cheek teeth are arranged in a straight line. The maxillary cheek teeth are similarly arranged, except that the intermediate premolars and molars are wider than the first premolar and the last molar giving the buccal side of the alignment a convex shape (b). The first and last teeth of the lower jaw are larger than the opposing tooth of the upper jaw. All the teeth, except the first and last of the upper jaw, possess an enamel fold which runs across the middle of the tooth from the vestibular to lingual surface. Because of the enamel fold, each tooth appears to consist of two parts. If viewed in this manner there are 10 molariform 'tooth parts' in each jaw, each one occluding with an opposite part. The teeth are arranged in staggered manner so that the enamel fold of one tooth corresponds to the mesial or distal surface of the opposing tooth. This relationship of the occlusal surfaces is illustrated in (d).
This arrangement forms an effective grinding surface that is used to sever tough fibrous plant material. The grinding effect of the teeth is enhanced by the enamel that forms the circumference of the tooth and the enamel fold in the centre of the tooth. The central ridge of enamel in the upper molariform teeth is convoluted and has the appearance of a serrated edge. This serrated edge corresponds to the enamel ridges of the distal part of one tooth and the mesial part of the next. The lingual aspect of the occlusal surface of the cheek teeth forms two raised 'horns'. These horns are greater on the lower cheek teeth than on the upper cheek teeth.
The grinding occlusal surface of the teeth is maintained by attrition. Attrition is tooth wear caused by rubbing or grinding against the opposing tooth in the absence of food material. Dental wear is affected by the abrasive nature of the diet. The effect of attrition and abrasion can be seen by examining the occlusal surfaces. Dental wear caused by attrition can be seen as polished facets on the occlusal surfaces of the teeth. Abrasion is characterized by scratched surfaces on the tooth. In healthy rabbits, polished facets can be seen on the occlusal surfaces. During mastication, the cheek teeth grind food by moving the lower jaw laterally. The mandibular movements are guided by the ridges and valleys in the teeth and are unidirectional. The occlusal configuration and the forces that occur during the chewing move the jaw back to the midline during contact with food (see Figure 7.4).

bone anchoring the tooth into the alveolar socket. Like the incisors, the cheek teeth are kept in shape by a continual process of growth and attrition. The soft cementum and dentine of the occlusal surface are worn away before the enamel, which survives as sharp edge, both at the circumference and across the centre of the tooth. This gives the molar and premolars an effective shredding surface (Michaeli *et al.*, 1980). The enamel fold forms a ridge across the centre of the occlusal surface that interlocks with the interdental space between the two occluding teeth (see Figure 7.2). This occlusal pattern results in a rostroau-

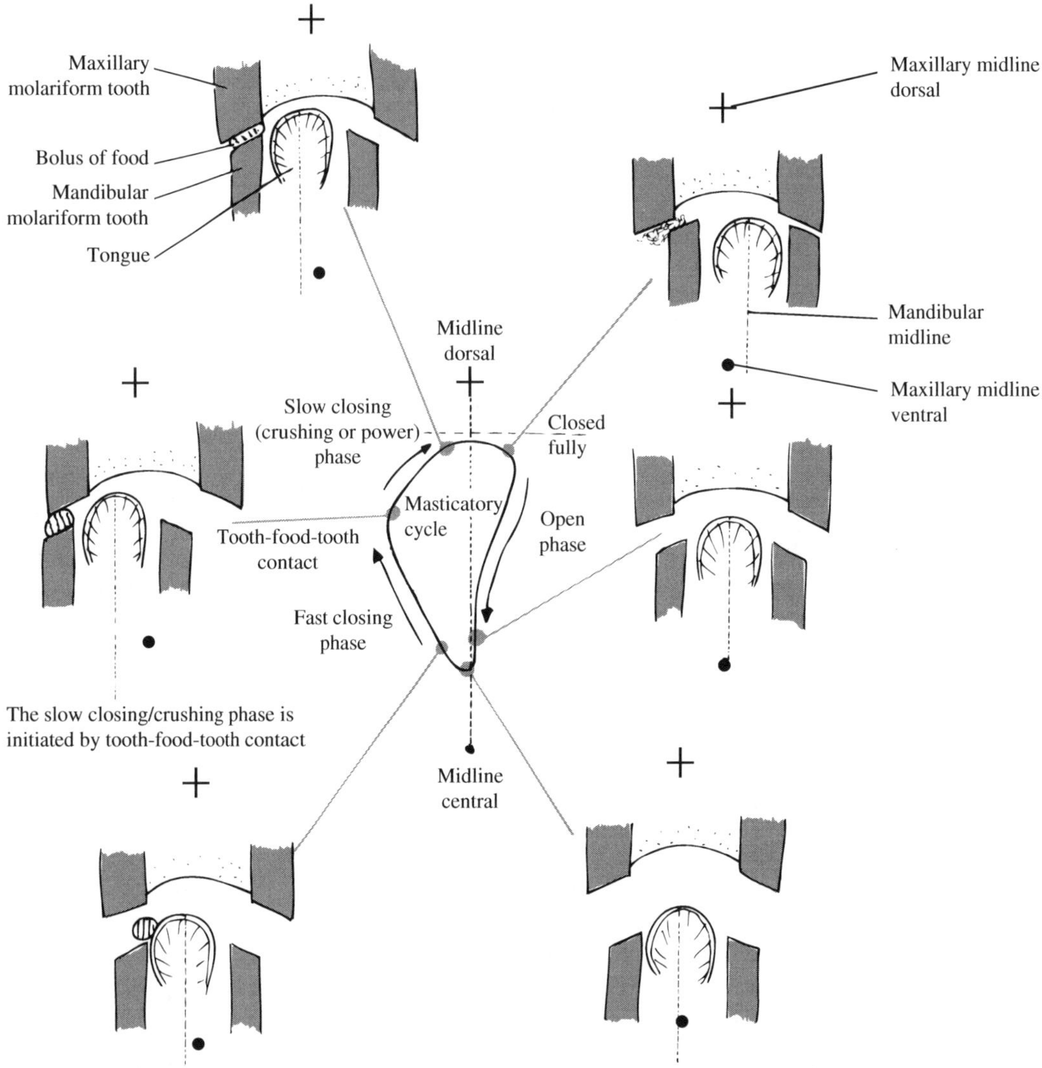

Figure 7.4 Movement of jaw during grinding of food between cheek teeth (Type II masticatory cycle). The jaw movement trajectory of rabbits has been traced using magnetic sensors placed at various sites on the head (Schwartz *et al.*, 1989; Yamada and Yamamura, 1996). Masticatory actions can be divided into three sequences or 'types'. These are described in Section 7.2. Type 1 is the preparatory masticatory sequence in which the incisors cut through food to reduce it to manageable pieces that are transported by the tongue to the posterior teeth for reduction. Type II is the sequence of jaw movements that take place during grinding of food between the cheek teeth. Type III is the masticatory sequence that takes place before the bolus of food is swallowed. This is a more complex cycle that has five phases.

Figure 7.4 summarizes the movement of the mandible during the Type II chewing cycle. Jaw movement follows a unidirectional crescent shaped movement. Either side of the mouth may be used to chew food, but only one side can be used at a time. The mandible is always moving towards the midline when food is crushed between the teeth. The force with which the food is crushed is directly proportional to the hardness of the food. The crushing phase is initiated by contact with food between the teeth. Sensory input to the feedback mechanism is transmitted through the trigeminal nerve from pressoreceptors in the periodontal ligament and muscle spindles in the muscles of mastication.

dal succession of transverse ridges and valleys along the surface of the cheek teeth. Upper ridges are reciprocal with lower valleys and vice versa. The pattern gives a characteristic zigzag pattern on lateral radiographs (see Figure 7.7).

The occlusal pattern of the cheek teeth is anisognathic, i.e. the mandible is narrow relative to the maxilla (see Figure 7.4). When the jaws are closed, the mandibular cheek teeth lie inside those of the upper jaw with the buccal edge of the lower cheek teeth just touching the palatal edge of the upper cheek teeth.

7.2 Mastication

Mastication has been studied extensively in rabbits. The masticatory sequence can be divided into three sequences or 'types'. During each type of masticatory cycle there are several phases of jaw movement.

Type I is the preparatory masticatory sequence that has two phases: a jaw opening phase and jaw closing phase. During this sequence, the incisors cut through food to reduce it to manageable pieces that are transported by the tongue to the posterior teeth for reduction. Jaw movement is predominantly in the sagittal plane with small lateral excursions away from the midline.

Type II is the reduction sequence of masticatory movements that occurs when food is ground down between the cheek teeth. During type II mastication, chewing can only take place on one side of the mouth at a time. Lateral excursion is wide and the jaw follows a unidirectional crescent-shaped movement throughout the chewing cycle (see Figure 7.5). There are three phases in the type II masticatory sequence, a jaw opening phase, a fast closing phase and a slow closing phase during which food is crushed between the teeth (see Figure 7.5). Although the upper and lower cheek teeth often do not come in contact during mastication (Schwartz *et al.*, 1989), the mandibular movements are guided by the ridges and valleys in the teeth (Langenbach *et al.*, 1991). The occlusal configuration and the medially directed forces that occur during chewing drive the jaw back to the midline during contact with food. The basic chewing rhythm is not affected by the food texture (Yamada and Yamamura, 1996) although the force that is applied by the teeth during crushing increases in proportion to the hardness of the food. Sensory input to the feedback mechanism comes from pressoreceptors in the periodontal ligament and muscle spindles in the muscles of mastication.

The third (type III) masticatory sequence is the preswallowing series of jaw movements that includes an additional two opening phases during which the bolus of food is swallowed.

7.3 Factors that affect tooth shape in rabbits

In healthy rabbits, the teeth are kept in shape by continual growth and attrition. Attrition is the occlusal wear of tooth against tooth. The soft dentine is worn away more quickly than the hard enamel that remains as sharp-edged ridges that cut against each other like scissors (see Figures 7.2, 7.3). Dental wear is affected by contact with food and the abrasive nature of the diet.

Rabbits can be seen grinding their teeth when they are at rest. There is evidence of dental wear from bruxism (tooth grinding) on the non-functional deciduous teeth of neonatal rabbits (Wiggs and Lobprise, 1995). Early zoologists believed that rabbits were animals that chewed cud (Shadle, 1936; Taylor, 1940), a characteristic which deemed rabbits to be 'unclean' in the Bible (Leviticus XI, v. 6) and included them in the Jewish list of unclean meats: The phrase '...as the camel and the hare and the coney, for they chew the cud but divide not the hoof, therefore they are unclean to you' appears in the Bible (Deuteronomy XIV, v.7). It is not clear whether this belief arose from observations of chewing behaviour or from the presence of caecotrophs in the stomach.

The rate of growth and attrition is variable between individuals and is also influenced by pregnancy, age and diet (Shadle, 1936; Ness, 1956; Lowe, 1998). The constant process of growth and attrition demands a supply of calcium and other minerals and nutrients for the formation of dentine and enamel. The periodontal space contains a capillary network that provides ameloblasts with nutrients (Okada *et al.*, 1990). The upper incisors do not grow as quickly as the lower incisors. Hamidur Rahman *et al.* (1983) recorded a rate

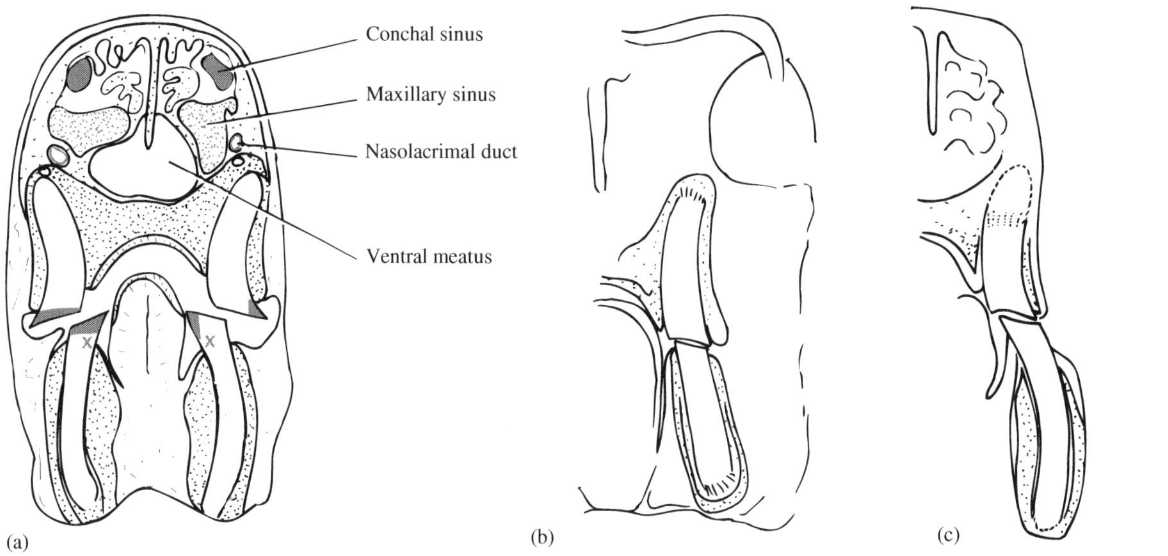

Figure 7.5. Cheek tooth malocclusion and root elongation (the position of the conchal and maxillary sinuses is also illustrated). (a) **Trimming cheek teeth.** This illustration was drawn from a transverse section of a decalcified head of a rabbit that was euthanased because it had developed molar malocclusion. Cheek tooth malocclusion and root elongation are part of the syndrome of acquired dental disease that affects pet rabbits. The whole structure, shape and position of the teeth alter. The teeth become long and curved. Sharp spurs develop on the mandibular molars that impinge on the tongue and interfere with chewing, licking and grooming. In advanced cases, these spurs can lacerate the tongue and cause substantial tissue damage (see Plates 20 and 21). The effect of trimming these spurs is illustrated in (a). Although, logically, it would seem that reducing the crowns to gum level should increase the time it takes for sharp spurs to regrow, this is not the case. In (a), the letter X marks the part of the tooth that will grow into in a spur. It can be seen from the diagram that trimming off the spur, and leaving an occlusal surface on the teeth has the same effect on X as removing the crown completely. Grinding the teeth down to gum level is counterproductive for several reasons:

(i) taking teeth out of occlusion can hasten their rate of eruption (see Section 7.2).
(ii) removing the crown exposes innervated dentine.
(iii) taking teeth out of occlusion prevents grinding of fibrous food and consumption of indigestible fibre. If teeth are trimmed down to the gum in the later stages of dental disease, when the teeth are no longer growing, loss of occlusion between the cheek teeth is permanent and the rabbit will never be able to grind fibrous vegetation again.

Figure 7.5a also shows the position of the conchal and maxillary sinuses. The anatomical relationship of the paranasal sinuses with the nasal passages is also illustrated in Figure 13.1a. The conchal and maxillary sinuses have a common entrance in the caudal nasal cavity. The rostral end of both sinuses is blind ending, which prevents drainage of exudate from the sinuses if they become infected (see Figure 13.1).

Figure 7.5b and c show how alterations in the shape of the teeth affect the occlusal forces that are placed on them during chewing. In order to grind food, the lower jaw is moved laterally and only one side of the mouth is used at any one time (see Figure 7.4). In (b) and (c) the mandible has been moved laterally to bring the teeth into occlusion. Figure 7.5b shows the occlusion of the cheek teeth during mastication in a healthy rabbit. Figure 7.5c shows the occlusion of the cheek teeth during mastication in a rabbit with cheek tooth malocclusion. Increased force is applied to the lingual edge of the lower cheek teeth and to the buccal edge of the upper cheek teeth. These illustrations are drawn from actual *post mortem* specimens.

of approximately 12.7 cm (5 inches) per year in the upper incisors and 20.3 cm (8 inches) per year in lower ones. These findings are similar to those of Shadle (1936) who recorded a growth rate of approximately 2 mm per week for the upper incisors and 2.4 mm per week for lower ones.

The speed at which crowns grow is not only determined by the rate of attrition but also the rate of eruption. Taking teeth out of occlusion and preventing attrition hastens the rate of eruption. Incisors were found to erupt at a rate of 280 µm/day (0.28 mm/day) in a study by Ness (1956) in which amalgam markers were placed in the labial surfaces of the teeth. Shortening the teeth and taking them out of occlusion increased the eruption rate to 700 µm/day (0.7 mm/day).

Dental wear is affected by the abrasive nature of the diet. Dental abrasion is caused by silicate phytoliths that are present in the skeleton of grasses. Cellulose and lignin are also abrasive. Abrasion results in microscratches on the occlusal surface of the tooth, whereas dental wear by attrition results in polished facets (Hillson, 1986). The diet of wild rabbits is naturally abrasive and requires grinding down to small particles before it can be swallowed and digested. By nature, rabbits are destructive creatures that strip bark off trees and chew through tree roots in addition to grazing and browsing. The abrasive nature of the diet is an important factor in the maintenance of normal occlusion. Wolf *et al.* (1993) studied the effect of diet on incisor growth and attrition. Groups of rabbits were fed on pelleted rations, cereal mixtures, green forages with or without hay and gnawing blocks. They found the biggest difference between the rate of tooth eruption and rate of attrition occurred in rabbits fed on a complete pelleted diet and the lowest difference occurred in rabbits fed on a diet of green forage. They concluded that the duration of feed intake might be more important than the hardness of feed as a determining factor in the rate of growth and attrition.

Key points 7.1

- Rabbits have a secondary pair of small incisors ('peg teeth') that are positioned behind the large upper primary incisors. These 'peg teeth' are a characteristic of lagomorphs
- Rabbits have a deciduous set of teeth that are shed just before or just after birth
- The crown and root of lagomorph teeth are morphologically indistinct
- All the teeth grow continually throughout life. There is germinal tissue at the apex of the tooth
- Rabbits' teeth are precisely arranged so the occlusal surface is maintained by wearing against the opposing teeth
- The cheek teeth have a central fold of enamel that occludes with the interdental space of the opposing teeth
- Dental wear is affected by the abrasive nature of the diet
- The incisors are worn to a fine cutting edge that is used to slice through vegetation
- There are no canines and a wide diastema
- The premolars and molars are indistinguishable from each other and form a row of cheek teeth that are used to grind food
- The rate of tooth growth is approximately 2 m per week. Calcium is required for the continual formation of dentine and enamel
- There is individual variation between the rate of tooth growth and attrition. The rate of growth and attrition is affected by age, pregnancy, diet and occlusal pressure.

7.4 Dental disorders of pet rabbits

Dental disorders have been recognized as a cause of disease in rabbits for many years. Excessive salivation in association with abnormal teeth was described as 'slobbers' by Pollock in 1951 and this term is still used in many texts. Until recently, dental disorders were considered to be congenital but it has now become evident that other factors are involved, although congenital malocclusion does occur. Rabbits' teeth are precisely arranged and aligned to wear against each other to maintain their shape and occlusion (see Figure 7.3). Any factor that alters the relative position of a tooth, even by a fraction, can result in the development of malocclusion and the formation of elongated crowns.

There is a progressive syndrome of acquired dental disease and malocclusion in rabbits that is characterized by elongation of the roots of the teeth. Although this syndrome is very common in pet rabbits, it is scarcely reported in laboratory or commercial rabbits. Weisbroth and Ehrman in 1967 recognized that ectopic tooth roots could penetrate the bones of the skull and result in abscessation. They believed the condition to be inherited and included no details of the diet and husbandry in their description of affected rabbits. A request was made for *'reasons, suggestions or comments by interested persons'* on the development, pathology and inheritance of malocclusion in rabbits. There is a subsequent individual case report (Ireson, 1968) in which elongation of the maxillary tooth roots is noted.

Acquired malocclusion was recognized and described by Zeman and Fielder in 1969 who wrote 'the nature of premolar and molar malocclusion seems to defy at this time any positive determination of the cause'. Speculation and debate on the aetiology of acquired dental disease and malocclusion in rabbits has continued ever since. Rabbit breeders have attributed 'slobbers' to a faulty diet, sudden changes in food, lack of sunlight or cold and damp hutches (Pollock, 1951). Some authors believe that cheek tooth malocclusion is a result of abnormal wear caused by incisor malocclusion (Jenkins, 1997) or that diseases of the temporomandibular joint may be responsible (Wiggs and Lobprise, 1995). Jenkins (1997) suggested ageing as a cause of cheek teeth malocclusion and Brown (1992) cited inflammation of the molar roots as a cause of primary molar malocclusion leading to secondary incisor malocclusion. Westerhof and Lumeij (1987) suggested that lack of hard food might be a predisposing factor for cheek teeth problems. Harcourt-Brown (1995) described a number of clinical conditions in rabbits that were caused by dental problems. The skulls of affected rabbits had a visual osteodystrophic appearance suggestive of metabolic bone disease.

7.5 Acquired dental disease in pet rabbits

There is a syndrome of acquired dental disease in pet rabbits that is a progressive condition and can be staged (Harcourt-Brown, 1997) (see Box 7.1). The disease is characterized by deterioration in tooth quality, acquired malocclusion and elongation of the tooth roots. Periapical abscesses frequently occur. The progression of acquired dental disease is described in Box 7.1 and illustrated in Figures 7.8, 7.11 and Plates 12–21. The exact aetiopathogenesis of this syndrome is not clear and several factors are probably involved, including metabolic bone disease, dietary texture and genetic predisposition. Experimentally, poor bone quality will exacerbate the effect of abnormal loads on rabbits' teeth, making them more susceptible to displacement and distortion. Ashcraft *et al.* (1992) found that orthodontic tooth movement was three to four times greater in rabbits with corticosteroid-induced osteoporosis than in the untreated control group. In rats, hypocalcaemia leads to enhanced alveolar bone resorption and an increased susceptibility to root resorption in response to a moderate orthodontic force (Engstrom *et al.*, 1988).

Acquired dental disease typically occurs in pet rabbits that are housed indoors, bedded on hay and fed on mixed cereal rations, with or without occasional vegetables and sporadic access to the lawn. Wild rabbits and pet rabbits that live outside all year round with unrestricted access to grazing and browsing do not develop this syndrome, whatever their breed. Housed pet rabbits that eat well, and consume a diet rich in grass, hay and vegetables are less likely to develop acquired dental disease than those rabbits that select certain ingredients from mixed rations and consume a diet that is low in indigestible fibre.

7.5.1 Causes of acquired dental disease in pet rabbits

Acquired dental disease in rabbits is usually attributed to lack of dental wear. Many handbooks and leaflets suggest that twigs and branches should be given to pet rabbits for them to gnaw on and wear their teeth down. There is a variety of artificial chews and blocks available from pet shops for this purpose. Lack of dental exercise and uneven wear has been suggested as a cause of enamel spurs on the cheek teeth (Crossley, 1995a). Although a fibrous diet and long periods of chewing keep tooth crowns short, the lack of an abrasive diet and dental exercise cannot be the only cause of acquired dental disease in rabbits. The progressive syndrome of acquired dental disease has only been described in pet rabbits and has not been described in laboratory or commercial rabbits. Instead, congenital defects that affect occlusion have been reported (Okerman, 1988; Lindsey and Fox, 1994). Laboratory and commercial rabbits are usually fed on a complete pelleted ration. Additional hay is not always provided and the diet of these animals is not always abrasive. Laboratory rabbits have been maintained for one year on a complete liquid diet without mention of dental problems (Latour *et al.*, 1998). A complete purified diet based on agar gel was fed to a group of laboratory rabbits for up to 2 years with no gross or histopathological lesions attributable to nutritional disease being observed during autopsy (Hunt and Harrington, 1974).

7.5.1.1 Metabolic bone disease as a cause of dental disease in rabbits

Evidence for metabolic bone disease as a cause of acquired dental disease in pet rabbits is given in Box 7.2. Metabolic bone disease includes a range of inter-related conditions such as rickets, osteoporosis, nutritional osteodystrophy and nutritional secondary hyperparathyroidism. Metabolic bone disease is defined by Fowler (1986) as '*a disease caused by dietary and husbandry mismanagement characterised by metabolic defects affecting the morphology and functioning of bones. The clinical, radiographic and pathological manifestations vary with the age of the animal, species of the animal, degree of deficiency, duration of the deficiency and presence of concurrent diseases*'. Metabolic bone disease occurs in many species whose natural characteristics and lifestyle involve exposure to sunlight. Problems develop with calcium metabolism when they are housed indoors and fed on foods that do not match their natural diet in the wild. The effects of metabolic bone disease vary with species and can be manifested in a variety of ways. For example, shell deformities in growing tortoises, pathological fractures of iguanas or hand-reared birds, dental malocclusion in monkeys (Fowler, 1986) or reduced bone density in ponies (El Shorafa *et al.*, 1979). Nutritional osteodystrophy has been described as a cause of acquired dental malocclusion in species such as sheep and monkeys (Duckworth *et al.*, 1961; McRoberts *et al.*, 1964; Fowler, 1986). Demineralization of supporting alveolar bone results in tooth movement and the development of malocclusion. In calcium deficient rats, demineralization of alveolar bone occurs before changes are seen in other bones, such as the femur (Abe *et al.*, 1989).

Mineral deposition in the teeth is affected by the availability of calcium, phosphate and vitamin D (Guyton, 1991). The fast rate of growth of rabbits' teeth means that there is a high demand for calcium for the continual formation of dentine and enamel. In other species with continually erupting teeth, such as rats, a diet deficient in calcium and vitamin D results in enamel hypoplasia after only 4 weeks (Engstrom and Noren, 1986) and hypomineralized enamel develops on the incisors of juvenile rats weaned on to a calcium deficient diet (Lozupone and Favia, 1989). Growth and reproduction increase susceptibility to calcium and/or vitamin D deficiency. Young rabbits have a higher demand for calcium during the growing period and dietary imbalances can have lifelong effects on the shape and structure of the skeleton, including the bones of the skull. At the other end of the scale, ageing may also affect tooth and bone quality. Pregnancy and lactation have a considerable influence on bone density in rabbits (Julius, 1997).

Poor bone calcification in pet rabbits was reported in 1978 by Wood, who recommended that treatment of fractures should include vitamin D and calcium therapy. A feature of acquired dental disease in rabbits is poor calcification of the bones of the skull, especially the alveolar bone that surrounds and supports the teeth. Loss of alveolar bone at the apex of the tooth allows the continually growing roots to elongate and eventually penetrate the periosteum (see Figure 7.8 and Plates 16 and 17). Loss of surrounding alveolar bone that supports the teeth results in distortion and loosening of the teeth, which causes uneven wear on the occlusal surfaces. The relative position of the teeth changes, which also alters occlusion. Enamel is lost both from the circumference and the centre of

Box 7.1 Grading the progression of acquired dental disease in rabbits

Grade 1: Normal

Grade 2: Root elongation and deterioration in tooth quality

At this stage, there may be no symptoms associated with dental disease, although examination of the teeth and surrounding structures reveals abnormalities. The incisors may or may not have horizontal ribs in the enamel although the shape of the teeth and occlusion can be normal. Hard swellings may be felt along the ventral border of the mandible. These are associated with elongated roots of the mandibular cheek teeth. Epiphora may be present that is caused by obstruction of the nasolacrimal duct by elongated roots of the upper primary incisors.

Grade 3: Acquired malocclusion

Loss of supporting bone and alterations in the position, shape and structure of the teeth changes the direction of growth and results in malocclusion. The mandibular incisors tend to tip forward. The maxillary incisors curl and rotate laterally. The mandibular cheek teeth tip towards the tongue and the maxillary cheek teeth flare towards the buccal mucosa. There is a range of clinical signs that may be seen at this stage:

- Incisor malocclusion that can cause grooming difficulties or problems prehending food. Secondary problems such as cheyletiellosis, fly strike and perineal soiling may be the result
- Sharp spurs on the lower cheek teeth can lacerate the tongue causing anorexia, salivation and pain
- Secondary bacterial infections can invade blocked nasolacrimal ducts resulting in dacryocystitis
- Abscesses can form in the cheek as a result of penetration of the buccal mucosa by elongated crowns, especially of the upper cheek teeth
- Loss of alveolar bone results in widening of the periodontal space. The teeth loosen, which exacerbates malocclusion, and allows periodontal infection to set in. Periapical abscesses can occur
- Plant material can become wedged between the teeth causing abscesses or exacerbating alterations in the position of the teeth.

  The changes in shape, structure and position do not take place in all teeth simultaneously. It is possible to have healthy incisors and major changes in the cheek teeth or vice versa.

Grade 4: Cessation of tooth growth

Eventually, the teeth become so diseased that destruction of germinal tissue at the apex of the tooth results in slowing and cessation of tooth growth. The crowns of the teeth may remain *in situ* as stumps or break off altogether and the gums heal. Affected rabbits can manage to eat, albeit slowly, with any teeth that remain in occlusion. Soft or shredded food may be required. The rabbit's overall condition may improve at this stage as long as there are no sharp spurs penetrating soft tissue. There can be permanent grooming difficulties and recalcitrant epiphora and dacrocystitis.

Many cases do not progress from this stage. It is not unusual to examine the cheek teeth of a healthy looking middle-aged rabbit and find that some crowns are missing. Periapical abscesses can occur at any stage although the risk is reduced by ensuring adequate dietary calcium and vitamin D to improve bone quality.

Grade 5: Endstage dental disease

Grade 5a: Osteomyelitis and abscess formation

Abscesses in rabbits are described in Chapter 8. Abscesses often develop at the sites where elongated roots have penetrated the periosteum. Multiple abscesses can be present. Microabscesses and osteomyelitis can be present throughout the bone. Occasionally tooth roots that have penetrated the periosteum continue to grow and curl round within the abscess cavity. Abscesses can occlude the nasolacrimal duct causing severe dacryocystitis, or form within the nasal passages causing rhinitis, respiratory noise and increased respiratory effort. Abscesses are often found along the border of the mandible in association with the roots of the mandibular cheek teeth. Affected rabbits often continue to eat and drink.

Grade 5b: Calcification of the teeth and surrounding bone

In some cases the remnants of the teeth become progressively calcified and embedded in the surrounding bone. It becomes increasingly difficult to distinguish between tooth and bone both radiographically and on visual examination of prepared skulls. Sometimes the crowns break off and roots remain embedded in the bone. Affected rabbits are usually debilitated. Epiphora, chronic dacrocystitis or rhinitis are often seen. Large rhinoliths can develop at the apex of the maxillary incisors (see Plate 17).

Box 7.2 Evidence for metabolic bone disease as a cause of acquired dental disease in pet rabbits

- The visual appearance of the skulls of rabbits affected by dental disease shows thin osteopaenic bone in comparison with unaffected rabbits (see Plates 12–15)
- There is radiographic evidence of a progressive osteodystrophic disease affecting the teeth and bones of the skull (see Figure 7.8)
- The visual and radiographic features are typical of nutritional secondary hyperparathyroidism, i.e. resorption of the lamina dura, osteoporosis of the calvarium and mandible, with thinning of the cortices
- Observation of the feeding habits of pet rabbits and analysis of their diet has shown that dietary calcium concentrations can be as low as 0.11% (see Figure 2.3 and Table 2.2). A dietary calcium level of 0.44% has been determined for bone mineralization in laboratory rabbits
- Determination of serum vitamin D concentrations in pet rabbits has shown undetectable levels, especially in housed rabbits during the spring
- Parathyroid hormone levels are significantly lower in rabbits that live outside than in housed rabbits suffering from advanced dental disease (see Figure 6.1)
- Total serum calcium levels are significantly lower in rabbits with advanced dental disease than in rabbits that live outside with unrestricted access to grazing and exercise (see Figure 6.1)
- In the early stages of dental disease, horizontal ridges in the enamel of the upper primary incisors will grow out if the diet is modified to increase calcium levels
- Acquired dental disease is uncommon in laboratory rabbits, wild rabbits and those pet rabbits that live outside all year round. Laboratory rabbits are usually maintained on a balanced pelleted ration.

the cheek teeth so the shredding occlusal surface cannot be maintained. The whole shape, structure and position of all the teeth is affected by the syndrome of acquired dental disease (see Figures 7.6–7.8, Plates 18 and 19).

In domestic animals metabolic bone disease is usually nutritional. The term 'nutritional secondary hyperparathyroidism' is often used. Nutritional secondary hyperparathyroidism can be caused by insufficient dietary calcium deficiency or a relative excess of phosphate. Vitamin D plays an integral part because of its effects on intestinal absorption, renal excretion and the mobilization of calcium to and from bone. There is a complex inter-relationship between calcium, phosphorus, vitamin D, parathyroid hormone (PTH) and calcitonin, which maintain calcium homeostasis. Parathyroid hormone (PTH) is released from the parathyroid glands, in response to a fall in blood calcium concentrations. PTH stimulates bone resorption and conversion of 25-hydroxycholecalciferol (25-OH-D) to dihydroxycholecalciferol (1,25$(OH)_2$D) in the kidney. A rise in PTH concentrations indicates the presence of metabolic bone disease. PTH concentrations have been measured in pet rabbits in a study by Harcourt-Brown and Baker (2001). Rabbits were assigned to one of four categories according to their husbandry and the state of their teeth. Rabbits that lived outside in free-range conditions had PTH levels that were significantly lower than rabbits suffering from clinical disease associated with dental problems (see Figure 6.1).

Radiography is an important part of diagnosis of metabolic bone disease. The radiographic signs of nutritional secondary hyperparathyroidism in any species have been described and include: resorption of the cortex of the tooth socket (*lamina dura*), osteoporosis of all bones, especially the calvarium and mandible, folding fractures of the long bones, compression fractures of the vertebrae and abnormalities of the pelvis (Morgan, 1972). Many of the radiographic changes that take place in rabbits with acquired dental disease are typical of metabolic bone disease. Resorption of the lamina dura is seen, especially on *post-mortem* radiographs of hemi-mandibles (see Figure 7.8) and osteoporosis of the mandible and calvarium are characteristic findings in prepared skulls (see Plate 16).

Rabbits have an unusual calcium metabolism (see Section 1.6.7). They absorb dietary

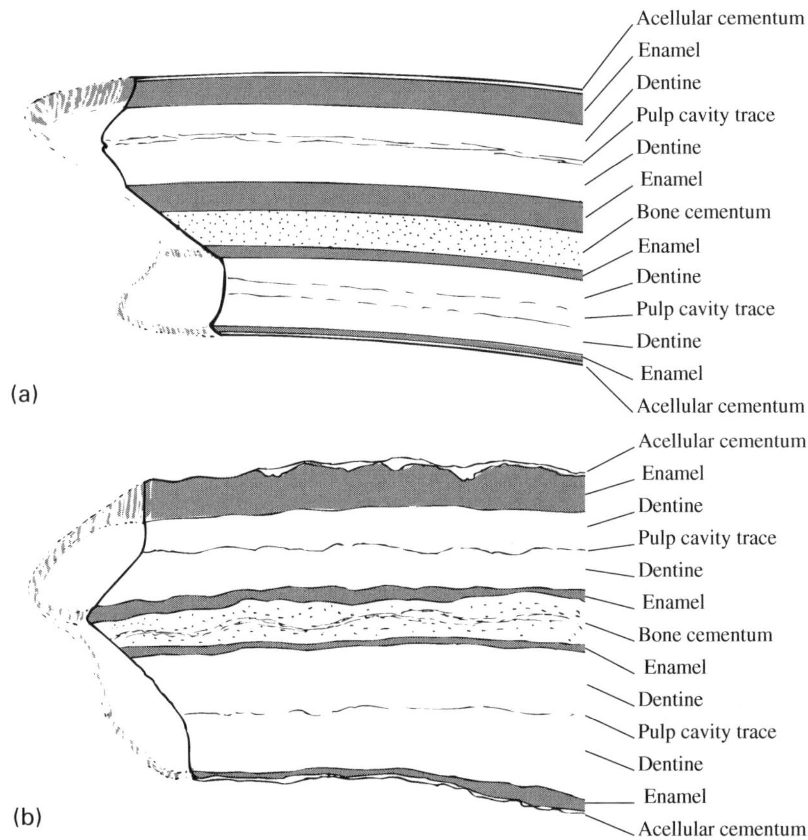

Figure 7.6. Comparison of the structure of healthy (a) and diseased (b) mandibular cheek teeth.

Figure 7.6a was traced from a longitudinal section through a healthy mandibular molar from an adult pet rabbit unaffected by dental disease; Figure 7.6b was traced from a longitudinal section through a first mandibular molar from an adult rabbit suffering from acquired dental disease. A comparison of the two illustrations shows that there are changes to the enamel, dentine and cementum throughout the diseased tooth. These changes have reduced the hardness of the tooth and altered the pattern of dental wear on the occlusal surface. These alterations in the strength and structure of the cheek teeth of rabbits with acquired dental disease leads to uneven wear and the development of 'step mouth' (see Figure 7.11b).

calcium efficiently from the gut and excrete large quantities in the urine. However, despite their efficient absorption, rabbits do have a minimum requirement for calcium (Chapin and Smith, 1967) and the diet of pet rabbits can be calcium deficient. Mixed rations permit selection of calcium deficient items such as maize and peas and rejection of the vitamin and mineral supplement. The supplement is usually incorporated into pellets that are not as palatable to rabbits as the other ingredients (see Figure 2.3). Analysis of the selected diet has shown that it can be severely deficient in calcium (see Table 2.2) (Harcourt-Brown, 1996). Selective feeding has been reported as a cause of metabolic bone disease in other species. For example, selection of cereals and bread from a mixed diet including pellets resulted in fractured vertebrae in the necks of emus and rheas (Wolf *et al.*, 1996). Dietary calcium deficiency has been shown to cause poor mineralization of the skeleton in rabbits. Laboratory rabbits are used as models of human osteoporosis. Reduced bone density is

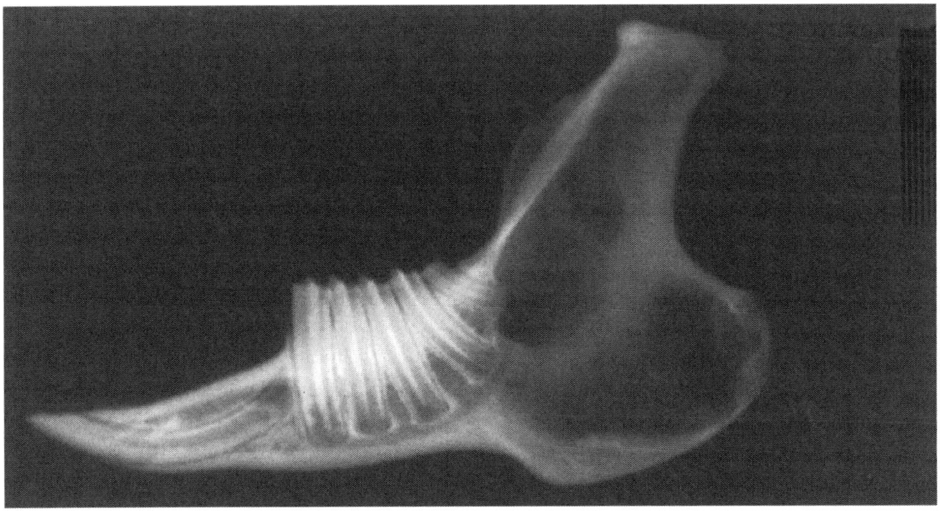

(a)

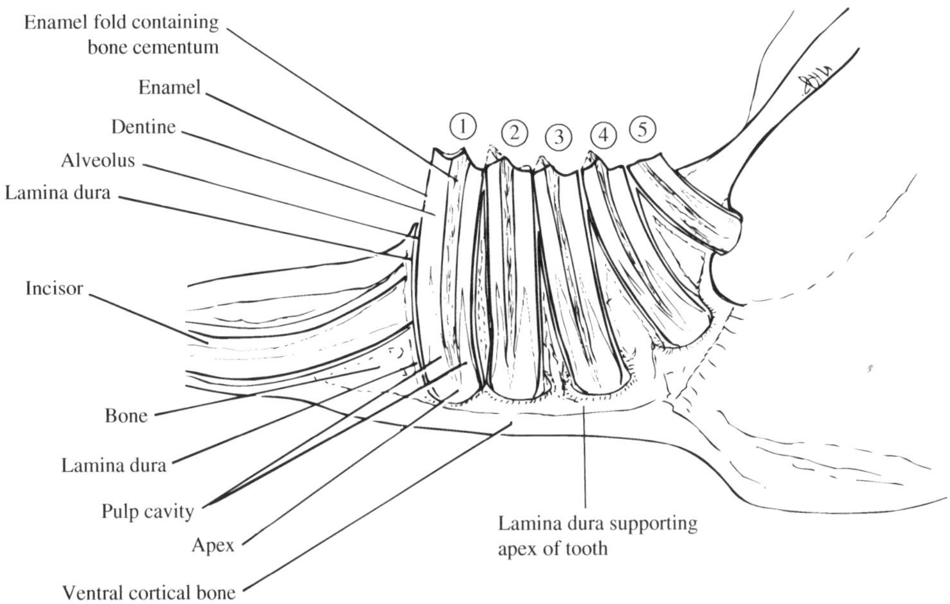

(b)

Figure 7.7. Radiographic anatomy of teeth and surrounding jaw. The figure is a radiograph (a) and a diagram (b) of the lateral view of a prepared hemi-mandible taken from an adult rabbit that was unaffected by dental disease. The radiographic anatomy of the tooth and surrounding structures can be seen.

Each alveolus (tooth socket) is bordered by the *lamina dura*, which is a line of radiodense bone that contains highly calcified cementing substance into which the periodontal ligament binds. The *lamina dura* and the wall of the tooth are separated by a space that contains the periodontal ligament. Each tooth has a central dense line formed by the enamel fold and the bone cementum that lies within it. Towards the apex of the tooth, on either side of the enamel fold, two tapering longitudinal radiolucent areas are formed by the pulp cavity. These areas become wider towards the apex, where they join to form a single radiolucent area that consists of blood vessels, nerves and germinal tissue. This area is also bordered by *lamina dura*. The ventral aspect of the normal mandible is a smooth bar of cortical bone.

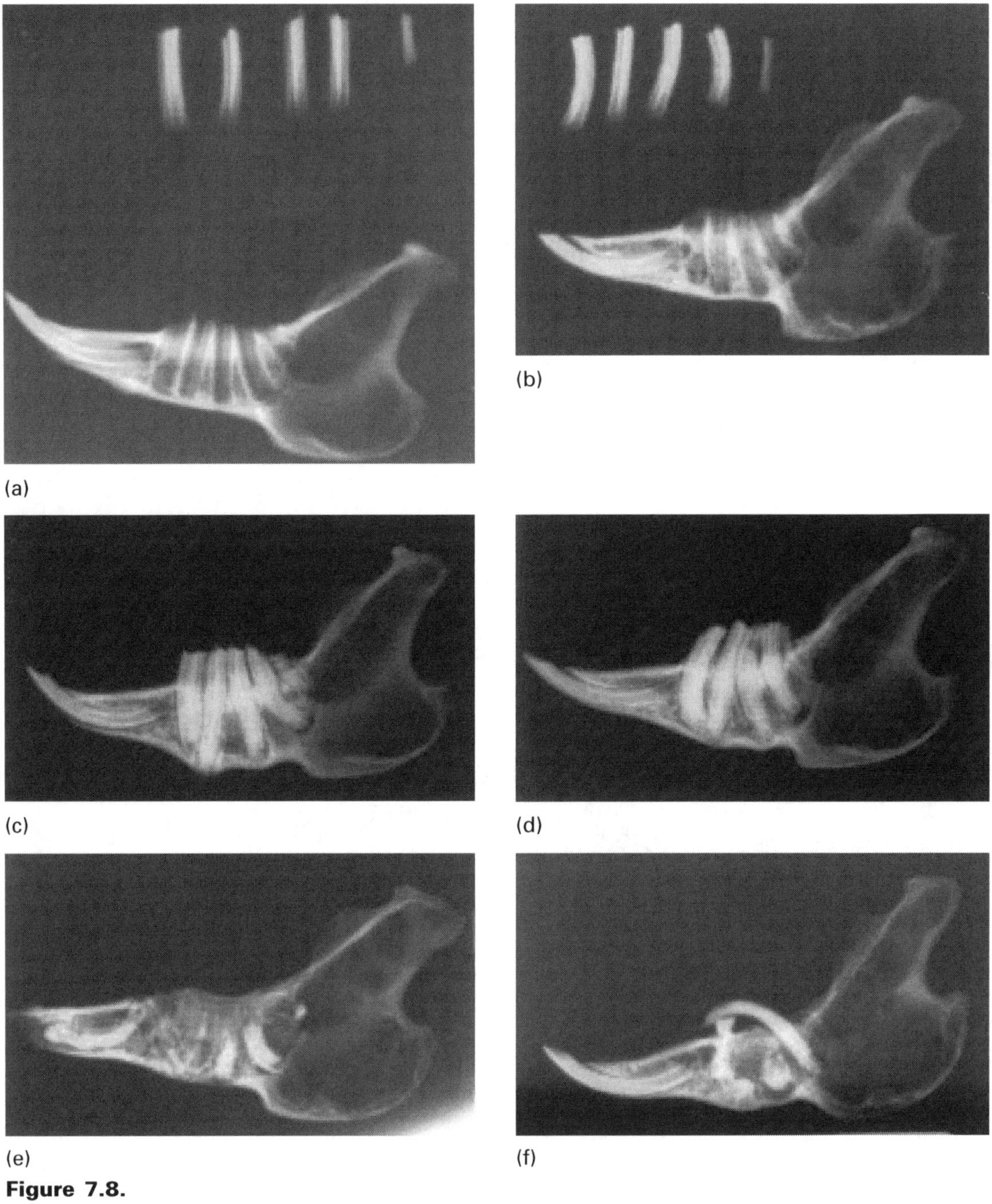

Figure 7.8.

induced by feeding a calcium deficient diet (Gilsanz *et al.*, 1991). In a study by Wu *et al.* (1990), mature rabbits suffered a 20% vertebral bone loss after only 14 weeks on a calcium deficient diet.

In addition to its inter-relationship with PTH and blood calcium levels, vitamin D also has a direct effect on the structure of teeth and in modelling and remodelling of bone. Fracture healing in laboratory rabbits is improved with vitamin D supplementation (Omeroglu *et al.*, 1997) and vitamin D influences the organization and mineralization of rabbit cartilage *in vitro* (Plachot *et al.*, 1982).

Figure 7.8. Progression of acquired dental disease. The changes that take place within the teeth and surrounding jaw of rabbits with acquired dental disease can be monitored radiographically: (a)–(f) are radiographs of the lateral view of prepared hemi-mandibles taken from pet rabbits at different stages of acquired dental disease. The radiographs were taken at the same exposure.

(a) A hemi-mandible and cheek teeth of a pet rabbit that was unaffected by dental disease (Grade 1, see Box 7.1). The rabbit was kept outside under free-range conditions. The *lamina dura* and calcified structures of the teeth can be seen.

(b) A hemi-mandible of an adult pet rabbit in the initial stages of acquired dental disease. There is loss of supporting alveolar bone, especially at the apex of the tooth. The *lamina dura* is not visible at the base of the alveolus that has extended into the cortical bone. The structure and shape of the teeth has changed. The enamel cannot be seen on the teeth as clearly as in 7.8a.

(c) A hemi-mandible with the teeth *in situ* of an adult pet rabbit. The rabbit showed signs of early dental disease (Grade 2, see Box 7.1). Hard swellings could be palpated along the ventral border of the mandible. Radiographically, the enamel on the edge of the teeth and in the central enamel fold is indistinct. The *lamina dura* is only evident in a few places. The shape of the tooth roots has altered although the occlusal surfaces are still in alignment. There is widening of the interdental space. There are radiolucent areas of bone, particularly at the apex of the second molar (cheek tooth 4).

(d) A hemi-mandible with the teeth *in situ* of an adult rabbit with acquired malocclusions (Grade 3, see Box 7.1). The enamel fold is not evident in most of the teeth. Pulp cavities cannot be seen. The teeth have moved and rotated within the sockets. Elongated roots have penetrated the cortical bone. There are areas of radiolucent bone.

(e) The hemi-mandible of a rabbit with advanced dental disease (Grade 5, see Box 7.1). The crowns have broken off and the roots are almost completely resorbed. This hemi-mandible was from an aged rabbit that had spent its life confined to a hutch. It had been eating until shortly before death and was not thin.

(f) The hemi-mandible of an adult rabbit that developed an abscess on the cheek (Grade 5, see Box 7.1). The elongated molar crown had penetrated the buccal mucosa. The crowns of most of the cheek teeth have broken off and the roots have resorbed. There are radiolucent areas of osteomyelitis. The shape of the lower incisor appears relatively normal but there is no pulp cavity.

The direct effect of vitamin D or bone and tooth structure could also be a factor in the development of dental disease in rabbits. In humans, vitamin D resistant rickets is associated with defective calcification of the teeth and periapical infections (Archard, 1971; Goodman *et al.*, 1998).

Radiographs of rabbit mandibles taken during a study of 'calcification processes' by Mellanby and Killick in 1926 showed demineralization of the bone and root elongation in rabbits fed on a diet that would induce rickets. The changes showed a great similarity to the changes seen in the mandibles of present-day pet rabbits suffering from acquired dental disease.

In rabbits, although vitamin D does not appear to be required for intestinal absorption of calcium if there is sufficient quantity in the diet, vitamin D is required to increase intestinal absorption if dietary calcium concentrations are restricted (Brommage *et al.*, 1988). Vitamin D will increase intestinal absorption of calcium in rabbits (Tvedegaard, 1987). Rabbits kept indoors or housed in hutches and carports away from sunlight cannot synthesize endogenous vitamin D. Supplemented vitamin D is not ingested by rabbits that leave the pellet portion of mixed rations uneaten. Blood vitamin D assays have demonstrated undetectable 1,25-$(OH)_2D_3$ concentrations in pet rabbits, especially in samples taken during the spring (Fairham and Harcourt-Brown, 1999).

Hay that has been artificially dried without exposure to sunlight may not contain much vitamin D. Calcium can also be leached out of poor quality hay. Calcium levels in hay can be as low as 0.25%, which is below the 0.44% that is required for bone calcification in rabbits (Chapin and Smith, 1967; McDonald *et al.*, 1996).

7.5.1.2 Diet and dental wear

Lack of dental exercise and tooth wear appear to play a role in the development of aquired dental disease, although the exact mechanism still remains unclear. Rabbits that live in the wild and those pet rabbits that have unlimited access to grazing do not develop acquired dental disease. Pet rabbits that eat well and consume large amounts of hay are much less likely to develop dental disease than those rabbits that are finicky in their eating habits.

Crossley *et al.* (1998) attribute root elongation in species with continually growing teeth to lack of dental wear, which results in coronal elongation, stretching of the masseter muscles and an increase in resting intraocclusal pressure. The authors postulate that the increased resting intraocclusal pressure places an intrusive load on the teeth that results in 'negative growth' and elongation of the tooth roots. This theory is based on experimental studies of occlusal pressure in laboratory rabbits. Because of their continually erupting teeth, laboratory rabbits are often used in investigations of resting intraocclusal pressure that could be relevant to tooth eruption and occlusion in humans. The investigations are carried out on anaesthetized rabbits, in which a measurable force is applied to the maxillary incisors over a period of several hours. The rate of tooth eruption is measured simultaneously (Steedle *et al.*, 1983; Proffitt and Sellers, 1986). It has been discovered that forces as light as 1 g can cause 'negative growth' or 'intrusion' of the teeth. However, it is difficult to extrapolate the results of experiments on anaesthetized rabbits to the situation in conscious rabbits without considering the effect of forces that occur during chewing. In order to understand the exact aetiopathogenesis of root elongation and dental disease in rabbits, the condition would have to be induced under experimental conditions with a limited number of variable factors.

7.5.1.3 Other causes of acquired dental disease

Apart from dental wear, dietary texture and nutritional hyperparathyroidism, there are other factors that could affect tooth quality and bone strength and play a part in the development of dental disease in pet rabbits. In humans, bone quality is affected by many factors including genetic predisposition, oestrogens, thyroid hormone, corticosteroids, drugs and systemic conditions, such as renal diseases or disorders of the gastrointestinal tract, liver and pancreas that affect calcium uptake and vitamin D absorption and metabolism (Rao and Honasage, 1996). In other animal species, the rate of development and speed of eruption of teeth can be accelerated by both thyroid and growth hormone.

In rabbits, there appears to be a genetic susceptibility to the development of dental disease. Dwarf Lop males appear most susceptible. Turner (1997) noted an over-representation of dwarf breeds of rabbit presented for dental treatment (68%) in comparison with the incidence of dwarf breeds presented in general (30%).

There could be other dietary factors, apart from dental wear, calcium and vitamin D, which play a role in the development of dental disease. Other nutrients, such as vitamin A and magnesium, are required for tooth and bone growth. Selective feeding from cereal rations and the rejection of the supplemented pellets will result in dietary deficiencies of a range vitamins and minerals. Protein deficiency is another potential cause of osteoporosis (Morgan, 1972).

Key points 7.2

- Dental problems in rabbits can be caused by congenital defects, trauma, foreign bodies, tumours and incorrect diet
- There is a progressive syndrome of acquired dental disease in pet rabbits that is common and is linked to diet and husbandry
- The visual and radiological appearance of the skull and teeth of affected rabbits is suggestive of metabolic bone disease
- Acquired dental disease can be staged. The syndrome starts with a deterioration in enamel quality and elongation of the roots. Subsequent alterations in the structure, shape and position of the teeth result in the development of malocclusion. Eventually the teeth stop growing. Abscesses are common.

Disuse atrophy caused by insufficient chewing and lack of dental exercise has been suggested as a cause of periodontal weakness and osteoporosis in pet rabbits (Crossley, 1995b). This suggestion does not fit with the visual, radiological or serological findings in rabbits with acquired dental disease. Disuse osteoporosis occurs in bone that is not subjected to stress or strain. It can be the result of weightlessness (astronauts in space) or prolonged immobilization of bone, e.g. after a fracture. Bone resorption results in hypercalcaemia and reduced levels of circulating PTH (Yang and Stewart, 1996). This is the exact reverse of the findings of rabbits suffering from acquired dental disease, which is associated with low serum calcium levels and elevated PTH (Harcourt-Brown and Baker, 2001) (see Figure 6.1). Visual osteopaenia is evident in all areas of the skull, including the area above the diastema that is not subjected to forces incurred by chewing (see Plates 16 and 17).

7.6 Clinical conditions associated with dental problems in rabbits

The extent of bone pain and toothache is difficult to evaluate in rabbits. Reduced appetite, lassitude, an unkempt coat and uneaten caecotrophs are often seen in association with dental disease. The sensory innervation of the teeth is from the inferior alveolar and maxillary branches of the trigeminal nerve that runs close to the tooth roots (see Figure 7.9). Elongated roots impinge on these nerves and it is probable that affected rabbits experience pain when occlusal pressure is applied during mastication. In humans, metabolic bone disease causes deep unrelenting bone pain (Holick, 1996) and it is possible that similar bone pain occurs in rabbits. Analgesics can be effective in restoring appetite and improving the demeanour of rabbits affected by dental disease, especially in the early stages. In the later stages, the degenerative changes that take place in the tooth affect the pulp cavity and nerve supply. It is likely that these changes are accompanied by a loss in sensation.

7.6.1 Lack of grooming

Rabbits spend a lot of time grooming themselves and their companions. They use their incisor teeth like pincers to remove skin debris and parasites from the coat. They lick their fur and sharp spurs on the molars can prevent licking and grooming (see Plate 20). Rabbits with dental problems often have a poorly groomed coat that contains matted fur, dead hair and skin debris. Skin disease is often seen in conjunction with dental disease (see Section 9.1).

7.6.2 Digestive disorders

Rabbits with dental problems can find chewing hay and fibrous vegetation painful. Indigestible fibre is necessary for optimal gut motility (see Box 2.2) and the pain and stress associated with dental problems increases the risk of gastrointestinal hypomotility. Intestinal obstruction can also be linked to dental disease. Rabbits with poor teeth cannot groom properly and mats develop easily, especially in rabbits with a fine, fluffy coat. Felts of matted hair are a common cause of small intestinal blockage (section 10.5). A possible association has also been made between dental disease and intestinal obstruction by hard locust bean seeds (Harcourt-Brown and Friggens, 1999).

7.6.3 Uneaten caecotrophs

The diet that predisposes to dental problems also predisposes to problems with caecotrophy. A healthy rabbit on a high fibre diet will usually ingest caecotrophs straight from the anus. Only the hard faecal pellets are found in the bedding. Rabbits on a low fibre diet that are fed on cereal rations have a reduced appetite for caecotrophs. Uneaten caecotrophs are soft and sticky and tend to stick to the fur around the anus. Dental problems, especially spurs on the cheek teeth (see Plate 20), can interfere with a rabbit's ability to lick up and ingest caecotrophs or groom the perineum. Uneaten caecotrophs stick to the fur and contain volatile fatty acids that give them a characteristic, unpleasant odour. Owners often incorrectly interpret the large

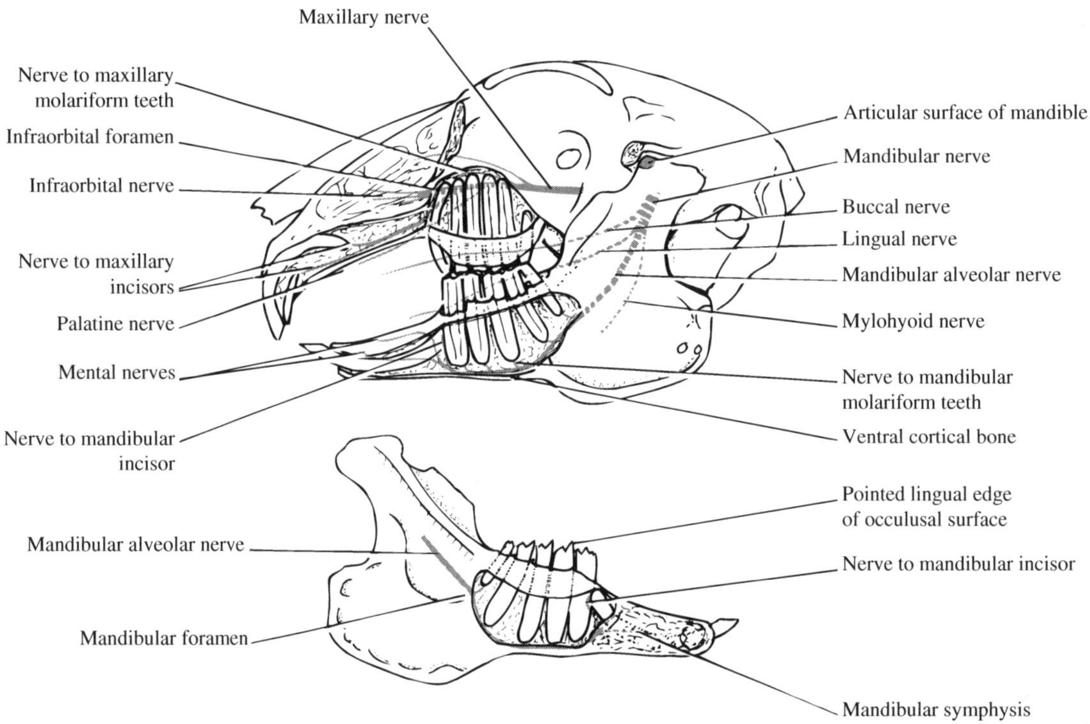

Figure 7.9. Innervation of the teeth. Figure 7.9 is drawn from a dissection of a decalcified head of a rabbit using Barone *et al.* (1973) as a reference source. The sensory innervation of the teeth is from the mandibular and maxillary branches of the trigeminal nerve. Elongated roots impinge on these nerves and it is probable that affected rabbits experience pain when occlusal pressure is applied during mastication.

Sympathetic and sensory axons extend into the dentine in tubules. Dentine becomes increasingly atubular towards the occlusal surface where the axons retract from the tubules and degenerate. Shortening the crowns of the teeth exposes innervated dentine.

In the later stages of acquired dental disease, degenerative changes take place in the tooth that affect the pulp cavity and nerve supply. It is likely that these changes are accompanied by a loss in sensation and interferes with the feedback mechanism that controls masticatory force during crushing of food between the cheek teeth (see Figure 7.4).

mound of foul smelling, soft faecal material under their rabbit's tail as diarrhoea. Sometimes the perineal skin beneath the uneaten caecotrophs becomes inflamed and sore. Urination then becomes painful and urinary incontinence can develop (Section 9.7.3). Urine scalding exacerbates the condition further and sets up a vicious circle.

7.6.4 Ribbed teeth

Developmental disturbances in enamel production result in enamel hypoplasia and the appearance of visual defects on the surface of the teeth. The condition is the result of disturbances to the ameloblasts in their enamel matrix production. Enamel hypoplasia results in the development of horizontal ridges giving the teeth a ribbed or 'washboard' appearance. Interference with calcium and phosphorus metabolism is among the causes of enamel hypoplasia in any species. In rats, dietary calcium deficiency at weaning results in a dramatic reduction in mineralization of enamel on the continually growing incisors. The changes are reversed within 60 days by providing a diet containing the requisite amount of calcium (Lozupone and Favia, 1994). In humans,

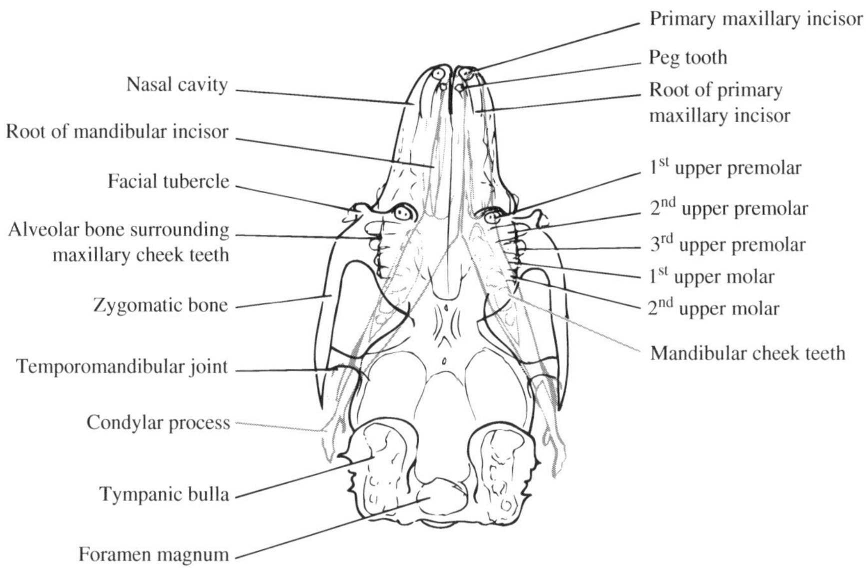

(a)

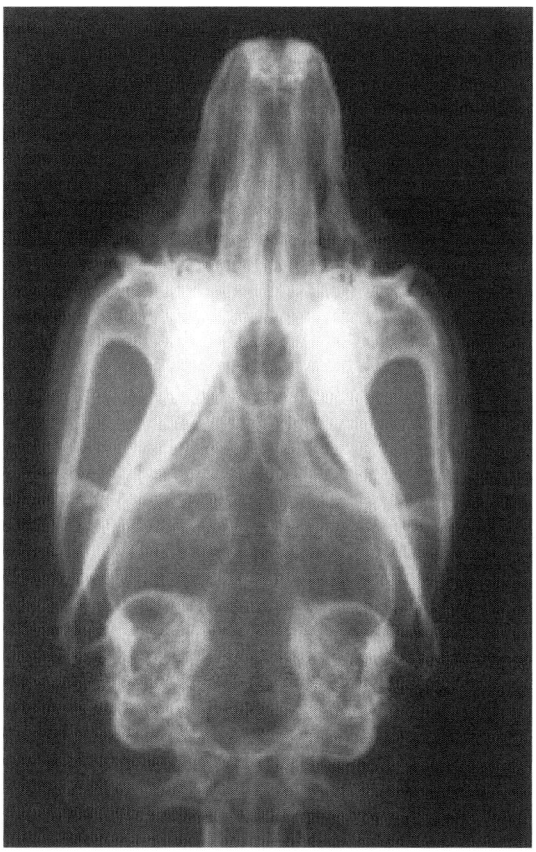

(b)

Figure 7.10. Interpretation of dorsoventral skull radiographs. Normal radiographic features of the skull are summarized in Box 7.4. This dorsoventral view is of the same rabbit in Figure 7.11. Careful positioning is necessary to obtain a true dorsoventral view. The angular process of the ramus, the incisors and the cleft in the upper lip are useful positioning landmarks.

congenital defects, infectious disease, toxicities, metabolic diseases and endocrinopathies are also listed as causes of enamel hypoplasia (Hillson, 1986).

In rabbits, the continual process of growth and attrition of the teeth demands a constant supply of calcium for the formation of dentine and enamel. Calcium deficiency can cause a deterioration of enamel quality.

In a healthy rabbit, the upper incisors have a clear vertical groove running longitudinally down the labial aspect. The enamel on the incisors is smooth and shiny. Early changes in the enamel can be detected by running a fingernail down the teeth. Horizontal ridges on the upper incisors are among the first signs of the acquired dental disease syndrome. Initially the tooth shape is retained and the teeth continue to grow, but the enamel is ribbed. The vertical groove in the enamel on the upper incisors becomes less distinct and can disappear completely as dental disease progresses. In the early stages, the horizontal ribs will grow out and be replaced by normal thick shiny enamel if the diet is changed or supplemented to provide extra calcium. More often, this stage goes unnoticed until teeth stop growing or permanent changes have taken place in the germinal layer at the apex of the tooth. Once tooth growth ceases, the ribbing is permanent. Ridges can also be seen in the enamel of the cheek teeth (see Figure 7.6).

7.6.5 Epiphora and dacrocystitis

Elongated roots of the upper incisors often impinge on the nasolacrimal duct that runs close to the apex of the upper primary incisor (see Figure 11.1). Blockage of the duct results in epiphora. Epiphora is often one of the first signs of acquired dental disease. Secondary bacterial infection can invade the nasolacrimal duct and lead to dacrocystitis (Section 11.6.4).

7.6.6 Abscesses

Elongated roots of the lower premolars can be felt as hard lumps along the ventral border of the mandible. Periapical abscesses can develop at these sites, particularly at the root of the first lower premolar that is situated alongside the root of the lower incisor. The cheek over the mandibular ramus is the site of abscess formation associated with last molar that emerges on the lateral aspect of the ramus under the masseter muscle (see Figure 7.1).

Elongated roots of the upper first premolar can penetrate the nasal cavity and cause abscessation. Occasionally the nasolacrimal duct is involved at this site. Elongated roots of the second upper premolar curl through the bone before penetrating the periosteum, usually at the base of the zygomatic prominence of the maxilla. Dorsoventral radiographs often show the position of this root clearly (see Figure 7.10). Periapical abscesses associated with these tooth roots appear just below the medial canthus of the eye (see Plate 16). Elongated roots of the upper molars penetrate the alveolar bulla into the zygomatic gland in the retrobulbar space and can cause retrobulbar abscesses (see Plate 16).

7.6.7 Incisor malocclusion

Incisor malocclusion in rabbits can be congenital or acquired. Typically the upper incisors curl outwards and the lower incisors grow forwards like tusks, hence the term 'walrus teeth' that is sometimes used to describe the condition. Incisor malocclusion is visually obvious and is associated with surprisingly few clinical signs. Usually the rabbit is presented for treatment because the owners have noticed the overgrown teeth protruding from the mouth. Most rabbits learn to prehend food despite elongated incisors. Sometimes the teeth become so long that they catch on the cage bars or water bottles. Hair can become entwined on the elongated mandibular incisors. The curled crowns of the maxillary incisors sometimes grow into the lips or gums and damage the soft tissue.

Congenital incisor malocclusion is usually due to mandibular prognathism or a disproportionately long mandible in relation to the maxilla. It is a common inherited disease of rabbits and few laboratory or commercial breeding stocks are free of the problem (Lindsey and Fox, 1994). The upper and lower incisors fail to meet correctly, if at all, and grow abnormally. The condition is obvious from an early age, sometimes as young as 3 weeks. Congenital incisor malocclusion has been shown to be an inherited autosomal recessive trait (Chai 1970; Fox and Crary, 1971). The underlying defect appears to be a short maxilla rather than a long mandible (Huang, 1987). Two surveys of malocclusion in pet rabbits have demonstrated a breed disposition towards rabbits under 1.5 kg, especially Netherland Dwarfs, although any breed or type of rabbit can be affected (Abbott, 1997; Turner, 1997). Rabbits with congenital incisor malocclusion should not be bred from.

Incisor malocclusion can also be the result of traumatic injury to the teeth or jaw. Fractured jaws or broken teeth are often the result of an accident, particularly being dropped or leaping from owners' arms on to a hard surface. Paradoxically, tooth trimming can cause malocclusion and dental disease. Healthy teeth do not require trimming but, occasionally, misguided owners believe that tooth trimming is an essential part of their pet's healthcare and clip healthy incisors.

Although conformational abnormalities and traumatic injuries occur, most pet rabbits acquire incisor malocclusion as adults. The development of malocclusion is insidious and is not associated with trauma. It is accompanied by visual changes in the structure and shape of the teeth. Incisor malocclusion develops as part of the syndrome of acquired dental disease and may be the first sign that the owners see. Some rabbits develop malocclusion of both the incisors and the molars. The condition usually develops in mature rabbits, typically about 1 year old or older.

7.6.8 Malocclusion of the cheek teeth

Alterations in the position, shape and structure of the molars leads to malocclusion of the cheek teeth. The development of molar malocclusion is also part of the syndrome of acquired dental disease characterized by deterioration of tooth and bone quality and root elongation. The shape of the tooth changes. Initially, the teeth tend to curl before becoming progressively distorted (see Figure 7.4, Plate 19). Typically the crowns on the upper cheek teeth flare laterally and the mandibular molars tip towards the tongue (see Figure 7.4 and Plates 19, 20 and 21). Loss of alveolar bone leads to widening of the periodontal space and loosening of the teeth, which increases the risk of foreign material entering the socket. Foreign material such as grass seeds, stems of hay or other fibrous material can become wedged between teeth and alter the alignment further. Periodontal disease, bone tumours or periapical abscesses can also loosen or distort teeth and result in malocclusion of the cheek teeth. There is only a few millimetres difference between the normal sharp zigzig occlusal points that are vertically aligned and do not impinge on the tongue and the sharp spurs that develop on the molars that are tipped towards the tongue, lacerating it and causing pain (see Plate 20). The situation can develop rapidly. In rabbits that have had their cheek teeth trimmed, the tongue is often scarred at the site of previous lacerations and is not as sensitive when the spurs re-grow.

7.6.9 Pain and anorexia

A reduced appetite is a characteristic of dental disease in rabbits. The razor sharp spurs that can develop on the lower cheek teeth lacerate the tongue and are acutely painful for the rabbit. Affected animals are sometimes totally anorexic and often salivate profusely. The salivation may be unilateral and occurs on the side of the tongue damage. A general anaesthetic is necessary to see these spurs which cannot always be seen in the conscious animal, especially if they have developed on the back molars. Affected animals usually resent auriscopic examination of the cheek teeth. Laceration of the tongue seriously interferes with its function and prevents licking and grooming as well as eating.

A reluctance to drink from a drinking bottle may be one of the first symptoms of molar malocclusion that owners notice. The rabbit has trouble licking water from a sipper bottle and prefers to drink water from a bowl. Sometimes dehydration and electrolyte imbalances result from the profuse salivation that accompanies oral pain and an inability to swallow. If sharp spurs are not removed from the teeth, secondary gastrointestinal stasis develops that eventually leads to hepatic lipidosis and death (see Section 10.3.2)

7.7 Examination of the teeth

Before embarking on examination of the face and oral cavity, the coat, especially the perineum, should be examined for the presence of matted fur or uneaten caecotrophs. The area dorsal to the base of the tail and the area between the shoulder blades are other sites where dead hair, scurf and evidence of cheyletiellosis can be seen in rabbits that are not grooming effectively.

For dental examination, a rabbit can be satisfactorily restrained by wrapping it in a towel and giving it to the owner or an assis-

Key points 7.3

- Dental disease underlies many of the clinical conditions that affect pet rabbits
- Grooming is necessary to remove dead hair and skin debris from the coat. Rabbits with tooth problems cannot groom effectively
- Matted hair around the perineum can become soiled. As a result, the underlying skin can become inflamed, infected and ulcerated
- Some rabbits with dental problems are unable to ingest caecotrophs that become entangled in the fur under the tail
- Fly strike can occur
- *Cheyletiella parasitovorax* numbers can build up in the ungroomed fur and cause disease
- Salivation in association with dental disease can cause superficial pyoderma under the chin and on the forelegs
- Felts of matted hair can be swallowed and cause intestinal obstruction
- The nasolacrimal duct can become blocked by elongated tooth roots causing epiphora and secondary dacrocystitis
- Acquired incisor malocclusion often results in grossly elongated crowns that interfere with the prehension of food
- Cheek tooth malocclusion results in the development of sharp spurs that lacerate the tongue and cause pain. Pain can result in gastrointestinal hypomotility that can be fatal
- Spurs can develop on the cheek teeth that prevent the rabbit from eating, causing anorexia, weight loss and general debility
- Facial abscesses are often related to dental problems. Periodontal and perapical infections occur. Elongated crowns penetrate buccal mucosa and introduce infection. Osteomyelitis occurs at the sites where elongated roots have penetrated the bone.

tant to hold on the consulting table. The sites that are commonly affected by root elongation should be examined and the eyes looked at carefully for signs of exophthalmus, epiphora, keratitis, conjunctivitis or dacrocystitis. Pressure on the medial canthus will sometimes squeeze purulent material from the nasolacrimal duct into the conjunctival sac in rabbits suffering from dacrocystitis. Root elongation of the lower cheek teeth causes swellings along the ventral border of the mandibles that can be palpated and may be painful. Signs of ptyalism are seen under the chin, on the dewlap and on the forelegs, especially the inner aspect of the carpus where the fur may be matted and soiled.

Examination of the teeth starts with the incisors that can be seen by carefully retracting the lips. The shape and bite of the incisors is noted in addition to the appearance of the enamel and the presence of the vertical groove running down the centre of each upper incisor. Running a fingernail over the labial aspect of the incisors can reveal horizontal ridging that is not obvious on visual examination.

The cheek teeth are examined with an auriscope by sliding it down each side of the mouth. If the head is held with the thumb around the mandible, the lower jaw can be moved from side to side to give a clearer view of the alignment and quality of the teeth. Most rabbits tolerate auriscopic examination of the molars and premolars, although a rabbit with spurs on the cheek teeth may resist. Excessive amounts of saliva in the mouth or the presence of blood or pus are indicative of a dental problem. General anaesthesia is required in these patients to enable a thorough examination of the oral cavity.

Acquired dental disease is common and many pet rabbits show some degree of dental abnormality. Although clinical disease results from the development of malocclusion, root elongation or abscessation, not all rabbits with abnormal teeth develop these problems and it is not unusual to find poorly aligned, uneven cheek teeth in a rabbit that shows no sign of pain. Some teeth show signs of cessation of growth such as dull discoloration or evidence of dental caries. If the rabbit is eating well and there is no evidence of associated health problems, then treatment is not necessary although dietary advice may be required and the owner warned of potential complications. If there is any suspicion that there are elongated crowns penetrating soft tissue then the rabbit must be anaesthetized for a thorough examination of the oral cavity. Acquired dental disease may not affect all teeth simultaneously and it is possible to have healthy incisors and major changes in the cheek teeth.

Once the rabbit is anaesthetized, good illumination is required to see inside the mouth. There is a variety of gags and cheek dilators available that facilitate examination of the oral cavity although insertion of the gag can stimulate the rabbit to make chewing movements if it is only lightly anaesthetized. It is sometimes difficult or impossible to place a gag if the incisors are absent, broken or abnormal. It may be necessary to shorten the incisors to enable visualization of the premolars and molars. It is possible to examine the mouth under anaesthetic without a gag by pulling the tongue out and placing a finger in the diastema to prop the mouth open. Good illumination from an operating light directed into the mouth is required. Gags and cheek dilators are essential if crowns are to be shortened using dental burrs.

7.8 Radiography

Radiography is a valuable tool in the assessment of dental disease. The indications for radiography are summarized in Box 7.3. Radiography gives useful information about the position and condition of the tooth roots. In order to interpret skull radiographs, consideration needs to be given to normal anatomy and the effects of superimposition and positioning on the image that is given. It is worth preparing some skulls, including one from an unaffected rabbit to compare with the radiograph. A set of normal radiographs is also necessary but one of the major problems in radiological assessment of rabbits is the decision of what constitutes normality. Wild rabbits generally have perfect teeth but are usually immature. The best option is to obtain radiographs from aged rabbits that show no gross abnormality of their teeth. These rabbits are hard to find and are usually individuals that are kept outside with unrestricted access to grazing and exercise in conditions close to a wild existence. The radiographs that are used in this book to make normal comparisons are of the author's own Dutch rabbit that was 7 years old and had lived outside in a parrot aviary all her life when the radiographs were taken. She is still alive at the time of writing (18 months later). There is breed and individual variation between the shapes of the skulls of pet rabbits.

Box 7.3 Indications for radiography of the skull

Skull radiography yields information about the roots of the teeth and is therefore indicated in conditions that result from tooth root problems. Abnormalities of the crowns can be seen by visual examination. The main indications for skull radiography are:

- Cases of recurrent dacrocystitis, conjunctivitis or epiphora
- Facial abscesses. Radiography is essential to assess the condition of the skull and teeth and to identify tooth roots that may be involved in abscessation
- Prior to surgical removal of the incisors in cases of acquired malocclusion in order to identify any lesions that may be present at the roots
- Recurrent malocclusion of the cheek teeth. Radiographic examination of the roots gives an idea of whether the teeth are growing or not and allows a prognosis to be given.

7.8.1 Positioning for radiography

Sedation or anaesthesia is generally required for radiography of the skull in order to position the rabbit correctly (see Box 5.3).

Positioning the patient correctly is important when taking radiographs. The skull on the dorsoventral view must be perfectly symmetrical to make a valid assessment of the roots. The head needs to be extended. Sternal recumbency for a dorsoventral view can result in the mandible being moved to one side and not being perfectly aligned with the maxilla. This does not pose a problem as long as the viewer is aware of the positioning. The cleft in the upper lip and the division between the upper incisors make good landmarks to align the head correctly. A tie can be tied around the upper incisors to extend the neck and anchor the head in position while the X-ray is being taken. The dorsoventral view is often more informative at a slightly higher exposure than the lateral view if it is the cheek teeth that are of interest. If the incisors are the important feature, the same exposure as the lateral view can be used.

A true lateral radiograph requires careful positioning and is difficult to obtain. Perfect positioning on the lateral view is not as critical as the dorsoventral view. Landmarks such as the borders of the mandible, the zygomatic prominences, the cleft in the upper lip or the division between the incisors can be used to align the head correctly. Foam wedges may be required. An almost lateral view, or slightly oblique view is informative, as the individual ventral borders of the hemimandibles can be viewed and the zigzag occlusal line between the molars on each side can be assessed more easily than on a true lateral. Different exposures and views including a dorsoventral, a true lateral, a slightly oblique view and an open mouth view can be taken to obtain as much information as possible. It is not possible to expose all areas of the skull correctly on one film as there is a big difference in thickness of the tissues around the incisors and cheek teeth. Intraoral views on dental film are useful and give information about individual teeth that cannot be gained from whole skull views because of superimposition (Crossley, 1995b). For most cases, however, a well-exposed, carefully positioned lateral and dorsoventral view gives a fair assessment of the teeth and bones of the skull.

7.8.2 Contrast studies

Contrast studies are a valuable part of the assessment of nasolacrimal duct infections and can also be used in the investigation of abscesses. It is relatively straightforward to introduce a cannula into the punctum lacrimale and fill the nasolacrimal duct with contrast medium before taking X-rays. The duct is outlined and the anatomical association with the tooth roots can be seen (see Figure 11.2). Nasolacrimal duct flushing is described in Section 11.6.4.1. Contrast material can be used to fill abscess cavities after lancing and flushing to ascertain the extent of the abscess cavity and to aid identification of the tooth roots that are involved.

A water-soluble iodine preparation can be used for contrast studies. The choice of contrast material is a matter of personal preference. Dilute preparations such as sodium/meglumine iothalamate (Conray 280) have the advantage of being cheap and easy to inject in comparison with more concentrated formulations that are more viscous and are more difficult to inject through the small duct. However, concentrated solutions give a clearer image and are retained in the duct for longer.

7.8.3 Interpretation of skull radiographs

The important radiological features are described in Box 7.4. Abnormalities of the crowns can be seen during visual examination of the oral cavity and radiographic findings can only be considered alongside a careful visual examination. Radiography does not give three-dimensional information and will not show tipping of the crowns or their position in relation to soft tissue structures such as the tongue. Malocclusion of the cheek teeth cannot be diagnosed radiographically. It is also difficult to assess the crown length of the cheek teeth as they often curve during the development of dental disease.

The lateral view gives a good view of the roots of the lower cheek teeth (see Figure 7.8). The alveolar sockets consist of a radiodense line called the *lamina dura*, which is seen as a series of parallel horizontal lines alongside the teeth. The enamel on the teeth and the longitudinal enamel fold down the centre of each cheek tooth are also seen as a series of vertical lines (see Figure 7.7). This 'parallel line effect' is lost during the course of acquired dental disease. An area of radiolucency should surround the apex of the teeth. This is the germinal layer from which the ameloblasts and odontoblasts originate. The mottled appearance of the parietal bone is a normal finding.

The occlusal surfaces of the cheek teeth should exhibit a symmetrical zigzag pattern (see Figure 7.11). An open-mouth lateral view (obtained by wedging the thick end of a cotton bud between the incisors) shows this feature more clearly than the closed-mouth lateral view. At rest, the medial zigzag edges of lower cheek teeth are situated inside the labial edges of the upper cheek teeth and only just occlude (see Figure 7.4). This results in slight superimposition of the occlusal surfaces on lateral radiographs unless the

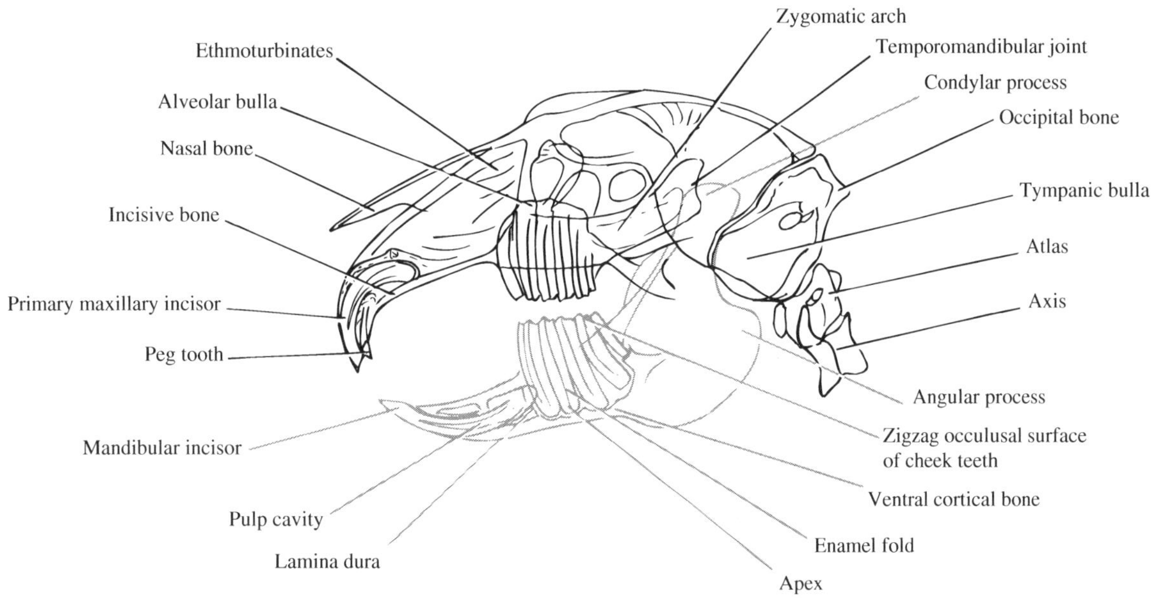

(a)

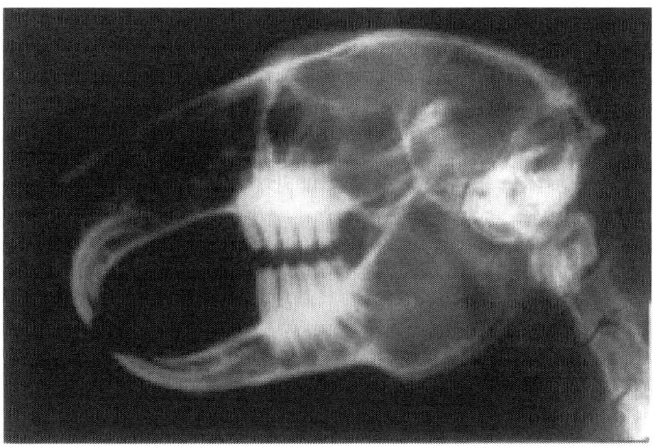

(b)

Figure 7.11. Interpretation of lateral skull radiographs. Normal radiographic features of the skull are summarized in Box 7.4. The lateral skull radiograph in a. is of a 7-year-old neutered female Dutch rabbit that has lived outside throughout the year in free-range conditions for the last 6 years. In order to show the occlusal surfaces of the cheek teeth, the mouth has been wedged open with a cotton bud between the incisors.

mouth is opened slightly (see Figure 7.10). The dorsoventral view is less informative (see Figure 7.12). The position of the maxillary incisor roots is visible and *lamina dura* can be seen encircling the upper first premolar if the positioning is good. In normal rabbits, the roots of the upper cheek teeth form symmetrical curves in the maxilla. The mandible is superimposed on the maxilla and the outline can be examined for any abnormalities. The overall appearance of the skull and tympanic bullae can be seen on this view.

Box 7.4 Normal radiographic features of the skull

Incisors

- The tips of the primary incisors should be worn to a fine cutting edge. The lower incisors occlude against the peg teeth, just behind the upper incisors
- The enamel on labial aspect of upper primary incisors should be thick and smooth. The pulp cavity in the upper and lower incisors can be seen in normal incisors
- The roots of the upper incisor end at least 1 mm away from the incisive bone, which is seen as a straight uninterrupted line at this point
- The root of the lower incisor should be seen at the level of the first lower premolar.
- The upper incisors can be seen as two slightly curved structures within the maxilla on DV view.

Cheek teeth

- The occlusal surfaces of the cheek teeth have a characteristic zigzag occlusal pattern in a normal rabbit
- The crowns of the first mandibular premolar should not be excessively curved
- The roots of lower cheek teeth should not penetrate the cortical bone along the ventral border of the mandible
- A thin layer of bone may be seen overlying the apices of the upper molars. These roots should not be excessively long
- A layer of enamel should be visible on the edge of any premolars that are not superimposed
- There is a radiolucent halo at the apex of each tooth signifying the presence of germinal tissue. This area is more pronounced in juvenile rabbits
- Each cheek tooth should have a longitudinal radiopaque line of enamel down the centre
- The radiodense lines of the alveolar bone and the enamel on the edge and in the centre of each tooth should be almost parallel to one another
- On the dorsoventral view, the roots of the cheek teeth, except the first premolar, form an arc within the maxillary bone. The bone overlying the apices is thinnest at the level of the second upper premolar.

Bone

The overall appearance of the skull should be of mineralized bone: 'Spongy' areas of parietal bone can be seen as a normal finding.

There should be clear contrast between lines of cortical bones and the rest of skull. The areas of interest are:

- The *lamina dura* can be seen on dorsoventral view as a fine line encircling the first upper premolars
- On the lateral view, the incisive bone should be a thick, straight, clear, uninterrupted line
- There should be a thick layer of maxillary bone at the angle where the line from the incisive bone meets the first upper premolar
- On the dorsoventral view, in the diastema between the incisors and the cheek teeth, the outline of the bone of the lateral aspect of the maxilla should be clear and smooth
- On the lateral view, the ventral border of the mandible should be smooth, straight and radiodense
- On the lateral view, a complete outline of the ramus of the mandible should be visible.

7.9 Radiographic progression of acquired dental disease

As dental disease progresses, the radiographic anatomy of the teeth and supporting bone changes (see Figure 7.8). The structure of the teeth alters. The formation of enamel is affected and the characteristic vertical line of enamel in the centre of the cheek teeth is lost. Initially, the teeth become curved and the roots elongate. As the disease progresses, the teeth become increasingly distorted and bizarre. Radiographically, the normal structure of the roots and surrounding bone is lost (see Figure 7.8). The lines of cortical bone on the ventral border of the mandible and along the incisive bone become thinner. Curved, elongated roots can be seen penetrating the cortex. Incisor malocclusion may develop as the shape of the incisors changes. The upper incisors become more curled and lower incisors tend to tip forward. The occlusal surfaces of the cheek teeth lose their characteristic zigzig pattern and become uneven. A site where alveolar bone loss assessed is the circle of *lamina dura* that surrounds the first upper premolar on the dorsoventral view, where superimposition does not occur. Elongated roots of the second upper premolar are often seen on this view and may grow in a distorted manner in or through the zygomatic prominence of the maxilla (see Figure 7.12g). Eventually the appearance of the roots becomes grossly abnormal. Loss of radiopaque alveolar bone and tooth enamel gives the teeth a blurred appearance. The shape of the teeth becomes distorted. Chronic alveolitis results in dystrophic calcification. At this point the teeth are no longer growing. Degenerative changes do not take place in all teeth simultaneously and it is possible to have one or two healthy growing teeth amidst grossly abnormal ones. The bones of the skull become radiolucent. There is less contrast between cortical and trabecular bone and the edges of the bones, particularly the mandibular ramus, become indistinct. There may be radiolucent areas of lytic bone around the apices of the teeth. Abscesses can develop during any stage of dental disease and appear as radiolucent areas, sometimes with evidence of new bone formation round the edge of the abscess cavity. Some abscesses appear as a mottled, radiolucent mesh of proliferative bone. Occasionally tooth roots that have penetrated the periosteum continue to grow and can be seen curling round within the abscess cavity.

Endstage dental disease is characterized radiographically by one of three syndromes. The crowns can remain as non-growing stumps that can be used to grind food. This is the best option for the rabbit. Or the crowns can break off completely leaving roots that resorb within the bone. This syndrome is more apparent in the mandibular cheek teeth than in the maxillary ones. The gums heal and the rabbit can usually manage to eat, especially if the food is softened or shredded. Occasionally a single tooth will continue to grow and form a sharp spur that grows into the tongue, gums or buccal mucosa. Or, the alveolus becomes calcified and the degenerative distorted teeth are effectively welded in the sockets with radiopaque proliferation around the roots. Rabbits that have had their diet modified to include sufficient calcium and vitamin D appear more likely to be left with functional stumps and less likely to develop abscesses.

Key points 7.4

- The whole rabbit should be examined for signs of dental disease. The coat and the area around the perineum are especially important
- The incisors can be examined by wrapping the rabbit in a towel and gently retracting the lips
- Hard swellings along the ventral border of the mandible are associated with elongation of the roots of the cheek teeth
- Rabbits with dental disease often resent palpation of the face, especially of the cheek overlying the cheek teeth. Abscesses may be felt in this area
- The cheek teeth can be examined by restraining the rabbit in a towel and gently sliding an auriscope into either side of the mouth. Anaesthesia is required for a thorough examination
- Good illumination is essential for examination of the cheek teeth in an anaesthetized rabbit. Rodent gags and cheek dilators can be helpful
- Skull radiography gives information about the roots of the teeth. The crowns can be seen by visual examination
- Skull radiography is indicated for facial abscesses, epiphora and dacrocystitis, and to offer a prognosis. Radiography of the roots gives an idea of whether the teeth are still growing.

7.10 Treatment of dental disorders of rabbits

Malocclusion is treated by shortening, reshaping or removing maloccluding teeth. Generally, realignment is not possible, although digital pressure for at least one hour a day to realign maloccluded incisors has been proposed (Emily, 1991). This is impractical for most cases and trimming elongated crowns is the usual form of treatment.

Rabbits' teeth are innervated by both sympathetic and sensory axons that arise from the pulp cavity and extend into the dentine in tubules (see Figure 7.9). Sensory axons are either myelinated or unmyelinated. Sympathetic axons are unmyelinated so it is possible to distinguish between sensory and sympathetic innervation by myelination of the nerve fibres. Species with continually

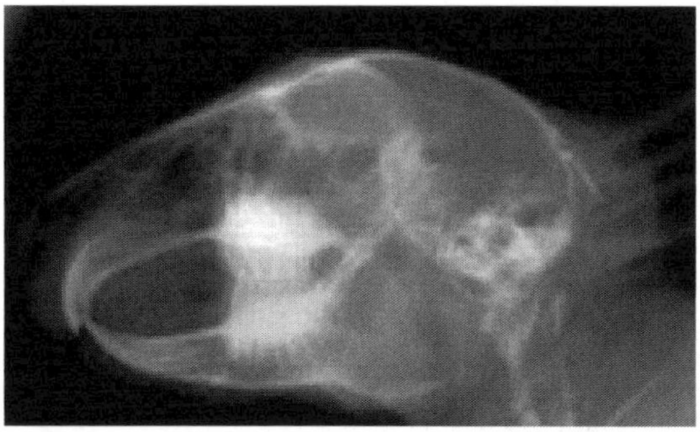

(a) Grade 1

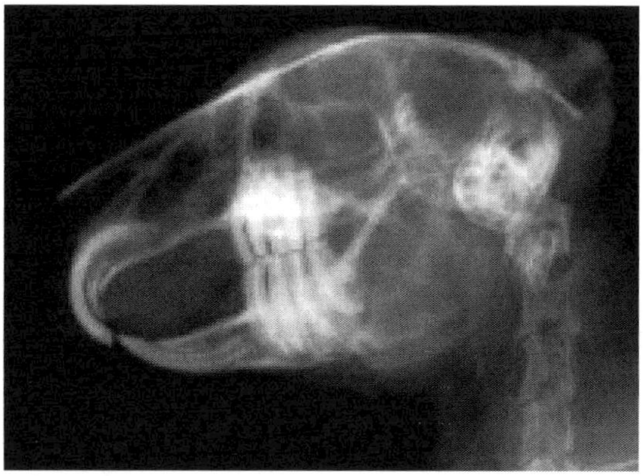

(b) Grade 2

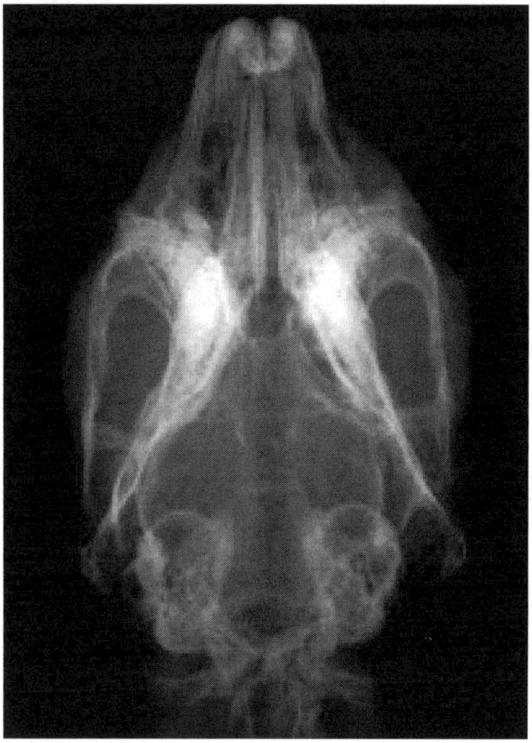

(c) Grade 2

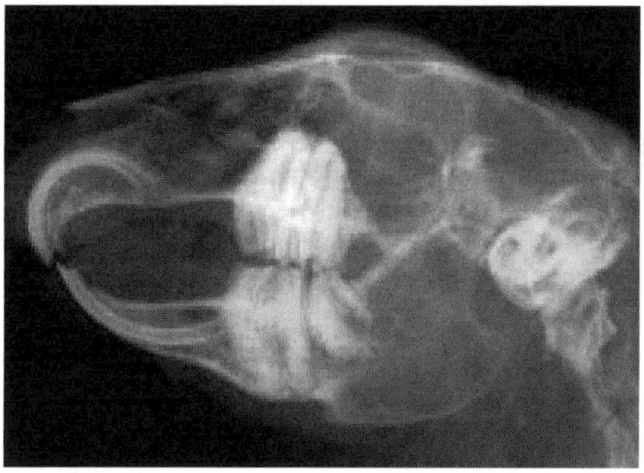

(d) Grade 4

Figure 7.12 a–d.

erupting teeth have smaller and fewer sensory axons than other species (Byers, 1984). In rat incisors, the pulpal nerve supply is almost exclusively unmyelinated and nerve endings remain in the pulp cavity and do not extend into the dentine. In contrast, histological and electron microscopic studies of rabbit premolars and molars have demonstrated the presence of innervated tubules in the dentine. Some axons are myelinated, which suggests the nerves are sensory and nociceptive (Bishop, 1995). Dentine becomes increasingly atubular towards the occlusal surface of the teeth where the axons retract from the tubules and degenerate. Therefore, the shorter the crowns are reduced during tooth trimming, the greater the likelihood of exposing innervated dentine. However, these studies were conducted on rabbits with healthy teeth. The extent of the pulp cavity is variable in rabbits with acquired dental disease so the sensory innervation could also be affected.

There are two options for tooth trimming. Elongated crowns can be shortened with

Figure 7.12. Radiographic progression of acquired dental disease.

(a) **Lateral view of the skull of an immature wild rabbit (Grade 1).** 7.12a shows the radiographic features of the normal skull are summarized in Box 7.4. The smooth radiodense lines of the enamel folds and the *laminae durae* can be seen, although because of superimposition, the individual roots cannot be seen clearly. X-Rays taken on dental film can be used to show changes in individual tooth roots.

(b) **Lateral view of a skull of a rabbit showing early signs of dental disease (Grade 2).** 7.12b shows a lateral view of the skull of an 18-month-old mixed breed male rabbit showing signs of epiphora. There is elongation of the roots and the crowns of the upper primary incisors. These teeth have become increasingly curved. The alteration in the shape of the incisors has changed the way in which they occlude and wear against each other. The lower incisors no longer occlude with the peg teeth. The root of the primary maxillary incisor is elongated so the apex is starting to penetrate the incisive bone. The line of the incisive bone is interrupted. The nasolacrimal duct makes an abrupt mediodorsal bend at the apex of the primary maxillary incisor and elongation of the incisor root blocks the duct at this point. Epiphora is the result. The crowns of the cheek teeth have lost their zigzag occlusal pattern. Changes in the structure and hardness of the cheek teeth have led to uneven wear. The apices of the lower cheek teeth are growing into the cortical bone along the ventral border of the mandible causing swellings that can be palpated along the jaw in this area. The roots of the upper cheek teeth have penetrated the alveolar bone. Radiographically, it is difficult to differentiate Stage 2 from Stage 3 of acquired dental disease (see Box 7.1). Molar malocclusion and the development of spurs may not be evident radiographically. Elongated crowns curve in a three dimensional manner that cannot be seen on a two dimensional radiographic image. The crowns must be examined visually.

(c) **Dorsoventral view of a rabbit showing early signs of dental disease (Grade 2).** 7.12c shows a dorsoventral view of the same rabbit as in (b). The dorsoventral view is not as informative as the lateral view of the skull in evaluating dental disease because superimposition of the mandible obscures most of the cheek teeth. The roots of the maxillary cheek teeth can be seen to be elongated. The root of the upper second premolar has penetrated the periosteum of the zygomatic prominence of the maxilla. The *lamina dura* that encircles the upper first premolar is becoming thin and indistinct.

(d) **Lateral view of a skull of a rabbit showing cessation of tooth growth (Grade 4).** 7.12d shows a lateral view of the skull of an aged male mixed breed pet rabbit that had a previous history of epiphora and spurs on the cheek teeth. At the time of radiography, the cheek teeth had stopped growing and dental treatment had not been required for several months, although the rabbit was suffering from dacryocystitis. On visual examination, the crowns of the cheek teeth could be seen as misshapen, yellowish stumps. However, the stumps were in occlusion and could be used to grind food. There were no sharp points growing into surrounding soft tissue so trimming was unnecessary. Pulp chambers can be seen within the incisors, which are continuing to grow. There is increased curvature of the upper primary incisors. The crowns and roots are elongated. The apex of the upper primary incisor is growing through the incisive bone at the point of contact with the nasolacrimal duct (see Figure 11.1). There is elongation of the crowns of the mandibular incisors, which are in abnormal occlusion with the maxillary incisors. The apices of the elongated mandibular incisors are superimposed on the roots of the lower premolars. There are radiological changes in the structure of the mandibular cheek teeth. The outline of each tooth is blurred and indistinct. The longitudinal line of the enamel fold in the centre of the teeth is not evident. There is erosion of the enamel of the crown on one of the first lower premolars indicating the presence of dental caries. The presence of caries indicates that tooth eruption has either ceased or has slowed down in order for the condition to have time to develop. The shape of the root is distorted and the *laminae durae* are not evident. The tooth roots are elongated and have penetrated the periosteum of the ventral border of the mandible. The maxillary cheek teeth are long. The roots are indistinct and radiodense indicating cessation of growth and the start of abnormal mineralization.

continued

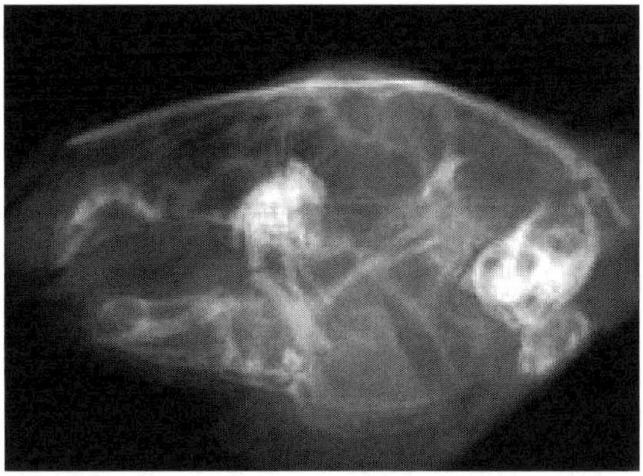

(e) Grade 5a

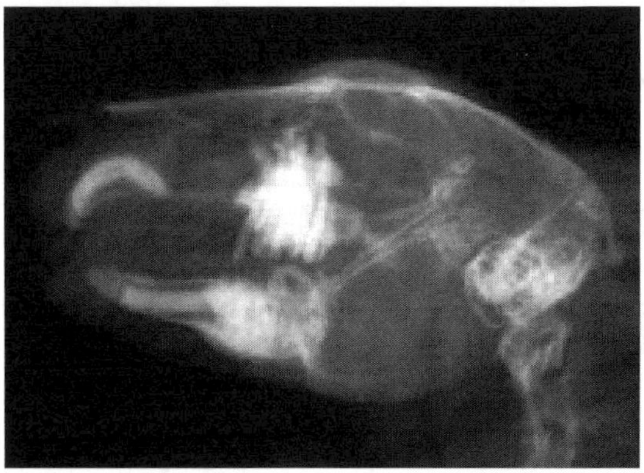

(f) Grade 5b

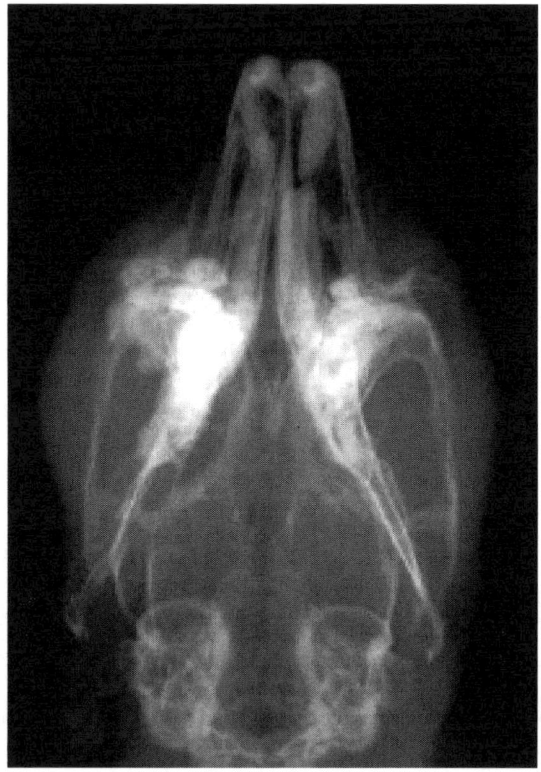

(g) Grade 5b

Figure 7.12 e–g.

hand-held clippers, or with dental burrs or cutting discs powered by a dental drill. Both techniques have advantages and disadvantages. The choice depends on personal preference and will vary between individual cases. Hand-held clippers are cheap, quick and available and are unlikely to cause iatrogenic soft tissue damage. They are satisfactory for trimming of thin slivers or weak, soft teeth. However, it is possible to shatter teeth, leaving sharp edges and exposed pulp cavity, especially if the enamel is strong. Teeth are less likely to shatter if the crowns are not shortened excessively and a strong sharp set of clippers is used. It is not possible to reshape teeth using hand-held clippers. Burring or cutting teeth with power equipment gives greater control of the final shape and size of the teeth but carries a risk of iatrogenic soft tissue damage and thermal injury to the pulp cavity. Both techniques cause discomfort to the conscious rabbit and firm restraint or sedation is always necessary. General anaesthesia is required to trim the cheek teeth. Whichever method is used, it is not possible to restore normal position, shape and structure to abnormal teeth that are growing in an abnormal direction. The aims of tooth trimming are to remove sharp points that cause soft tissue damage and, if possible, to leave the rabbit with a set of functional teeth.

7.10.1 Incisor elongation and malocclusion

The interval between incisor trimming depends on the cause of malocclusion, the condition of the teeth and their rate of growth. Rabbits with congenital malocclusion but otherwise healthy teeth require lifelong tooth trimming every 4–6 weeks unless the incisors are removed. For rabbits with acquired dental disease the situation is more

Figure 7.12. *Continued*
(e) **Lateral view of a skull to show osteopaenia, root resorption and osteomyelitis (Grade 5a).** 7.12e shows the same rabbit as (b) and (c). The radiograph shown was taken three years after those shown in (b) and (c). In the interim the rabbit had been maintained on a mixed cereal ration with *ad lib* hay. He was given some vegetables each day. He was kept in a hutch with a run attached during the summer months. The radiograph shows generalized loss of bone density. Most of the crowns of the teeth have broken off and the roots have been absorbed. There is an abscess in the mandible associated with the remnants of the lower incisor. The line of the incisive bone is barely visible. A single mandibular molar had continued to grow and penetrated the gum on the opposing jaw. A large abscess had developed on the side of the face that originated from the right upper first premolar. An area of radiolucency can be seen in this area.
(f) **Lateral view of a skull to show demineralization of the bone and mineralization of the tooth roots (Grade 5b).** 7.12f shows a lateral view of the skull of a 4-year-old Dwarf Lop male rabbit that had a long history of dental problems. The crowns of the most of the teeth have broken off. The roots are mineralized and radiodense. The roots of the cheek teeth cannot be differentiated from the surrounding jaw. Two skulls from rabbits showing similar changes are shown in Plates 16 and 17. There is generalized demineralization of the skull. There is little contrast between cortical and cancellous bone. This radiograph was taken at the same exposure as the other lateral skull radiographs illustrated in this figure.
(g) **Dorsoventral view of a skull to show demineralization of the bone and mineralization of the tooth roots (Grade 5b).** 7.12g shows the dorsoventral view of the same rabbit as (f). The apices of the roots of the maxillary premolars teeth are grossly abnormal, especially on the left side. The roots have penetrated the zygomatic prominence of the maxilla, the lacrimal bone and the nasal cavity. The nasolacrimal duct is blocked at this site. The roots of the maxillary molars have penetrated the alveolar bulla. This is a common site for abscess formation. Periapical infection of the upper molars results in the formation of pus in the retrobulbar space and exophthalmus. On this dorsoventral view, the calcified roots of the lower incisors can be seen in the mandible. The crowns have broken off. This radiograph illustrates the potential difficulties associated with identifying and removing an infected tooth root.

complex. In advanced cases, the incisors eventually stop growing and no longer need to be trimmed. The crowns can break off completely and fail to regrow. In other cases, some or all of the incisors continue to grow and require regular trimming, although the rate of growth is variable. Surgical removal of the incisors affords a permanent cure but in older rabbits, with acquired malocclusion, the procedure carries a higher risk of complications.

Clipping incisor teeth with nail clippers is the traditional approach to shortening overgrown incisors (Rosskopf and Woerpel, 1982; Eisele 1986). Some people consider the use of hand-held clippers to be cruel because of the excessive force that is applied to the teeth and favour the use of power equipment. Some practitioners have become adept at burring incisors in the conscious animal and find that wrapping the rabbit in a towel or restraining the animal on its back is satisfactory. Others will only use power equipment on a rabbit that has been sedated. Wooden tongue depressors, syringe cases or some other type of gag is necessary to keep the soft tissues of the lips and tongue away from the burr or cutting disc. Opinions vary as to whether high speed or low speed drills are preferable or whether burrs or cutting discs should be used. Water is necessary to cool the teeth during burring. The heat generated from burring through the teeth can result in sterile pulpitis or even pulp necrosis if the equipment is used incorrectly (Gorrel and Robinson, 1995). A water spray is used in conjunction with high-speed drills. Application of water-soaked cotton wool before and after the procedure can be used in conjunction with low speed burrs. Cutting discs are effective but should be used with care. Guards are available that protect surrounding tissue and the operator from damage.

7.10.1.1 Surgical removal of the incisors

Brown (1992) described surgical removal of the incisors as a permanent solution to the recurrent problem of incisor malocclusion. In addition to slicing through food, rabbits use their incisors like pincers to pull out dead hair from their coat. Although rabbits without their incisors quickly adapt and learn to prehend food with their lips, they can experience grooming problems, especially the fluffy breeds such as Dwarf lops. Hard foods such as apples, carrots or broccoli that would have been sliced by the incisors need to chopped or grated.

Surgical removal of the incisors is the treatment of choice for congenital malocclusion. In young rabbits, the procedure is generally straightforward. Older rabbits with acquired malocclusion are more likely to have complications associated with the surgery. The teeth can be brittle and prone to fracture. There can be gross deformities of the teeth and the roots can be long, curved or even twisted. Some roots are embedded in the socket by periosteal reaction around the apex. Preoperative radiography can be helpful in assessing the condition of the teeth and surrounding structures. Teeth that have gross changes at the apex are unlikely to be growing. The pulp cavity of the incisors can be assessed radiographically.

Periodontal or periapical infection can result in postoperative infections and the development of abscesses after incisor removal, especially on the mandible. A sterile technique and postoperative antibiotics reduce the risk of infection.

In adult rabbits with acquired dental disease, it is important to warn owners that incisor malocclusion may only be part of their rabbit's dental problems and that molar malocclusion can still develop. The cheek teeth must be assessed. However, there are only three options for rabbits with maloccluded incisors that are growing – euthanasia, incisor removal or continual tooth trimming. Incisor removal is often the best of the three.

Good anaesthesia is essential for incisor removal and a recommended technique is described in Box 5.4. Pre-emptive analgesia is advisable and postoperative analgesia is essential. Owners must be told to bring the rabbit back for treatment promptly if it does not eat postoperatively. Further analgesia and motility stimulants can be required as postoperative gastrointestinal hypomotility can easily develop after this procedure.

7.10.1.2 Surgical technique for incisor removal

The periodontal ligament around the incisors is broken down using an elevator or large hypodermic needle (16–18 g). A purpose-made elevator has been manufactured especially for this technique (Crossley elevator, Veterinary Instrumentation, Sheffield). The elevator is gently pushed into the periodontal space maintaining pressure to tear the fibres of the periodontal ligament. Bleeding within the ligament aids destruction of the periodontal tissue and loosens the tooth so the ligament around each tooth can be worked on a little at a time, in rotation, to allow alveolar haemorrhage to occur. Once the tooth is loose, it is gently rocked in the socket until it can be extracted by gently pulling along the line of the tooth using forceps. It is important not to rush the procedure or attempt to twist the tooth or it will fracture. Occasionally weakened teeth do fracture. If this occurs, it may be possible to remove the tooth fragment using a root pick, or the root can be left *in situ* and removed at a later date if the regrowth takes place. It is often the peg teeth that fracture. The roots of these teeth can usually be located and removed easily. Fractured root fragments of teeth do not always regrow.

The extracted teeth should be examined to make sure they are complete and that the pulp tissue has been removed with the tooth. Regrowth occurs either because the tooth has fractured during extraction leaving a viable root or because the tooth has been removed so atraumatically that the pulp tissue remains in the socket. If the tooth is extracted without tissue in the pulp cavity, a bent hypodermic needle can be used to curette the socket and destroy the pulp tissue. Alternatively, gently intruding and pressing the loosened incisor into the socket and rocking it for 20–30 seconds should crush and disrupt the apical soft tissue and prevent regrowth (Steenkamp and Crossley, 1999). Despite these precautions, it is advisable to warn owners in

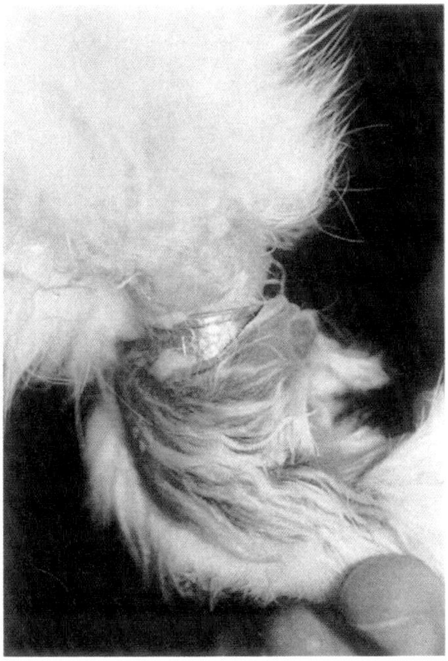

Plate 1. Identification ring occluding the blood supply to the hind foot. Pedigree rabbits are identified by aluminium rings slipped over the hock when the rabbit is 8–10 weeks old. The rings are supplied by the British Rabbit Council in a range of sizes. Each ring has the year of birth and a unique number from which the rabbit can be identified. Occasionally, rabbits with identification rings are sold as pets. It is advisable to remove the rings because hair can become entrapped beneath the ring and occlude the blood supply to the foot. This rabbit was euthanased.

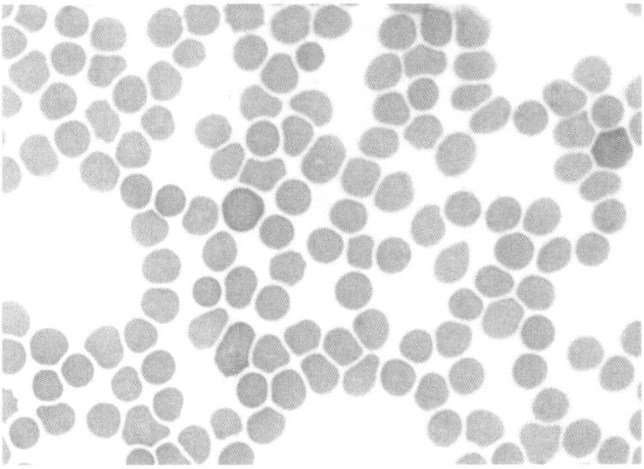

Plate 2. Anisocytosis and polychromasia. The red blood cells of rabbits vary in diameter within a range of 5.0–7.8 µm. This variation in diameter (anisocytosis) is a feature of blood smears from rabbits and is not a significant finding. There is also variation in erythrocyte colour (polychromasia) in normal rabbits. The blood smear illustrated was from a normal rabbit and was stained with Rapi-diff. Interpretation of haematology results is discussed in Section 6.2.2. (Photograph taken by Dr Joan Duncan, Idexx Laboratories, Wetherby.)

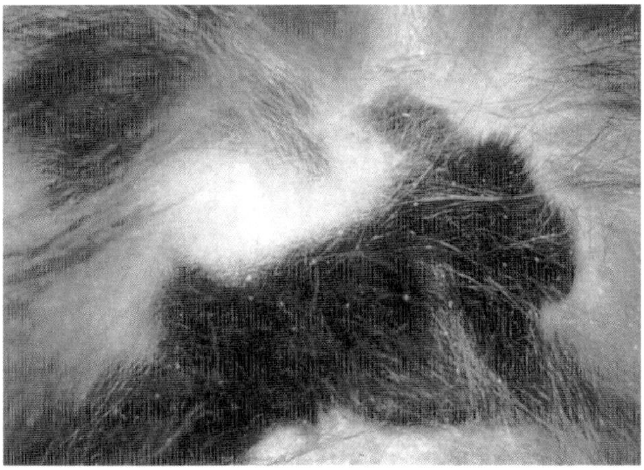

Plate 3. Patchy hair loss. Some breeds of rabbit with fluffy coats, notably Dwarf lops and Minilops, develop hairless patches of skin during moulting. The alopecic areas often cause concern to owners. The bald skin is not inflamed. A typical lesion is illustrated. Regrowth of hair is rapid. Dense fur starts to grow at the centre of the lesion within 7–10 days and takes place simultaneously with hair loss at the periphery of the lesion. This is a self-limiting physiological process.

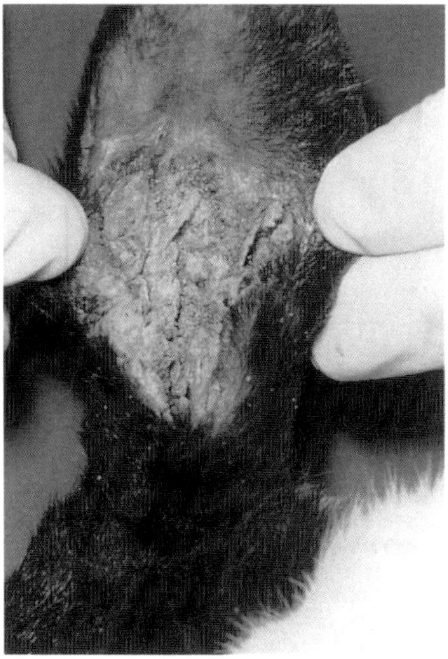

Plate 4. Ear mites (*Psoroptes cuniculi*). Otitis externa caused by ear mites (*Psoroptes cuniculi*) in rabbits is characterized by a crusty exudate within the external ear canal, which often extends up the pinna. Occasionally, only one ear is affected. The condition is intensely pruritic and painful. A typically affected ear is illustrated. The skin beneath the exudate is ulcerated and sore. The condition responds well to treatment with ivermectin or selamectin. Cleaning the ear is painful for the rabbit and unnecessary. Further discussion of *Psoroptes cuniculi* infestation can be found in Section 9.14.2.1.The mite is illustrated in Figure 16.1.

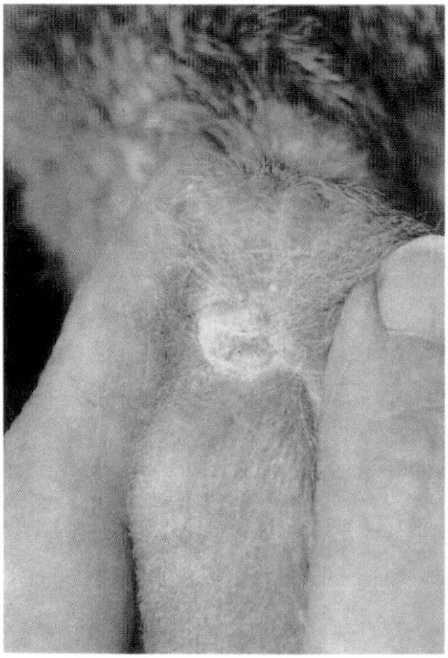

Plate 5. Initial stage of ulcerative pododermatitis. The area of skin on the point of the hock of rabbits is prone to pressure necrosis. A small area of hairless skin can often be found in adult pet rabbits although it is usually concealed by the fur that lies across it. Hard flooring, lack of exercise and long periods of inactivity increase the pressure over the hock. Plate 5 shows a circular patch of hairless skin on the hock of a rabbit that was presented for vaccination. It was an incidental finding.

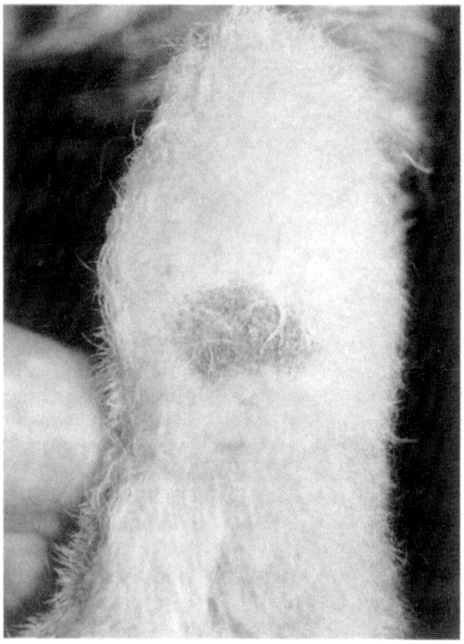

Plate 6. Ulcerative pododermatitis in a Rex rabbit. Pressure sores develop in the thin skin over the bony prominence of the central tarsal bone, especially in rabbits with sparse hair coating such as the Rex. This plate shows the hock of a 4-year-old neutered male Rex house rabbit. The hairless area of reddened skin that does not blanch on pressure is an early sign of ulcerative pododermatitis. Once the area has lost its protective fur, the skin is subject to increased mechanical trauma and pressure. The lesions can progress to form decubital skin ulcers. Occasionally the medial plantar vein or artery, which lie just beneath skin, is eroded and causes haemorrhage.

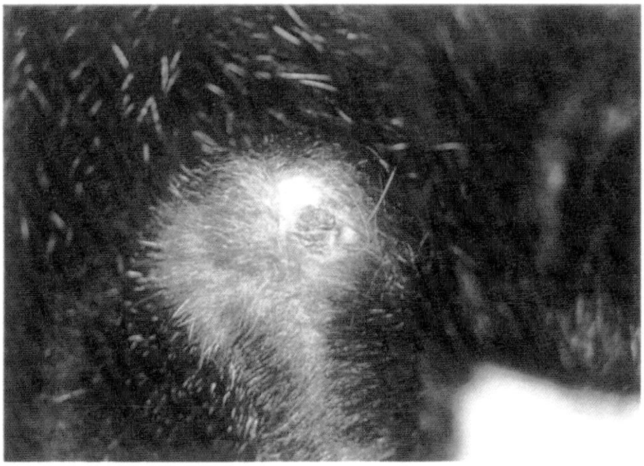

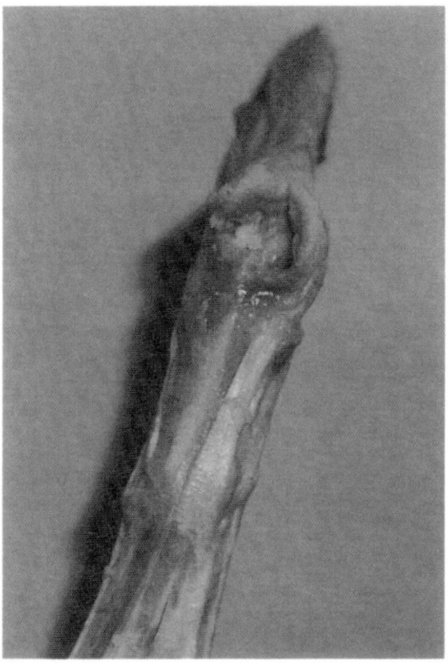

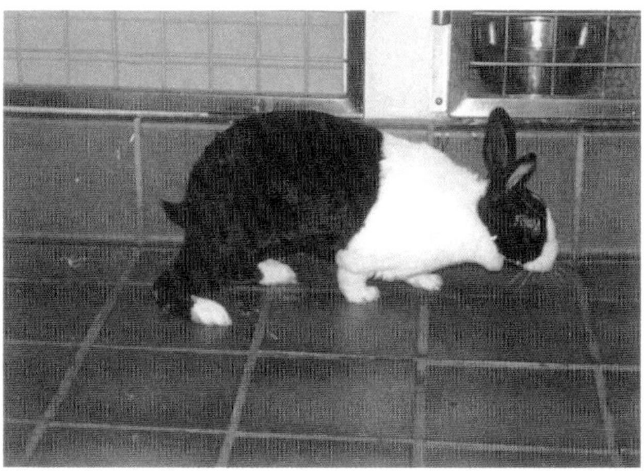

Plate 7. Advanced ulcerative pododermatitis. In the later stages of ulcerative pododermatitis, the ulcer extends through the dermis and epidermis. Devitalized skin over the lesion is lost and infection spreads into the deeper tissues, including bone and synovial structures. An abscess develops around the hock. This plate shows the hock of a 3-year-old Silver Fox breeding buck that had spent his entire life confined to a small hutch. Pus could be expressed from the ulcerated area. The rabbit was unable to hop. He was euthanased. A *post-mortem* preparation of the hock is illustrated in Plate 8. The anatomy of the hock in diseased and healthy rabbits is illustrated in Figures 9.3 and 9.4. Ulcerative pododermatitis is discussed in Section 9.10.

Plate 8. Dissection of an infected hock to show displacement of the superficial flexor tendon. In advanced cases of ulcerative pododermatitis, osteomyelitis and infection erodes the bone and the tendon of insertion of the superficial digital flexor tendon. The superficial digital flexor tendon displaces medially from the hock. The rabbit is unable to flex the digits to adopt a digitigrade stance. The foot is no longer supported and extension of the hock is impaired. The rabbit is permanently disabled. Displacement of the tendon can be diagnosed by observing the gait of the patient as it attempts to hop around the floor (see Plate 9) and by flexing the hock and observing the toes (see Figure 9.4).

Plate 9. Typical gait of a rabbit with advanced pododermatitis and displacement of the superficial flexor tendon. Once the superficial flexor tendon is displaced, the hock drops and the rabbit can no longer take its weight on its claws. It is forced to weight bear on the ulcerated infected tissue of the hock. The rabbit becomes increasingly disabled and reluctant to move, which exacerbates the problem further. The prognosis at this stage is grave. This plate shows a 5-year-old Dutch female house rabbit with advanced pododermatitis. The rabbit was treated with long-term antibiotic therapy, non-steroidal analgesics and a change of bedding from carpet to a deep bed of hay covering a layer of newspaper with thick towelling beneath. The abscesses on the hocks were lanced and flushed, taking care to preserve weight-bearing skin. The cavities were filled with Manuka honey twice daily (see Section 8.3.2). When the infection subsided, the rabbit became more mobile and was able to lead a reasonable quality life although she was permanently disabled. Once the infection was under control, the hairless areas of the hock were treated with a liquid bandage preparation (Nu-skin, Germolene) painted on once or twice daily as necessary.

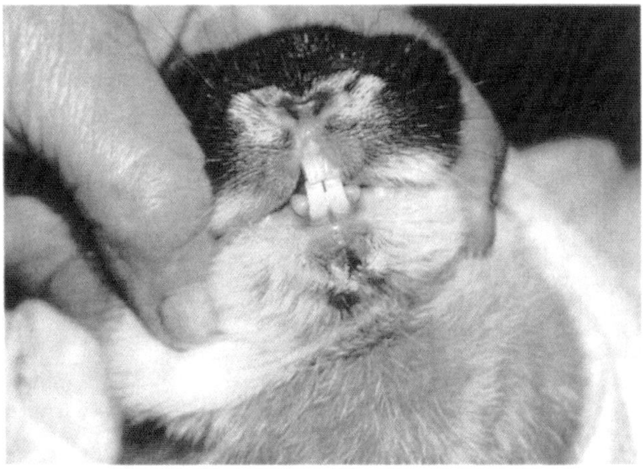

Plate 10. *Treponema cuniculi* ('rabbit syphilis'). This plate shows the lips of a 6-month-old Netherland Dwarf female rabbit. There are crusty lesions originating from the mucocutaneous junction. There were similar crusty lesions affecting the mucocutaneous junction of the vulva. The lesions had been present for some weeks. The rabbit was injected with a long-acting penicillin preparation. The lesions regressed rapidly. Treponematosis is discussed in Section 9.13.

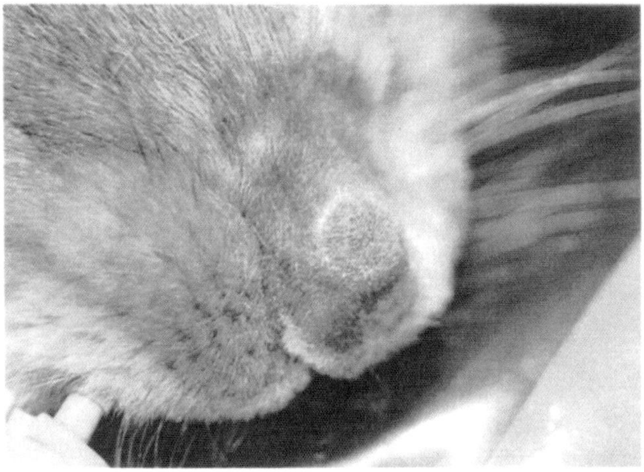

Plate 11. Atypical myxomatosis. Multiple benign fibromas sometimes develop on rabbits that have been vaccinated against myxomatosis and are subsequently exposed to natural infection. This plate shows a lesion on the nose of a mature female rabbit that was recently rehomed to a garden that was visited by wild rabbits. She had been vaccinated against myxomatosis previously but 15 months had elapsed since the last dose. There were several similar lesions around the body. Histology confirmed the diagnosis of atypical myxomatosis. She was treated with antibiotics and the nodules eventually regressed.

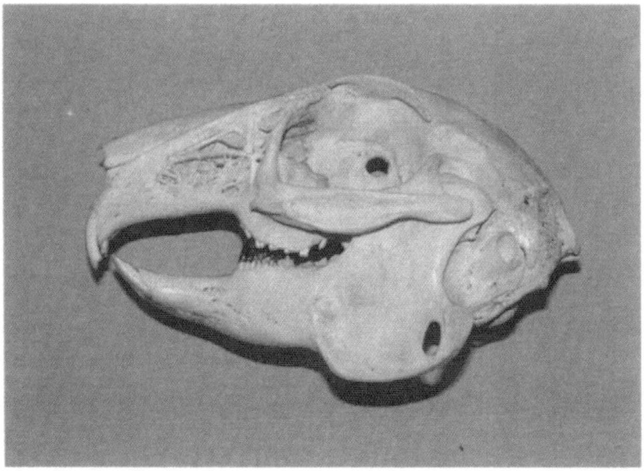

Plate 12. Wild rabbit skull: lateral view. A prepared skull of an adult wild female European rabbit (*Oryctolagus cuniculus*) that was found dead in Menorca, a limestone Mediterranean island with plenty of sunshine. The skull is well calcified. The teeth show brown staining that often occurs in rabbits that eat grass and other natural vegetation.

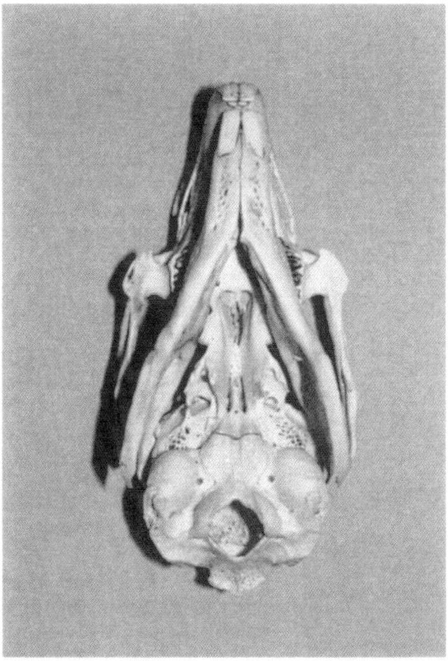

Plate 13. Wild rabbit skull: ventrodorsal view. A ventrodorsal view of the same skull as in Plate 12. These views can be used to identify radiographic landmarks illustrated in Figures 7.9–7.11.

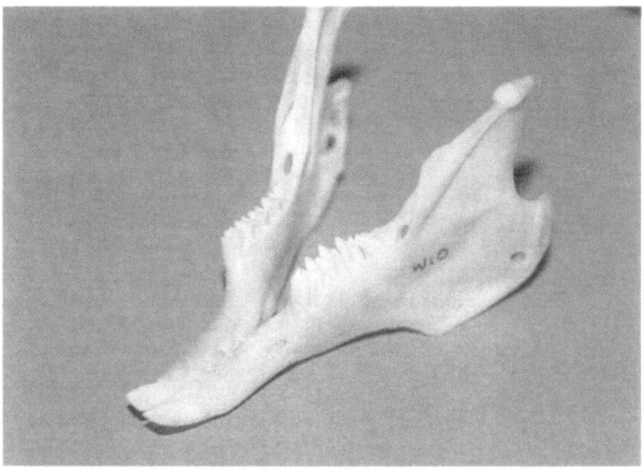

Plate 14. Healthy mandible to show points on the cheek teeth. A prepared mandible from a wild rabbit. Sharp points on the lingual edge of the lower cheek teeth is a normal finding. They do not require removal.

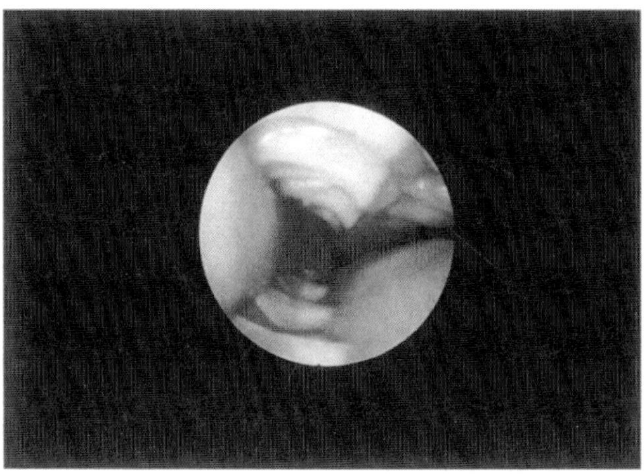

Plate 15. Auriscopic view of normal cheek teeth. The cheek teeth can be examined using an auriscope (otoscope). Auriscopic examination gives a guide to the condition of the cheek teeth. General anaesthesia is required for a thorough examination. This plate is a view of the cheek teeth of a conscious healthy 3-year-old female rabbit taken through a rigid endoscope. The normal zigzag pattern of the points on the lingual edge of the occlusal surface on the lower cheek teeth can be seen. Most rabbits tolerate the auriscopic examination of the oral cavity well, unless there is a painful lesion within the mouth.

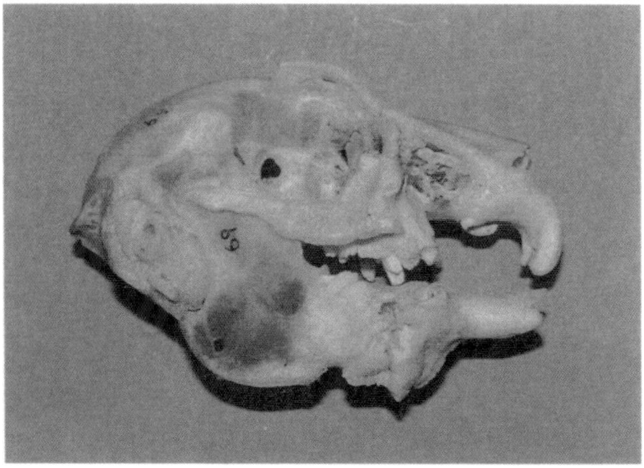

Plate 16. Prepared skull of a rabbit with advanced dental disease; lateral view. This is a skull of a 4-year-old Netherland Dwarf female rabbit that was presented for euthanasia. She had spent her entire life confined to a hutch and was fed on *ad lib* 'rabbit food' consisting of a mixture of maize, peas, wheat, oats, pellets and extrusions. Hay was available although she didn't eat it. No vegetables were offered because the owner believed they would cause 'diarrhoea'. She was suffering from dacryocystitis and inappetance. The skull shows generalized osteopaenia. The roots of all the teeth are elongated and penetrating periosteal bone. Calcification around the roots has resulted in large bony reactions that are effectively welding the teeth into the skull. There is a large bony reaction in the orbit around the site of the lacrimal sac and nasolacrimal duct. The crowns of most of the teeth have broken off.

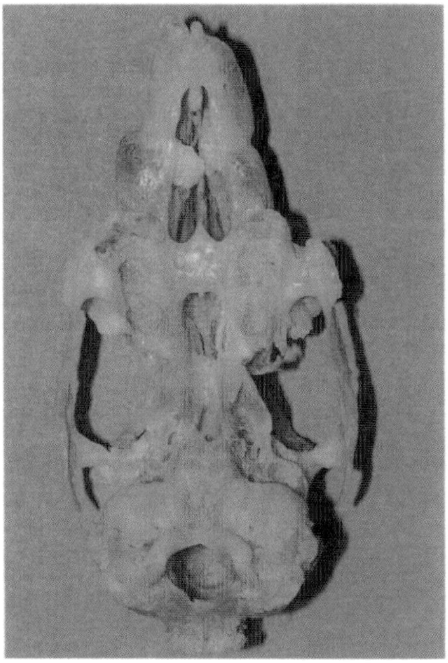

Plate 17. Prepared skull of a rabbit with advanced dental disease; ventrodorsal view. A ventrodorsal view of a prepared skull of a 4-year-old male Dwarf lop rabbit. He was kept in a hutch for most of the year but was placed in a run in the garden on fine days during the summer months. The rabbit was always a finicky eater, he would (or could) not eat hay or hard vegetables. He lived on bread and selected ingredients from mixed rabbit food. He would eat watercress and the occasional dandelion leaf. During his life, the rabbit had suffered from a range of clinical conditions related to his teeth: epiphora, dacrocystitis, molar malocclusion and incisor malocclusion. The progression of dental disease is summarized in Box 7.1. The rabbit was euthanased because he became dyspnoeic. The skull shows osteopaenic bone and dilation of the maxillae. Abscesses have developed at the roots of the primary incisors, which are occluding the nasal passages. The crowns of the cheek teeth have disintegrated.

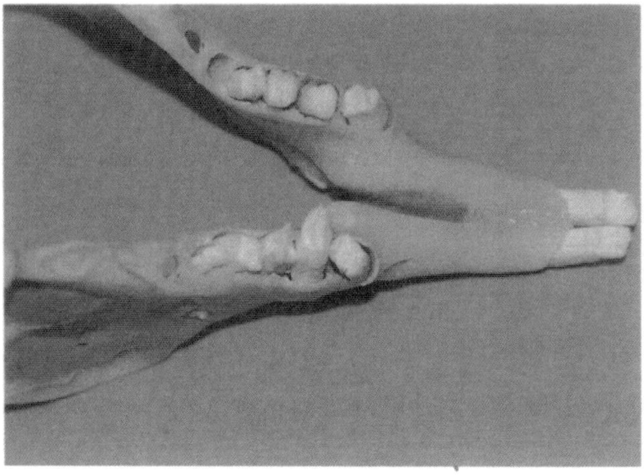

Plate 18. Mandible from a rabbit showing early signs of dental disease. This mandible is from a 2-year-old castrated Dwarf Lop house rabbit that died due to intestinal obstruction caused by a felt of ingested hair. Although swellings could be palpated along the ventral border of the mandible, no other signs of dental disease were evident. The crowns were not long. The structure, shape and position of the teeth has changed so they are no longer in alignment. Loss of alveolar bone has resulted in wide periodontal spaces. The second right premolar is starting to tip towards the tongue.

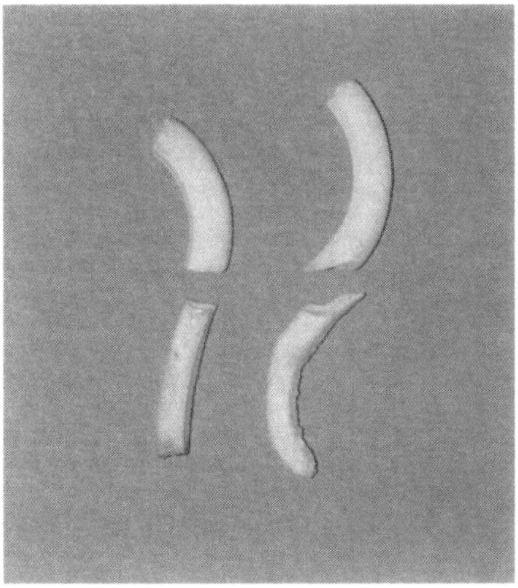

Plate 19. Comparison of the structure of healthy and maloccluded cheek teeth. This plate shows an upper and lower premolar taken from the skull of a healthy rabbit (left) and a rabbit suffering from molar malocclusion (right). The maloccluded teeth are curved and elongated. The enamel is poor. Curvature of the teeth has altered the direction of the biting force on the teeth. The changes in tooth shape are irreversible and show that it is impossible to restore normal occlusion by corrective dentistry.

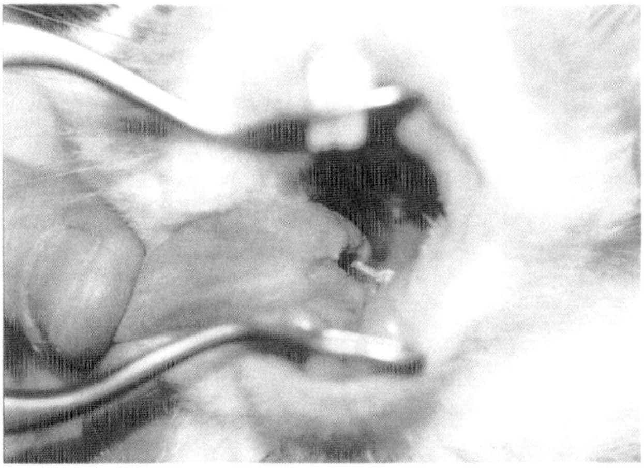

Plate 20. Spur on lower cheek tooth. A sharp spur has developed on a lower cheek tooth of this 2-year-old male Dwarf lop rabbit. The spur has lacerated the tongue. The rabbit was not grooming. He had cheyletiellosis and there were caecotrophs caked to the fur under the tail. He was salivating and unable to eat. The spur was trimmed using a set of long handled molar clippers. The rest of the teeth were checked and trimmed or smoothed with a diamond rasp where necessary. He was given a non-steroidal analgesic. The rabbit started to eat as soon as he regained consciousness. Two months later, he was presented because a spur had developed on a different cheek tooth. The spur on the tooth illustrated had not regrown. Trimming cheek teeth is described in Section 7.10.2. (Image reproduced with kind permission from Waltham Focus.)

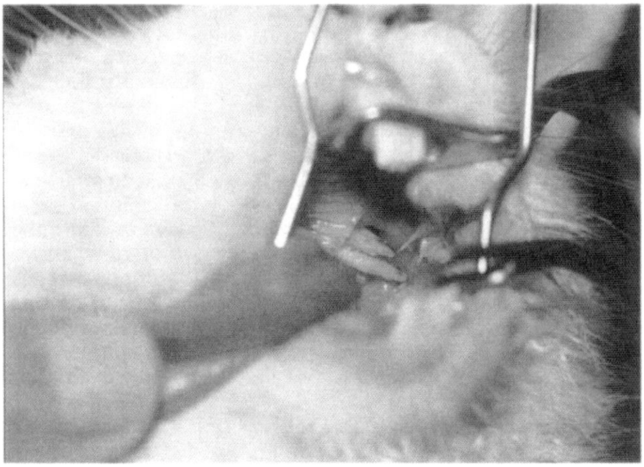

Plate 21. Spurs on the upper premolars. Sharp spurs had developed on the upper premolars of this mature mixed breed male rabbit. He was adopted from a rescue centre 1week before this photograph was taken. He had spent 6 months in the rescue centre and had been passed as 'fit for rehoming'. The rabbit was able to eat but was not grooming well and was thin. The spur had penetrated the buccal mucosa inside the cheek and an abscess was beginning to form. The crowns look dull and discoloured. There is erosion of the gum around the first premolar resulting in a cavity that could entrap food material. These spurs were easily trimmed off using molar clippers. A dental burr was not used because of the risk of soft tissue damage.

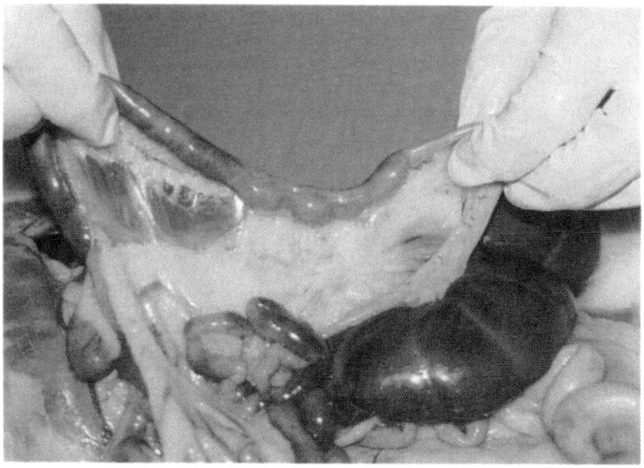

Plate 22. *Fusus coli.* The *fusus coli* is a highly innervated, vascular, muscular section of the ascending colon (see Section 1.5.3). The *fusus coli* acts as a pacemaker for colonic motility that alters with the type of faeces that are passing through the colon. It is influenced by the autonomic nervous system and hormones such as aldosterone and prostaglandins. The mucosa of the *fusus coli* is deeply folded and contains many goblet cells. This plate shows the *fusus coli* of a rabbit that died during the morning when the colon was in the soft faeces phase. Pasty caecal material is passing into the *fusus coli* from the proximal colon (left). In the *fusus coli*, the intestinal contents are squeezed into pellets that become encapsulated in mucus before being excreted as soft caecotrophs.

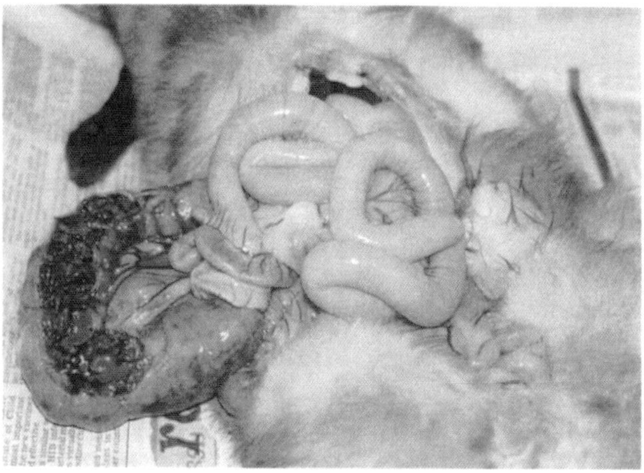

Plate 23. Mucoid enteropathy. This plate shows the abdominal contents of a 14-week-old Dwarf lop male rabbit that was euthanased. He had passed no faeces for 3 days and had become bloated. He was inappetant and could be seen grinding his teeth. A hard impacted caecum was palpable. On *post-mortem* examination, the caecum was found to be filled with hard impacted material. The colon was distended and quantities of gelatinous mucus spilled out when it was incised. Mucoid enteropathy is discussed in Section 10.9.

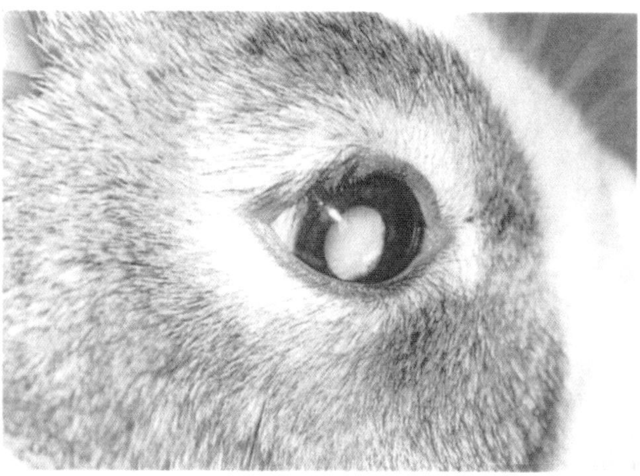

Plate 24. Phacoclastic uveitis caused by *Encephalitozoon cuniculi.* This plate shows the eye of a 9-month-old Dwarf lop male rabbit. The owner had noticed an opacity in the lens. The rabbit was eating, happily and showing no apparent signs of discomfort. He was seropositive for *E. cuniculi.* Encephalitozoonosis is a cause of ocular disease. Lens rupture, uveitis and cataract formation in young rabbits is associated with *Encephalitozoon cuniculi* infection. It is believed that vertical transmission results in *E. cuniculi* organisms invading the developing lens of rabbits *in utero* when the lens capsule is very thin or absent. After birth, the parasite causes the lens to rupture at its thinnest point on the anterior surface, releasing lens material into the anterior chamber that causes phacoclastic uveitis. Ocular disease caused by *E. cuniculi* is discussed in Section 11.7.3.1. The life cycle of the parasite is described in Section 16.4.2.

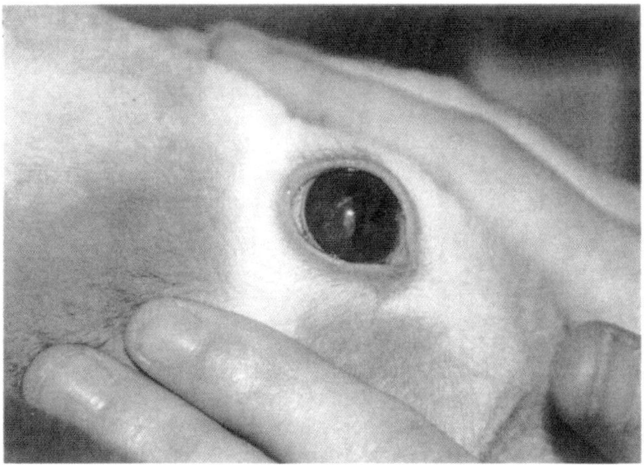

Plate 25. Lymphosarcoma in the anterior chamber. This plate shows the eye of a 2-year-old Rex male rabbit. Lesions were present in both eyes. The rabbit had suddenly become thin and inappetant. His condition deteriorated rapidly and he was euthanased 48 h after this photograph was taken. *Post-mortem* examination showed generalized lymphomatous lesions throughout the body, especially in the liver, intestines and lymph nodes. Histopathology confirmed generalized lymphosarcoma. Lymphosarcoma is the second most commonly encountered neoplastic disease affecting *Oryctolagus cuniculi*. Uterine adenocarcinoma is the most common.

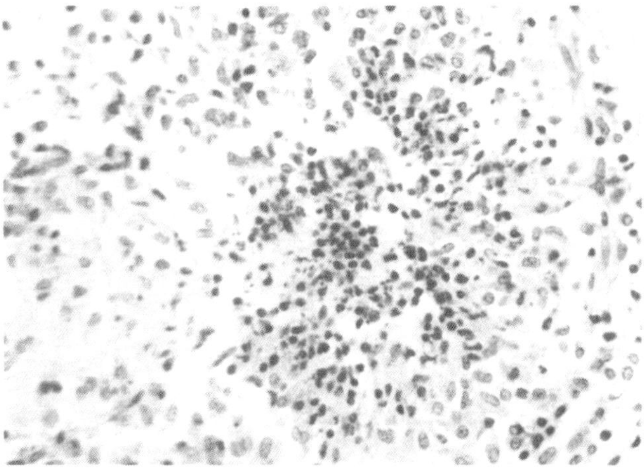

Plate 26. Granulomatous encephalitis caused by *Encephalitozoon cuniculi*. This plate is a section of brain taken from an immature mixed breed female rabbit that suddenly developed seizures and became blind. The rabbit died. Histologically, there was moderate disseminated granulomatous encephalitis throughout the brain with lymphoplasmacytic perivascular cuffing and meningitis. The granuloma illustrated consists of a defined collection of histiocytes, occasional multinucleated cells and peripherally located lymphocytes and plasma cells. Small numbers of gram-positive spherical *E. cuniculi* spores can be seen in cells within the granuloma. (Photograph supplied by Malcolm Silkstone, Abbey Veterinary Services, Newton Abbot.)

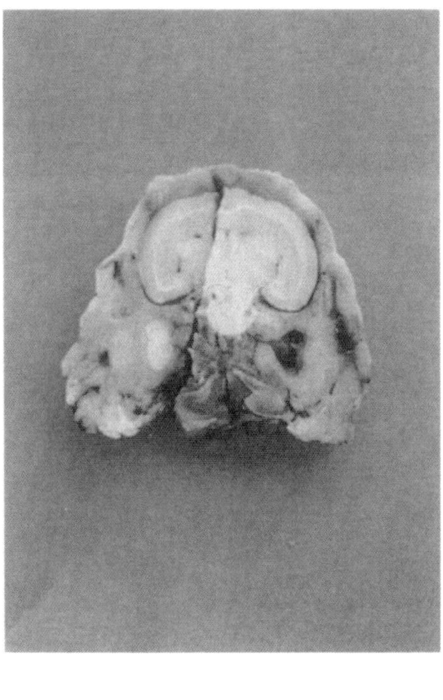

Plate 27. Pus in tympanic bulla. This plate is a cross-section of a decalcified head. There is also a sagittal section through the specimen. The skull is from a Netherland Dwarf male rabbit that developed a head tilt. Despite an initial response to antibiotic therapy, the rabbit relapsed and was euthanased. The skull has been sectioned at the level of the tympanic bullae. The left tympanic bulla is filled with pus.

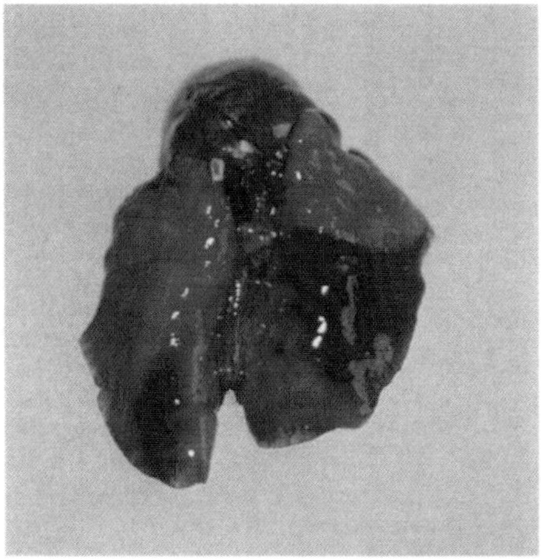

Plate 28. Pneumonia. This plate shows the lungs of a juvenile mixed breed male rabbit that was found dead after not eating for 24 h. The lungs showed evidence of acute pneumonia typical of *Pasteurella multocida* infection.

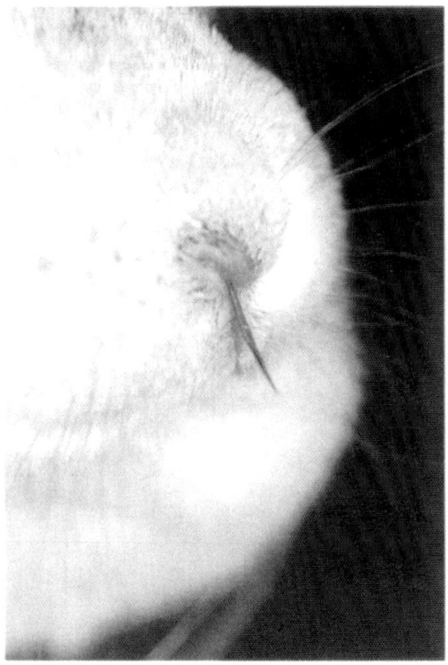

Plate 29. Nasal foreign body. This plate shows the nostrils of a mature Dwarf lop male rabbit that was presented because he was sneezing. In this case, a blade of hay could clearly be seen protruding from the nostril and the foreign body was easy to remove. Seeds and stems of hay can make their way into a number of sites and cause disease in rabbits. Nasal foreign bodies are relatively common. Sometimes stems of hay can lodge in or around the larynx and cause choking. Foreign bodies can become wedged in the periodontal space. Both these conditions are linked with dental disease. Grass seeds can also lodge in the inguinal skin folds that are situated on either side of the genital orifice.

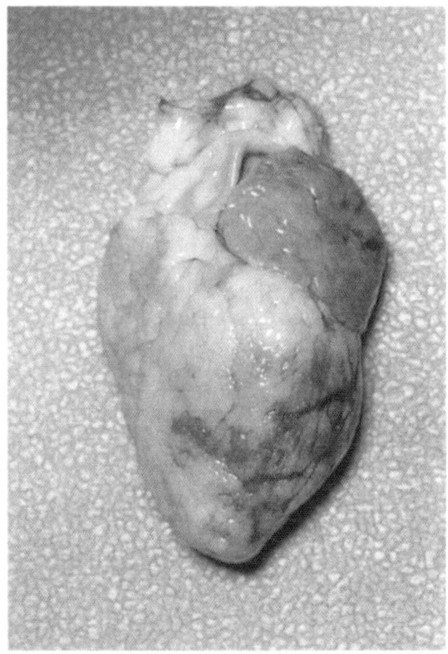

Plate 30. Cardiomyopathy. This plate shows the heart of an adult neutered male French lop (> 6 kg) that died suddenly following a period of lethargy but no other obvious clinical signs. Histopathological and gross *post-mortem* examination showed no lesions in other organs apart from congestion. Sections of heart muscle showed myocardial fibrosis.

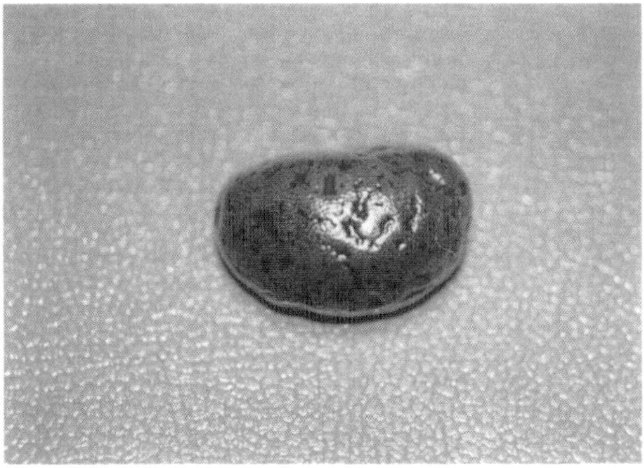

Plate 31. Kidney showing gross lesions associated with *Encephalitozoon cuniculi* infection. This plate shows the kidney of a 4-year-old male Dwarf lop rabbit that was known to be seropositive for *Encephalitozoon cuniculi* although he showed no obvious clinical symptoms. Both kidneys showed irregular, depressed areas. *E. cuniculi* causes granulomatous interstitial nephritis. Long-standing lesions show interstitial fibrosis and collapse of the parenchyma. Early lesions show focal granulomatous inflammation. Lesions are present in the renal tubule and spores are shed in the urine, which is infective to other rabbits.

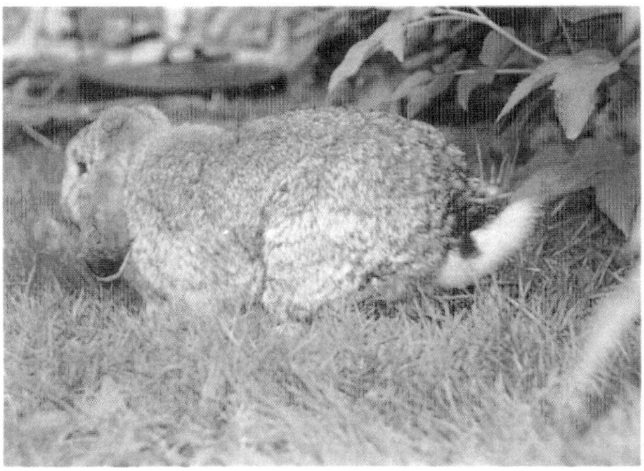

Plate 32. Normal urination stance. Rabbits that are given the freedom to exercise and mark their territory urinate frequently. In order to direct the jet of urine away from the body, the rabbit lifts its hindquarters and raises its tail. Failure to adopt the correct stance for urination can result in urine contaminating the fur around the genitalia and scalding the skin.

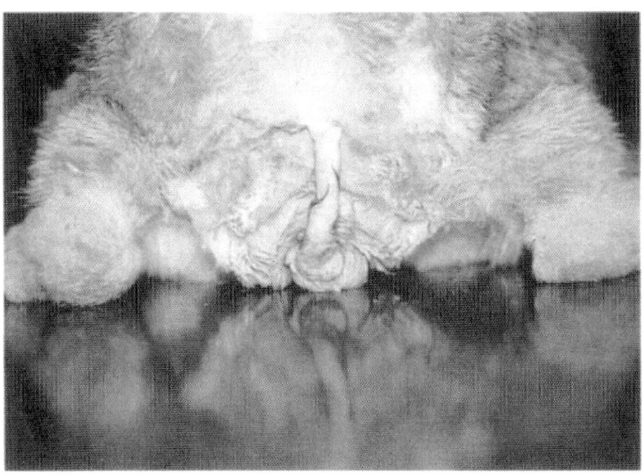

Plate 33. Urine scalding. Any condition that prevents a rabbit from adopting the correct stance for urination can result in urine retention or urine scalding of the perineal skin. Once the skin is inflamed, urethritis makes urination painful and a vicious circle begins (see Figure 14.2). The rabbit illustrated is a 3-year-old neutered male Dwarf lop house rabbit that was suffering from urine scalding of the perineum and inner thighs. He had urine retention and 'sludgy urine' (see Figure 14.1). Radiography revealed a displaced 7th lumbar vertebra and a narrowed lumbosacral disc space. As a result of the spinal lesion, the rabbit could not adopt the correct position to urinate. Plate 34 shows the urine from this rabbit.

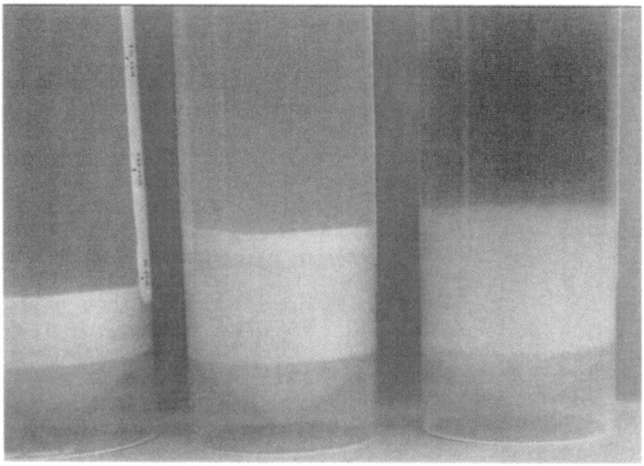

Plate 34. A comparison of normal urine with 'sludgy' urine. There are differences in the way in which sediment forms in sludgy and normal urine. The two samples on the left of the picture are 'sludgy' urine that was expressed from the rabbit illustrated in Plate 33 and Figure 14.1. The far left sample was the urine that was initially expressed from the bladder. The middle sample was thick viscid urine that had apparently been retained in the bladder for some time. It had the consistency of toothpaste. A fine sediment that set like concrete formed in both these samples after they were left standing for a few hours. The sediment could only be broken up by shaking the sample vigorously. The sample on the right is urine from a normal rabbit that also contains sediment. However, the sediment in the normal sample easily forms a suspension with gentle shaking, even after it is left undisturbed for 48 h or more. Analysis of both samples is similar. They both contain calcium carbonate and some calcium oxalate crystals which give urine its radiodense appearance on radiographs.

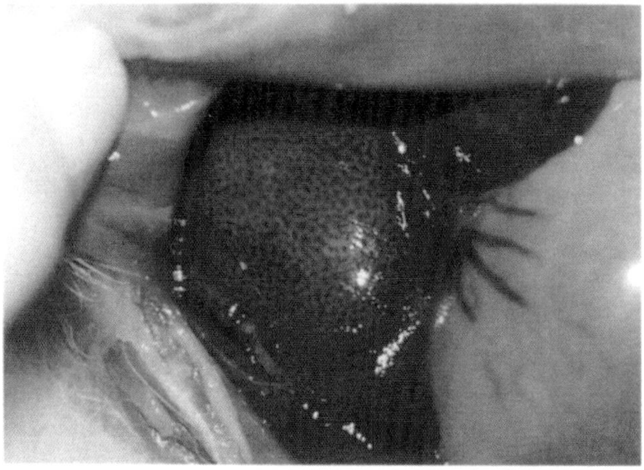

Plate 35. The liver of a rabbit that had died from viral haemorrhagic disease (VHD). The typical appearance of the liver of a rabbit that has died from viral haemorrhagic disease is shown. The liver is enlarged, although not strikingly so, and friable and pale with a distinct lobular pattern. The liver is always affected in cases of viral haemorrhagic disease although the gross appearance may not reflect the severe histopathological changes. The histological appearance of the liver is often diagnostic. It is severely congested with marked hepatocyte necrosis involving extensive areas of most lobules.

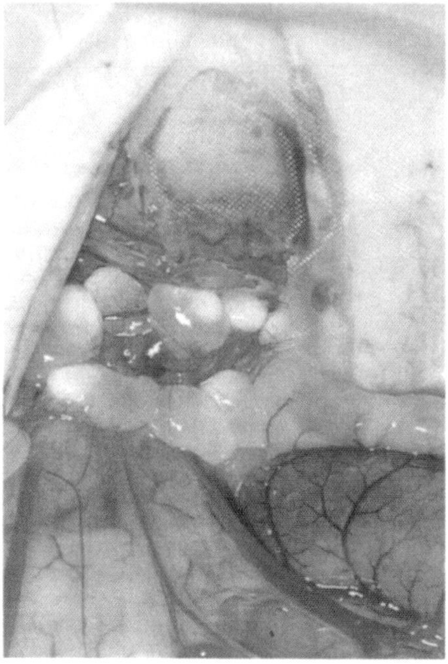

Plate 36. *Cysticercus pisiformis.* *Cysticercus pisiformis* is the larval stage of *Taenia pisiformis,* which is a tapeworm that affects dogs and foxes with rabbits acting as the intermediate host. Multiple oval cysts are found in the mesentery. The cysts contain the inverted scolex of the tapeworm. This plate shows some of the cysts that were found during an exploratory laparotomy of an anorexic rabbit that was showing signs of abdominal discomfort. No faeces had been passed for 48 h. The rabbit was a mature Angora male that had recently been adopted by a rescue centre. The cysts were most abundant in the mesentery between the stomach and the distal colon. The cysts had become so large that they had obstructed the large intestine.

advance of the small risk of regrowth. Removal of a regrown tooth at a later date is usually straightforward. Non-growing root fragments can be left *in situ* unless problems develop.

7.10.2 Trimming cheek teeth

Congenital malocclusion of the cheek teeth is rare but acquired malocclusion is a common condition of pet rabbits. The position, shape and structure of the cheek teeth are altered so normal occlusion is lost. The teeth become misaligned and the direction of growth is changed. In the early stages of acquired dental disease, the lower cheek teeth tend to curve and tip towards the tongue (see Figure 7.4). Sharp spurs form that lacerate the lingual mucosa. These spurs are extremely painful for the rabbit and prevent eating and grooming.

Corrective dentistry cannot restore normal occlusion to maloccluded cheek teeth because of the altered position, shape and structure of the teeth (see Figure 7.4 and Plate 19). Changes in the direction of growth mean that malocclusion recurs and the spurs regrow, often in a matter of a few weeks. However, acquired dental disease is progressive and eventually the germinal layer at the roots is destroyed and the teeth stop growing so trimming is no longer required. The crowns may break off altogether so the gum heals, or the crowns remain and the rabbit is left with misshapen stumps that are used to grind food. The number of times that the teeth require trimming is variable.

General anaesthesia is required to trim the cheek teeth. A gag and cheek dilators are required, especially if the cheek teeth are to be shortened using power equipment. Good illumination and competence at using the equipment are essential. In common with incisor trimming, there is debate about the use of hand-held versus power equipment to shorten cheek teeth. Special long handled molar clippers are available (Veterinary Instrumentation, Sheffield) that can be used to trim spurs and nibble away at crowns to shorten them. Diamond rasps can then be used to smooth off any sharp points. The advantage of hand-held equipment is that it is unlikely to cause serious soft tissue damage if it is used carefully. The disadvantage is that it is not possible to shape the teeth precisely. Alternatively, dental burrs can be used to remove spurs and carefully reshape the teeth. Some type of guard, such as a wooden tongue depressor is required to protect and retract surrounding soft tissue. Some vets use a combination of the two techniques and 'debulk' the teeth with clippers before smoothing and shaping them with a low speed burr. Whichever method is used, it is not possible to restore the complex occlusal surface of the cheek teeth (see Figure 7.3) either by clipping with hand-held clippers or by using dental burrs.

Superficial blood vessels within the mouth can be punctured during cheek teeth trimming, either with hand-held or power equipment. The lingual artery is in close proximity with the mandibular cheek teeth (see Figure 3.6). Serious life-threatening haemorrhage can occur. Packing the area with cotton wool is usually successful in controlling the bleeding. Rabbit blood clots very quickly. Dental burrs can also cause serious iatrogenic soft tissue damage. A common injury is a penetration of the mucosa, just labial to the first upper premolar where the drill has 'walked off' the tooth. This injury can result in a chronically infected cavity that collects food material and does not heal. Treatment is difficult or impossible. Iatrogenic injury can also be caused by thermal damage during lengthy burring procedures without cooling the teeth. Affected rabbits do not eat or drink postoperatively and develop generalized periodontal infection. Pus can be seen surrounding the teeth a few days after the procedure. The condition is usually fatal.

There is debate about the extent to which the crowns of cheek teeth should be shortened. Some practitioners burr the teeth down to gum level to take them out of occlusion. Others simply trim off the spurs and reshape the teeth. Shortening the teeth to gum level increases the risk of exposing innervated dentine. Burring the cheek teeth down to gum level also takes them out of occlusion and prevents the rabbit from grinding fibrous food, such as grass or hay, postoperatively. Some rabbits are unable to eat at all if all the cheek teeth have been burred down to gum level. This is temporary if the teeth are growing, but permanent if they are not. The ability to chew fibrous food is important to maintain optimum digestive function. Reducing crowns to gum level does not significantly increase the interval between tooth trimming (see Figure 7.4). Trimming off the spurs and leaving the teeth in occlusion allows the rabbit to eat fibrous food postoperatively.

The occlusion of the incisors is also an important consideration. If the incisors are long, the cheek teeth do not occlude until the crowns are quite long. The incisors may also require trimming and shaping.

Postoperative analgesia is always required after cheek teeth trimming (Section 5.9.2). Antibiotics are indicated if there is soft tissue damage.

7.10.3 Extraction of cheek teeth

Owners often request removal of cheek teeth to prevent regrowth of spurs that require regular trimming. Unless periapical abscesses are present, extraction of the cheek teeth is inadvisable and often unnecessary. Extraction of the whole length of molars and premolars is a difficult procedure. The bone overlying the cheek teeth is thin, even in a healthy rabbit, and prone to fracture. Access to the periodontal space to break down the periodontal ligament is almost impossible through the oral cavity because of the anatomical impossibility of opening the mouth widely. Buccotomy is feasible but requires surgical damage to the muscles of mastication and is painful postoperatively. Also, in many cases, it is not a single tooth that is causing problems but a generalized condition affecting several cheek teeth. Most cases of cheek tooth malocclusion eventually resolve as the teeth stop growing. Therefore it is preferable to leave the teeth *in situ* rather than attempt removal.

Sometimes crowns from diseased cheek teeth can be pulled off through the oral cavity. As dental disease progresses the tooth quality deteriorates and the crowns can fracture, usually just below the gingival margin. These teeth are found to be loose during examination under anaesthesia and are easily removed without ill effect. It is not uncommon to examine aged rabbits and find that they have no crowns at all on the lower cheek teeth. The crowns have broken off and the gums have healed with no apparent problems.

Cheek teeth affected by perapical abscesses can be removed by dissecting out the root within the abscess cavity. The pus is removed from the abscess cavity, taking care to minimize contamination of the surrounding tissues (see Section 8.3.1). A Volkmann's scoop is a useful instrument for removing pus. The cavity is flushed and the roots identified. The roots of neighbouring teeth may be seen within the cavity. These can be left alone providing all necrotic and infected tissue is removed. However, if the periodontal attachments of adjacent teeth have eroded and the teeth are loose, they will also require removal to prevent recurrence of the abscess. Residual periodontal attachments are broken down before removing the tooth, either through the mouth or through the abscess cavity. A set of instruments has been designed specifically for loosening and extracting molars. The Crossley molar luxator and molar extraction forceps are very useful pieces of equipment (Veterinary Instrumentation, Sheffield).

It is a commonly held misconception that if a cheek tooth is removed, then the opposing tooth should also be removed. This is not true for several reasons. First, examination of the occlusal pattern of the cheek teeth shows that an upper tooth occludes with two lower teeth and vice versa. Secondly, adjacent teeth tend to tip towards any gap that is left and thirdly, the teeth probably are not occluding normally anyway because they are growing in a distorted fashion.

Once the teeth have stopped growing and the symptoms of molar malocclusion no longer occur, it is important to check the cheek teeth periodically as, occasionally, one or two crowns continue to grow, albeit slowly, and can penetrate surrounding soft tissue and cause an abscess. It is often the molars at the back of the mouth that cause problems (see Figure 7.8e)

7.11 Dietary advice for rabbits with dental disease

Prevention of dental disease in pet rabbits is summarized in Box 7.5.

Key points 7.5

- Elongated crowns can be shortened using hand-held clippers or power driven burrs and cutting discs. There are advantages and disadvantages with both methods. It is unlikely that either method will restore occlusion for more than a few weeks if the teeth are still growing
- The aim of tooth trimming is to remove sharp points that are growing into surrounding soft tissue and, if possible, to restore occlusion
- It is not possible to restore the normal shape, occlusion and position of maloccluded teeth by trimming them
- Clipping teeth with hand-held clippers is quick and easy. It can be a satisfactory method of trimming poor quality, weakened teeth. It is not satisfactory for healthy teeth with strong enamel
- Hand-held clippers exert an unnatural force on the tooth that may be painful to the rabbit. The teeth can shatter and expose the pulp cavity. It is not possible to shape the teeth accurately and sharp points can remain
- Special clippers with long handles are available for trimming cheek teeth. These are useful for removing sharp spurs. They can also be used to shorten cheek teeth by nibbling them away gradually. A diamond rasp can be used to smooth the teeth afterwards
- The alternative to hand-held clippers is power driven equipment such as dental burrs or cutting discs. These give greater control in shaping the teeth and do not shatter the teeth
- Power driven equipment poses a risk of soft tissue damage, especially if the rabbit moves during the procedure or the burr 'walks off' the tooth into neighbouring tissue
- Although cutting discs are very good for trimming incisors, they pose a risk to both rabbit and operator. Sedation or anaesthesia is indicated and some type of guard is required to protect the soft tissue
- Diamond burrs can be used to shorten incisors in the conscious, well-restrained rabbit
- Thermal damage of the pulp cavity can occur if the teeth become too hot during burring. Water is required for cooling
- Rabbit dentine is innervated. Histological studies suggest a sensory innervation that decreases towards the occlusal surface of the tooth. Excessive shortening of the tooth exposes the pulp cavity and potentially sensitive dentine
- Excessive shortening of the cheek teeth takes them out of occlusion and prevents mastication of fibrous food that is essential for optimum gut motility. This will be permanent if the teeth are no longer growing
- Excessive shortening of the teeth can result in postoperative anorexia. Flaps of gum or buccal mucosa can grow across the remnants of teeth that have been burred down to the gum. These can become inflamed and painful when the rabbit attempts to eat
- Postoperative anorexia and pain can result in fatal hepatic lipidosis in rabbits
- It is possible to remove maloccluded incisors. Removal of maloccluded cheek teeth is not so easy
- Surgical removal of the incisors is the treatment of choice for hereditary malocclusion
- Surgical removal of the incisors may be the treatment of choice for malocclusions that have resulted from accidental fractures of the teeth or jaws
- Young, immature rabbits are less likely to develop complications associated with incisor removal
- Older rabbits with weakened teeth and acquired dental problems are prone to tooth fracture during incisor removal
- Postoperative analgesia is essential for all rabbits undergoing surgical removal of the incisors
- Endotracheal intubation is required for removal of the incisors, otherwise satisfactory anaesthesia can be difficult. Nasal intubation can be used in small rabbits that are difficult to intubate endotracheally
- Removal of the incisors will not prevent malocclusions developing on the cheek teeth and may not mean the end of the rabbit's dental problems.

Although there is debate about the aetiopathogenesis of acquired dental disease in pet rabbits, there is agreement about the general dietary advice that is given to rabbit owners to prevent and to treat tooth problems. There is no doubt that rabbits that

Box 7.5 Prevention of dental disease in pet rabbits

- Select breeding stock without congenital incisor malocclusion and with no history of the disease in their pedigree
- Ensure breeding stock and growing rabbits have sufficient calcium and vitamin D. Growing rabbits are most susceptible to metabolic bone disease. Mixed cereal rations are not suitable for groups of juvenile rabbits as it impossible to prevent selective feeding
- Provide *ad lib* fibrous food. Grass and hay are ideal to provide dental wear
- Provide a diet that contains sufficient calcium for mineralization of the continually growing teeth and surrounding bone – 0.5–1.0% is ideal. Excessive amounts could contribute to urinary tract disease
- Choose good quality hay. The calcium content of poor quality hay can be as low as 0.25%, which is lower than the 0.44% dietary requirement for bone mineralization. Sun dried hay is a good source of vitamin D. Barn dried hay may not contain vitamin D
- If possible, feed a variety of weeds and wild plants. In general, weeds and wild plants are balanced sources of calcium and are good sources of indigestible fibre
- Feed at least three types of fruit or vegetable each day, including one type of fibrous vegetable such as broccoli, cabbage, spring greens, spinach or cauliflower leaves. Root vegetables and fruit, such as carrots and apples, are poor sources of calcium
- If possible, allow exercise outside each day. This not only provides the opportunity to graze, but also enables the rabbit to bask in the sun, which prevents vitamin D deficiency
- Feed a well-balanced concentrated food to iron out any deficiencies in the rest of the diet. A small bowlful should be offered once a day and should be eaten completely within 2 h
- Do not allow the rabbit to select low calcium cereals and legumes from cereal mixtures. If the rabbit does not eat all the mixture, switch brands to a more palatable one. Palatable extruded or pelleted diets are preferable as they prevent selective feeding.

are fed mainly on cereal mixtures with little or no supplementary hay or grass are high-risk candidates for the development of malocclusion and other dental problems. Rabbits have evolved to eat grass and fibrous vegetation and those individuals that are maintained on a natural diet do not develop dental disease (Harcourt-Brown and Baker, 2001). However, there is reluctance among rabbit owners to feed hay, grass and wild plants to their pets. Hay is messy. Owners often believe that grass and wild plants may be poisonous or contaminated with weedkillers, lead from exhaust fumes, diseases from wild rabbits, dog urine or other unseen dangers. Rabbits are often kept in cities where grass and weeds are unavailable. Advertising strategies and marketing by rabbit food manufacturers encourage rabbit owners to buy food from pet shops or supermarkets and engender the belief that rabbits should be fed on cereal mixtures. There is conflicting advice from breeders and pet shops about the advisability of feeding vegetables to rabbits which confuses owners. As a result, many rabbit owners continue to feed cereal mixtures because they believe them to be safe and find them convenient. It is common practice to leave a bowl of food in the cage at all times.

To prevent dental disease, owners should be encouraged to feed grass and other fibrous weeds such as dandelions, bramble and tree leaves when they are available. The opportunity to exercise and graze in the garden, perhaps confined to a pen or large enclosure is to be encouraged. Good quality hay must be available to all pet rabbits at all times. A selection of vegetables can be offered daily. A moderate amount of a balanced cereal ration is acceptable as it provides vitamins and minerals and is a convenient method of supplementing food when grass and greens are scarce or expensive during the winter months. It is important to ensure the rabbit eats the entire ration. Extruded diets are ideal for this purpose as they prevent selective feeding and ensure the provision of a balanced diet. Concentrated rations should not be offered *ad libitum* to adult rabbits. A small bowlful once a daily is all that is required, if plenty of hay and other food is available.

Correcting the diet will not reverse changes that have already taken place to the structure and position of the teeth, although it will improve bone quality and reduce the risk of abscess formation. Rabbits that have already developed dental problems often do not accept dietary changes readily. They may be reluctant to chew hay or grass because their teeth are painful. Often, they have been given the same diet for years and will steadfastly refuse to eat anything new. These cases require a vitamin and mineral supplement to improve bone quality, but supplements do not re-align teeth and cannot be viewed as a quick fix to dental problems. High calcium supplements are to be avoided because of the risk of urolithiasis. Care must be taken to ensure the rabbit is actually ingesting the supplement. Simply sprinkling it onto the food is not sufficient. Mixing it with palatable foods or sprinkling it on bread can be effective. Routine vitamin and mineral supplements are not required by rabbits eating a balanced diet.

References

Abbott, M. (1997). A study of the prevalence of malocclusion in pet rabbits. Survey conducted at Cottontails Rabbit Sanctuary, Bristol, UK.

Abe, J., Yoshikawa, M., Makamura, M. (1989). Effect of high protein low calcium diet on rat alveolus. 7 day diet (English abstract, article in Japanese). *Meikai Daigaku Shigaku Zasshi*, **18**, 267–275.

Archard, H.O. (1971). The dental defects of vitamin D-resistant rickets (Abstract). *Birth Defects Orig Artic Ser.*, **7**, 196–199.

Ashcraft, M.D., Southard, K.A., Tolley, E.A. (1992). The effect of corticosteroid-induced osteoporosis on orthodontic tooth movement. *Am J Orthodontic Dentofacial Orthopaed.*, **102**, 310–319.

Bishop, M.A. (1995). Is rabbit dentine innervated? A fine-structural study of the pulpal innervation in the cheek teeth of the rabbit. *J Anat.*, **186**, 365–372.

Brommage, R., Miller, S.C., Langman, C.B. *et al.* (1988). The effect of chronic vitamin D deficiency on the skeleton in the adult rabbit. *Bone*, **9**, 131–139.

Brown, S.A. (1992). Surgical removal of incisors in the rabbit. *J Small Anim Exotic Med.*, **1**, 150–153.

Byers, M.R. (1984). Dental sensory receptors (Abstract). *Int Rev Neurobiol.*, **25**, 39–94.

Chai, C.K. (1970). Effect of inbreeding in rabbits. Skeletal variations and malformations. *J Heredity*, **61**, 2–8.

Chapin, R.E., Smith, S.E. (1967). Calcium requirement of growing rabbits. *J Anim Sci.*, **26**, 67–71.

Crossley, D.A. (1995a). Clinical aspects of lagomorph dental anatomy: The rabbit (*Oryctolagus cuniculus*). *J Vet Dentistry*, **12**, 137–140.

Crossley, D.A. (1995b). Dental disease in rabbits. *Vet Rec.*, **137**, 384.

Crossley, D.A., Jackson, A., Yates, J., Boydell, I.P. (1998). Use of computed tomography to investigate cheek tooth abnormalities in chinchillas (*Chinchilla laniger*). *J Small Anim Pract.*, **39**, 385–389.

Duckworth, J., Benzie D., Cresswell E. *et al.* (1961). Dental malocclusion and rickets in sheep. *Res Vet Sci.*, **2**, 375–380.

Eisele, P.H. (1986). Dental problems in rabbits and rodents. In *Current Veterinary Therapy IX* (Kirk, R.W. ed.) pp 759–762. W.B. Saunders.

El Shorafa, W.M., Feaster, E., Ott, E.A., Asquith, R.L. (1979). Effect of vitamin D and sunlight on growth and bone development of young ponies. *J Anim Sci.*, **48**, 882–886.

Emily, P. (1991). Problems peculiar to continually erupting teeth. *J Small Exotic Anim Med.*, **1**, 56–59.

Engstrom, C., Noren, J.G. (1986). Effects of orthodontic force on enamel formation in normal and hypocalcaemic rats (Abstract). *J Oral Pathol.*, **15**, 78–82.

Engstrom, C., Granstrom, G., Thilander, B. (1988). Effect of orthodontic force on periodontal tissue metabolism. A histologic and biochemical study in normal and hypocalcaemic young rats (Abstract). *Am J Ortho Dentofacial Orthop.*, **93**, 486–495.

Fairham, J., Harcourt-Brown, F.M. (1999). Preliminary investigation of the vitamin D status of pet rabbits. *Vet Rec.*, **145**, 452–454.

Fowler, M.E. (1986). Metabolic bone disease. In *Zoo and Wild Animal Medicine*, 2nd edn. (M.E. Fowler, ed.) pp 69–90. W.B. Saunders.

Fox, R.R., Crary, D.D. (1971). Mandibular prognathism in the rabbit. *J Heredity*, **62**, 163–169.

Gilsanz, V., Roe, T.F., Antunes, J. *et al.* (1991). Effect of dietary calcium on bone density in growing rabbits. *Am J Physiol.*, **260**, E471–E476.

Goodman, J.R., Gelbier, M.J., Bennett, J.H., Winter, G.B. (1998). Dental problems associated with hypophosphataemic vitamin D resistant rickets (Abstract). *Int J Paediatr Dent.*, **8**, 19–28.

Gorrell, C., Robinson, J. (1995). Endodontics in small carnivores. In *Manual of Small Animal Dentistry* (D.A. Crossley, S. Penman, eds). pp 168–181. British Small Animal Veterinary Association.

Guyton, A.C. (1991). *Textbook of Medical Physiology*, 8th edn. W.B. Saunders.

Hamidur Rahman, A.S.M., Al-Mahmud, K.A., Nashiru-Islam, K.M. (1983). Dental malocclusion in New Zealand White rabbit. *Bangladesh Vet J.*, **16**, 85–88.

Harcourt-Brown, F.M. (1995). A review of clinical conditions in pet rabbits associated with their teeth. *Vet Rec.*, **137**, 341–346.

Harcourt-Brown, F.M. (1996). Calcium deficiency, diet

and dental disease in pet rabbits. *Vet Rec.*, **139**, 567–571.
Harcourt-Brown, F.M. (1997). Diagnosis, treatment and prognosis of dental disease in pet rabbits. *In Practice*, **19**, 407–421.
Harcourt-Brown, F.M., Friggens, M.T. (1999). Intestinal obstruction in rabbits by locust bean seeds. *Vet Rec.*, **145**, 203.
Harcourt-Brown, F.M., Baker, S.J. (2001). Parathyroid hormone, haematological and biochemical parameters in relation to dental disease and husbandry in pet rabbits. *J Small Anim Pract.*, **42**, 130–136.
Hillson, S. (1986). *Teeth*. Cambridge University Press.
Hirschfield, Z., Weinrab, M.M., Michaeli, Y. (1973). The incisors of the rabbit: anatomy, histology and post-natal development. *J Dent Res.*, **52**, 377–384.
Holick, M.F. (1996). Vitamin D and bone health. *J Nutr.*, **126**, 1159S–1164S.
Huang, C.M. (1987). Morphometric relationships between skull traits and malocclusion in the domestic rabbit. *Bull Inst Zool Acad Sin.*, **26**, 123–131.
Hunt, C.E., Harrington, D.D. (1974). Nutrition and nutritional diseases of the rabbit. In *The Biology of the Laboratory Rabbit*. (S.H. Weisbroth, R.E. Flatt, A.L. Kraus, eds). pp 403–428. Academic Press.
Ireson, H. (1968). A preliminary report on an abnormal dental condition in rabbits. *J Inst Anim Tech.*, **19**, 36–39.
Jenkins, J.R. (1997). Rabbit dentistry. *Rabbit Medicine and Procedures for Practitioners, Veterinary Conference Program and Abstracts*. pp 35–37. House Rabbit Society, USA.
Julius, C. (1997). Untersuchungen zur Knochendichte bei weiblichen ZIKA-Zuchtkaninchen an Calcaneus sowie am distalen tibiaende über einen Zeitraum von mehreren Reproduktionszyklen mittels peripherer Quantitativer Computertomographie (pQCTtm). *Doctoral Thesis*, (with English summary).
Langenbach, G.E., Weijs, W.A., Koolstra, J.H. (1991). Biomechanical changes in the rabbits masticatory system during postnatal development. *Anat Rec.*, **230**, 406–416.
Latour, M.A., Hopkins, D., Kitchens, T. *et al.* (1998). Effects of feeding a liquid diet for one year to New Zealand White rabbits. *Lab Anim Sci.*, **48**, 81–83.
Lindsey, J.R., Fox, R.R. (1994). Inherited diseases and variations. In *The Biology of the Laboratory Rabbit*, 2nd edn. (P.J. Manning, D.H. Ringler, C.E. Newcomer, eds). pp 293–313. Academic Press.
Lozupone, E., Favia, A. (1989). Effects of a low calcium maternal and weaning diet on the thickness and microhardness of rat incisor enamel and dentine (Abstract). *Arch Oral Biol.*, **34**, 491–498.
Lozupone, E., Favia, A. (1994). Morphometric analysis of the deposition and mineralization of enamel and dentine from rat incisor during the recovery phase following a low-calcium regimen (Abstract). *Arch Oral Biol.*, **39**, 409–416.
Lowe, J.A., (1998). Pet rabbit feeding and nutrition. In *The Nutrition of the Rabbit*, (C. de Blas, J. Wiseman, eds). pp 309–332. CABI Publishing.
McDonald, P., Edwards, R.A., Greenhalgh, J.F.D., Morgan, C.A. (1996). *Animal Nutrition*, 5th edn. Longman.
McRoberts, M.R., Hill, R., Dalgarno, A.C. (1965). The effects of diets deficient in phosphorus, phosphorus and Vitamin D or calcium, on the skeleton and teeth of growing sheep. *J Agric Sci.*, **65**, 1–18.
Mellanby, M., Killick, E.M. (1926). A preliminary study of factors influencing calcification processes in the rabbit. *Biochem J.*, **20**, 902–926.
Michaeli, Y., Hirschfield Z., Weinreb M.M. (1980). The cheek teeth of the rabbit; Morphology, histology and development. *Acta Anat.*, **106**, 223–239.
Morgan, J.P. (1972). *Radiology in Veterinary Orthopaedics*. Lea and Febiger.
Ness, A.R. (1956). The response of the rabbit mandibular incisor to experimental shortening and prevention of its eruption. *Proc Roy Soc.*, **146**, 129–154.
Okada, S., Ohta, Y., Nishimura, *et al.* (1990). Microvascular architecture of the enamel organ of the upper major incisor in the rabbit (Abstract). *Okajimas Folia Anat Jpn.*, **67**, 231–241.
Okerman, L. (1988). *Diseases of Domestic Rabbits*, Blackwell.
Omeroglu, H., Ates, Y., Akkus, O. *et al.* (1997). Biomechanical analysis of the effects of single high-dose vitamin D3 on fracture healing in a healthy rabbit model. *Arch Orthopaed Trauma Surg.*, **116**, 271–274.
Plachot, J.J., Du Bois, M.B., Halpern, S. *et al.* (1982). *In vitro* action of 1,25-dihydroxycholcalciferol and 25-dihydroxyxholecalciferol on matrix organization and mineral distribution in rabbit growth plate. *Metabolic Bone Dis Rel Res.*, **4**, 135–142.
Pollock, S. (1951). Slobbers in the rabbit. *J Am Vet Med Assoc.*, **119**, 443–444.
Proffitt, W.R., Sellers, K.T. (1986). The effect of intermittent forces on eruption of the rabbit incisor. *J Dent Res.*, **65**, 118–122.
Rao, D.S., Honasoge, M. (1996). Metabolic bone disease in gastrointestinal, hepatobiliary and pancreatic disorders. In *Primer on the Metabolic Bone Diseases and Disorders of Mineral Metabolism* (M.J.Favus, ed.) pp 306–310. Lippincott-Raven.
Rosskopf, W.J., Woerpel, R.W. (1982). Malocclusion in pet rabbits. *Mod Vet Pract.*, **63**, 482.
Schwartz, G., Enomoto, S., Valiquette, C., Lund, J.P. (1989). Mastication in the rabbit: a description of movement and muscle activity. *J Neurophysiol.*, **62**, 273–287.
Shadle, A.R. (1936). The attrition and extrusive growth of the four major incisor teeth of domestic rabbits. *J Mammol.*, **17**, 15–21.
Steedle, J.R., Proffitt, W.R., Fields, H.W. (1983). The effects of continuously axially-directed intrusive loads on the erupting rabbit mandibular incisor. *Arch Oral Biol.*, **28**, 1149–1153.
Steenkamp, G., Crossley, D.A. (1999). Incisor tooth regrowth in a rabbit following complete extraction. *Vet Rec.*, **145**, 585–586.

Taylor, E.L. (1940). Pseudo-rumination. *Vet Med.*, **35**, 481.

Turner, T. (1997). The incidence of dental problems in pet rabbits. *Proceedings of the 5th World Veterinary Dental Congress.* Birmingham.

Tvedegaard, E. (1987). Arterial disease in chronic renal failure. An experimental study in the rabbit. *Acta Pathol Microbiol Immunol Scand.Section A. Suppl 290*, **95**, 3–28.

Weisbroth, S.H., Ehrman, L. (1967). Malocclusion in the rabbit; a model for the study of the development, pathology and inheritance of malocclusion. I. Preliminary note. *J Heredity*, **58**, 245–246.

Westerhof, I,. Lumeij, S.J. (1987). Dental problems in rabbits, guinea pigs and chinchillas. *Tijdschrift voor Diergeneeskunde*, **12**, 6S–10S.

Wiggs, R.B., Lobprise, H. (1995). Dental anatomy and physiology of pet rodents and lagomorphs. In *Manual of Small Animal Dentistr.*, 2nd edn. (D.A. Crossley, S. Penman, eds). pp 68–73. British Small Animal Veterinary Association.

Wolf, P., Bucher, L., Kamphues, J. (1993). A study on the influence of feeding on growth and attrition of rabbit's incisors. *Proceedings of 8th Symposium on Diseases of Rabbits, Furbearing and Fancy Pet Animals.* Germany.

Wolf, P., Kummerfeld, N., Mischok, D. (1996). Animal nutrition in veterinary medicine-actual case reports. Nutritionally related bone development in emus and rheas (Abstract, Article in German). *Dtsch Tierarztl Wochenschr.*, **103**, 519–512.

Wood, C. (1978). The pet rabbit – veterinary problems. *Vet Rec.*, **102**, 304–308.

Wu, D.D., Boyd, R.D., Fix, T.J., Burr, D.B. (1990). Regional patterns of bone loss and altered bone remodelling in response to calcium deprivation in laboratory rabbits. *Calcif Tissue Int.*, **47**, 18–23.

Yamada, Y., Yamamura, K. (1996). Possible factors which may affect phase durations in the natural chewing rhythm. *Brain Res.*, **706**, 237–242.

Yang, K.H., Stewart, A.F. (1996). Miscellaneous causes of hypercalcaemia. In *Primer on the Metabolic Bone Diseases and Disorders of Mineral Metabolism* (M. Favus, ed.) pp 213–216. Lippincott-Raven.

Zeman, W.V., Fielder, F.G. (1969). Dental malocclusion and overgrowth in rabbits. *J Am Vet Med Assoc.*, **155**, 1115–1119.

Abscesses

8

The definition of an abscess is 'a localised collection of pus in a cavity formed by the disintegration of tissue' (Blood and Studdert, 1999). Pus is the product of suppuration, which is the inflammatory process that occurs in the presence of pyogenic organisms that resist phagocytosis. Pus consists of dead phagocytes, predominantly neutrophils, inflammatory exudate, bacteria and cellular debris. Neutrophils contain lysosomal granules that contain degradative enzymes, which play a major role in the destruction of bacteria. The life span of the neutrophil is short (3–4 days). Dead or dying neutrophils release lysosomal enzymes that not only autolyse the neutrophil but also digest dead tissue cells around them. As the suppurative process continues a cavity forms that becomes walled off from the surrounding tissue. The wall is composed of young connective tissue containing collagen fibres and blood vessels. Neutrophils and other leucocytes continue to migrate into the abscess from blood vessels in the wall. Antibodies that can neutralize toxins and kill bacteria arrive at the site. Eventually the abscess becomes enclosed in a fibrous capsule that is composed of fibroblasts and inflammatory cells, with an inner layer of degenerating neutrophils (Chaffee *et al.*, 1975). The abscess expands along the line of least resistance and can rupture through the skin or into a body cavity, discharging pus, bacteria and toxins. Surgical intervention to provide drainage can resolve the suppurative process or it may persist to become chronic.

Chronic abscesses are refractory to treatment. Resorption of water from pus results in thick, caseous material within the abscess cavity. The presence of any type of foreign material within the abscess harbours bacteria that have an inhibitory or toxic effect on neutrophils. Antibiotics cannot penetrate abscess cavities because of the poor vascularity. Binding with purulent material inactivates some antibiotics. Failure of an abscess cavity to heal after rupture or surgical drainage may occur because the fibrous wall of the capsule has become so rigid that it cannot collapse. Residual microorganisms can then lead to renewal of inflammation.

Chronic suppuration is common in rabbits and slow growing, well-encapsulated, relatively painless abscesses develop readily. *Pasteurella multocida* is frequently isolated. This bacterium has capsular polysaccharides that resist phagocytosis (Deeb, 1993). *Pasteurella multocida* can reside in the nasal flora of asymptomatic rabbits and spread to other sites during grooming. Other pyogenic bacteria such as staphylococci, *Pseudomonas* spp. and *Fusiformis* spp. can also be isolated from rabbit abscesses (Chaffee *et al.*, 1975; Dominguez *et al.*, 1975; Ward *et al.*, 1981). Secondary infections in tissues damaged by other causes such as surgical incisions, bite injuries, trauma, penetrating wounds or foreign bodies often result in abscess formation. Once a primary abscess has become established, haematogenous spread to other sites or local spread along the lymphatics can result in the formation of secondary abscesses. Venereal transmission and injuries to the genital tract can result in abscesses developing in the reproductive system of breeding does.

Chronic abscesses in rabbits are notoriously difficult to cure. In other species, acute inflammation due to pyogenic bacteria is associated with leucocytosis, due to an increase rate of production of neutrophils from the bone marrow. This response is not marked in rabbits (Toth and Krueger, 1989). Lymphopaenia is associated with any chronic disease in rabbits including abscesses (Hinton *et al.*, 1982; Harcourt-Brown and Baker, 2001). In other species, abscesses often burst and providing drainage alone can be sufficient to effect a cure (Knight *et al.*, 1980). Abscesses in rabbits seldom 'point' and rupture spontaneously, although large areas of skin can become necrotic and slough if the abscess is particularly large. In rabbits, lancing and flushing is seldom curative, even in combination with aggressive antibacterial therapy, and relapse is common.

The immune response of rabbits affected by abscesses has been investigated. Rabbits that have an existing chronic abscess show reduced neutrophil influx into a new acute abscess in comparison to rabbits without an existing abscess (Bamberger *et al.*, 1989). *In vitro* studies have demonstrated that blood neutrophils from rabbits with long-standing abscesses show a decreased chemotaxis to *S. aureus* in comparison with neutrophils from rabbits with acute abscesses. Bamberger and Herndon (1990) also found that neutrophils from rabbits with chronic abscesses (2 weeks old) have diminished bactericidal capacity and superoxide function. Superoxide is a free radical that is involved in the destruction of bacteria within the neutrophil. The rabbits with chronic abscesses did not produce serum opsonic factors. Opsonins are substances such as antibody or complement that render bacteria more susceptible to phagocytosis. The abscess fluid from the rabbits with chronic abscesses was inhibitory to neutrophil function.

In pet rabbits, abscesses are often related to underlying dental disease. Periapical abscesses are common and result in extensive osteomyelitis. Microabscesses form within the bone. Malnourishment is associated with dental problems and can delay wound healing and exacerbate abscessation. Commercial rabbits kept in intensive conditions for meat or fur commonly develop abscesses in association with poor ventilation and sanitation (Cheeke *et al.*, 1982) where particularly pathogenic strains of *Staphylococcus aureus* or *Pasteurella multocida* can exist.

8.1 Causes of abscesses in pet rabbits

The causes of abscesses in pet rabbits are summarized in Table 8.1. It is important to ascertain the cause of abscess formation in order to institute appropriate therapy and remove the underlying cause. In dogs and cats, abscesses are usually due to penetrating injuries, especially bite wounds. Fights between rabbits can result in abscess formation or bite wounds can be inflicted on rabbits by dogs, cats, foxes or other predators. Penetrating wounds can also be caused by foreign bodies, such as seeds or pieces of hay that penetrate the skin or mucosal surfaces of the mouth. Haematogenous spread to distant sites can occur from any primary abscess and internal abscesses may develop in the thoracic cavity or abdomen.

In pet rabbits, most abscesses occur around the head and face and are associated with dental disease. They can be caused by overgrown crowns of maloccluded teeth that have penetrated the buccal mucosa or the skin on the lips. Alternatively, facial abscesses may be associated with infection at the apex of the teeth (see Figures 8.1–8.3). Acquired

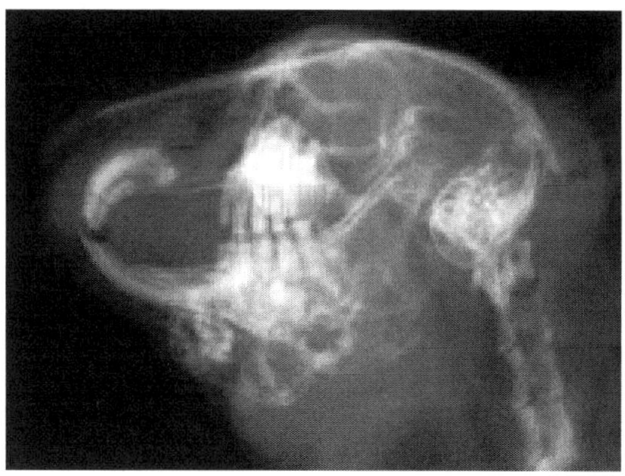

Figure 8.1. Lateral view of the skull of a rabbit with advanced osteomyelitis of the mandible. The figure shows a lateral view of the skull of a 3-year-old, female Netherland Dwarf. There is extensive osteomyelitis involving the roots of the mandibular cheek teeth and surrounding bone of one hemi-mandible. A large abscess was evident in which proliferative bone could be seen radiographically. This type of abscess carries a poor prognosis.

Table 8.1 Types of abscesses, treatment and prognosis. Any long-term therapy of abscesses in rabbits should include supportive care, i.e. good diet, opportunity to exercise, clean bedding, companionship, etc.

Appearance	*Site*	*Possible cause*	*Treatment*	*Prognosis*
External abscesses				
Superficial, encapsulated, mobile structures in skin	Anywhere	Puncture wounds of penetrating foreign bodies such as grass seeds Haematogenous spread	**Options** 1. Excision and postoperative systemic antibiotic 2. Or no treatment if abscess is longstanding and not causing problems	Good
	In scruff Close to another abscess	Following injections Lymphatic spread		
	On plantar aspect of feet	Associated with pressure and poor posture	Soft bedding is also required	
Subcutaneous swelling involving deeper tissue	Anywhere	Fight wounds	**Options** 1. Excision 2. Lancing and expressing pus prior to thorough debridement and placement of antibiotic beads 3. Marsupialization and topical treatment, e.g. honey and gentamicin drops Systemic antibiotics, e.g. enrofloxacin, are also indicated	Good
	On cheek	Elongated crowns, especially upper premolars penetrating buccal mucosa	Above treatment needs to be combined with tooth trimming	Good, although repetitive dental work may be necessary
Large, fast growing, soft subcutaneous swelling associated with skin necrosis	Anywhere, often on cheek or submandibular	Penetrating wounds, especially from teeth Flare up of long-standing abscesses involving deeper structures	• Culture and sensitivity, as unusual organisms may be involved • Surgical drainage in initial stages. Surgical investigation after antibiotic therapy may be required • Sytemic antibiotics with good tissue penetration, e.g cephalexin or enrofloxacin • Analgesia. NSAIDS, e.g. carprofen or meloxicam and opioids such as buprenorphine	Prognosis is variable and depends on cause Follow up radiography and treatment may be necessary

continued

dental disease in pet rabbits is characterized by demineralization of the alveolar bone supporting the teeth. The periodontal space widens and the teeth become loose. Extraneous plant material can become impacted in the periodontal space. Periodontal disease can progress to allow periapical abscesses to develop. Once infection has reached the apex

Table 8.1 *Continued*

Appearance	*Site*	*Possible cause*	*Treatment*	*Prognosis*
External abscesses				
Firm encapsulated swellings adherent to underlying bone on face May be multiple Can be associated with other symptoms caused by abscesses within the skull, e.g. nasal discharge, dacrocystitis	Along ventral border of mandible On zygomatic prominence	Periapical infections of mandibular cheek teeth Usually associated with acquired dental disease May be caused by impacted food material or splinters entering periodontal space	Consider euthanasia **or** • Skull radiology • Culture and sensitivity • Oral examination • Exploration, thorough debridement and curettage • ?Apicectomy or tooth extraction • Antibiotic impregnated beads into abscess cavity • ?Calcium hydroxide in bony cavities (**Care with soft tissues**) • Systemic antibiotics with good penetration into bone, e.g. cephalexin, enrofloxacin • Analgesia. NSAIDS, e.g. carprofen or meloxicam and opioids such as buprenorphine	Variable Depends on extent and severity of underlying dental disease Cure is possible Relapse is common Expensive to treat Alterations of alignment of teeth can result in associated malocclusion
Chronic discharging sinus from abscess deep within the tissue	On cheek or submandibular Anywhere	Associated with dental disease, e.g periapical infection or due to advanced dental disease Chronic infection	**Options** 1. ?Euthanasia 2. Surgical removal and placement of antibiotic impregnated beads (unlikely to effect a cure, but may give period of remission) 3. Topical therapy with antiseptics such as chlorhexidene or povidone iodine **or** application of honey plus gentamicin twice daily 4. Long-term antibiotics, e.g oral enrofloxacin or parenteral oxytetracycline Long-term analgesia may be required, e.g. meloxicam ?Periodic culture and sensitivity	Cure is unlikely but not impossible Rabbits will require constant care and nursing from owners Rabbits can lead a relatively normal life for some months or even years Abscesses need assessing periodically to ensure that a new problem such as elongated crowns has not developed
Swollen, painful joints associated with lameness	Any joint can be affected but most common is the tarsus in association with ulcerative pododermatitis	Haematogenous spread Ulcerative pododermatits is predisposed by immobility due to cramped housing, illness, obesity or pain from another condition such as	• Consider euthanasia **or** • Radiography • Culture and sensitivity • Long-term systemic antibiotic • Clean, dry soft bedding. ?weight reduction. • Analgesia. NSAIDS and opioids	Poor prognosis May be permanent damage to structure of joint causing permanent disability even if infection is controlled

continued

		spondylosis. The condition is exacerbated by poor conformation, thin exposed skin, hard floorings and dirty conditions	**Options** 1. Lance and flush (aggressive flushing can disseminate infection further) 2. Surgical debridement (may cause further damage) 3. Amputation	Amputation may not solve the underlying problem and can add to immobility and increased pressure on remaining joints
Internal abscesses				
Abscesses caused by penetration of nasal passages or retrobulbar space by elongated roots of the maxillary teeth	May be manifested by exophthalmos, severe purulent dacrocystitis, nasal obstruction or nasal discharge	Acquired dental disease Abscesses may have been developing for some time before symptoms appear	• Consider euthanasia **or** • Identify and extract affected teeth if possible • Supportive care, long-term antibiotics and analgesics • ?Enucleation to expose and drain abscess cavity and place antibiotic impregnated bead or treat as draining abscess • Drainage of retrobulbar space by aspiration, followed by flushing and placement of antibiotic impregnated bead • ?Nasolacrimal duct flushing	Poor prognosis Usually associated with generalized advanced dental disease Abscesses in nasal cavities are inaccessible
Abdominal masses	Abscesses associated with uterus or ovaries or as masses in peritoneal cavity that are adherent to surrounding structures	Bacteraemia Pasteurellosis Abdominal surgery	**Options** 1. Euthanasia 2. Surgical removal and systemic antibiotics (Ovariohysterectomy may be required) 3. Leave alone and give long-term antibiotic therapy	Poor due to adhesion formation with surrounding structures that makes surgical removal difficult or impossible
Abscesses along vestibular tract	Brain (causing vestibular disease)	Ascending pasteurellosis from nasal cavity via eustachian tube and middle ear	**Options** 1. Euthanasia 2. Supportive care, long-term antibiotics and analgesics 3. Bulla osteotomy	Poor
Abscesses in thoracic cavity		Haematogenous spread Pasteurellosis Penetrating bite wounds	**Options** 1. Euthanasia 2. Supportive care, long-term antibiotics and analgesics	Poor

of the tooth, the structure of the root is destroyed and the surrounding alveolar bone becomes infected. Microabscesses can form throughout the surrounding bone (see Figure 8.1). Once osteomyelitis has become established, the prognosis is poor (Westerhof and Lumeij, 1987; Bohmer and Kostlin, 1988; Harcourt-Brown, 1995; Jenkins, 1997).

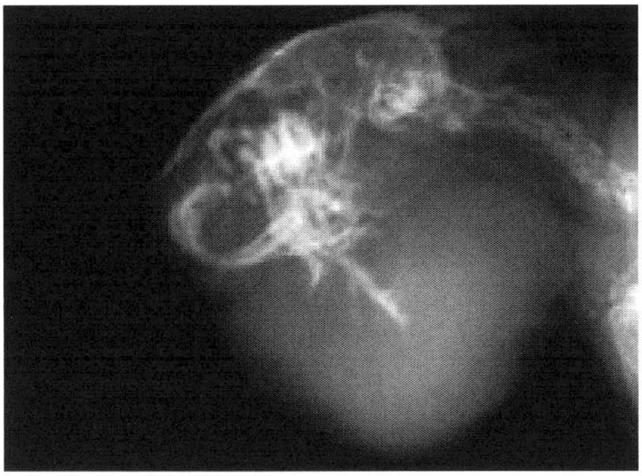

Figure 8.2. Lateral view of the skull of a rabbit with multiple abscesses associated with tooth roots that have penetrated the bone and continued to grow (image reproduced with kind permission from Waltham Focus). The figure shows a lateral view of the skull of a rabbit suffering from advanced dental disease. Several tooth roots are growing into abscess cavities. The abscess under the chin contained a tooth root that was several centimetres long and was curling round in the cavity. The root of an upper second premolar is also elongated and curling round in an abscess involving the nasal cavity. Multiple abscesses in association with advanced dental disease carry a poor prognosis.

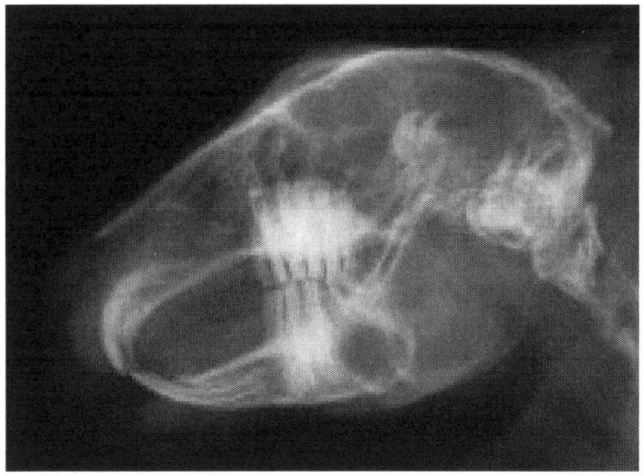

Figure 8.3. Lateral view of the skull of a rabbit with an abscess to show radiolucency. The figure shows an area of radiolucency in the mandible associated with periapical infection of the second mandibular molar (fourth cheek tooth). This 1-year-old female mixed breed rabbit had developed a palpable abscess over the lateral ramus 6 months prior to the radiograph. A large splinter of wood was wedged in the alveolar socket. The tooth was removed and the abscess successfully treated with antibiotic impregnated beads. The rabbit subsequently developed an abscess in exactly the same place on the contralateral jaw. She spent her life in the garden where she would dig holes and chew through twigs and tree roots. The area of lytic bone shows clearly because there is no superimposition of the contralateral tooth.

8.2 Diagnosis of abscesses in rabbits

Abscesses in rabbits can be classified according to their clinical appearance and characteristics (Harvey, 1997). The prognosis varies with the type of abscess and each type requires a different approach (see Table 8.1). In most species, the development of an abscess is characterized by pain, accompanied by malaise and pyrexia. In rabbits, abscesses often do not appear to be painful and the animal may be eating well and not depressed. Pyrexia is not a feature of abscesses in rabbits.

Perapical abscesses are the most common type and occur at typical sites in association with elongated tooth roots (Harcourt-Brown, 1995) (see Figure 7.1). Abscesses affecting the apex of the mandibular teeth can be palpated along the mandible and present as slow growing subcutaneous swellings that may be mobile or may be adherent to deeper tissue. Neoplasia is a differential diagnosis. Osteogenic sarcoma has been recorded in the jaw in rabbits (Walberg, 1981) but is rare. Periapical abscesses of the maxillary teeth invade the nasal passages or periorbital space and cannot be palpated unless they have distorted the surrounding bone. Retrobulbar abscesses cause exophthalmos and can require enucleation of the eye to make a definitive diagnosis, although it is sometimes possible to aspirate the abscess by inserting a needle into the periorbital space. Tumours and cysts can also occur at this site. Abscesses within the nasal cavity require endoscopic confirmation, although a presumptive diagnosis can be made radiologically (see Plate 17). Affected rabbits may or may not show signs of respiratory tract obstruction such as a purulent nasal discharge, laboured breathing or upper respiratory noise. Nasal foreign bodies cause similar symptoms, which are usually unilateral (see Section 13.3). Chronic pasteurellosis also causes chronic purulent nasal discharge and upper respiratory tract disease (see Section 13.2.3). Abscesses around the apex of the maxillary incisors or premolars can obstruct the nasolacrimal duct and cause chronic dacrocystitis. Bony swellings of the zygomatic prominence can be palpated in association with abscesses at this site (see Plate 16). Occasionally they will burst and discharge pus. The cheek is also the site of an abscess caused by penetration of the buccal mucosa by elongated crowns of the upper cheek teeth. Elongated crowns can be detected on careful examination of the oral cavity.

Superficial abscesses around the body can be palpated easily. Abscesses caused by bite wounds or penetrating injuries are usually associated with a history of a fight and may have a visible skin wound at the site of penetration. Abscessed joints are swollen and painful and the rabbit is lame. Internal abscesses can be difficult to diagnose. Large abscesses can develop within the abdomen without obvious clinical signs. They may involve the reproductive tract or be associated with adhesions. Symptoms only develop if adhesions interfere with digestive function. Lung abscesses impair respiratory function and cause dyspnoea, although symptoms may not be evident in the early stages of the disease when the rabbit is at rest.

Haematology is seldom diagnostic. Rabbits with abscesses do not seem to show a leucocytosis and neutrophilia, although a left shift is occasionally seen. Instead, non-specific signs of ill heath such as mild anaemia and lymphopaenia are encountered (see Figure 6.1). An increased monocyte count may be found in rabbits affected by abscesses, although monocyte counts within the laboratory reference do signify the absence of an abscess (see Section 6.2). Ultrasound scanning is a useful diagnostic aid to differentiate between internal abscesses and neoplasms. Radiology can also be useful. Some abscesses contain gritty, calcified material that shows up radiologically or ultrasonographically.

8.2.1 Radiology

Radiology can be used to determine the underlying cause of abscesses in rabbits and to ascertain the extent of bone destruction in cases of osteomyelitis. Radiography is indicated for any abscess involving underlying bone, i.e. facial abscesses or those affecting limbs or joints. Radiology of the skull is described in Section 7.8. Periapical abscesses may be a localized entity or part of a more serious disease process affecting the whole skull (see Figure 8.1). Abscessation is often the end point of acquired dental disease in rabbits (see Box 7.1). Lateral and dorsoventral skull radiographs are necessary to assess the general state of the teeth and surrounding bone and to offer a prognosis. If the abscess is localized, it may be possible to identify the infected tooth from skull radiographs. Affected roots are often long and distorted (see Figure 8.2) or an area of radiolucency around the root may be seen (see Figure 8.3). Intraoral views on dental film are useful to assess changes that have taken place in association with infection of a specific tooth root. Flushing the cavity and instilling contrast medium can yield additional information about the extent of an abscess cavity.

Radiography is necessary for the assessment of abscesses involving joints or long bones. If there is extensive bone destruction or multiple limbs are involved the prognosis is poor. Although amputation can be an option if a single joint is involved, it increases the pressure on the remaining limbs and can result in ulcerative pododermatitis (see Section 9.10)

8.2.2 Bacteriology

Wherever possible, swabs should be taken for bacteriology and sensitivity. Although *Pasteurella multocida* is often believed to be the pathogen in rabbit abscesses, this is not always the case. *Staphylococcus aureus* is often found and other bacteria such as *Bacteroides*, *Pseudomonas* or *Proteus* can also be isolated

Key points 8.1

- Abscesses consist of a thick fibrous capsule containing pus that is composed of neutrophils, fluid and cellular debris
- Abscesses in rabbits tend to be slow growing, relatively painless and contain thick caseous pus
- Lancing and flushing abscesses in rabbits is seldom curative
- In order to cure abscesses in pet rabbits, it is important to identify and treat the underlying cause
- Neoplasia is a differential diagnosis
- Periapical abscesses occur frequently.
- Periapical abscesses of the mandibular teeth can be palpated
- Periapical abscesses of the maxillary teeth cannot be palpated. Tooth roots invade the nasal cavity or retrobulbar space and can cause secondary clinical signs such as exophthalmos, dacryocystitis, occlusion of the nasal cavity and purulent nasal discharge
- Malnourishment and stress associated with dental disease can delay wound healing
- Nasal foreign bodies, usually pieces of hay, can lodge in the nasal cavity and can be a differential diagnosis. Chronic pasteurellosis can cause chronic nasal discharge
- Radiology is necessary to assess the extent of tissue damage in abscesses that involve bone, i.e. facial abscesses or those involving a joint
- Radiology and ultrasonography are useful diagnostic aids for diagnosis of internal abscesses
- Haematology is seldom diagnostic
- Culture and sensitivity identifies the causative organism and aids antibiotic selection although sterile cultures may be obtained
- Bacteria are more likely to be cultured from a swab taken from the wall of an abscess than from the contents
- A variety of organisms can be cultured from abscesses in rabbits including *Pasteurella multocida, Staphylococcus aureus.*

(Hillyer, 1997). Swabbing the interior wall of the capsule of an abscess cavity is less likely to give a sterile culture than swabbing purulent contents.

8.3 Treatment of abscesses

The factors that improve success in treating rabbit abscesses are summarized in Box 8.1. Treatment is directed at removing as much exudate, necrotic debris and infected tissue as possible and mopping up residual infection with antibiotics. Removal of the underlying cause and improving the health status of the rabbit are required to prevent recurrence. Treatment can prove expensive because of the need for repeated anaesthetics and the cost of diagnostic workup, surgical exploration and long-term antibacterial therapy. Many different treatments for abscesses in rabbits have been described. Placing gentamicin soaked collagen material into the abscess cavity was described by Bohmer and Kostlin (1988). Implantation of punctured clindamycin capsules into the cavity was described by Chappell (1994). Remeeus and Verbeek (1995) recommended packing abscess cavities with calcium hydroxide. Brown (personal communication) has had some success with injecting the abscess capsule in multiple sites with

Box 8.1 Basic principles of treatment for abscesses in rabbits

- Identify underlying cause. Thorough visual examination of the crowns of the teeth and radiological examination of the roots is required for all facial abscesses
- Remove focus of infection, e.g. trim elongated crowns, remove infected tooth roots, foreign bodies or infected bone
- Remove as much exudate and infected tissue as possible. Excise the whole abscess or explore cavities thoroughly and debride away all necrotic tissue
- Minimize contamination of surrounding tissues. Aspirate pus through a syringe or remove with a scoop. Vigorous flushing can spread infection deeper into tissues
- Use antibiotic therapy to mop up residual infection. An effective antibiotic against the causal organism that reaches infected tissue at therapeutic levels is required. Culture and sensitivity are indicated
- Improve the general health status of the patient. Dietary modification, opportunity to exercise, companionship, comfortable bedding, etc.

gentamicin. Other authors recommend long-term or permanent systemic antibiotic therapy (Hillyer, 1997) while others suggest the placement of drains in the abscess cavity (Malley, 1995). Setons were used by Hinton (1979). The use of creams and sprays containing digestive enzymes (trypsin) is described by Jenkins (1997). Blackwell (1999) describes the use of intramammary suspensions to pack abscess cavities after flushing the cavity with saline. As there is such a wide range of treatment options, it is obvious that there is no universal cure for abscesses in rabbits and each case has to be judged on its own merit. The prognosis depends on the underlying cause (see Table 8.1).

In some cases, owners may opt for no treatment at all. Not all rabbits with abscesses are ill and many do not appear to be in pain. The abscess may be well encapsulated and slow growing. There can be multiple abscesses present. Although it is not ideal, these cases can be left alone or treated conservatively with long-term antibiotic therapy. The abscess can remain as an encapsulated swelling, during which the rabbit can lead a relatively normal life. Occasionally, the abscess will become completely walled off or even regress altogether, although this is unusual.

Providing optimum nutrition and raising the patient's general health status is an important part of any treatment protocol for abscesses in rabbits. Many abscesses are associated with dental problems that are debilitating. Underlying metabolic bone disease is often present. If possible, dietary modification to include sufficient calcium and vitamin D and plenty of indigestible fibre is beneficial. In advanced cases of dental disease, it is not always possible to introduce abrasive foods such as hay or fibrous vegetables and the patient may need to be maintained on shredded or pureed vegetables and softened foods. Companionship from another rabbit, daily exercise and the opportunity to browse and lie in the sun is mentally and physically beneficial.

8.3.1 Surgical exploration or removal of abscesses

Surgical removal of the entire abscess, including the fibrous capsule is the treatment of choice for rabbit abscesses, although it is not always possible. For example, surgical removal is not possible if the abscess originates from osteomyelitic bone, infected tooth roots, septic joints or multiple sites. Remnants of dead bone can impair bacterial clearance from the site (Masem *et al.*, 1990). Attempting to remove an abscess in its entirety also helps to identify the source of infection.

Prior to surgical exploration of an abscess, the hair is clipped and the skin prepared for surgery. It is important to minimize contamination of surrounding tissues as far as possible. The skin over the abscess is incised before dissecting through the underlying tissues to expose the capsule. If the abscess is freely mobile then it can be dissected out in a similar fashion to a tumour. If the abscess is attached to surrounding tissue, the pus can be drained through a tiny incision in the capsule using a syringe. After most of the pus has been removed and the capsule is no longer under pressure, the incision can be extended to expose the interior of the cavity, which is then debrided thoroughly. A Volkmann's scoop is a useful instrument for removing pus and debriding and removing infected tissue. It is important to remove all necrotic and diseased tissue. Some abscesses have fibrous tracks that connect with other abscesses deep in the tissue. Catheters can be used as probes to flush pus from deeper cavities. Loose infected teeth need to be removed from periapical abscesses (see Section 7.10.3). In some cases, elongated roots that are still growing are found within abscess cavities, curling around in the midst of the pus. Occasionally, it is possible to perform an apicectomy, remove infected tooth roots, and leave the healthy portion of the tooth including the crown *in situ*. This procedure is only successful if there is healthy bone between the gingival margin and the abscess cavity. After debridement, it may be possible to dissect out and remove the abscess capsule. All tracks and sinuses should be explored to ensure that no pockets of infection remain and that all infected bone and foreign bodies, such as hayseeds, are removed. The abscess can then be packed and stitched or left open to drain. Packing the cavity with antibiotic impregnated beads provides high concentrations of antibiotic at the abscess site, the wound is stitched and is aesthetically more pleasing to the owner than an open abscess cavity that is treated topically.

8.3.2 Topical treatment

In other species, lancing, flushing and instilling some kind of topical treatment into an abscess is often the only treatment that is required to cure an abscess. In rabbits, it is unlikely that lancing and flushing will effect a permanent cure, although it can be effective for some superficial abscesses caused by penetrating injuries. Usually, once a hole is made through the capsule, purulent material continues to drain and contaminates the surrounding skin and fur. The wound does not heal quickly, if at all, and requires constant cleaning and bathing. Some owners are prepared to cope with a chronic discharging abscess and will clean and dress the cavity daily rather than opt for surgery or euthanasia. Draining abscesses can be managed by daily flushing and the instillation of some type of antiseptic solution. The selection of a safe antibiotic is important because rabbits can ingest the compound during licking and grooming and develop antibiotic-associated diarrhoea. Sinuses from periapical abscesses into the mouth are a potential route for oral ingestion of instilled antibiotic preparations. The most useful non-toxic topical antibiotics are gentamicin, tobramicin, fluoroquinolones, chloramphenicol and metronidazole.

Although abscess cavities can be treated with antiseptic preparations such as chlorhexidene or povidone iodine solutions, they are seldom curative. Strong sugar solutions are an alternative, safe topical remedy, which is effective and sometimes curative. Concentrated sugar solutions have hygroscopic and bactericidal properties. The sugar molecules 'tie up' water molecules so that bacteria have insufficient water to support growth. In humans, *'even the most offensive wounds are usually fully deodourised within three days'* if they are treated with strong sugar solutions (Morgan, 1988). Malodour in wounds is due to ammonia, amines and sulphur compounds that are produced by bacterial degradation of proteins in serum and necrotic tissue. If glucose is available as a substrate, lactic acid is produced as an end product rather than the malodorous compounds (Molan, 1999).

In addition to its hygroscopic effects, honey has other antibacterial properties and also stimulates wound healing. It has been used to treat infected wounds in humans for centuries. Recent studies have shown that honey is effective against a range of bacteria, including antibiotic-resistant, coagulase-positive *Staphylococcus aureus* infections. Honey promotes wound healing. It is a mixture of bees' saliva and glucose and fructose that have been converted from sucrose. Bees' saliva contains enzymes such as glucose oxidase that converts glucose to gluconic acid, which is antibacterial. Glucose in honey is also enzymatically converted to hydrogen peroxide, which is also antibacterial. The potency of honey varies with the flower that it is made from. Some flowers provide additional antibacterial components, such as flavonoids and aromatic acids in the nectar (Molan, 1999). Honey from the New Zealand tea tree, called manuka, is reputed to have the most antibacterial properties. Australian honey from the jelly bush (also a tea tree) also has a good reputation (Lord, 2000).

Honey promotes the formation of clean, healthy granulation tissue. It acidifies the wound and promotes healing. Animal studies have confirmed that the application of honey accelerates wound healing in rabbits (Bergman *et al.*, 1983). Controlled studies in infected wounds in rabbits showed that treated lesions showed less oedema, fewer polymorphonuclear and mononuclear cell infiltration, less necrosis, better wound contraction, improved epithelialization and lower glucosaminoglycan and proteoglycan concentrations postoperatively (Oryan and Zaker, 1998).

Owners can be shown how to instill clear unboiled honey into an abscess through a syringe. Prior to treatment, surgical drainage, debridement and removal of all pus and necrotic tissue from the abscess cavity are necessary. The honey has to be introduced into the cavity and not just on to the external wound. It may be combined with an application of a topical antibiotic such as gentamicin drops. Twice daily application is satisfactory. Most rabbits find honey palatable and will constantly clean and lick the wound, which provides additional drainage that is beneficial. The honey dries to a thick plug that needs to be removed prior to each application. Like any treatment protocol for rabbit abscesses, this method is not universally successful but can be curative, even for some intractable abscesses. Treatment can be continued for weeks. Honey has the added advantage of being cheap and non-toxic.

8.3.3 Antibacterial therapy

The use of antibiotics in rabbits is not as straightforward as in other species. The correct balance of microorganisms in the caecum is important for digestion and good health. Oral antibiotics can upset the balance of bacteria permitting overgrowth of pathogenic species such as clostridia and result in enterotoxaemia (see Section 4.1.3). Parenteral antibiotics are less likely to interfere with caecal microflora than oral preparations. In rabbits, the selection of an antibiotic for the treatment of abscesses not only depends on the sensitivity of the causative organism but also its effect on the gut flora and its distribution in infected tissue. Some of the antibiotics that are indicated for osteomyelitis in other species are likely to interfere with the gut flora in rabbits. For example, clindamycin and lincomycin are high-risk antibiotics and can cause a fatal enterotoxaemia. *Pasteurella multocida* is usually resistant to clindamycin and lincomycin anyway (Manning *et al.*,1989). Effective antimicrobial therapy for *Pasteurella* spp. includes cephalosporin, ampicillins and gentamicin with tetracyclines as a second choice (Knight *et al.*, 1980). Penicillin-related antibiotics are effective against staphylococci. The efficacy of some antibiotics, such as potentiated sulphonamides, is limited because they are inactivated by exudate and debris (Whittem and Gaon, 1998). A summary of antibiotic therapy for rabbits is given in Table 4.1.

Enrofloxacin is a broad-spectrum antibiotic that is licensed for use in rabbits and does not appear to cause digestive problems, even when administered over long periods. It is available as an oral preparation and can be administered by owners. Tissue levels two to three times higher than that found in serum have been demonstrated in laboratory animals. Organs in which high levels can be expected are the lungs, liver, kidney, skin, bone and lymphatic system (Product datasheet). In order to maintain minimum inhibitory concentrations of enrofloxacin for

Key points 8.2

- Successful treatment of abscesses in rabbits can be time consuming and expensive. Anaesthesia and surgery are necessary and most cases require radiology and bacteriology. Relapse is common and surgery may need to be repeated on several occasions
- Many rabbit abscesses require surgical removal or debridement
- Antibiotic therapy is only part of the treatment protocol for abscesses
- Most antibiotics that are effective in the treatment of sepsis in other species will cause enterotoxaemia in rabbits. Clindamycin and lincomycin are high-risk antibiotics in rabbits
- Tissue penetration and efficacy against the causative organism are considerations when selecting antibiotics to treat abscesses. Trimethoprim combinations are inactivated by purulent material
- Enrofloxacin is licensed for use in rabbits and can be given for prolonged periods, even by the oral route
- Long-acting injectable preparations of oxytetracycline or penicillin can be used to control infection in cases that cannot be cured
- Cephalosporins are effective against *Pasteurella multocida* and can be given parenterally. Oral cephalosporin preparations are not suitable for rabbits
- Clear unboiled honey can be used as a cheap, effective, topical therapy for abscesses in rabbits. It is sterile, non-toxic and has hygroscopic and antiseptic properties
- Australian honey or New Zealand (manuka) honey is reputed to have greater antibacterial properties than other honeys
- Topical treatment with honey can be combined with instillation of a 'safe' antibiotic such as gentamicin, tobramicin, enrofloxacin, chloramphenicol or metronidazole
- Conservative treatment with long-term antibiotics and analgesics may be indicated for rabbits with incurable abscesses. Dedicated owners may opt for cleaning and dressing discharging abscesses rather than euthanasia
- Perapical abscesses usually require tooth extraction. Apicectomy is occasionally possible if there is healthy bone between the gingival margin and the abscess cavity
- A Volkmann's scoop is useful to scoop pus from the abscess cavity and to debride the cavity.

Pasteurella multocida, 12 hourly dosing of 5 mg/kg is required (Broome *et al.*, 1991). Even this regimen may not achieve sufficient tissue concentrations to eliminate infection from the nasal cavity, trachea, middle ear and outer ear where *Pasteurella multocida* resides (Mähler *et al.*, 1995). Oral administration of 10 mg/kg twice daily can be given for long periods to rabbits and is more likely to achieve therapeutic tissue levels. Tilmicosin has been advocated as treatment for recalcitrant abscesses but the antibiotic carries a risk of causing a fatal adverse reaction in rabbits (see Section 4.2.1.11)

A variety of techniques can be used to deliver high levels of antibiotic to an abscess site without long-term systemic administration. These techniques include instillation of drops, injecting the abscess capsule with antibiotic or implanting antibiotic capsules, impregnated beads or collagen into the cavity.

8.3.4 Antibiotic impregnated polymethylmethacrylate (PMMA) beads

Polymethylmethacrylate (PMMA) is a high-density plastic formed by combining a fluid monomer and powdered polymer. The plastic is used as bone cement in a variety of orthopaedic operations including hip replacement in humans and in dogs. PMMA does not significantly affect the immune response of the body (Henry and Galloway, 1995) but has a slight long-term bacteriostatic effect (Chapman and Hadley, 1976). Freeze dried gentamicin was incorporated into PMMA bone cement for hip replacement after it was discovered that local concentrations of the antibiotic exceeded minimum inhibitory concentrations (MIC) of most pathogens for a prolonged period. Gentamicin impregnated beads of PMMA have also been used in the treatment of chronic osteomyelitis in humans (Klemm, 1993). Antibiotics leach out of PMMA beads in a bimodal fashion. Elution is rapid during the first few days after which the antibiotic elutes slowly over a period of weeks to months. Approximately 5% of the total amount of antibiotic is released into the surrounding tissue in the first 24 h. The initial concentration of antibiotic in local tissue is very high but is low systemically thereby avoiding some of the complications that can occur with systemic antibiotic therapy. The diffusion rate of an antibiotic from PMMA beads is determined by the type of cement, the antibiotic's diffusion coefficients, the concentration of the antibiotic and the size, surface area and roughness of the bead. Diffusion is also affected by the amount of fluid that moves past the bead (Calhoun and Mader, 1989). Vascular tissue such as muscle or granulation tissue has higher absorption and removal of antibiotic from the implantation site. Serum and urine concentrations of gentamicin in human patients with implanted PMMA are low and beads can be placed in patients with renal insufficiency. In a study by Chapman and Hadley (1976), no detectable antibiotic was found in tissue and serum samples from rabbits with gentamicin impregnated PMMA beads implanted in the tibia. The entire antibiotic had eluted from the beads over a period of 37 days. Negligible serum levels of antibiotic are also found after implantation of impregnated beads in vascular sites such as muscle (Alpert *et al.*, 1989).

Not all antibiotics are suitable for PMMA bead impregnation. Tetracyclines, chloramphenicol and erythromycin do not elute well from polymethylmethacrylate. The exothermic heat that is generated during the hardening process has an adverse effect on these antibiotics. Conversely, penicillins, cephalosporins, aminoglycosides and lincosamides have shown good release rates during *in vitro* testing. Combining two or more antibiotics affects the rate of elution from the bead (Tobias *et al.*, 1996).

Gentamicin is the most frequently used antibiotic in bone cement in human medicine. Ready-made beads can be purchased already impregnated with the antibiotic (Septopal, Merck). In the USA, tobramycin has been used successfully as an alternative to gentamicin due to problems in obtaining gentamicin beads (Tobias *et al.*, 1996). No information about the suitability of fluoroquinolones in impregnated beads could be found at the time of writing.

8.3.4.1 Use of antibiotic impregnated beads in veterinary medicine

Antibiotic impregnated PMMA beads have been used in veterinary medicine for the treatment of a variety of diseases. For example, septic arthritis and osteomyelitis in the digit of a bull (Trostle *et al.*, 1996), infective synovitis in horses and cattle (Butson *et al.*, 1996), chronic osteomyelitis and cellulitis in a juvenile bald eagle (Wheler *et al.*, 1996) and in 185 cases of bumblefoot in raptors (Remple and Forbes, 2001).

Osteomyelitis is a serious complication of compound fractures in humans. For many years, the possibility of treating the condition with local administration of high concentrations of antibiotics has been explored, often using rabbits as experimental models of the disease. Typically, *Staphylococcus aureus* is inoculated into a metaphysis or fracture site in a bone such as the tibia or a dorsal spinous process to induce osteomyelitis. Various antibiotics and methods of delivery have been tested in rabbits including ampicillin, gentamicin, clindamycin, cefazolin, cephalothin and tobramycin in beads made from PMMA, hydroxyapatite (bone graft substitute) or biodegradable poly-DL-lactide-coglycolide (Chapman and Hadley, 1976; Keogh *et al.*, 1989; Jacob *et al.*, 1991; Seligson *et al.*, 1992; Cornell *et al.*, 1993). Results from one study showed a 100% success rate for combined systemic cephalosporin and implanted gentamicin impregnated beads (Septopal, Merck) in rabbits with experimentally induced osteomyelitis. The wounds contained devascularized bone contaminated with *Staphylococcus aureus* (Evans and Nelson, 1993).

8.3.4.2 Manufacturing antibiotic impregnated polymethylmethacrylate (PMMA) beads

Antibiotic impregnated PMMA beads can be purchased in small quantities already impregnated with gentamicin or they can be made by hand. Ready-made beads (Septopal, Merck) measure 7 mm in diameter, which is quite large for some abscess cavities but has the advantage of convenience and sterility. Making beads by hand is time consuming but has the advantage of producing a range of size and shape of bead. Beads can be made from gentamicin impregnated bone cement that is available as a pack of the powdered polymer and liquid monomer designed to be mixed together just before use. Bone cement can be purchased from suppliers of orthopaedic equipment (Veterinary Instrumentation, Sheffield). Once the pack is opened, all the cement must be mixed, as unused portions do not keep. The cement takes approximately 15 minutes to harden so it is important to be prepared to work quickly to make all the cement into small beads before it sets. In human surgery, the beads are made on a thread to form a chain. It is not easy to do this when hand manufacturing beads. Individual ones are just as useful. A 20 g pack of sterile bone cement (CMW1Gentamicin Bone Cement, DePuy) makes a large number of beads.

Plain cement can be used to incorporate different antibiotics, if required. Ideally, a pre-sterilized monomer and methacrylate powder should be used, although the liquid monomer is effective in killing most bacteria including *Staphylococcus aureus*, *Escherichia coli*, β-haemolytic streptococci and *Staphylococcus pyogenes*. Some *Bacillus* spp. can survive (Chapman and Hadley, 1976). The exothermic reaction, which takes place during the curing process, has some effect on bacterial viability. In order to avoid sterilization, the beads can be prepared from sterile bone cement in an aseptic manner by personnel who have scrubbed up. Batches of beads can then be stored in sterile universal containers. If sterilization is necessary, the beads require cold sterilization with ethylene oxide because autoclaving can cause a loss in antimicrobial potency (Wheler *et al.*, 1996). Beads that have been sterilized with ethylene oxide should be aerated for 24 h to ensure the gas has dissipated. Beads can be stored for several months in sterile universal containers.

The ratio of powdered monomer to liquid is 2:1 to make up PMMA for use as bone cement. If antibiotics are to be added to the mixture, a ratio of 3:1 may be preferable because it produces a lower peak temperature during the curing process. The 2:1 mixture heats to approximately 75°C in comparison with 65°C generated by the 3:1 mixture. The amount of antibiotic that is used in bead manufacture is empirical; 1–2 g of antibiotic powder are added to 40–60 g of PMMA powder, although larger quantities have been used (Wheler *et al.*, 1996). Liquid antibiotics can be used but affect the hardness of the cement. The ratio of antibiotic to PMMA and how the beads are formed affect the diffusion of antibiotic into the surrounding tissue. High concentrations of antibiotic powder result in large pores in the cement and increase the rate of elution of antibiotic from the bead. Homogeneous distribution of the antibiotic is achieved by mixing it with the liquid monomer prior to adding it to the polymethacrylate powder. A maximum ratio of 1:5 of powdered antibiotic:powdered polymer has been recommended for bead fabrication (Calhoun and Mader, 1989). If more antibiotic is used, the cement will not harden properly.

8.3.4.3 Antibiotic impregnated plaster of Paris beads

Alternatives to polymethylmethacrylate have been investigated *in vitro* (Miclau *et al.*, 1993) including bone graft, demineralized bone matrix and plaster of Paris. PMMA is used as bone cement because of its mechanical properties. Strength or shrinkage are not important for antibiotic impregnated beads that are only used as vehicles for local antibiotic administration. Plaster of Paris is cheaper than bone cement and is readily available. Small quantities can be used to make up beads containing antibiotic to which the organism is known to be sensitive. Plaster of Paris is well tolerated when implanted into infected bone cavities and is absorbed over a period of weeks to months. It effectively obliterates much of the dead space, leaving little room for haematoma formation and is replaced by bone of normal architecture (Mackey *et al.*, 1982). Modelling grade plaster of Paris can be sterilized by heating to 100°C in an dry oven for 4 h. Under sterile conditions, 10 g of powder is mixed with 7 ml of sterile water and the antibiotic that is to be incorporated. The mixture is either hand rolled into small beads or squeezed into a sterile mould from a syringe. Pellets of approximately 3–5 mm diameter are suitable for most abscess cavities. When the pellets have hardened, they can be stored in a cool place with silica gel desiccant.

Elution rates from plaster of Paris beads are significantly higher than from PMMA beads in the first 48 h (Bowyer and Cumberland, 1994) but are much lower than PMMA after this period.

Plaster of Paris beads have not been evaluated in the treatment of osteomyelitis in rabbits but may offer a cheaper, more convenient alternative to polymethylmethacrylate. They are unlikely to be successful in the treatment of chronic bone infections such as osteomyelitis or periapical infections but may be useful for initial or temporary treatment of abscesses.

8.3.4.4 Choice of antibiotic for impregnated beads in rabbits

Potentially, a wide range of antibiotics can be incorporated into antibiotic impregnated beads but the choice is severely limited in rabbits because of the risk of antibiotic-associated diarrhoea. Although antibiotics such as cephalosporins, penicillin, ampicillin, cloxacillin, clindamycin, amoxycillin and flucloxacillin are suitable to incorporate into beads, they must not be used in rabbits in sites where there is a risk of oral ingestion. Rabbits will groom and lick exudate from the wounds on the face, limbs or other parts of the body. Antibiotics that are placed in facial abscesses can enter the oral cavity through fistulae.

Antibiotics that do not work well in PMMA beads include tetracyclines, chloramphenicol, polymixin, erythromycin and fusidic acid (Wheler *et al.*, 1996). Fusidic acid elutes well from plaster of Paris beads over a long period of time.

Gentamicin is the antibiotic of choice for impregnated beads because it withstands the heat generated during the curing process, elutes well from PMMA, is unlikely to cause antibiotic-associated diarrhoea and is effective against many species of *Pasteurella multocida*. Tobramycin also elutes satisfactorily from PMMA (Flick *et al.*, 1987).

8.3.4.5 Implantation of antibiotic impregnated beads

Antibiotic impregnated beads are only effective if the area has been thoroughly debrided and all necrotic tissue removed. Purulent material binds and inactivates some antibiotics including aminoglycosides such as gentamicin (Elliott, 1998). Simply lancing and flushing an abscess and placing a bead in the cavity is unlikely to be effective. Following surgical debridement of the abscess and implantation of the impregnated bead, antibiotic is leached from the PMMA into the haematoma and wound secretions. The antibiotic is only effective for 2–3 mm around the bead (Tobias *et al.*, 1996). Closure of the wound is required to keep the beads in place but the presence of suture material in wounds carries a risk of secondary abscess formation because buried suture material can form a nidus for infection. Therefore, it is advisable to use as few sutures as possible, especially in deeper tissues. If possible, skin sutures alone should be used to keep the beads in place. If buried sutures are necessary, the risk of infection can be minimized by using fine suture materials and small knots. Monofilament suture materials withstand contamination better than multifilament sutures so materials such as polydioxanone (PDS, Ethicon) or poliglacaprone (Monocryl, Ethicon) are preferable to braided or multifilament materials. Bacteria can persist within the interstices of the braided fibre where they are resistant to removal by macrophages (Niles and Williams, 1999). Alternatively, rapidly absorbable materials such as catgut can be used that are degraded and removed from the wound along with any associated bacteria.

Polymethylmethacrylate beads should be left in place for at least 4 weeks. Occasionally, beads are discharged through the skin, in which case further debridement and placing another bead may be necessary. In most cases the beads become encased in fibrous tissue and can be left in place permanently. In unsuccessful cases, beads that have been in place for several months can act as a nidus for abscess formation and will require removal prior to further treatment of the abscess.

8.3.5 Calcium hydroxide

Calcium hydroxide is a substance that has been used in dentistry for many years for its astringent properties. It is available from veterinary wholesalers and suppliers of veterinary dental products in several forms including a powder that reacts with carbon dioxide in the air to form calcium carbonate. Calcium hydroxide powder should be kept in an airtight bottle with a silica gel bag and the surface layer discarded before use. In dentistry, calcium hydroxide is used to encourage mineralization and deposition of secondary dentine. It has bactericidal properties due to its high pH (12) and the alkaline environment it creates. However, calcium hydroxide does not penetrate necrotic tissue and only kills surface bacteria (Foreman and Barnes, 1990). Therefore, debridement and removal of diseased tissue is required before its application. Calcium hydroxide not only damages bacteria by its alkalinity but any other living tissue that it comes in contact with. It can cause serious soft tissue necrosis and should be used with care. It should not come in contact with soft tissues such as blood vessels, nerves, muscle or skin.

Calcium hydroxide has been used to treat facial abscesses in rabbits with some success. Remeuus and Virbeek (1995) described the procedure. The authors used artificial tears (Hypromellose, non-proprietary) or lignocaine to mix with the calcium hydroxide to form a paste which was loaded into a syringe and extruded into the abscess cavity after debridement and extraction of any associated loose teeth. The wound was left open. The calcium hydroxide hardened over time and the authors suggested removal after a week.

Calcium hydroxide can be useful to fill bony abscess cavities. It can be used to fill empty sockets after loose teeth have been removed to prevent fistula formation into the mouth. Any excess calcium hydroxide that enters the mouth must be removed promptly and thoroughly. Calcium hydroxide may also be used in conjunction with antibiotic impregnated beads. Calcium hydroxide was found to potentiate the effectiveness of tobramycin in polymethylmethacrylate beads in a study by Murakami *et al.* (1997), possibly by pH regulation or by its effects on bone metabolism.

The main problem with calcium hydroxide is its effects on soft tissue. It causes tissue necrosis and nerves, blood vessels and muscle can be seriously damaged. It is not universally effective as a remedy for abscesses but can be included in the treatment regimen for some cases, especially those that involve bone.

Key points 8.3

- Antibiotic impregnated beads can be implanted into abscess cavities to provide local high tissue concentrations of antibiotic. Polymethylmethacrylate, a substance that is used as bone cement, can be used to manufacture beads
- Gentamicin-impregnated beads can be purchased ready made (Septopal, Merck) or made by hand from gentamicin-impregnated bone cement
- If different antibiotics are required, they can be incorporated into plain bone cement or plaster of Paris for bead manufacture
- Plaster of Paris is not as satisfactory as polymethylmethacrylate but may be used as a short-term measure. It is cheaper and easier to use
- Tetracyclines, chloramphenicol and eythromycin are not suitable for impregnation of polymethylmethacrylate
- Penicillins, cephalosporins, aminoglycosides and lincosamides are suitable for polymethylmethacrylate bead manufacture although some of these antibiotics can cause fatal enteroxaemia if they are accidentally ingested. Gentamicin is one of the safest
- Antibiotic can enter the oral cavity through fistulae from perapical abscess cavities
- Antibiotic impregnated beads release antibiotic into tissue 2–3 mm around implantation site. They are only effective if all infected tissue has been thoroughly debrided and all the pus removed
- Antibiotic-impregnated beads may be left *in situ* or removed. Experimental studies with gentamicin-impregnated polymethylmethacrylate beads suggest that all the antibiotic has eluted by 37 days after implantation
- Some sutures are required to keep implanted antibiotic impregnated beads in place. The sutures can act as a nidus for abscess formation. Fine monofilament sutures and small knots minimize the risk
- Calcium hydroxide is an alkali with astringent properties. It can be used to kill surface bacteria within an abscess cavity and stimulate mineralization
- Calcium hydroxide has been used successfully to treat abscesses but should be used with great care as it can cause extensive soft tissue necrosis.

8.4 Prognosis for facial abscesses in rabbits

Facial abscesses in rabbits frequently recur and are often associated with dental disease. The prognosis for facial abscesses is more dependent on the extent of the underlying dental disease than on the choice of antibiotic or the species of bacteria present. Facial abscesses that have arisen from penetrating wounds caused by elongated crowns, fight wounds or foreign bodies carry a more favourable prognosis than periapical abscesses, as the initiating cause can be removed. However, abscesses that involve the jaw alter the alignment of the teeth and cause malocclusion, which becomes a further complication.

Periapical abscesses usually require thorough debridement and tooth removal for treatment to be effective and the potential complications of this procedure change according to the stage of dental disease. In the early stages, when the teeth are still growing, extraction of a tooth may result in distortion of an opposing tooth that can subsequently develop a long crown which can cause soft tissue damage. In the advanced stages, there is often extensive periosteal reaction around the tooth roots and surrounding bone that effectively welds the root into the bone making extraction impossible (see Plates 16 and 17). Conservative treatment is the only option. The position of the affected tooth also influences the prognosis. Mandibular abscesses involving the roots of the lower cheek teeth are easier to treat than abscesses involving the upper cheek teeth that have invaded the nasal cavity or retrobulbar space. The roots of the mandibular teeth are more accessible so that it is easier to provide effective drainage.

In the later stages of dental disease, there are often multiple abscesses and extensive pathology of the bones and teeth. Many of these animals are unable to chew and require softened food in order to survive. Euthanasia is probably the best option for these cases although some rabbits with chronic or multiple abscesses do not appear to be 'suffering' and still seem to enjoy life, so their owners may resist euthanasia. These cases will never be cured, although they can be managed conservatively with topical treatment, antibiotics and analgesics. They require life-long treatment.

References

Alpert, B., Colosi, T., von Fraunhofer, J.A., Seligson, D. (1989). The *in vivo* behavior of gentamicin-PMMA beads in the maxillofacial region (Abstract). *J Oral Maxillofac Surg.*, **47**, 46–49.

Bamberger, D.M., Herndon, B.L., Bettin, K.M., Gerding, D.N. (1989). Neutrophil chemotaxis and adherence *in vitro* and localisation *in vivo* in rabbits with *Staphylococcal aureus* abscesses (Abstract). *J Lab Clin Med.*, **114**, 135–141.

Bamberger, D.M., Herndon, B.L. (1990). Bactericidal capacity of neutrophils in rabbits with experimental acute and chronic abscesses (Abstract). *J Infect Dis.*, **162**, 186–192.

Bergman, A., Yanai J., Weiss J. *et al.* (1983). Acceleration of wound healing by topical application of honey. An animal model (Abstract). *Am J Surg.*, **145**, 374–376.

Blackwell, N.J. (1999). Abscesses in rabbits. *Vet Rec.*, **144**, 540.

Blood, D.C., Studdert, V.P. (1999). *Saunders Comprehensive Veterinary Dictionary*, 2nd edn. W.H. Saunders.

Bohmer, E., Kostlin, R.G. (1988). Dental disease of rabbits and rodents. *Der praktische Tierarzt*, **69**, 37–50.

Bowyer, G.W., Cumberland, N. (1994). Antibiotic release from impregnated pellets and beads. *J Trauma*, **36**, 331–335.

Broome, R.L., Brooks D.L., Babish J.G. *et al.* (1991). Pharmacokinetic properties of enrofloxacin in rabbits. *Am J Vet Res.*, **52**, 1835–1841.

Butson, R.J., Schramme, M.C., Garlick, M.H., Davies, J.V. (1996). Treatment of intrasynovial infection with gentamicin-impregnated polymethylmethacrylate beads. *Vet Rec.*, **138**, 460–464.

Calhoun, J.H., Mader, J.T. (1989). Antibiotic beads in the management of surgical infections. *Am J Surg.*, **157**, 443–449.

Chaffee, V.W., James, E.A., Montali, R.J. (1975). Suppurative mandibular osteomyelitis associated with *Pasteurella multocida* in a rabbit. *Vet Med/Small Anim Clin.*, **70**, 1411–1473.

Chapman, M.W., Hadley, K. (1976). The effect of polymethylmethacrylate and antibiotic combinations on bacterial viability. *J Bone Joint Surg.*, **58**, 76–81.

Chappell, S. (1994). The rabbit abscess and antirobe. *Antirobe In-Focus. Magazine.* Upjohn Ltd, Animal Health Division, Crawley, West Sussex, RH10 2LZ.

Cheeke, P.R., Patton, N.M., Templeton, G.S. (1982). *Rabbit Production.* Interstate Publishers.

Cornell, C.N., Tyndall D., Waller S. *et al.* (1993). Treatment of experimental osteomyelitis with antibiotic-impregnated bone graft substitute (Abstract). *J Orthop Res.*, **11**, 619–626.

Deeb, B. (1993). Update for veterinary practitioners on Pasteurellosis in rabbits. *J Small Exotic Anim Med.*, **2**, 112–113.

Dominguez, J., Crase, D., Soave, O. (1975). A case of pseudomonas osteomyelitis in a rabbit. *Lab Anim Sci.*, **25**, 506.

Elliott, J. (1998). Logical antibacterial drug prescribing – the theory behind the practice. *CPD Vet Med.*, **1**, 55–60.

Evans, R.P., Nelson, C.L. (1993). Gentamicin impregnated polymethyl methacrylate beads compared with systemic antibiotic therapy in the treatment of chronic osteomyelitis. *Clin Orthopaed Rel Res.*, **295**, 37–42.

Flick, A.B., Herbert, J.C., Goodell, J., Kritiansen, T. (1987). Non commercial fabrication of antibiotic impregnated polymethylmethacrylate beads. *Clin Orthopaed.*, **223**, 282–286.

Foreman, P.C., Barnes, L.E. (1990). A review of calcium hydroxide. *Int Endodontic J.*, **23**, 283–297.

Harcourt-Brown, F.M. (1995). A review of clinical conditions in pet rabbits associated with their teeth. *Vet Rec.*, **137**, 341–346.

Harcourt-Brown, F.M., Baker, S.J. (2001). Parathyroid hormone, haematological and biochemical parameters in relation to dental disease and husbandry in pet rabbits. *J Small Anim Pract.*, **42**, 130–136.

Harvey, C. (1997). Abscesses in rabbits. In *Rabbit Medicine and Procedures for Practitioners Program and Abstracts.* pp 87–92. House Rabbit Society.

Henry, S.L, Galloway, K.P. (1995). Local antibacterial therapy for the management of orthopaedic infections. Pharmacokinetic considerations (Abstract). *Clin Pharmacokinet.*, **29**, 36–45.

Hillyer, E.V. (1997). Dermatological diseases. In *Ferrets, Rabbits and Rodents, Clinical Medicine and Surgery* (E.V. Hillyer, K.E. Quesenberry, eds). pp 212–219. W.B. Saunders.

Hinton, M. (1979). Mandibular osteomyelitis in the rabbit. *Vet Rec.*, **103**, 263–264.

Hinton, M., Jones D.R.E., Festing M.F.W. (1982). Haematological findings in healthy and diseased rabbits, a multivariate analysis. *Lab Anim.*, **16**, 123–129.

Jacob, E., Setterstrom, J.A., Bach, D.E. *et al.* (1991). Evaluation of biodegradeable ampicillin anhydrate microcapsules for local treatment of experimental staphylococcal osteomyelitis (Abstract). *Clin Orthop.*, **267**, 237–244.

Jenkins, J.R. (1997). Soft tissue surgery and dental procedures. In *Ferrets, Rabbits and Rodents, Clinical Medicine and Surgery* (E.V. Hillyer, K.E. Quesenberry, eds). pp 227–239. W.B. Saunders.

Keogh, B.S., Triplett, R.G., Aufdemorte, T.B., Boyan, B.D. (1989). The effect of local antibiotics in treating chronic osseous Staphylococcus aureus infection (Abstract). *J Oral Maxillofac Surg.*, **47**, 940–945.

Klemm, K.W. (1993). Antibiotic bead chains. *Clin Orthopaed Rel Res.*, **295**, 63–76.

Knight, H.D., Hietala, S.K., Jang, S. (1980). Antibacterial treatment of abscesses. *J Am Vet Med Assoc.*, **176**, 1095–1098.

Lord, A. (2000). Sweet healing. *New Scientist*, 7 October, p. 32.

Mackey, D., Varlet, A., Debeaumont, D. (1982). Antibiotic loaded plaster of Paris pellets: an *in vitro* study of a possible method of local antibiotic therapy in bone infection (Abstract). *Clin Orthop.*, **167**, 263–268.

Mähler, M., Stunkel, S., Ziegowski, C., Kunstyr, I. (1995). Inefficacy of enrofloxacin in the elimination of *Pasteurella multocida* in rabbits. *Lab Anim.*, **29**, 192–199.

Malley, A.D. (1995). Rabbits. *Lecture notes for BSAVA Continuing Education Course.*

Manning, P.J., Digiacomo, R.F., Delong, D. (1989). Pasteurellosis in laboratory animals. In *Pasteurella and Pasteurellosis* (C. Adlam, J.M. Rutter, eds). pp 264–289. Academic Press.

Masem, M., Greenberg, B.M., Hoffman, C. *et al.* (1990). Comparative bacterial clearances of muscle and skin/subcutaneous tissues with and without dead bone: a laboratory study (Abstract). *Plast Reconstr Surg.*, **85**, 773–781.

Miclau, T., Dahners, L.E., Lindsey, R.W. (1993). *In vitro* pharmacokinetics of antibiotic release from locally implantable materials (Abstract). *J Orthop Res.*, **11**, 627–632.

Molan, P. (1999). The role of honey in the management of wounds. *J Wound Care*, **8**, 415–418.

Morgan, D.A. (1988). *Formulary of Wound Management Products*, 3rd edn. D.A. Morgan.

Murakami, T., Mutakami H., Ramp W.K. *et al.* (1997). Calcium hydroxide ameliorates tobramycin toxicity in cultured chick tibiae. *Bone*, **21**, 411–418.

Niles, J., Williams, J. (1999). Suture materials and patterns. *In Practice*, **21**, 308–320.

Oryan A., Zakar S.R. (1998). Effects of topical application of honey on cutaneous wound healing in rabbits (Abstract). *Zentralbl. Veterinarmed.*, **45**, 181–188.

Remeeus, P.G.K., Verbeek, M. (1995). The use of calcium hydroxide in the treatment of abscesses in the cheek of the rabbit resulting from a dental periapical disorder. *J Vet Dent.*, **12**, 19–22.

Remple, J.D., Forbes, N.A. (2000). Antibiotic-impregnated polymethylmethacrylate beads in the treatment of bumblefoot in raptors. In *Raptor Biomedicine II* (Lumeij, J.T., Remple, J.D., Redig, P.T., Lierz, M., Cooper, J., eds) pp. 255–263, Zoological Educational Network.

Seligson, D., Mehta, S., Voos, K. (1992). The use of antibiotic polymethylmethacrylate beads to prevent the evolution of localised infection. *J Orthop Trauma*, **6**, 401–406.

Tobias, K.M., Schneider, R.K., Besser, T.E. (1996). Use of antimicrobial-impregnated polymethyl methacrylate. *J Am Vet Med Assoc.*, **208**, 841–845.

Toth, L.A., Krueger, J.M. (1989). Haematological effects of exposure to three infective agents in rabbits. *J Am Vet Med Assoc.*, **195**, 981–985.

Trostle, S.S., Hendrickson, D.A., Stone W.C., Klohnen, A.A. (1996). Use of antimicrobial-impregnated polymethyl methacrylate beads for the treatment of chronic refractory septic arthritis and osteomyelitis in a bull. *J Am Vet Med Assoc.*, **208**, 404–406.

Walberg, J.A. (1981). Osteogenic sarcoma with metastasis in a rabbit. *Lab Anim Sci.*, **31**, 407–408.

Ward, G.S., Crumrine, M.H., Mattloch, J.R. (1981). Inflammatory exostosis an inflammation associated with *Fusobacterium nucleatum* in a rabbit. *Lab Anim Sci.*, **31**, 459–464.

Westerhof, I,. Lumeij, S.J. (1987). Dental problems in rabbits, guinea pigs and chinchillas. *Tijdschrift voor Diergeneeskunde*, **12**, 6S–10S.

Wheler, C.L., Machin, K.L., Lew, L. (1996). Use of antibiotic-impregnated polymethyl methacrylate beads on the treatment of chronic osteomyelitis and cellulitis in a juvenile bald eagle. *Proc Assoc Avian Vet.*, 187–194.

Whittem, T., Gaon, D. (1998). Principles of microbial therapy. *Vet Clin N Am.*, **28**, 197–211.

Skin diseases

9

9.1 Underlying causes of skin disease in rabbits

Skin disease is common in pet rabbits but apparently rare in their wild counterparts. The wild rabbit has a short dense coat that it grooms regularly using the incisors to pull out dead hair. The coat is short and dense and does not knot and mat easily like the fluffy coats of many pet rabbits. Wild rabbits live in groups where mutual grooming is an important part of their social behaviour. During periods of rest, they lie together and groom each other, especially around the face and head. Wild rabbits are not confined to a small space and do not sit for hours on end on a bed contaminated by urine or faeces. They do not become obese and disabled individuals are quickly caught by predators.

Many pet rabbits have underlying problems that prevent them from grooming effectively. Solitary rabbits have no companion to groom them. The fast growing, fine fluffy coat of breeds such as the Angora is impossible for a rabbit to groom. Incisor malocclusion removes the pincer like action of the teeth making removal of dead hair difficult. Cheek tooth malocclusion results in the formation of sharp spurs that grow into the tongue, making licking and grooming painful. Effective grooming requires flexibility, which is impaired by obesity, arthritis or spondylosis. Kyphosis, scoliosis and spondylosis are often found in pet rabbits (see Section 12.7). Underlying neurological problems, such as encephalitozoonosis affects the ability to balance and adopt the correct posture to reach inaccessible parts of the body. Rhinitis makes it hard to breathe and groom at the same time. Hard flooring, inactivity, obesity and poor conformation predispose to avascular necrosis of the skin over the bony prominences of the feet and the development of sore hocks. Abrasive surfaces such as wire cages or tough carpets can traumatize the skin and predispose to infection. Damp, dirty bedding encourages bacterial contamination of skin and the array of chemicals, such as disinfectants and shampoos that pet rabbits are exposed to increases the incidence of contact dermatitis and allergies. Some present day breeds, such as the French lop, develop huge skin folds under the chin or around the genitalia, which are prone to moist dermatitis.

Therefore, it is important to identify and, if possible, treat the underlying reasons for skin conditions in rabbits in addition to treating the condition itself. Many skin diseases can be alleviated or prevented by the provision of a soft clean bed, the opportunity to exercise, a high fibre diet and a companion, maybe human, who will diligently groom the coat, keeping it free from mats and debris.

9.2 Examination of the skin

The approach to skin disease follows the same principles as in other species. The owners need to be asked about diet and husbandry regimens and in-contact animals. Some owners know whether their rabbit is pruritic, others may not. A full clinical examination, including the mouth, perineum and hocks may reveal underlying conditions that interfere with normal grooming activity and result in skin disease. The skin of mature entire male rabbits can become thickened along the dorsum from the neck to the rump. Histologically, the skin shows prominent, thick, dermal collagen similar to the cheek skin from entire male cats (Hargreaves and Hartley, 2000; Mackay, 2000). This is a secondary sexual characteristic.

The conformation of the rabbit is important. Some rabbits develop large skin folds under the chin or around the perineum, which can become infected. Large, loose eyelids can interfere with the protective mechanism of the precorneal tear film and result in epiphora and facial dermatitis. Some rabbits develop a large 'skirt' of skin around the thighs that is in constant contact with the ground and prone to mechanical trauma and contact dermatitis. Poor conformation or mobility problems due to spondylosis or obesity can lead to pressure sores or the inability to adopt the correct position for urination, which results in urine scalding.

The rabbit needs to adopt a variety of postures to reach all areas of the body. The face and ears are groomed using the front legs. The area between the tail and the dorsum and the area between the shoulder blades at back of the neck are the most difficult parts of the body for a rabbit to reach (see Figure 3.8). A bonded companion will groom its mate, especially around the head and face but seldom around the tail. Combing through the coat with a fine toothed flea comb gives an idea of whether the rabbit is grooming effectively. If dead hair can be groomed or pulled out of all areas of the body then it can be assumed that the rabbit is hardly grooming at all and is suffering from a generalized condition. If some areas are well groomed and the 'difficult to reach' areas are not, then a flexibility problem may be present. The amount of dead hair increases during periods of moulting.

Good illumination and a magnifying glass facilitate close examination of the fur. Broken hairs, flea dirt or mites may be seen, especially in white fur. Infestation with *Leporacus gibbus* (fur mite) gives the impression that the coat has been dusted with 'salt and pepper'. Evidence of trauma, alopecia, erythema, etc. can be seen on close examination of the skin. Some rabbits start to lick and chew at the area under the neck or may lick the handler in response to being combed, especially along the dorsum at the base of the tail. This response can indicate an underlying pruritic condition in an inaccessible site. For example, obese rabbits or those that cannot reach their perineum due to spondylosis may start to lick their dewlap, in response to being combed, especially if they are affected by perineal dermatitis or cheyletiellosis at the base of the tail.

There are many laboratory aids to diagnosis of skin conditions in rabbits (see Section 6.9). Mites can be seen by examining skin brushings under low magnification. Acetate tape strips applied to the skin before microscopic examination can be used to look for cheyletiella, bacteria and yeasts. Microscopic examination of the hair can be used to differentiate between alopecic conditions. Barbering caused by a dominant cage mate chewing the hair is characterized by the presence of broken, but healthy hair shafts. Ringworm can be diagnosed by the presence of spores in broken hairshafts. Fungal culture confirms dermatophysosis and identifies the causal organism. Smears can be taken for dark ground microscopy from lesions in which *Treponema pallidum* is suspected. Bacterial culture can be used in cases of bacterial skin disease to identify the organism and give an antibiotic sensitivity. Skin scrapings may be necessary in pruritic animals or those that are suspected of suffering from sarcoptic or demodectic mange. Skin biopsies may be required to differentiate between some skin conditions or to obtain a diagnosis and prognosis in cases of neoplasia.

9.3 Grooming and dematting rabbits

Grooming is important in rabbits to keep the coat free from debris and dead hair, and to prevent the formation of mats. Fluffy and long-haired breeds are especially prone to developing mats between the hind legs and around the base of the tail. Dirty bedding, urine or faecal contamination can result in the skin beneath these mats becoming infected and inflamed. Clipping away the soiled, matted hair and treating the underlying skin breaks a vicious circle that occurs when the coat is too matted and the skin too painful for the rabbit to groom properly, but lack of grooming allows mats to form and become

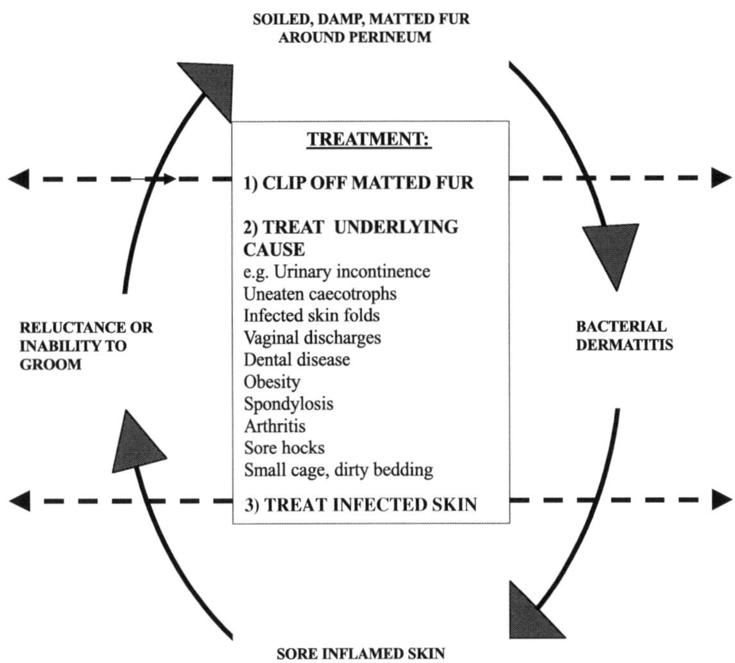

Figure 9.1. Vicious circle of perineal dermatitis.

soiled (see Figure 9.1). Some mats can be teased apart and the dead hair gently pulled out before combing through the remaining fur. It is important to be gentle when pulling mats out of the fur as the skin can be torn easily. Solid mats need to be cut out. A sharp pair of curved scissors can be used, taking care to cut close to the mat without cutting the skin. Time, patience and good illumination are required. Many rabbits require sedation and fentanyl/fluanisone is most effective (see Box 5.3). Clippers can be used to remove matted fur, but are often unsatisfactory for the removal of consolidated mats. The fine hair quickly becomes trapped in the blades. Stretching the skin out in front of the clippers and running them slowly over the skin reduces the risk of traumatizing the skin.

Bathing soiled rabbits is seldom satisfactory without clipping away the soiled fur first. It is almost impossible to cleanse the dense, fine fur of a rabbit, which usually becomes matted as a result of bathing. A mass of soiled, damp fur overlying infected skin is counterproductive. Bathing rabbits can be stressful and there are reports of shock and death of rabbits following the use of insecticidal baths or dips (Harvey, 1995). Clipping and cleansing affected areas is often effective without the use of baths. Hair needs to be removed as it is a barrier between the skin and any topical preparations that are applied.

9.4 Moulting

Rabbit hairs arise singly or in multiples from the hair follicles (Sandford, 1996) giving the characteristic dense coat. Hair grows quickly on newborn rabbits and initially consists of guard hairs that are followed by the soft undercoat over a matter of a few days. The baby coat is replaced at 5–6 weeks of age by the intermediate coat that persists until the rabbit is 4–5 months old. This intermediate pelt is free from moulting hairs and is used in the fur industry.

Moulting in adult rabbits follows a seasonal pattern and there are usually two complete coat changes per year. During moulting, there are areas of fur in various stages of growth throughout the body. The moult usually starts on the head and works down the neck and back with the stomach being the last area to shed the coat. Environmental stimuli, hormones and nutrition affect the moulting process. The density of the coat is also affected by environmental temperature and nutrition. The summer coat is generally shorter than the winter coat and may vary in colour. Colour point breeds such as Californian or Siamese Sable show a similar pigment response to exposure as Siamese cats, where hair regrowth in shaved areas may be coloured black (Cheeke *et al.*, 1982).

9.5 Alopecia

Hair loss in rabbits can be physiological. Some rabbits are naturally thin coated in the area at the nape of the neck. The modified coat texture of breeds such as the Angora, Dwarf and Miniature lop has resulted in fluffy, fine fur that knots and mats easily. It is often shed in patches rather than in the typical pattern that occurs in wild rabbits or coarser coated breeds such as the Dutch or English. Alopecic areas appear that can concern owners (see Plate 3), but regrowth is usually rapid with areas of dense new hair appearing within 7–10 days. This phenomenon of patchy hair growth appears to be a variant of normal moulting. It may be more apparent after an area has been clipped for surgery (Hoyt, 1998).

In pregnant does the hair loosens and is plucked to line the nest during late pregnancy. This behaviour can result in large bald areas appearing on the chest and ventral abdomen. Pseudopregnant does also pluck hair from these areas. A dominant companion can chew the fur of its cage mate to a stubble, especially on the lateral flanks. This process is known as barbering. Microscopic examination of the fur shows broken hair shafts.

Poor nutrition can underly alopecia. Sulphur-containing amino acids are required for keratin production and wool growth. Rabbits have a nutritional requirement for essential amino acids despite amino acid synthesis in the caecum (Cheeke, 1987).

Key points 9.1

- Many skin conditions in rabbits are associated with underlying diseases such as dental disease, obesity or spondylosis, that affect the animal's ability to groom effectively
- Coat texture can also affect the ability to groom. For example, the fine fluffy coat of the Angoras is often impossible for the rabbit to lick and groom effectively
- Mutual grooming is an important part of social behaviour and another rabbit will spend hours licking and grooming its companion especially around the head and face
- Combing through the fur with a fine-toothed flea comb to see how much dead hair is in the coat gives an idea of whether a rabbit is grooming effectively or not
- Mites, fleas and flea dirt may be seen in skin brushings
- Loose skinned rabbits can develop large skin folds especially under the chin and around the genitalia. These skin folds easily become infected
- Clipping away soiled fur is a vital part of treating skin infections in rabbits, especially in the perineal area and around the base of the tail
- The thin skin is easily torn and traumatized. Time, patience, good illumination and a sharp pair of curved scissors are required. Some rabbits require sedation, others can be 'tranced' by lying them on their back
- Rabbit's fine fur easily becomes trapped in clipper blades. Stretching the skin out in front of the blade and running the clippers slowly over the skin can reduce trauma and facilitate clipping. A good quality set of clippers is an advantage
- Although bathing rabbits is sometimes necessary, it can be counterproductive if the fur is not clipped off. It is difficult to cleanse and dry rabbit's fur effectively, and damp, soiled mats over infected skin can increase infection. Bathing can be stressful for rabbits
- Rabbits moult twice a year. Moulting is a continuous process that starts on the head and progresses to the neck, back and abdomen
- Some fluffy coated breeds such as the Angora, Dwarf Lop or Miniature lop develop alopecic patches on the back during moulting
- Pregnant or pseudopregnant does may pull hair from their chest or abdomen, leaving large bald areas
- Debility or a poor diet can be reflected in the coat. Essential sulphur-containing amino acids are required for keratin formation. Cereals are deficient in lysine.

Keratin is characterized by its high content of cystine that is synthesized from the essential amino acid methionine (McDonald *et al.*, 1996). Lysine is also important in the formation of keratin as well as fibrin and collagen. In general, cereals are deficient in lysine and methionine, whereas legumes are good sources. Sulphur amino acid deficiency can be reflected in poor coat quality in rabbits that are debilitated or are fed on a high cereal diet. Selective feeding from mixed rations results in a diet consisting almost entirely of cereals. Magnesium deficiency has also been linked with alopecia and alterations in fur texture in rabbits (Cheeke, 1987).

Areas that have been traumatized, e.g. by injection reactions or fight wounds, can remain hairless for some weeks after the lesion has healed. Repetitive trauma and contact dermatitis can result in patches of alopecia in areas of skin that are in contact with flooring, especially the hocks. If a contact reaction is present, the skin is thickened, inflamed, hyperaemic and pruritic.

9.6 Injection reactions

Rabbits are prone to injection reactions. A lesion is found at the site of the injection a few days later. In some individuals, the reaction is extensive and areas of epidermis can slough. Viral haemorrhagic disease vaccine, carprofen and enrofloxacin injections are common culprits. Injection reactions can be avoided by ensuring that the product is delivered subcutaneously and not intradermally and dispersed by gently massaging the skin. Although injection reactions are unsightly, most heal quickly. If necessary, topical antiseptic creams can be applied.

9.7 Dermatitis

Rabbit skin is thin and easily traumatized. It is reactive and easily irritated. Primary irritant contact dermatitis can result from the application of chemical agents such as topical iodine washes (Wilkinson and Harvey, 1994). Superficial pyoderma is common and is often secondary to underlying causes such as epiphora, ptyalism, urine scalding, bite wounds, injection reactions or infected skin folds. Deep skin folds accumulate debris and provide the correct environmental conditions for bacteria and yeasts to grow. Some rabbits have excessively large folds of skin around the anus and genitalia.

Staphylococcus aureus is a common pathogen in infected skin conditions in rabbits (DeLong and Manning, 1994). *S. aureus* can be isolated from all body sites in rabbits, but is present in greater numbers in the ear and perineum. There are several different biotypes and phage types that are related to virulence (Hermans *et al.*, 1999). Other bacteria such as *Fusobacterium necrophorum* or *Pseudomonas aeruginosa* are also associated with skin infections, especially in farmed rabbits in intensive conditions. 'Schmorls disease' or necrobacillosis is caused by *Fusobacterium necrophorum* and is characterized by necrosis, ulceration and abscessation. *P. aeruginosa* is associated with moist dermatitis of the dewlap in rabbits kept in damp conditions. The infection is characterized by a blue/green discoloration of the fur and is associated with intensive husbandry, wet bedding and contaminated water bottles (Scott *et al.*, 1995). This type of infection is rare in the pet rabbit. *Pasteurella multocida* is the most common pathogen in purulent skin conditions. The organism can be found in the nares of healthy rabbits and can be spread to other sites during grooming. *P. multocida* is often cultured from abscesses (see Section 8.1) and is a cause of respiratory tract infections (see Section 13.2.1).

Superficial pyoderma is treated by clipping hair away from the lesion, cleaning the skin and applying an antiseptic or antibiotic cream. Bathing may be necessary to remove any exudate or faecal contamination but is counterproductive unless the overlying fur is clipped off. The dense coat of rabbits mats easily, dries slowly and moist conditions encourage bacterial growth. If bathing is necessary, chlorhexidene or povidone/iodine preparations are suitable skin cleansers and are effective against yeasts that inhabit skin folds. Treatment with topical preparations containing antibiotic and corticosteroid are effective. Corticosteroids are absorbed from these preparations, especially if the skin is inflamed (see Section 4.10). Prolonged administration of topical corticosteroids can result in thinning of the skin. Fuciderm (Leo Laboratories Ltd) is a useful product that contains fusidic acid and only needs to be applied once daily. Fusidic acid does not interfere with the gut flora and is effective against the staphylococci spp. that are often present in infected skin conditions.

Systemic antibiotics are indicated in severe cases of bacterial skin infections. Culture and sensitivity may be required. Enrofloxacin or trimethoprim combinations are safe antibiotics in rabbits and can be used to treat bacterial skin infections. Usually, systemic corticosteroids are not necessary and may be contraindicated due to their immunosuppressive effects (see Section 4.4). If the skin is particularly painful or inflamed, non-steroidal preparations such as carprofen can be effective. NSAIDs are also beneficial in treating any underlying or painful condition that is restricting grooming.

9.7.1 Moist dermatitis of the dewlap

The skin under the chin and throat can become infected and sore, especially if it is continually wet. Conditions that cause ptyalism increase the risk of moist dermatitis in this region. Dental disease, especially spurs on the cheek teeth, can cause excessive salivation. Saliva runs down the chin and throat, especially on the side of the affected teeth.

Dirty water bottles and damp conditions cause outbreaks of moist dermatitis of the dewlap in rabbits kept in intensive conditions. Some rabbits cannot drink from a water bottle without immersing their dewlap in it. Large breed females are the most susceptible. Substituting sipper bottles for water bowls is recommended as a preventative measure. Licking and chewing the dewlap can be a displacement activity for irritation at another site. For example, obese does that cannot reach their perineum or dorsum may chew their dewlap, which then becomes infected and sore. Removing the primary source of irritation, e.g. perineal dermatitis or cheyletiellosis is required to cure the dewlap.

Loose-skinned rabbits, especially females, develop huge skin folds under the chin and around the dewlap. These skin folds can easily become infected. Daily cleansing with an antiseptic solution can be used to control the condition. Alternatively, surgical removal of the skin folds may be required (see Section 9.7.3).

9.7.2 Facial dermatitis

Superficial bacterial skin infections around the face can be the result of excessive drooling, fight wounds or chronic epiphora. Epiphora may be due to infection, trauma or blockage of the nasolacrimal duct (see Section 11.6.3). Epiphora is often the first sign of acquired dental disease (see Section 7.6.5). The nasolacrimal duct curls around the apex of the upper primary incisor and becomes blocked by the root if it is elongated (see Figures 11.1 and 11.2). Tears flow down the face instead of down the nasolacrimal duct. The fur under the eye becomes continually wet and mineral deposits cause matting of the fur, encouraging bacterial growth on the skin beneath. Although topical preparations can be helpful in controlling the infection, this condition is difficult to cure (see Section 11.6.3). It is important to keep the area clean and dry. Often, the best solution is a bonded companion who will constantly lick and clean this area of the face.

9.7.3 Perineal dermatitis

Perineal dermatitis is usually caused by secondary bacterial infection of the skin around the anus and genitalia. Grooming difficulties and a fine coat texture often result in mats of fur accumulating in the genital region and on the ventral aspect of the tail, especially when the animal is moulting. These mats of fur absorb urine, adhere to faeces, and exacerbate bacterial infection. Areas of inflamed skin can extend down the inside of the thighs to the hocks and are exacerbated by either urine scalding or contamination of the skin by caecotrophs or both. Uneaten caecotrophs often become entangled in the fur under the tail, especially if they are soft and sticky. Volatile fatty acids in caecotrophs irritate the skin and cause inflammation. There are several conditions that prevent caecotroph ingestion, such as dental disease, obesity, spondylosis, arthritis, sore hocks and inadequate fibre intake (see Figure 10.6). Conditions that can cause urinary incontinence and urine scalding include cystitis, urolithiasis, neurological disease and penile disorders, etc. (see Section 14.4.3).

Large perineal skin folds can develop in obese animals and will persist even after the animal has lost weight. Females are more often affected than males. These folds of skin entrap hair, discharges, urine, faeces and necrotic debris. They are prone to chronic infection. Occasionally *Psoroptes cuniculi* are found in the perineal skin fold of rabbits suffering from ear mite infestation. A crusty exudate forms and mites can be seen on smears taken from the area.

The perineal area is extremely sensitive in rabbits and pain associated with inflamed, infected skin can, in itself, prevent a rabbit from grooming the perineum or ingesting caecotrophs. Lack of grooming starts a vicious circle (see Figure 9.1). Fly strike can be the end point of the disease. Rabbits with painful, infected perineal skin are prone to urethritis. They are reluctant to adopt the correct stance for urination and consequently retain urine and may develop cystitis. Urethritis causes rabbits to dribble urine and dirty wet bedding compounds the situation by scalding the perineal skin. Polydypsic/polyuric rabbits produce copious quantities of urine, which also wets the bedding and exacerbates perineal dermatitis.

Any condition that alters the direction of the jet of urine on to the skin during urination can result in constant urine soaking of the fur and subsequent infection. Conditions of the prepuce or penis, such as scars from fight wounds, can cause penile deviations or partially occlude the urethral opening and alter the direction of urine flow. Rabbits with spinal problems or sore hocks are unable to lift their hindquarters into the correct position to lift their tail and spray urine which dribbles down the inside of the legs instead.

Treatment of perineal dermatitis is aimed at breaking the vicious circle of inflammation, pain, lack of grooming and secondary bacterial infection. Clipping and cleaning the perineum, treating secondary infection and providing analgesia is effective in most cases. Most rabbits require sedation for the clipping and cleaning, which also offers the opportunity for radiography that may provide a diagnosis. Sludgy urine, urolithiasis, spinal problems or arthritic joints are conditions that can be seen on X-ray and predispose to urine scalding or faecal contamination of the perineum. In order to cure perineal dermatitis and prevent recurrence, the underlying reason for faecal or urinary incontinence needs to be addressed. For example, a high fibre diet may be required to encourage ingestion of caecotrophs or for weight reduction (see Section 3.4). NSAIDs are indicated for chronic arthritic conditions such as spondylitis. NSAIDs interfere with prostaglandin synthesis and have the added advantage of reducing caecotroph production (Pairet *et al.*, 1986). Dental diseases that prevent grooming require treatment. Space to exercise and urinate away from the bedding is also necessary.

Rabbits that have developed large folds of skin around the genitalia will benefit from surgical removal of these folds which encourage infection (see Section 9.7.3.1). Entire female rabbits with underlying reproductive disorders that cause vaginal discharges will also need to be spayed. Paraplegic patients nearly always develop a degree of perineal dermatitis and require constant nursing to keep the perineal skin clean, dry and free from matted hair.

9.7.3.1 Perineal dermoplasty

Surgical removal of perineal skin folds is a simple, effective remedy for chronic perineal dermatitis providing other predisposing factors have been resolved. In some cases it is not possible to cure the underlying cause, but removal of infected skin folds will improve the situation, for example rabbits with spondylitic problems that are unable to groom properly.

Perineal dermosplasty is performed by making a crescent-shaped incision cranial to the genital opening. The crescent includes the infected and inflamed skin. In male animals, the scrotum and testicles are included so the rabbit is castrated. The amount of skin that needs to be removed varies in each individual. Insufficient skin removal will result in relapse of the condition. Excessive removal will alter the position of the genital orifice and affect the direction of urine flow. There should be no tension on the skin sutures. The incision can be repaired with a soft suture material such as 4/0 Polyglactin 910 (Vicryl Rapide, Ethicon) that does not require suture removal and is comfortable and well tolerated postoperatively. The inflammatory response to polyglactic acid in rabbits is mild (see Section 15.3).

9.8 Fly strike (myiasis)

During the summer months, pet rabbits that are housed in hutches can be affected by maggot infestation. Healthy rabbits are not affected by fly strike. Obese rabbits are especially prone to the condition.

There is always a reason for the perineal fur to be contaminated by urine or faeces. Bluebottles *(Calliphora.)* and greenbottles *(Lucilia)* are attracted to soiled fur or infected skin to lay their eggs. The commonest site for fly strike in rabbits is the area at the base of the spine, between the tail and the dorsum. This is a difficult area for rabbits to groom effectively, especially if they are overweight or have a flexibility problem due to spondylosis or arthritis (see Figure 3.8). Dental disease also prevents effective grooming and allows mats to form. Uneaten caecotrophs (see Section 10.6) or damp dirty bedding increase the risk of fly strike. When the eggs hatch out, the maggots are concealed by matted, soiled fur and may not be obvious until the rabbit becomes unwell. The skin lesions exude a characteristic smell. Maggots can be intensely irritating for affected rabbits that are restless and inappetant.

Key points 9.2

- Bacterial skin infections are common in rabbits. They are usually secondary to some other condition that either prevents grooming or causes wetness and bacterial contamination of the skin
- *Staphylococcus aureus* is a common pathogen although other organisms such as yeasts, *Fusobacterium necrophorum, Pseudomonas aeruginosa* or *Pasteurella multocida* may be involved
- Bacterial skin infections are treated by clipping away soiled fur, cleansing the area and applying topical creams. Systemic antibiotics and non-steroidal analgesic drugs (NSAIDS) may be indicated
- Bacterial infections of the chin and neck can be caused by ptyalism associated with dental disease or be associated with large dewlaps and skin folds
- Some rabbits will lick their dewlap as a displacement activity caused by irritation in a remote site such as the dorsum or perineum that is inaccessible to them. Pruritic conditions such as perineal dermatitis or cheyletiellosis may cause rabbits to chew the dewlap and make it sore.
- Chronic epiphora can cause dermatitis on the face. Epiphora is often associated with dental disease and can be difficult to cure. The provision of a bonded companion constantly to lick and groom the face can be an effective remedy.
- Perineal dermatitis is often associated with mats of damp, soiled fur around the tail and genitalia
- Fluffy breeds such as Angoras, Dwarf lops or Miniature lops are prone to developing mats in the perineal region
- Uneaten caecotrophs, urine and vaginal discharges can contaminate the fur and allow superficial pyoderma to develop around the perineum
- Perineal dermatitis is painful and can prevent a rabbit from licking and grooming the area or adopting the correct stance for urination. A vicious circle is created that can be broken by treating the dermatitis and providing analgesia
- The underlying cause of perineal dermatitis needs to be addressed to cure the condition without recurrence
- Fly strike may be the end point of the disease
- Fly strike is treated by clipping and cleaning the affected area and picking out all the maggots. A hair dryer can be used to draw the maggots to the surface as they are attracted by heat
- Ivermectin, antibiotics and analgesics are also indicated in the treatment of fly strike
- Obese rabbits are particularly prone to fly strike and require aggressive treatment, including fluid therapy, syringe feeding and analgesia to prevent hepatic lipidosis
- Although flyscreens and environmental treatment with insecticides can help prevent fly strike, prevention and treatment of the underlying causes of perineal soiling are also necessary.

Sedation is usually required to clip away soiled fur from the lesion and pick out the maggots. Fentanyl/fluanisone provides sedation and effective analgesia. All the maggots must be removed from the affected area, which can then be bathed with a medicated shampoo or an antiseptic preparation such as povidone-iodine (Pevidene Surgical Scrub). An insecticidal shampoo can be used, although this is not necessary if all the maggots have been removed. Drying the area with a hair dryer brings out any remaining maggots as they are attracted by the heat. A precautionery dose of ivermectin can be administered. Antibiotic therapy is indicated. Enrofloxacin or trimethoprim combinations are safe choices. A non-steroidal analgesic such as carprofen is necessary. Inappetant, obese rabbits are at risk of rapidly developing fatal hepatic lipidosis and it is important to provide aggressive treatment for these patients. Fluid therapy, syringe feeding, analgesia and motility stimulants are necessary. Addressing the underlying cause of perineal soiling is required to prevent further episodes of fly strike, although providing some type of fly screen and ensuring a clean dry bed are beneficial. Prophylactic insecticidal preparations such as fiprinol (Frontline) are not advisable as rabbits can suffer adverse reactions and such preparations do not address the underlying cause.

In the USA, rabbits can be affected by a warble fly *Cuterebra cuniculi*. The incidence of infestation decreases with age, which correlates with the development of immediate and delayed-type hypersensitivity reactions to the larvae. Initial lesions include subcutaneous cystic structures. As the larvae enlarge, a breathing hole or fistula develops. The surrounding coat becomes moist and matted and secondary bacterial infection is common. The lesions are often painful. Treatment consists of surgical removal of the larvae without crushing or damaging them. The condition is prevented by eliminating contact with the warble fly (Scott *et al.*, 1995).

9.9 Otitis externa

There is natural diverticulum in the vertical ear canal of rabbits and both the diverticulum and the external ear canal require auriscopic examination. A waxy deposit is often seen during auriscopic examination, which obscures the view of the horizontal canal and eardrum. Lop eared breeds appear most susceptible to forming this deposit. A thick, creamy exudate in the horizontal canal can also obscure the view of the eardrum. This exudate is a common finding during *post-mortem* examination of rabbits (Harcourt-Brown, unpublished data). In a small proportion of cases, the exudate extends through the eardrum into the tympanic bulla. Affected rabbits have usually shown no obvious signs of otitis externa or otitis media during life. It is possible that the exudate affected hearing but hearing loss is difficult to quantify in rabbits. In a survey by Flatt *et al.* (1977), otitis media was found in 4% of young rabbits and 32% of adults slaughtered for human consumption in a study of 2001 rabbits. The animals were clinically healthy on *ante-mortem* inspection.

It is difficult to clear wax and debris in the external ear canal of rabbits with any degree of long-term success. Wax forms an effective barrier against any ear preparations that are used to treat it and general anaesthesia or sedation is usually required to clean the horizontal ear canal. Relapse is common. As a rule, it is better not to embark upon treatment unless clinical signs are present. Erythema, pruritus, head shaking, malodour or the presence of pus are indications for treatment, which follows the same principles as for dogs and cats. Ear preparations that are produced for other species can be used.

Ear mites (*Psoroptes cuniculi*) cause otitis externa in rabbits. Infestation is characterized by a crusty exudate that forms within the external ear canal and extends up the pinna (see Plate 4). Occasionally, only one ear is affected. The condition is intensely pruritic. Diagnosis is confirmed by microscopic examination of exudate from the ear in which mites can be seen. *Psoroptes cuniculi* mites are just visible to the naked eye (see Figure 16.1). The mite is transmitted by direct contact between rabbits. Crusts dislodge into the environment and contain many mites that can survive for up to 21 days off the host. Survival is greatest at low temperatures and high humidity (Arlian *et al.*, 1981). The mites pierce the skin to feed and hypersensitivity to mite-related antigens might be important in the pathogenesis of the dermatitis and pruritus (Scott *et al.*, 1995). Subcutaneous ivermectin is an effective treatment for this condition. It is not necessary to attempt to remove the crusts. Severely affected animals have ulcerated ear canals and attempts to remove debris and clean the ear canal can be intensely painful and leave the ear canal raw and bleeding.

Any residual debris can be removed when the inflammation and ulceration have subsided after ivermectin treatment (Flecknell, 1998). Ivermectin does not kill *Psoroptes cuniculi* eggs, but the persistence of the drug in the tissues is sufficiently long to kill new generations of mites as they hatch. The eggs hatch after 4 days. Dosages of 400 μg/kg are required; 200 μg/kg was found to be inadequate in the elimination of ear mites in a study by Wright and Riner (1985). Topical treatment with selamectin (Stronghold, Pfizer) can also be used to eliminate earmite infestations in rabbits. In a study by Hack *et al.* (2001), selamectin was found to be effective against *Psoroptes cuniculi* at dose rates of 6 mg/kg and 18 mg/kg. No adverse effects were seen.

Psoroptes cuniculi can be spread from the ears to other parts of the body during grooming (Cutler, 1998). The mites may be found in the perineal area where they cause crusting and exudative skin lesions (Yeatts, 1994).

Key points 9.3

- There is a natural diverticulum in the vertical ear canal of rabbits
- A waxy deposit in the external ear canal is a common finding in normal rabbits, especially in lop eared breeds
- Visualization of the horizontal ear canal and ear drum can be difficult
- Purulent exudate in the horizontal ear canal is a common *post-mortem* finding in asymptomatic rabbits. The exudate may extend through the ear canal to the tympanic bullae
- Otitis externa can be caused by ear mites, *Psoroptes cuniculi*
- Ear mite infestation is intensely pruritic. A crusty exudate forms within the ear canal and may extend up the pinna. The condition may be unilateral
- Ivermectin or selamectin is an effective remedy for ear mites. The ears do not require cleaning. Removal of the crusty exudate can be painful and is not necessary
- *Psoroptes cuniculi* can be spread from the ears to other parts of the body such as the perineal skin.

9.10 Ulcerative pododermatitis

'Ulcerative pododermatitis' is the term used to describe ulcerated infected areas of skin on the caudal aspect of the tarsus and metatarsus and occasionally the metacarpus of rabbits. Sometimes the term 'sore hocks' is used instead. Neither term is a satisfactory description of the condition as it is not always inflammatory and can sometimes affect the forefeet. Avascular necrosis of the plantar aspect of the feet would be a more accurate term, but 'ulcerative pododermatitis' is succinct and is universally understood. Many authors shorten the term to 'pododermatitis'. The condition is essentially a pressure sore (Bergdall and Dysko, 1994). Pressure sores develop in focal areas over bony prominences. Pressure, shearing forces, friction and moisture are predisposing factors in the development of bedsores in people and the predisposing causes of ulcerative pododermatitis in rabbits appear to be similar.

Ulcerative pododermatatis in rabbits is a serious, painful condition that is progressive and difficult to cure once infection has set in. The lesions can bleed repetitively leading to anaemia. Death may be due to septicaemia or anorexia caused by the pain. Ulcerative pododermatitis has been attributed to primary pasteurellosis or to conformational defects (Hago *et al.*, 1987). In recent years, the condition has increasingly been recognized as a secondary disease to some other physical, conformational or husbandry problem. Large breeds kept in wire cages are particularly prone to the condition that poses a huge welfare problem in farmed rabbits (Drescher and Sclender-Böbbis, 1993). House rabbits are also prone to the condition.

9.10.1 Predisposing factors of ulcerative pododermatitis in rabbits

The development of ulcerative pododermatitis in rabbits is outlined in Figure 9.2. Rabbits

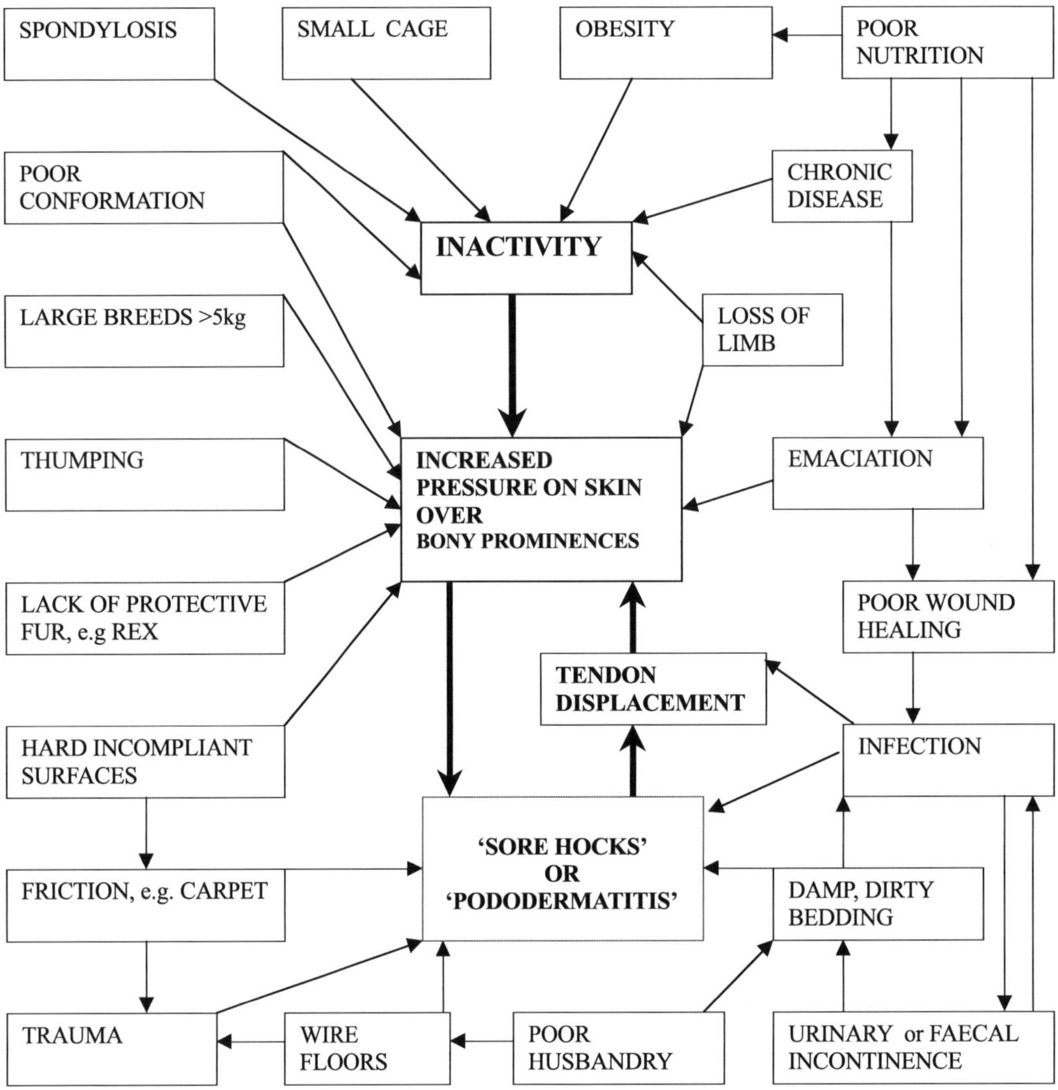

Figure 9.2. Development of ulcerative pododermatitis.

do not have footpads and their skin is very thin. When they hop, they are digitigrade. In healthy rabbits, the weight is taken by the claws during locomotion, especially on the hind feet. At rest, most of a rabbit's weight is distributed between the hind claws and the plantar aspect of the metatarsus (see Figure 9.3). This area is normally protected by thick fur. The skin in this area is adherent to the underlying tissues and forms a tarso-metatarsal skin pad. The superficial flexor tendon is constantly under tension so that the rabbit can spring up and flee readily. The rabbit has evolved to live on an earth substrate that the claws can grip into.

The type of substrate that a rabbit is housed on affects the distribution of weight between the metatarsus and claws. Wire flooring does not allow the rabbit to walk or rest on its claws so the weight is taken entirely by the hock and metatarsus. Hard flooring, such as concrete or vinyl, does not allow the claws to sink in to the subsrate so, again, most of the weight is borne by the metatarsus. Abrasive flooring, such as

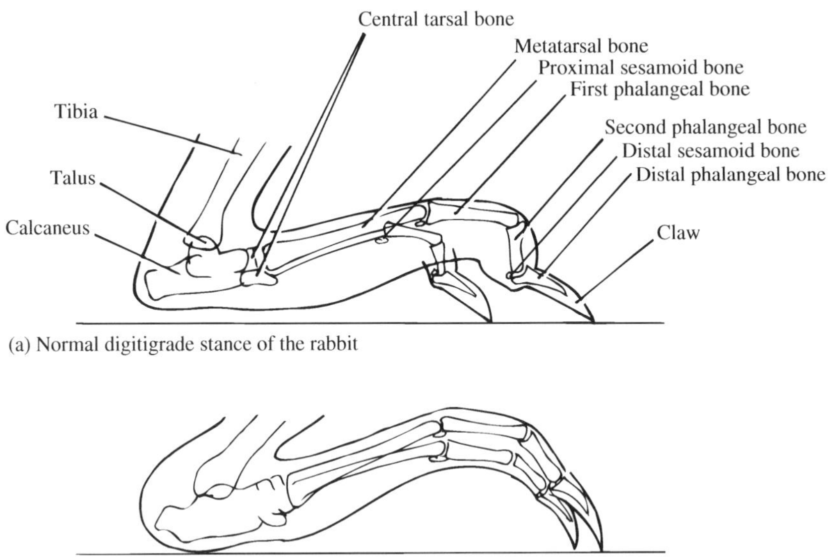

Figure 9.3. Normal digitigrade hindlimb stance (a) compared with abnormal stance due to displacement of the superficial digital flexor tendon (b).
(a) Figures 9.3a and b are drawn from standing lateral radiographs. During rest, most of the rabbit's weight is taken on the hind limb. The normal hindlimb stance of rabbits is digitigrade. In a healthy rabbit, the weight is distributed between the claws and the plantar aspect of the metatarsus (a). The superficial flexor tendon is constantly under tension, which allows the rabbit to spring rapidly into action to escape from predators. Floors that do not permit the correct distribution of weight between the claws and the metatarsus are a predisposing cause of ulcerative pododermatitis. Wire mesh floors pose a high risk because they prevent weight bearing on the claws. All the rabbit's weight is borne by the metatarsus and hock, which results in increased pressure and the development of pressure sores. In advanced cases, infection and erosion of the ligaments around the hock result in medial displacement of the tendon (see also Figure 9.4 and Plates 9 and 10). The redistribution of weight that occurs once the superficial digital flexor tendon has become displaced can be seen in Figure 9.4b.

carpet, predisposes to ulcerative pododermatitis by increasing the shearing forces and friction on the skin. Close confinement, lack of exercise, obesity, pregnancy and poor conformation all affect the weight distribution on the hind leg. Ulcerative pododermatitis is more commonly encountered in commercial rabbits that are confined to tiny wire mesh cages than in pet rabbits that are allowed exercise and are bedded on hay. House rabbits kept in houses with tough, rough carpeting are more susceptible than rabbits that spend most of their time sitting on grass. Lawns are softer and are more compliant than carpet, ceramic tiles or vinyl flooring.

Certain breeds, such as the Rex, have fine sparse hair on the metatarsus that offers little protection. Clipping hair from the hocks of fine coated Angoras also predisposes to ulcerative pododermatitis (Richardson, 2000). Large breeds and rabbits that are overweight are more susceptible. Many rabbit breeders believe that 'sore hocks' is a hereditary condition. Bare pads are considered a fault in show animals and broken skin merits disqualification (Sandford, 1996). In addition to the role of coat texture, the conformation of the animal and the weight distribution over the plantar aspect of the hock also play a part in the development of the disease. Some rabbits sit with their hind legs almost extended in front of them so that a disproportionate amount of weight is taken on the hock. Physical conditions, such as spondylosis, alter the

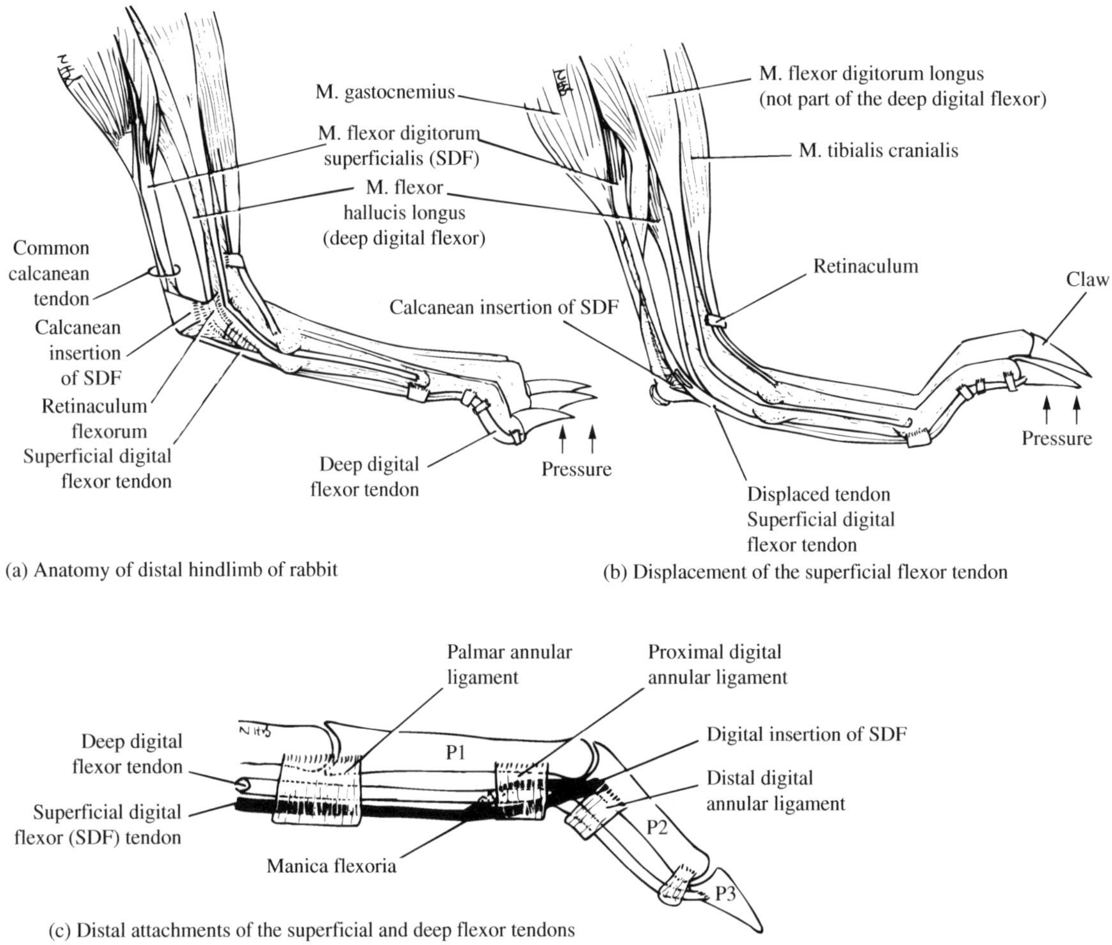

(a) Anatomy of distal hindlimb of rabbit

(b) Displacement of the superficial flexor tendon

(c) Distal attachments of the superficial and deep flexor tendons

Figure 9.4.

way that individual rabbits take their weight and decrease their level of activity. Loss of sensation and prolonged recumbency can result in the development of ulcerative pododermatitis. Nervous rabbits that stamp and thump repeatedly are reputed to be candidates for developing sore hocks. Dirty, wet bedding and constant faecal contamination increase the risk of bacterial infection. In the later stages, the condition becomes painful and prevents the rabbit from moving around, which exacerbates the condition further. Eventually, osteomyelitis and infection of the synovial structures of the hock joint result in displacement of the superficial flexor tendon so the rabbit can no longer adopt a digitigrade stance and has to sit back on its hocks permanently (see Figure 9.4 and Plate 9). Affected animals are disabled and tend to remain immobile, which increases the pressure on the skin over the bony prominences of the hock and exacerbates the condition further. Ulcerative pododermatitis is a vicious circle with the condition causing pain and disability and the pain and disability causing the condition. Decubital ulcers can develop in debilitated animals and ulcerative pododermatitis is itself debilitating.

9.10.2 Pathogenesis of pododermatitis

The development of pressure sores is well documented in other species and parallels can be made with rabbits. The primary pathological change in pressure sores is ischaemia and necrosis of the soft tissues that are compressed

Figure 9.4. Displacement of the superficial flexor tendon due to advanced ulcerative pododermatitis (drawn from dissections of the hindlimbs of a normal rabbit a rabbit with advanced ulcerative pododermatitis).

Figure 9.4a shows the normal anatomy of the distal hindlimb of the rabbit. The hock joint is superficially like that of the cow or sheep and is dissimilar to that of the horse and dog. The fibula is absent distally and the tibiotarsal articulation is formed between the tibia and both the calcaneus (fibular tarsal bone) and talus (tibial tarsal bone). The calcaneus has a single articulation and the talus a double articulation separated by a condylar groove.

The tendon of insertion of the superficial digital flexor muscle (*m. flexor digitorum superficialis*) winds medially around the tendon of insertion of the gastrocnemius muscle to become the most caudal tendon at the tuber calcanei. Although relatively movable over the tuber calcanei, the tendon of the superficial digital flexor broadens like a cap and inserts (initially) laterally and medially onto the tuber calcanei and is also united with the fascia from the other muscles. This insertion keeps the tendon in place throughout the full range of movements of the hock joint. The tendon also continues to the distal tarsal bones where it divides into four branches to digits II, III, IV, and V. It finally inserts on each of the phalanges at the proximal second phalangeal bone, having been perforated by the deep digital flexor tendon and restrained by the transverse ligaments forming cylinders (*manica flexoria*) to contain the flexor tendons (c).

The deep digital flexor tendons are formed from *m. flexor hallucis longus* alone. The tendon of insertion runs on the caudal and plantar aspects of the calcaneus in a groove in the bone being held in place by a retinaculum. The deep flexor tendon divides into four in the distal tarsal region and passes to each digit. On the plantar aspect of each digit one branch of the deep flexor tendon is contained by the *manica flexoria* and finally inserts on the distal phalangeal bone (c).

The normal stance of the hindlimb of the rabbit is digitigrade (see Figure 9.3). Tension in the superficial digital flexor tendon maintains the digits in a flexed position that suspends the metatarsus. Displacement of the superficial digital flexor tendon is the end-stage of ulcerative pododermatitis (see Plate 9). Infection of the deep structures of the tarsus erodes through the calcaneal insertion of the superficial digital flexor tendon and its retinaculum. The deep flexor tendon cannot be displaced at the hock as it is contained in the flexor groove. The superficial flexor can only be displaced medially. Lateral displacement is prevented by the tendons of the gastrocnemius and soleus muscles that insert on the calcaneus.

Once the superficial flexor tendon is displaced, it loses tension and the hock drops. The toes are no longer maintained in a flexed position so the weight of the rabbit is taken on the point of the hock instead of being distributed between the tarsometatarsal area and the claws. The rabbit becomes disabled and increasingly immobile. Immobility and increased pressure on the point of the hock exacerbate pressure necrosis and infection.

Displacement of the tendon can be diagnosed by observing the rabbit's gait and by applying pressure to the claws that cannot be flexed (b). The rabbit adopts a dropped hock gait that could be mistaken for sciatic nerve paralysis (see Plate 10).

between a bony prominence and the surface on which the animal is resting. The degree and severity of ulceration varies with the extent of vascular occlusion. Biochemical changes occur within the ischaemic skin that contributes to tissue necrosis. Intermittent reperfusion of ischaemic skin results in the release of oxygen-free radicals that damage the endothelium and results in vascular thrombosis that causes further dermal necrosis (Swaim *et al.*, 1996).

The area of skin on the point of the hock of rabbits is prone to pressure necrosis. A small area of hairless skin can be found in most adult pet rabbits, although it is concealed by the fur that lies across it. Pressure sores can also develop in the thin skin over the bony prominence of the central tarsal bone, especially in rabbits with sparse hair coating such as the Rex (see Figure 9.3). The lesions can progress eventually to form decubital skin ulcers in this area or on the point of the hock (see Plates 5–7). The first sign is a hairless area of reddened skin. Once the area has lost its protective fur, the skin is subject to increased mechanical trauma and pressure and the condition progresses to hyperkeratosis of the epithelium. Recognition of the disease and identification and treatment of the underlying cause at this stage can prevent progression to ulceration. Without treatment, a shallow ulcer develops that extends into the subcutaneous tissues. Occasionally the medial plantar vein or artery, which lie just beneath skin, is eroded and results in haemorrhage that can be alarming to owners. Bacterial infection, e.g. by *Staphylococcus aureus* or *Pasteurella multocida*, sets in and the wound becomes exudative. The surrounding hair becomes matted and adheres to the lesion, which increases pressure on the skin and exacerbates bacterial contamination further. Infection spreads into deeper tissues and is painful and debilitating. Affected rabbits are reluctant or unable to move about. Urinary and faecal incontinence and dirty bedding encourage infection in the areas of devitalized skin. Ulceration extends through the dermis and epidermis until a decubital ulcer develops. The devitalized skin over the lesion is lost and infection spreads into the deeper tissues, including bone and synovial structures. Erosion of the bone and ligaments of the hock results in displacement of the superficial digital flexor tendon which slips off the hock (see Figures 9.3, 9.4 and Plate 8). Extension of the hock is impaired and the rabbit permanently disabled. It is hamstrung. Displacement of the tendon can be diagnosed by observing the gait of the patient as it attempts to hop around the floor (see Plate 9) and by flexing the hock and observing the toes (see Figure 9.4). The prognosis at this stage is grave.

9.10.3 Treatment of ulcerative pododermatitis

Treatment of ulcerative pododermatitis is aimed at relieving pressure on the affected area and treating any secondary infection. The underlying cause should be addressed if possible. Dirty bedding must be changed, obese rabbits should lose weight and indolent animals encouraged to exercise. A bonded companion can encourage activity. A non-abrasive, soft, dry surface is required for exercise. In dry weather, a lawn is ideal as it is compliant and clean.

Smooth hard surfaces increase the pressure on bony prominences and the choice of bedding to reduce pressure is an important part of treatment. Foam rubber in a convoluted egg crate design is used in humans with pressure sores. In rabbits, a deep bed of hay or soft material must be provided in the place where the rabbit spends most of its time. Foam rubber or a thick towel placed under newspaper with hay on top provides a soft compliant bed. A deep layer of peat moss is used as a bedding for recumbent horses as a treatment for pressure sores and has also been advised for rabbits (Sandford, 1996). The moss reduces shear forces and friction and allows excessive moisture to be drawn away from the skin. It also provides a surface that the claws can grip into. Any ulcerated areas of skin must be kept clean and dry. Liquid bandages (Nu Skin, Germolene) that can be painted on to the lesion can be effective. This type of preparation is available from most chemists. Protective bandages can be advantageous but most rabbits will remove them. A variety of innovative bandaging techniques is used in other species for the treatment of pressure sores. For example, foot splints are used in birds of prey with bumblefoot and doughnut-shaped bandages, foam rubber insulation pipes with holes cut out and aluminium foot splints are used in dogs (Swaim *et al.*, 1996). The shape of a rabbit's hock does not lend itself to such techniques but the principle of padding the surrounding area and not the actual ulcer can still be applied to tolerant rabbits that will leave such dressings alone. Bandages need changing regularly, usually daily, by the owner, as they quickly become soiled and increase the risk of infection. Care must be taken to prevent any padding slipping out of position and increasing pressure on the affected area.

The hair surrounding the ulcer should be trimmed so that it does not extend over the wound, but should not be clipped down to the skin. The fur on the skin surrounding an ulcer can be used to take the weight of the rabbit and relieve the pressure on the ulcerated area in a similar manner to a corn plaster. Systemic antibiotics are indicated for infected wounds and will be required for long periods. Analgesics are required to treat the pain of the condition itself and to make the rabbit more mobile by treating any underlying spondylitic or arthritic condition that is making the rabbit reluctant to move. Meloxicam (Metacam, Boerhinger Ingelheim) is useful for these cases and can be given for prolonged periods.

Surgery should be avoided if possible. In other species, skin flaps and other surgical techniques are sometimes used to close the skin deficit created by a decubital ulcer. In rabbits, there is insufficient skin over the metatarsus to make this a feasible proposition. The skin in this area is naturally adherent to the underlying tissues and any attempt to move it around is likely to make matters worse. Curetting devitalized and infected tissue to allow healing by secondary intention is indicated in some cases but is only likely to be successful if the underlying cause of the ulcerative pododermatitis is addressed and additional methods of reducing pressure on the area are also instigated. Abscesses of the hock can be drained by incising skin that is not weight bearing and curetting out infected tissue. Honey is a useful topical treatment (see Section 8.3.2)

Many cases of ulcerative pododermatitis are incurable, although the condition can be alleviated with medical treatment. Mild cases can respond to bandaging and systemic antibiotics. Once the condition has progressed

Key points 9.4

- Ulcerative pododermatitis is a term used to describe avascular necrosis of the plantar aspect of the feet. Pressure, shearing forces, friction and moisture are predisposing causes of the condition, which is essentially a pressure sore
- Ulcerative pododermatitis is a progressive painful condition that can be fatal. It poses a huge welfare problem in farmed rabbits, especially those large breeds that are kept in wire cages
- At rest, healthy rabbits take most of their weight on their hind claws and the metatarsal skin pad that lies over the bony prominences of the tarsus. In most breeds, a thick pad of hair protects the skin in this region
- The protective layer of fur is absent in certain short furred breeds such as the Rex
- Hard, non-compliant flooring increases the pressure on the bony prominences. Carpet can cause friction and trauma to the area
- Obesity and long periods of inactivity increase the pressure on bony prominences and predispose to pododermatitis. Illness, arthritis and spondylosis can also reduce activity and lead to the development of sore hocks
- Poor conformation can alter the distribution of weight on the legs and increase pressure on the hocks
- Pressure sores can develop that erode through the skin and bleed intermittently
- Dirty wet bedding increases the risk of infection into the pressure sores
- A vicious circle is set up where pododermatitis causes inactivity and inactivity exacerbates pododermatitis
- Eventually, infection of the synovial structures of the tarsal joint and osteomyelitis set in. The tendon of the superficial digital extensor tendon can become displaced
- Displacement of the superficial digital extensor tendon prevents digitigrade locomotion. The rabbit is forced to walk on its hocks which increases the pressure in that area
- The area around the hock becomes infected. Abscesses often develop. The rabbit is in constant pain and may become debilitated and anorexic as a result
- Treatment is directed at relieving pressure on the plantar aspect of the metatarsus, treating infection and increasing mobility
- Clean, compliant surfaces such as lawns, foam rubber or a deep bed of hay can relieve pressure
- Weight reduction and increased opportunity to exercise are important
- Systemic antibiotic therapy and analgesia are also important parts of the treatment protocol
- Abscesses involving the area may be drained and treated topically. Care is required for antibiotic selection as any topical preparation will be licked off and ingested. Manuka honey is safe and non-toxic
- The prognosis for rabbits with a displaced superficial digital extensor tendon is grave. Euthanasia may be necessary.

to abscessation of the hocks or displacement of the flexor tendon, euthanasia should be considered.

9.11 Contact dermatitis

Contact dermatitis occurs as a result of repeated exposure to chemicals such as disinfectants, newsprint, wood shavings or topical creams and ointments. The distribution of lesions can be helpful in identifying the cause. Lesions around the face, head and ears can be caused by substances that are distributed over these regions during grooming. Lesions on the scrotum or hocks can be associated with contact reactions to the substrate.

9.12 Self-mutilation

Some rabbits are prone to self-mutilation. Lesions can occur anywhere, although lesions on the fore feet seem to occur most commonly. Self-trauma can be so severe that some of the digits are lost. The cause of self-mutilation is not clear and it is likely that a number of conditions may result in this type of behaviour. Obsessive/compulsive behaviour, hypersensitivity, harvest mite infection, atopy and contact dermatitis are among the causes that have been considered. Many rabbits carry *Cheyletiella parasitovorax* and/or *Leporacus gibbus* mites and hypersensitivity is a possibility. Treatment should always include a parasiticide such as ivermectin or selamectin. Sometimes hay seeds or grass awns can become embedded in the skin and cause intense irritation. This type of foreign body can usually be seen on close examination of the skin.

Self-mutilation sometimes appears to be a psychological disorder. Active, sociable animals seem most susceptible. Environmental enrichment, including the opportunity to exercise and a bonded companion can be successful in preventing the syndrome. Neutering is required to prevent frustration associated with the desire to find a suitable nesting site or receptive companion. A high fibre diet is important. Chewing through a mound of hay or grazing grass prevents boredom as well as providing indigestible fibre. Toys, such as cardboard boxes or branches of wood will also provide entertainment.

Compulsive self-mutilation has been reported in laboratory rabbits. A genetic predisposition has been identified in one particular strain of rabbits by Iglauer *et al.* (1995). The disease started as small areas of erythema on the digits of the front feet. The lesions appeared to be intensely pruritic and the rabbits would lick their feet and 'air box' frequently. The disease occurred at any age and there appeared to be a seasonal incidence in the late summer and autumn. The authors could find no causative agent on bacteriological, mycological or parasitological investigation or on histological examination of skin lesions or brains of affected animals. Treatment with haloperidol (0.2–0.4 mg/kg twice daily) was successful and a diagnosis of self-mutilation was made.

Self-mutilation and the removal of digits has also been reported in two laboratory rabbits as a sequel to intramuscular injections of ketamine and xylazine into the caudal thigh (Beyers *et al.*, 1991). The symptoms appeared 2–3 days post-injection. Though lameness was not observed, skin irritation was obvious. During ambulation the rabbits extended the leg posteriorly and shook the paw with each step. *Post-mortem* examination showed axonal degeneration in the sciatic nerve.

9.13 Treponematosis or 'rabbit syphilis'

Treponematosis is an infectious disease in rabbits that is sexually transmitted and may be called 'rabbit syphilis'. The disease is caused by a spirochaete, *Treponema cuniculi,* that resembles the causative organism of human syphilis, *Treponema pallidum.* The two organisms are antigenically similar. After the discovery of *Treponema cuniculi* in 1912, some investigators inoculated themselves with *T. cuniculi* in the hope that asymptomatic infection would occur that would convey protection against *T. pallidum* and lead to the development of a vaccine against syphilis (Delong and Manning, 1994). The investigators found that humans could not be infected with *T. cuniculi* but laboratory rabbits could be infected with *T. pallidum.*

Treponema cuniculi occurs in wild lagomorphs including hares. Vertical transmission can take place with young rabbits being infected during the passage through the birth canal of an infected dam. Treponematosis is sometimes encountered in the individual pet rabbit, especially in young animals within a few months of purchase. The disease is characterized by crusty lesions on the mucocutaneous junctions of the nose, lips or eyelids, or the external genitalia (see Plate 10). Lesions begin as areas of hyperaemia and oedema. Erythematous raised papules develop, which can progress to large papillary nodules that can become eroded on the surface, exude serum and become crusty. Chronic lesions can bleed sporadically. Hyperplasia of the regional lymph node can occur. The prepuce of males and the vulva in females are the usual sites of infection in breeding animals and the lesions can extend to the anus and into surrounding skin. Although the disease is most common in juvenile animals, it is occasionally encountered in an adult pet rabbit that has been kept on its own. Lesions can persist in untreated cases for long periods of time. The disease has a long incubation period. Studies on outbreaks have suggested a period of 10–16 weeks (DiGiacomo *et al.*, 1984). Subclinical infections can occur.

Positive diagnosis can be made by examination of material scraped from the lesion, skin biopsy or serology. Special silver staining techniques are required to stain the organism that is seen in the dermis and epidermis. Sometimes the organism can be seen under dark field microscopy. The lesion is abraded with a swab soaked in sterile saline and the exudate examined immediately. There is also a serological test available from some commercial laboratories in the UK. Lesions can occur before the development of positive serology so false negatives may occur in early infections. Rabbits can remain seropositive after lesions have resolved. Rabbits treated with antibiotic experience a gradual decline or disappearance of detectable antibody (Delong and Manning, 1994).

A presumptive diagnosis of treponematosis can be made from response to treatment. Penicillin is the treatment of choice and is usually curative. Other antibiotics are not as effective. The recommended protocol is three injections of penicillin at weekly intervals (Cunliffe-Beamer and Fox, 1981). Many reference sources give dosages of penicillin in international units (IU) and there are 1000 IU per milligram of penicillin. A dose rate of 42 000 IU/kg is often quoted. For pet rabbits, long-acting depot injections of penicillin can be used to treat treponematosis at a dose rate of 20–25 mg/kg procaine benzylpenicillin combined with benzathine benzylpenicillin. This translates to a dose of 0.15 ml/kg once a week for most preparations (e.g. Duplocillin

Key points 9.5

- Contact dermatitis can occur in rabbits as a result of repeated exposure to chemical agents such as disinfectants or topical creams and ointments
- Self-mutilation occurs in rabbits and can result in loss of digits. Hypersensitivity, atopy, obsessive/compulsive behaviour, harvest mite infestation and neurological disease have been suggested as possible causes
- *Treponema cuniculi* can affect pet rabbits. The organism causes 'rabbit syphilis' and is antigenically similar to *Treponema pallidum* that causes human syphilis. *T. cuniculi* cannot be spread from rabbits to humans
- Treponematosis is a sexually transmitted disease that is most commonly seen in breeding rabbits. It is sometimes seen in the newly acquired juvenile rabbit that has been infected during the passage through the birth canal of an infected dam. Occasionally, treponematosis is seen in the adult pet rabbit
- Treponematosis causes crusty lesions on the mucocutaneous junctions of the nose, lips and genitalia. Occasionally lesions can be seen on the eyelids. Without treatment, the lesions can persist for considerable periods of time
- Positive diagnosis of treponematosis can be made by dark ground microscopy and silver staining of the exudate. Serological tests are available
- Parenteral penicillin is the treatment of choice for *T. cuniculi*. Other antibiotics are not as effective. Although penicillin carries a small risk of antibiotic-associated diarrhoea, the risk is minimal if the antibiotic is administered parenterally. Three, weekly penicillin injections are usually effective.

Intervet, Lentrax Merial). There are reports of the death of kits when nursing does have received procaine penicillin. The deaths have been attributed to the toxic effects of procaine (Collins, 1995). Penicillin also carries a small risk of antibiotic-associated diarrhoea in rabbits but is generally safe when administered parenterally (see Section 4.2.1.8).

Lesions start to regress approximately 5 days after the first injection. Complete regression typically occurs within 2 weeks. Intractable cases may require skin biopsy and histopathology to differentiate them from other diseases. Differential diagnoses include infected wounds (bites or iatrogenic injuries from dental burrs), atypical myxomatosis, neoplasia and recurrent trauma from some repetitive action such as pushing the nose through the netting in a hutch. Rectoanal papillomas can resemble treponematosis. Histologically, treponematosis causes acanthosis of the epidermis with erosions or shallow ulcers covered by necrotic cellular debris. Plasma cells and macrophages are present in the underlying dermis (Kraus *et al.*, 1984).

9.14 Parasitic skin disease

Some common external parasites of pet rabbits are illustrated in Figures 16.1–16.3.

9.14.1 Fleas

The rabbit flea, *Spilopsyllus cuniculi*, has a predilection for the pinnae where they feed in clumps. The cat or dog flea *Ctenocephalides felis* or *Ctenicephalides canis* can also be encountered in rabbits that live with dogs or cats or in infested premises. The distribution of the dog and cat fleas differs from the rabbit flea that is found on the ears and face. *Ctenocephalides felis* or *Ctenicephalides canis* are found along the dorsum and at the base of the tail. Flea infestation is intensely pruritic in rabbits. The condition is easily diagnosed by examining the coat for the presence of fleas and flea dirt. Flea allergic dermatitis with hair loss along the dorsum can also occur. Imidacloprid (Advantage 40, Bayer) is an effective remedy, although it does not hold a product licence for use in rabbits. Selamectin (Stronghold, Pfizer) is an alternative. Dosages similar to cats are used.

9.14.2 Mite infestations

9.14.2.1 Ear mites

The ear mite *Psoroptes cuniculi* inhabits the auditory canal, although infection can spread to other areas such as the perineal skin folds (Yeatts, 1994) and ventral abdomen (Cutler, 1998). Otitis externa caused by ear mites has already been described (see Section 9.9). There is a report of *Psoroptes cuniculi* infestation of a guinea pig that was kept with a rabbit which had ear mites. The guinea pig was severely affected with generalized scaling and crusting and *Psoroptes cuniculi* mites were identified on the ears and legs (Yeatts, 1994).

9.14.2.2 Fur mites

Both *Cheyletiella parasitovorax* and *Leporacus gibbus* (formerly known as *Listrophorus gibbus*) can be found in the coat of most pet rabbits. The mites can just be seen with the naked eye, either in the fur or in skin brushings. Mites are easily seen on microscopic examination of skin brushings. Simply placing a small amount of fur that has been brushed out of the coat in a clear plastic bag and examining it under low power will give an indication of the number and type of mite that is present. The presence of mites may not be associated with disease and they can be considered to be commensal ectoparasites (Kirwan *et al.*, 1998). Although mites can be found on any part of the body, they are usually found along the dorsum, especially in the area at base of the tail and the area between the shoulder blades. These areas are difficult for the rabbit to reach and are not groomed as well as other parts of the body. Bonded companions do not groom these areas as much as the area around the face and head. Skin debris and parasites can build up. Large numbers of *Cheyletiella parasitovorax* cause pruritus, areas of alopecia and large amounts of white scale. *Leporacus gibbus* infestation is usually asymptomatic, although it may be associated with mild scurf and pruritus (Kirwan *et al.*, 1998). Grooming difficulties and hypersensitivity reactions could account for differences in pathogenicity of mites between individuals.

9.14.2.3 *Cheyletiella parasitovorax*

Cheyletiella parasitovorax is an obligate non-burrowing mite that lives on the keratin layer of the epidermis. The mites create pseudo-tunnels through the scale and debris on the skin surface. The entire life cycle of *C. parasitovorax* takes place on the host and is completed in about 35 days (Chomel, 1992). Ova are attached to hair shafts and there are two nymphal stages (Wilkinson and Harvey, 1994). Many rabbits harbour the mite with no sign of disease. In a survey of 220 laboratory rabbits, 43.2% had inapparent *Cheyletiella parasitovorax* infestations (Flatt and Weimers, 1976). Clinical signs may be seen in young and immunosuppressed individuals (Scarff, 1991) or in animals suffering from an underlying condition that prevents satisfactory grooming. Large flakes of white scale are associated with the disease and many affected rabbits are mildly pruritic. Underlying grooming problems due to dental disease, long fine coat texture (Angoras), obesity or spondylitis prevent the rabbit from removing parasites and debris from the coat and allow the parasites to proliferate. Mites can be seen by plucking or brushing some hair and debris from the dorsum or by applying clear acetate tape to the skin and looking for parasites under the microscope (see Figure 16.2). The mites are just visible to the naked eye. Scale combed out of lesions can be seen to be moving if viewed under bright illumination. As in other species, the term 'walking dandruff' can be applied to cheyletiellosis in rabbits.

Treatment of cheyletiellosis involves killing the mite, removing the scale and identifying and treating underlying grooming difficulties. The keratin that the mites feed on can be physically removed with a fine toothed flea comb. Treating the underlying cause, such as dental disease or obesity, and combing out skin debris can bring about a marked improvement in the condition. Bathing the rabbit in selenium sulphide shampoo (Seleen, Sanofi) is advocated by some authors. The shampoo has no insecticidal properties but removes the keratin that the mites feed on. Bathing rabbits is difficult due to their thick dense fur, restraint and the risk of chilling. Ivermectin or selamectin is effective in killing the mites. A second dose of ivermectin needs to be administered 10–14 days after the first. Although fipronil is effective in killing cheyletiella, the manufacturers warn that the product must not be used either as a spray or a spot-on preparation in rabbits. Fatal adverse reactions have occurred. Imidacloprid (Advantage 40, Bayer) is ineffective against cheyletiella.

Eggs and adult female *C. parasitovorax* mites can live off the host for 10 days without feeding (Timm, 1988). Larvae, nymphs and adult males are not very resistant and die in about 2 days in the environment (Chomel, 1992). Environmental control is required to eliminate infection. *Cheyletiella parasitovorax* is zoonotic. The mites can cause a mild pruritic dermatitis in humans that handle infested rabbits. Lesions are usually found on the forearms and neck.

9.14.2.4 *Leporacus gibbus*

The rabbit fur mite *Leporacus gibbus* (formerly *Listrophorus gibbus*) is a common inhabitant of rabbit fur. It is a pelage inhabiting mite with specially adapted legs that enable it to cling to the hair shaft. There is sexual dimorphism (see Figure 16.3). The female mite is large and oval with a characteristic thumb print pattern on the body. The male is slightly smaller and possesses two long adanal processes and distinct adanal suckers. Hatched eggs can be seen attached to hair shafts in a similar way to louse eggs (nits). The egg appears to split down the dorsal midline during larval emergence, giving the egg cases two wing-like structures (Kirwan *et al.*, 1998). Empty cuticles persist on hairs after moulting has taken place giving the fur a characteristic 'salt and pepper' appearance. The cuticles can also persist after the mites have been killed with acaricidal treatment. In contrast, dead *Cheyletiella parasitovorax* soon disappear from the host following treatment (Kirwan *et al.*, 1998). *L. gibbus* can just be seen with the naked eye and tends to move away from direct light. Infestation is usually asymptomatic, although hypersensitivity reactions have been reported (Patel and Robinson, 1993).

9.14.2.5 *Demodex cuniculi*

Demodex cuniculi has been found in skin scrapings taken from rabbits in the UK (Harvey, 1990). The mite appears to be able to exist on the skin of normal rabbits in the absence of associated clinical signs.

9.14.2.6 Sarcoptic mange

Sarcoptic mange has been reported in association with *Notoedres cati* and *Sarcoptes scabei* infestation in laboratory or commercial rabbits. Pruritic lesions are found, especially on the face, nose, lips and external genitalia (Percy and Barthold, 1993). Other areas such as the pinnae and neck may be affected (Lin *et al.*, 1984). The skin is covered in yellow scaly crust. Sarcoptic mange is rare in the UK, although it is common in other parts of the world such as Africa. (Scott *et al.*, 1995). Ivermectin is an effective remedy.

9.14.2.7 Harvest mites

Harvest mites can infest rabbits that have access to outdoor habitats where harvest mites are found. Adult mites lay their eggs in the soil and, on hatching, the larvae move onto low vegetation and await a suitable host. Larvae can survive for up to 30 days without a host. When a host is available, the larvae attach to the surface of the skin to feed. When engorged, the larvae drop to the ground and, after a period of quiescence, moult and emerge as non-parasitic nymphs that feed on insects and insect eggs. Unfed larvae are a deep red colour. Fully fed larvae are larger and a pale yellow colour (Hofing and Kraus, 1994).

In rabbits, harvest mite larvae are most commonly found on the ears, anus, canthi of the eyes, and feet. The feeding process induces intense pruritus and the formation of discrete macules and pustules. Treatment is difficult and the disease is seasonal and self-limiting. Removing the rabbit from the source of the harvest mites prevents further infestations.

9.14.3 Lice

The sucking louse, *Haemodipsus ventricosus*, can affect domestic rabbits. It may be found in breeding establishments, especially if husbandry standards are poor. It commonly affects wild rabbits and there has been discussion as to whether it can act as a mechanical vector for myxomatosis (Owen, 1992). Lice are known to be vectors for tularaemia. Lice may be found on the dorsal and lateral aspects of the body and around the perineum. The eggs are laid on the host and are firmly attached to the hair. They are oval in shape with a distinctive operculum from which the larvae emerge. The young are similar to the adult and undergo three ecdyses before they are adult. The entire life cycle takes 2–5 weeks depending on environmental conditions (Owen, 1992).

9.14.4 Tapeworm cysts

Taenia serialis is a tapeworm that affects dogs and foxes. The larval stage, *Coenurus serialis*, can be found in the subcutaneous and intramuscular tissues of rabbits. The onchosphere emerges from ingested eggs in the small intestine and makes its way to the subcutaneous tissue where it develops into a cyst that can reach 4–5 cm in diameter. *Coenurus serialis* cysts have been reported in a number of sites in pet rabbits including the retrobulbar space, the cheek and the axilla (Bennett, 2001; Wills, 2001). The cyst is filled with fluid and has secondary buds protruding to the inside, each with an inverted scolex (Owen, 1992). The cysts do not affect the rabbit and can be removed surgically. Alternatively the cyst can be punctured and the contents aspirated. Praziquantel can be used to kill the cestode.

9.15 Ringworm

Trichophyton mentagrophytes and *Microsporum canis* can affect rabbits causing circular, crusty, erythematous, alopecic areas that are pruritic. Lesions are usually found on areas that are frequently groomed, such as the base of the ears and muzzle, but can spread to other areas of the body such as the paws. Secondary lesions found on the feet can involve the nail beds (Franklin *et al.*, 1991). *M. canis* fluoresces under a Wood's lamp but *T. mentagrophytes* does not. *M. gypseum*, *M. audouinii*, *T. verrucosum* and *T. schoenleinii* have also been recorded (Scott *et al.*, 1995). Ringworm is most common in young rabbits

Key points 9.6

- Cat and dog fleas can infest rabbits. The distribution of dog or cat fleas is different from the rabbit flea that is normally encountered on the head, especially on the ears and around the eyes. Cat and dog fleas are usually found on the dorsum
- Flea infestation can be intensely pruritic. Imidacloprid is an effective remedy
- Both *Cheyletiella parasitovorax* and *Leporacus gibbus* (formerly *Listrophorus gibbus*) can be found in the fur of asymptomatic rabbits. These mites can be commensal
- Underlying grooming difficulties allow *Cheyletiella parasitovorax* to proliferate and cause disease. Typically, large areas of white scale are found along the dorsum, particularly between the shoulder blades and at the base of the tail
- *Cheyletiella parasitovorax* feeds on keratin. Physically removing dead skin and hair from the coat with a comb can help to reduce parasite numbers
- Treating the underlying cause, such as obesity, poor grooming or dental disease is as important as treating the mites
- Insecticidal treatment with selamactin or ivermectin is effective in killing mites. Fipronil is also effective but the manufacturers do not advocate its use in rabbits because fatal adverse reactions have occurred. Imidacloprid is ineffective
- *Cheyletiella parasitovorax* is zoonotic and can cause mild pruritic lesions in humans
- The rabbit fur mite *Leporacus gibbus* is usually asymptomatic although hypersensitivity reactions have been reported
- *Demodex cuniculi* has been reported in asymptomatic pet rabbits
- Sarcoptic mange can occur although it is rare in the pet rabbit
- The sucking louse *Haemodipsus ventricosus* may occasionally be found in pet rabbits. It is usually encountered in farmed rabbits kept in intensive conditions
- Dermatophyte infection, usually *Trichophyton mentagrophytes* and *Microsporum canis*, can affect rabbits causing circular, crusty, erythematous, alopecic areas that are pruritic. Lesions are usually found on the ears and face. Treatment is similar to other species.

especially where husbandry is suboptimal. Dermatophytosis has been associated with underlying stressors such as concurrent disease, poor nutrition or experimental manipulation (Franklin *et al.*, 1991). Ringworm is uncommon in pet rabbits. Asymptomatic infections have been reported (Vangeel *et al.*, 2000). Brushing the entire rabbit with a sterile toothbrush and culturing the brushings on selective media can be used to detect infected animals.

Treatment is similar to other species. Topical miconazole or clotrimazole can be used. Concurrent administration with cisapride should be avoided as there is potential for adverse drug interactions to occur. Griseofulvin is effective but may be teratogenic in breeding does. Spontaneous resolution of ringworm can occur (Wilkinson and Harvey, 1994).

9.16 Skin nodules

Small abscesses can present as skin nodules. They may be the result of fight wounds, injections, surgical incisions or haematogenous or lymphatic spread from other sites. Surgical excision is usually curative.

Skin nodules can also be caused by 'atypical myxomatosis' (see Plate 11). Multiple benign fibromas can sometimes be found in vaccinated pet rabbits that are exposed to natural infection. Vaccination against myxomatosis requires a small intradermal dose that is important to confer full immunity. It is thought that atypical myxomatosis is more likely to occur in rabbits that have not received the intradermal dose. Atypical myxomatosis nodules regress with time. Occasionally superficial ulceration and infection warrant treatment with antibiotics. Corticosteroids are contraindicated as they are immunosuppressive and delay the development of natural immunity and resolution of the lesions. Myxomatosis is covered in Section 16.2.1.

Localized and generalized cutaneous fibrosarcomas can occur in pet rabbits. Skin metastases from uterine adenocarcinomas also present as multiple hard nodules in the skin. As in other species, excision or biopsy and histopathological examination are required to make the differential diagnosis of skin tumours. EMLA cream (see Section 5.4.3) can be used as a local anaesthetic to biopsy lesions in the conscious rabbits. Papillomas, basal cell carcinomas, squamous cell carcinoma, sebaceous carcinoma, osteosarcoma and lymphoma have all been reported in rabbits (Scott *et al.*, 1995). Collagenous naevus has also been reported (Wilkinson and Harvey, 1994). Focal accumulations of collagen present as painless solitary or multiple dome-shaped papules or nodules which may be alopecic. The condition appears to be benign.

9.17 Papillomas

Papillomas can develop at the rectoanal junction. These small, friable tumours have a cauliflower-like appearance and bleed easily. They arise from the epithelium at the mucosal junction and can be seen protruding from the anus. In many instances the papillomas do not cause problems and will eventually be resolved with time. In other cases, surgical removal is required, ensuring that the base of the tumour is removed to prevent recurrence. It is not known if these tumours are transmissable. Transmission experiments with tumour tissue from two rectoanal papillomas in laboratory rabbits were unsuccessful. The papillomas were well differentiated and benign and inclusion bodies could not be demonstrated (Weisbroth, 1994).

Oral papillomatosis is manifested by wart-like growths on the ventral aspect of the tongue and on other parts of the oral mucosa. This condition is transmissable. Young rabbits are most susceptible and the papillomas grow slowly over a period of 6–9 months. The animals become immune at which point the base of the papilloma becomes inflamed causing sloughing of the tumour, ulcer formation and finally re-epithelialization. Oral papillomas of rabbits are not known to undergo carcinomatous transformation (Kraus *et al.*, 1984)

9.18 Diseases of the mammary gland

Diseases of the mammary gland are similar to other species and occur more frequently in the entire breeding doe than in the spayed family pet. Mammary development takes place in pregnant and pseudopregnant does and is manifested by several discrete mammary swellings in association with each nipple. Adenocarcinomas of the mammary gland can occur in does, usually over 3 years of age, and will metastasize. Cystic mastitis can progress to benign neoplasia and adenocarcinoma in laboratory rabbits. Early surgical removal of lumps in the mammary tissue is indicated. Ovarohysterectomy can be considered at the same time.

Mastitis can occur in lactating does and occasionally in non-lactating or pseudopregnant rabbits. The colloquial term 'blue breast' has been used to describe mastitis that is predisposed by heavy lactation, poor sanitation and injury to the mammary glands (Bergdall and Dysko, 1994). The condition is treated with antibiotics.

9.19 Connective tissue disease

A connective tissue disease similar to the genetic disorder Ehlers Danlos syndrome has been reported in two sibling rabbits. Ehlers Danlos syndrome is characterized by joint hyperextensibility, skin hypermobility and skin fragility. The condition was recognized after a hair pluck sample was taken from one

Key points 9.7

- Skin nodules may be caused by scar tissue, small abscesses, atypical myxomatosis or neoplasia, e.g. generalized fibromas or fibrosarcomas
- Atypical myxomatosis occurs when vaccinated rabbits are exposed to natural infection. The condition resolves with time although systemic antibiotics are sometimes indicated. Corticosteroids are contraindicated
- Mammary tumours occur in female rabbits. The mammary glands of pregnant or pseudopregnant does can sometimes be felt as discrete lumps
- A rare connective tissue disease similar to the genetic disorder Ehlers-Danlos syndrome has been reported in rabbits
- Sebaceous adenitis has been described in pet rabbits. The aetiology is unknown and the condition is refractory to treatment.

of the rabbits during clinical examination. In the process of epilation a piece of skin about 1 cm in diameter was removed and the wound had to be sutured (Harvey *et al.*, 1990).

9.20 Sebaceous adenitis

Sebaceous adenitis has been described in pet rabbits. A series of four cases was described by White *et al.* (2000) that showed histological skin changes comparable with the condition in other species. Affected rabbits showed progressive exfoliative, non-pruritic dermatosis that was refractive to treatment.

References

Arlian, L.G., Kaiser, S., Estes, S.A., Kummel, B. (1981). Infestivity of Psoroptes cuniculi in rabbits (Abstract). *Am J Vet Res.*, **42**, 1782–1784.

Bennett, H. (2001). Coenurus cyst in a pet rabbit. *Vet. Rec.*, **147**, 428.

Bergdall, V., Dysko R.C. (1994). Metabolic, traumatic, mycotic and miscellaneous diseases. In *The Biology of the Laboratory Rabbit*, 2nd edn. (P.J. Manning, D.H.Ringler, C.E.Newcomer, eds). pp 336–355. Academic Press.

Beyers, T.M., Richardson, J.A., Prince, M.D. (1991). Axonal degeneration and self-mutilation as a complication of the intramuscular use of ketamine and xylazine in rabbits. *Lab Anim Sci.*, **41**, 519–520.

Cheeke, P.R., Patton, N.M., Templeton, G.S. (1982). *Rabbit Production.* Interstate Publishers.

Cheeke, P.R. (1987). *Rabbit Feeding and Nutrition.* Academic Press.

Chomel, B.B. (1992). Zoonoses of house pets other than dogs, cats and birds. *Paediatr Infect Dis J.*, **11**, 479–481.

Collins, B.R. (1995). Antimicrobial drug use in rabbits, rodents and other small mammals. *Proceedings of Symposium on Antimicrobial Therapy and The North American Veterinary Conference.*

Cunliffe-Beamer, T.L., Fox, R.R. (1981). Venereal spirochaetosis of rabbits: epizootology. *Lab Anim Sci.*, **31**, 366–382.

Cutler, S.L. (1998). Ectopic *Psoroptes cuniculi* infestation in a pet rabbit. *J Small Anim Pract.*, **39**, 86–87.

Delong, D., Manning, P.J. (1994). Bacterial diseases. In *The Biology of the Laboratory Rabbit*, 2nd edn. (P.J. Manning, D.H. Ringler, C.E. Newcomer, eds). pp 131–170. Academic Press.

DiGiacomo, R.F., Lukehart, S.A., Talburt, C.D. *et al.* (1984). Clinical course and treatment of venereal spirochaetosis in New Zealand White rabbits. *Br J Vener Dis.*, **60**, 214–218.

Drescher, B., Sclender-Böbbis, I. (1993). Pododermatitis beim Kaninchen. (Article in German, English summary). *Kleinterpraxis*, **41**, 99–103.

Flatt, R.E., Deyoung, D.W., Hogle, R.M. (1977). Suppurative otitis media in the rabbit: prevalence, pathology and microbiology. *Lab Anim Sci.*, **27**, 343–347.

Flatt, R.E., Wiemers, J. (1976). A survey of fur mites in domestic rabbits (Abstract). *Lab Anim Sci.*, **26**, 758–761.

Flecknell, P.A. (1998). Developments in the veterinary care of rabbits and rodents. *In Practice*, **20**, 286–295.

Franklin, C.L., Gibson, S.V., Caffrey, C.J. *et al.* (1991). Treatment of Trichophyton mentagrophytes infection in rabbits. *J Am Vet Med Assoc.*, **19**, 1625–1630.

Hack, R.J., Walstrom, D.J., Hair, J.A. (2001). Efficacy and safety of two different dose rates of selamectin against naturally acquired infestations of *Psoroptes cuniculi* in rabbits. *Scientific Proceedings of British Small Animal Association Congress 2001*, p. 552.

Hago, B.E.D., Magid, O.Y.A., El Sanousi, S.M. *et al.* (1987). An outbreak of suppurative osteoarthritis of the tibiotarsal joint in rabbits caused by Pasteurella multocida. *J Small Anim Pract.*, **28**, 763–766.

Hargreaves, J., Hartley, N.J.W. (2000). Dermal fibrosis in a rabbit. *Vet Rec.*, **147**, 400.

Harvey, C. (1995). Rabbit and rodent skin diseases. *Sem Avian Exotic Pet Med.*, **4**, 95–204.

Harvey, R.G. (1990). *Demodex cuniculi* in dwarf rabbits (*Oryctolagus cuniculus*). *J Small Anim Pract.*, **31**, 204–207.

Harvey, R.G., Brown, P.J., Young, R.D., Whitbread, T.J. (1990). A connective tissue defect in two rabbits similar to the Ehlers Danlos syndrome. *Vet Rec.*, **126**, 130–132.

Hermans, K., De Herdt, P., Devriese, L.A. *et al.* (1999). Colonisation of rabbits with Staphylococcus aureus in flocks with or without chronic staphylococcus (Abstract). *Vet Microbiol.*, **67**, 37–46.

Hofing, G.L., Kraus, A.L. (1994). Arthropod and helminth parasites. In *The Biology of the Laboratory Rabbit.*, 2nd edn. (P.J. Manning, D.H.Ringler, C.E.Newcomer, eds). pp 231–258. Academic Press.

Hoyt, R.F. (1998). Abdominal surgery of pet rabbits. In *Current Techniques in Small Animal Surgery*, 4th edn. (M.J. Bojrab, ed.) pp 777–790. Williams and Wilkins.

Iglauer, F., Beig, C., Dimigen, J. *et al.* (1995). Hereditary compulsive self-mutilating behaviour in laboratory rabbits. *Lab Anim.*, **29**, 385–393.

Kirwan, A.P., Middleton, B., McGarry, J.W. (1998). Diagnosis and prevalence of *Leporacus gibbus* in the fur of domestic rabbits in the UK. *Vet Rec.*, **142**, 20–21.

Kraus, A., Weisbroth, S.H., Flatt, R.E., Brewer N. (1984). Biology and diseases of rabbits. In *Laboratory Animal Medicine.* pp 207–237. Academic Press.

Lin S.L., Pinson D.M., Lindsey J.R. (1984). Diagnostic exercise. *Lab Anim Sci.*, **34**, 353–354.

Mackay, R., (2000). Dermal fibrosis in a rabbit. *Vet Rec.*, **147**, 252.

McDonald, P., Edwards, R.A., Greenhalgh, J.F.D., Morgan, C.A. (1996). *Animal Nutrition*, 5th edn. Longman.

Owen, D.G. (1992). Parasites of laboratory animals. In *Laboratory Animal Handbooks No 12.* Royal Society of Medicine Services Ltd.

Pairet, M., Bouyssou, T., Ruckesbuch, Y. (1986). Colonic formation of soft feces in rabbits: a role for endogenous prostaglandins. (Abstract). *Am J Physiol.*, **250**, G302–G308.

Patel, A., Robinson, K.J.E. (1993). Dermatosis associated with *Listrophorus gibbus* in the rabbit. *J Small Anim Pract.*, **34**, 409–411.

Percy, D.H, Barthold, S.W. (1993). Rabbit. In *Pathology of Laboratory Rodents and Rabbits*, pp 179–223. Iowa State University Press.

Richardson, V. (2000). *Rabbits. Health, Husbandry and Diseases*. Blackwell Science.

Sandford, J.C. (1996). *The Domestic Rabbit*, 5th edn. Blackwell Science.

Scarff, D.H. (1991). Skin disorders of small mammals. *J Small Anim Pract.*, **32**, 408–412.

Scott, D.W., Miller, W.H., Griffin, C.E. (1995). Dermatoses of pet rodents, rabbits and ferrets. In *Muller and Kirk's Small Animal Dermatology*, 5th edn. pp 1127–1174. W.B. Saunders.

Swaim, S.F., Hanson, R.R., Coates, J.R. (1996). Pressure wounds in animals. *Compendium on Continuing Education*, **18**, 203–219.

Timm, K.I. (1988). Pruritus in rabbits, rodents and ferrets. *Vet Clin N Am: Small Anim Pract.*, **18**, 1077–1099.

Vangeel, I., Pasmans, F., Vanrobaeys, M. *et al.* (2000). Prevalence of dermatophytes in asymptomatic guinea pigs and rabbits. *Vet Rec.*, **146**, 440–441.

Weisbroth, S.H. (1994). Neoplastic diseases. In *The Biology of the Laboratory Rabbit*, 2nd edn. (P.J. Manning, D.H.Ringler, C.E.Newcomer, eds). pp 259–292. Academic Press.

White, S.D., Linder, K.E., Schultheiss, P. *et al.* (2000). Sebaceous adenitis in four domestic rabbits. *Vet Dermatol.*, **11**, 53–60.

Wilkinson, G.T., Harvey, R.G. (1994). *Color Atlas of Small Animal Dermatology – A guide to diagnosis*. Wolfe.

Wills, J. (2001). Coenurosis in a pet rabbit. *Vet. Rec.*, **148**, 188.

Wright, F.C., Riner, J.C. (1985). Comparative efficacy of injection routes and doses of ivermectin against Psoroptes in rabbits (Abstract). *Am J Vet Res.*, **46**, 752–754.

Yeatts, J.W.G. (1994). Rabbit mite infestation. *Vet Rec.*, **134**, 359.

Digestive disorders

10

A wide array of digestive disorders affects rabbits. Diarrhoea, bloat, scours, mucoid enteritis, enterotoxaemia, gut stasis, wool-block, trichobezoars, enteritis, gastroenteropathy, mucoid enteropathy are among the variety of non-specific terms used to describe the diseases that affect the gastrointestinal tract. Many of the digestive disorders that afflict pet rabbits are related to diet and only a few are caused by enteric pathogens. There is a complex inter-relationship between the predisposing factors and causes of digestive disease. This inter-relationship is summarized in Figure 10.1. Enteric disease is manifested by a disruption in normal faecal production. The consistency and frequency of hard and/or soft faeces are altered. There may or may not be mucus production. The term 'diarrhoea' can be confusing, both to owners and vets. A list of differential diagnoses of 'diarrhoea' is given in Table 10.1.

10.1 Digestive physiology

A detailed description of the rabbit's digestive physiology is given in Section 1.5. Briefly, the rabbit is a strict herbivore whose digestive system is adapted for the ingestion of a fibrous diet. Digestion in the stomach and small intestine is similar to monogastric animals and food that reaches the hindgut is mainly composed of fibre that cannot be broken down by the digestive enzymes of the stomach and small intestine. The rabbit has the ability to separate large fibre particles from small fibre particles in the proximal colon. The small particles and the large undigested particles are simultaneously sent in opposite directions. Large particles of undigested fibre pass distally and are excreted in hard faecal pellets. Small fibre particles are sent in a retrograde direction into the caecum where they undergo bacterial fermentation. Bacterial fermentation within the caecum releases volatile fatty acids that are absorbed as an energy source. The result of bacterial fermentation within the caecum is a fine paste containing amino acids, vitamins, enzymes, microorganisms and volatile fatty acids.

Therefore, the rabbit's colon has a dual function. For most of the day, it mixes and separates ingesta, simultaneously sending indigestible particles towards the anus, and fermentable particles towards the caecum. Periodically, the motility of the proximal colon alters completely, and pasty caecal contents are directed along the colon to be expelled as soft faecal pellets or caecotrophs. Caecotroph production follows a diurnal rhythm. Most rabbits produce soft faeces during the morning and evening approximately 4 h after feeding. These caecotrophs are re-ingested directly from the anus to be digested in the stomach and small intestine as an additional source of nutrients for the rabbit. The nature of the intestinal contents, muscular activity, transit time and exchange of water and electrolytes alter according to the type of faeces that are passing through the colon. Therefore, digestion and colonic motility can either be in the 'hard faeces phase' or the 'soft faeces phase' (see Figure 1.2). The amount of ingesta and gas in the various sections of the digestive tract alters according to the phase of excretion. The size and shape of the caecum also follows a diurnal rhythm, which is an important consideration during abdominal palpation or radiography of rabbits.

Separation of ingesta in the proximal colon is accomplished by a combination of

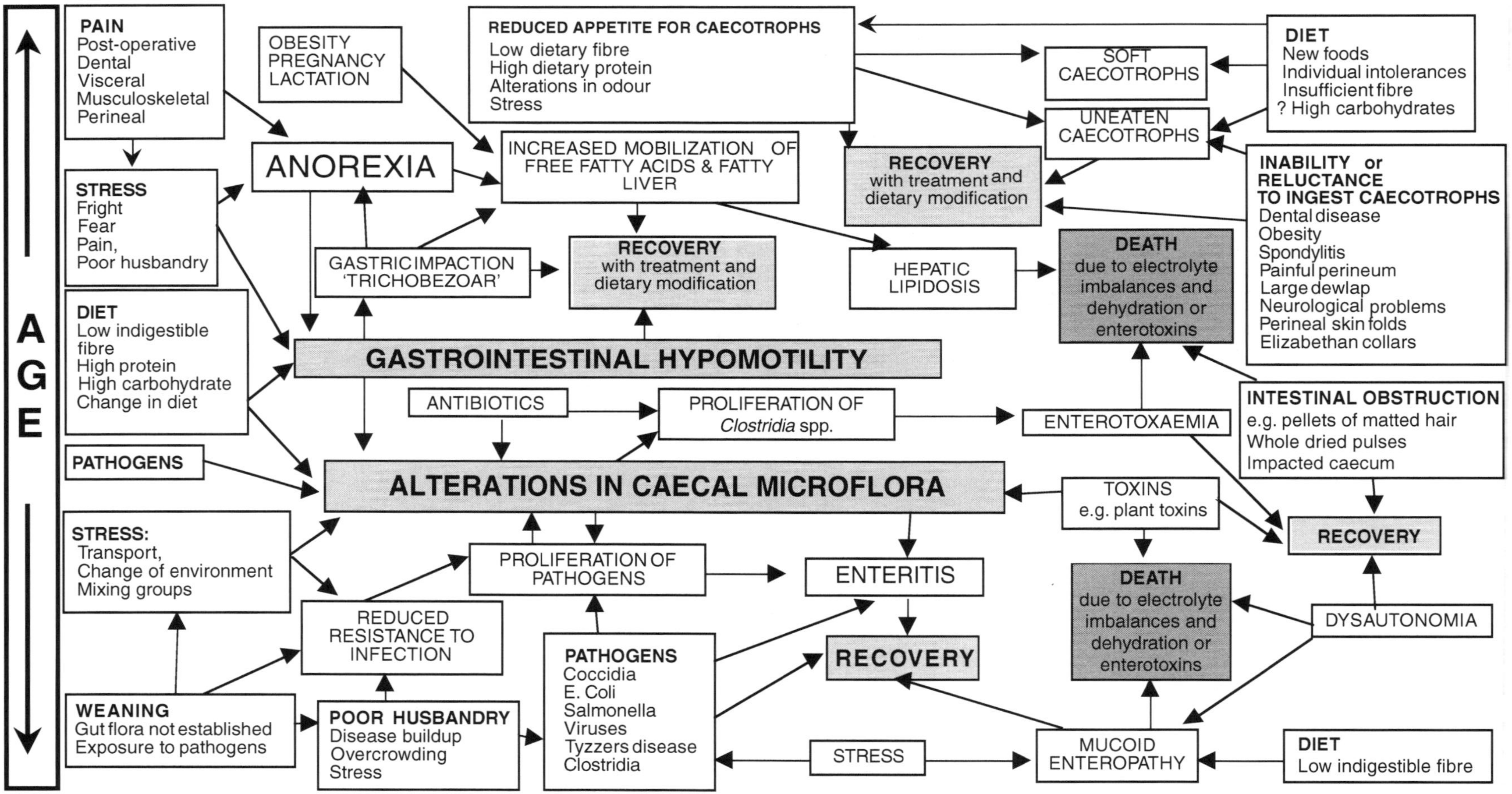

Figure 10.1. Inter-relationship of predisposing factors and causes of gastrointestinal disease in rabbits.

Table 10.1 Differential diagnosis of 'diarrhoea' in rabbits

Syndrome	*Incidence in pet rabbits*	*Hard faeces*	*Caecotrophs*	*Condition of rabbit*	*Causes*
Uneaten normal caecotrophs (Soft odorous faecal material that looks like diarrhoea to the owner)	Common	Copious quantities of hard faecal pellets	Normal consistency	Well Appetite good	Obesity Dental disease Spondylosis Arthritis Perineal dermatitis etc.
Uneaten soft caecotrophs	Common	Copious quantities of hard faecal pellets	Soft, liquid consistency	Well	Change of diet Lack of dietary fibre Succulent foods Stress + same causes as uneaten normal caecotrophs
Coccidiosis	Rare in adult Common in juvenile	Diarrhoea can range from haemorrhagic liquid faeces to bulky soft faeces	Indistinguishable from hard faeces	Depends on severity of condition	*Eimeria* species
Mucoid enteropathy	Rare in adult Associated with stress Sporadic outbreaks juveniles	Normal hard faeces are absent Mixed or interspersed mucus and diarrhoea No faecal output in later stages	Abnormal soft caecotrophs may be intermittently interspersed with mucus and diarrhoea	May be eating in early stages Bloated appearance Progresses to inappetance and tooth grinding	Still unclear Dysautonomia has been found in some cases
Caecal impaction	Sporadic incidence	Absence of hard faeces Can produce mucus which owners mistake for diarrhoea	None in later stages	May pick at food in early stages	Appears to be associated with pain or stress Caecal impaction is also part of mucoid enteropathy complex Can be caused by ingestion of materials that are moved into the caecum, absorb water and are not broken down by caecal microflora. Examples include clay litter, methylcellulose or other bulk laxatives
Enteritis	Rare in adults Enteritis caused by bacterial overgrowth/ imbalances are more	Normal hard faeces are absent Liquid diarrhoea	Not seen	Unwell Anorexic May crave fibre	Bacterial or viral pathogens such as *E. coli*, clostridia, rotaviruses etc. Can be induced by antibiotics Plant toxins

continued

Table 10.1 *continued*

Syndrome	*Incidence in pet rabbits*	*Hard faeces*	*Caecotrophs*	*Condition of rabbit*	*Causes*
	common in the suckling or growing rabbit				
Enterotoxaemia	Sporadic cases in adult rabbits More common in juveniles	Liquid faeces that may be tarry Rabbit may die before diarrhoea develops	Not seen	Unwell Rapidly progressive Maybe collapsed	Clostridial species Can be induced by antibiotics
Chronic inflammatory disease	Rare Only adults	Large amounts of bulky soft faeces	Indistinguishable from hard faeces	Thin, bloated Periods of ravenous appetite interspersed with periods of anorexia	Not known ? immune mediated Sometimes associated with adhesions ? post spay

In other species, diarrhoea is manifested by the frequent evacuation of watery droppings (Blood and Studdert, 1999). Rabbits produce two types of droppings, i.e. hard faeces and caecotrophs. Normal caecotrophs are soft in consistency and are often mistaken for diarrhoea. The nature and frequency of both types of faeces are an important consideration. In some conditions, there is also excessive mucus production that can be mistaken for diarrhoea.

functional anatomy and colonic motility. Sacculations in the wall of the proximal colon (*haustra*) retain small particles while the larger particles accumulate in the lumen. Haustral activity directs small particles towards the caecum, while segmental activity directs large particles towards the anus. Lagomorphs have a specially adapted muscular segment of the colon known as the *fusus coli* that contains a large number of mucus glands (see Plate 22). The *fusus coli* acts as pacemaker for colonic motility. It is highly innervated and vascular and is not only controlled by the autonomic nervous system but is also subject to the effects of metabolites and hormones such as aldosterone and prostaglandins. During the excretion of caecotrophs, haustral activity ceases and caecal material is moved swiftly along the large colon. In the *fusus coli*, the material is formed into pellets that become encapsulated in mucus (see Plate 22). The transit time for soft faeces through the colon is 1.5–2.5 timeS faster than for hard faeces (Fioramonti and Ruckesbusch, 1976).

Within the caecum lies a complex ecosystem of microflora nourished by water and digesta that arrive from the small intestine via the proximal colon. Water is secreted into the proximal colon during the process of mixing and separating and is sent into the caecum with the small particles. Water is absorbed from the caecum across the caecal wall into the circulation. The retention time of digesta within the caecum is affected by both caeco-colonic motility and the nature of ingesta that reaches it. Conditions within the caecum are affected by the type and amount of nutrients that supply the microflora and the products of bacterial fermentation. The balance of microorganisms in the caecum is of paramount importance to the health of the animal. A healthy microflora digests food efficiently. Any factor that upsets the balance of caecal microflora has the potential to result in the proliferation of pathogenic bacteria and cause disease.

10.2 Inter-relating factors in digestive disease

10.2.1 Intestinal microflora

The caecum is a finely balanced ecosystem composed of a variety of microorganisms nourished by a constant supply of water and nutrients from the small intestine. Changes in the amount and content of the ingesta that reaches the caecum have an effect on the

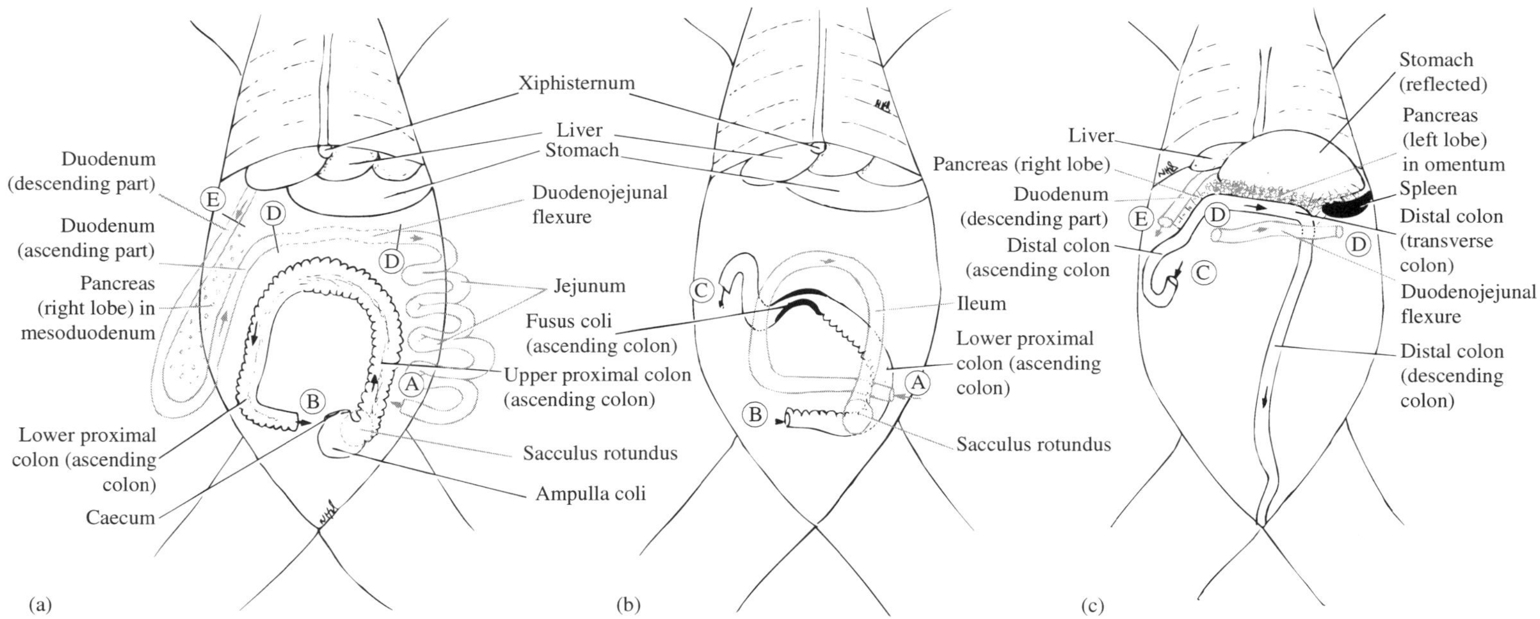

Figure 10.2. Three-dimensional topographical anatomy of the abdominal contents of the rabbit with the caecum removed. Figure 10.2 illustrates the topographical relationship of the liver, spleen, pancreas, small intestine and colon at three levels from superficial (ventral) to deep (dorsal). The diagrams were drawn from fresh dissections after removal of the caecum. Each of the three drawings shows the small intestine in green and the large intestine in black. Dotted lines show structures that are deeper (more dorsal) than the illustrated layer. The progression through the bowel from stomach to anus is shown by arrows. The intestines are held firmly in place by their mesenteric attachments.

balance of microorganisms, which are therefore dependent on diet and intestinal motility. *Bacteroides* spp. predominate in a microflora composed of aerobic and anaerobic gram-positive and gram-negative rods, cocci, filaments, coccobacilli and spirochaetes. In addition to the aerobic flora, over 74 strains of anaerobic bacteria have been isolated from the caecal mucosa and many of these species have not been cultivated (Straw, 1988). The microbial flora can contain small numbers of potential pathogens such as *Clostridium* spp. Stress has an effect on caecal microflora. Increased glucocorticoid levels increase coliform counts and narrow the aerobic to anaerobic bacteria ratio in the gut (Straw, 1988). Changes in the caecal microflora can be seen in gram-stained smears of caecal contents. In the healthy rabbits, high numbers of large anaerobic metachromatic bacteria (LAMB) and protozoa are present. In rabbits suffering from mucoid enteropathy, a drop in the number of LAMB and protozoa and an increase in coliforms are found (Lelkes and Chang, 1987).

The caecal microflora synthesize volatile fatty acids that are absorbed across the caecal wall into the circulation. Anaerobic *Bacteroides* are the principal source of butyrate that is used as an energy source for the caecal epithelium. The caecal epithelium is adapted for the efficient absorption of water and electrolytes. Butyrate is also important in the regulation of caecal pH, which has an optimim of 5.7–6.1. Changes in caecal pH alter the caecal microflora and can result in the proliferation of pathogens. The proportions of volatile fatty acids in the caecum influences appetite and gut motility. In healthy rabbits, acetates predominate, followed by butyrates and proprionates. Low fibre diets result in decreased acetates and increased proprionates and butyrates. An increase in caecal butyrate inhibits normal peristalsis of the gut (Lang, 1981).

The microflora of the rabbit's digestive tract changes according to the age and diet of the animal. In wild rabbits and those pet rabbits that eat a natural diet of grass and hay, a healthy gut flora becomes established that is resilient to any minor dietary changes that occur as the result of eating novel foods. In contrast, in intensive situations where large numbers of rabbits are kept in a small space and fed on artificial diets containing products that rabbits would not normally eat, alterations in the intestinal microflora can rapidly result in the proliferation of pathogens and the development of enteritis. Large numbers of pathogenic bacteria are most likely to be present in intensive situations. Commercial rabbits are young, growing animals, in which a healthy caecal microflora has not become established. Because of the financial importance of losses due to enteric disease in commercial units, extensive research has been carried out into the effects of varying dietary protein, carbohydrate and fibre levels on caecal microflora and volatile fatty acid production. These considerations are beyond the remit of this book, which is mainly concerned with the individual pet rabbit and not commercial rabbit production. The nutrition of the commercial rabbit is described in detail by P.R. Cheeke (*Rabbit Feeding and Nutrition*, 1987, Academic Press, Orlando) and reviewed in *The Nutrition of the Rabbit* (eds C. De Blas and J. Wiseman, 1998, CAB Publishing, Wallingford, Oxford).

10.2.2 Diet

It is not possible to consider any digestive problem in rabbits without examining the diet. The role of fibre and its 'digestibility' or 'indigestibility' is an important concept in the understanding of digestive disease in rabbits. Fibre digestion depends upon the presence of cellulolytic bacteria within the digestive tract. In rabbits the term 'digestibility' includes bacterial degradation or fermentation within the caecum, and not just digestion in the stomach and small intestine. For this reason, the term 'fermentable fibre' may be less confusing than 'digestible fibre'. Bacterial fermentation of fibre within the caecum varies according to the chemical structure and particle size (see Figure 2.2). For example, hemicellulose is more digestible than lignin. Small particles enter the caecum where their digestibility is affected by their size. Smaller particles of fermentable fibre have a relatively greater surface area for bacteria to adhere to and are digested more quickly than the larger particles. Very large particles (> 0.5 mm) do not enter the caecum and are expelled, undigested, in the hard faeces. Although it has no nutritive value, indigestable fibre is an essential part of the diet because it

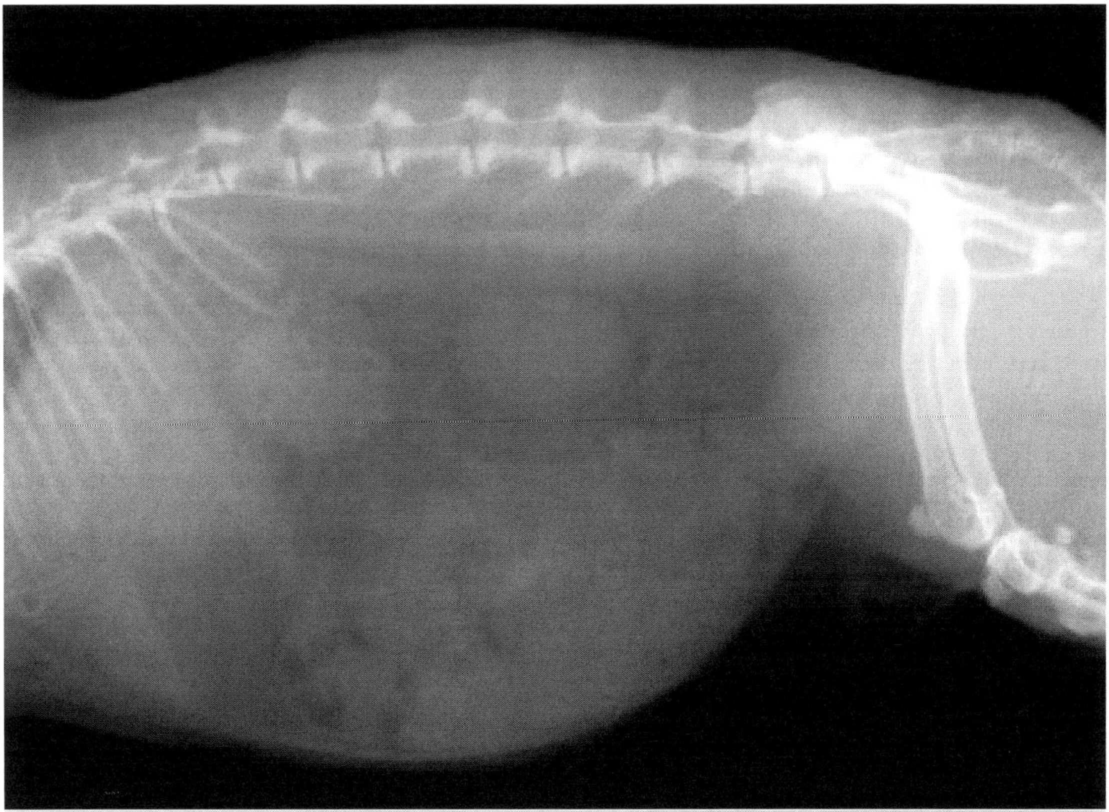

Figure 10.3. Radiographic anatomy of lateral view of normal abdomen. Interpretation of abdominal radiographs is summarized in Box 10.1. Figure shows a lateral radiograph of a healthy 2-year-old neutered male rabbit (no nipples are evident). The radiograph was taken during mid-morning and the colon is in the soft faeces phase. Hard faecal pellets are not evident in the rectum. The ileocaecocolic complex that occupies the caudoventral abdomen is relatively small and the contents amorphous. Gas shadows can be seen in the distal colon. Both kidneys, the stomach, liver and bladder can be seen.

stimulates gut motility, which sends nutrients and fluids into the caecum for bacterial fermentation. Insufficient indigestible fibre results in slow gut motility and retention of hair and ingesta in the stomach. Reduced motility in the proximal colon affects the separation of intestinal contents and reduces the supply of digesta and fluid to the caecum. Lack of both fermentable and indigestible fibre results in changes in caecal pH, volatile fatty acid distribution and the balance of microbial flora. Alterations in the populations of microorganisms can allow enteric pathogens to proliferate. Therefore, although a low level of dietary fibre may not actually cause disease, it is a major predisposing factor. Additional factors such as coccidiosis or treatment with ampicillin are needed to cause pathological disease in commercial rabbits fed on a low fibre diet (Licois and Mongin, 1980). The caecal appendix is larger in rabbits on a low fibre diet suggesting either an increased demand for the buffering effects of bicarbonate or an increase in lymphoid activity in response to greater production of bacterial toxins (Cheeke *et al.*, 1986).

The amount of indigestible (non-fermentable) fibre in the diet has an effect on appetite, both for food and for caecotrophs. High levels of indigestible fibre promote caecotroph ingestion whereas high protein levels reduce it. More food is consumed by rabbits on a diet high in indigestible fibre, i.e. large particles of lignified plant material.

However, processing the food to reduce the indigestible fibre down to particles small enough to enter the caecum will suppress appetite. Lignin is not digested by the caecal bacteria whereas cellulose, hemicellulose and pectin are. Excessive amounts of ground lignified material in the caecum increases retention time and decreases digestibility (Chiou *et al.*, 1998). Caecal impaction can be the result.

10.2.3 Age and husbandry considerations

The digestive disorders of the young rabbit, especially around the time of weaning, are very different from the adult pet. The stomach pH of suckling rabbits is approximately 5–6.5. Adult rabbits have a stomach pH of 1–2, except during digestion of caecotrophs when the pH rises. The high pH of suckling rabbits not only permits healthy bacteria to pass through the digestive tract and colonize the hindgut, but also permits the passage of pathogens, such as pathogenic strains of *E. coli*. Susceptibility to pathogenic strains of *E. coli* varies with age; rabbits of 3 weeks are more susceptible than rabbits of 6 weeks of age (Licois *et al.*, 1992). Weaning is a stressful period for rabbits when healthy caecal microflora is not yet established and juvenile rabbits are susceptible to disease. Ingestion of maternal caecotrophs aids the population of the caecum with a healthy gut flora and early weaning and separation from the dam increase susceptibility to bacterial enteritis.

After weaning, ammonia levels in the caecum decrease as the diet changes. Caecal pH becomes more acidic as volatile fatty acid concentrations increase. The proportions of individual volatile fatty acids alter with the change of diet from milk to solids. Proprionate, valerate and branched chain fatty acids predominate until the rabbit starts to eat solid food. The microbial flora changes in association with alterations in volatile acid production (Padilha *et al.*, 1995). Pathogenic strains of *E. coli*, *Clostridia* spp., coccidiosis or rotaviruses are likely to be present in the environment of newly weaned rabbits. Several animals sharing a small space increase faecal contamination and the risk of cross-infection. After weaning, rabbits are often stressed by change of housing and diet, transport and mixing with different individuals. Intercurrent disease such as pasteurellosis can be present. Minimizing stress and a diet containing sufficient indigestable fibre is especially important at this age to prevent enteric disease.

In the adult pet rabbit, infectious causes of enteritis are rare in comparison with the young commercial rabbit. Instead, it is far more common to see diet-related problems. Dietary changes can result in the production of soft caecotrophs that are left uneaten. Instead, the caecotrophs are deposited in the bedding or are found stuck to the fur under the tail. The smelly faecal mass is often mistaken for 'diarrhoea' by the owner, although it is not caused by infection (see Section 10.6).

10.2.4 Effect of digestive disease on water and electrolyte exchange

The effects of gastrointestinal disease on the water, electrolyte and acid–base balance of rabbits are complex. Disturbances in water, electrolyte and acid–base balance have a rapid and profound effect on health. Water and electrolytes are continually exchanged along the digestive tract and, in rabbits, any condition that affects this cycle of secretion and absorption also affects fluid and electrolyte balance (see Figure 1.2). Saliva is constantly produced by rabbits and, during the hard faeces phase, water is secreted into the stomach and proximal colon. It is then reabsorbed from the caecum and distal colon. Dehydration develops rapidly during intestinal disease, despite no obvious fluid loss in vomit or diarrhoea. Conditions that cause intestinal obstruction result in the accumulation of large amounts of fluid proximal to the site of obstruction. Conversely, gastrointestinal hypomotility reduces the secretion of water into the stomach and results in impaction of the contents. Dehydration is associated with gastrointestinal hypomotility, presumably due to decreased absorption of water from the stomach, caecum and distal colon.

Mucus is rich in potassium (Riley and Cornelius, 1989) and a feature of enteropathy in rabbits is the production of large amounts

Key points 10.1

- There is a complex inter-relationship between stress, diet, gut motility and infectious agents in the aetiopathogenesis of digestive disorders in rabbits
- Enteritis is more commonly encountered in the young, commercial rabbit kept in intensive conditions than in the adult, individual pet with an established gut flora
- A variety of non-specific terms are used to describe the array of digestive diseases that afflict rabbits. Examples include: bloat, mucoid enteritis, gut stasis, wool-block and gastroenteropathy
- Water and electrolytes are continually absorbed and secreted along the digestive tract. Dehydration and electrolyte imbalances occur readily as a result of intestinal disease
- The role of digestible (fermentable) and indigestible (non-fermentable) fibre in the digestive physiology is an important concept in the understanding of digestive disease. Fibre is composed of constituents of plant cell walls and includes cellulose, hemicellulose and lignin
- Indigestible fibre consists of large particles of lignified material that are directed into the colon and do not enter the caecum. It has no nutritive value but stimulates gut motility
- Fermentable fibre is composed of small particles that are directed into the caecum to act as a substrate for the caecal microflora. It is mainly composed of hemicellulose and cellulose. Fermentable fibre has no direct effect on gut motility
- The rabbit's caecum is an ecosystem containing a microflora that is essential to the health of the rabbit. A healthy caecal microflora requires a constant supply of nutrients and fluid. Alterations in the balance of microorganisms within the caecum can result in proliferation of pathogenic bacteria
- Optimal gut motility is important to maintain absorption and secretion of water and electrolytes along the digestive tract and to transport nutrients and fluid to the caecum
- The limited ability of the rabbit kidney to regulate acid–base disturbances makes this species vulnerable to acidosis and electrolyte imbalances. Fluid therapy is an essential part of treatment of many digestive disorders.

of mucus. Diarrhoea can result in hypokalaemia (Licois *et al.*, 1978).

The absorption and secretion of electrolytes along the digestive tract is also affected by changes in acid–base status. In a study by Charney *et al.* (1983), alkalosis in rabbits decreased the absorption of water, sodium and chloride whereas acidosis had the opposite effect and reduced bicarbonate secretion. Anorexia in rabbits can quickly lead to metabolic acidosis (see Section 10.3.2) and the limited ability of the rabbit kidney to correct acid–base disorders makes the species vulnerable to the effects of acidosis or alkalosis (see Section 1.6.5). Changes in acid–base status can affect the contractility of the proximal colon (Lofqvist and Nilsson, 1981) which, in turn, will affect the secretion of water and its absorption from the caecum.

Therefore, effective fluid therapy is a vital part of the treatment of many gastrointestinal diseases in rabbits (see Section 4.11). Intravenous or intraosseous fluid therapy is necessary for most cases. Although subcutaneous fluids can be used, they are not suitable for ill, dehydrated or hypotensive patients as absorption of fluids from under the skin is poor when peripheral tissue perfusion is reduced by shock or hypovolaemia.

10.3 Gastrointestinal hypomotility

10.3.1 Gastrointestinal hypomotility and formation of trichobezoars (hairballs)

Optimum gastrointestinal motility is important for digestion of food, absorption of water and electrolytes and maintenance of a healthy gut flora. Many factors influence gastrointestinal motility in rabbits (see Box 10.1). Reduced gastrointestinal motility leads to impacted food in the stomach or caecum, impaired glucose absorption and a reduction in the supply of nutrients and fluids to the caecal microflora.

For many years, the presence of impacted hair and food material in the stomach ('trichobezoars' or 'hairballs') was believed to be the cause of disease in rabbits. It was

Box 10.1 Interpretation of abdominal radiographs

The rabbit's digestive processes follow a natural circadian rhythm that affects the appearance of abdominal radiographs. It is important to consider the time of day that an X-ray was taken, and whether the rabbit had recently ingested food.

Hard faeces phase

During the phase of hard faeces formation and excretion, the stomach can contain large quantities of fibrous food. The caecum becomes progressively distended as ingested food passes down the small intestine and through the ileocolic junction. A full caecum and proximal colon gives the ventral abdomen a general mottled appearance. The outline of the caecum is sometimes visible. Hard faecal pellets are often seen in the distal colon. Small amounts of intestinal gas may be seen.

Soft faeces phase

The soft faeces phase is much shorter than the hard faeces phase and usually occurs during the morning. A small amount of food may be seen in the stomach. The caecal contents are expelled into the proximal colon so the caecum is reduced in size. The caecum may contain small quantities of gas. Hard faecal pellets are absent from the distal colon and rectum.

Radiographic findings

- The stomach is situated within the costal arch and normally contains some food, which gives the organ a mottled appearance
- The main body of the stomach lies on the left on the ventrodorsal view
- The liver can be seen in the anterior abdomen although the ventral border is not always clearly demarcated on the lateral view
- The spleen cannot be seen radiographically
- The small intestine cannot be distinguished from the long distal colon in the normal rabbit. Small pockets of gas may be seen in the intestines of normal rabbits
- Obstruction or slowing of gut motility results in the accumulation of gas in parts of the digestive tract. Distended loops of bowel can be identified by their anatomical position (see Figure 10.2)
- The ileocaecocolic segment occupies most of the ventral abdomen. The appearance of the ileocaecocolic segment varies with the phase of digestion
- Extraneous radiopaque material is sometimes seen in the digestive tract of rabbits that eat food that contains particles of soil or grit. Small particles are moved in a retrograde fashion into the caecum. Accumulations of sand or grit in the caecum should be differentiated from calcification in abscesses in organs such as the ovaries
- Radiopaque deposits in the bladders are due to the presence of calcium carbonate in the urine. This is a normal finding. A solid radiopaque bladder suggests the presence of 'sludgy urine' (see Figure 14.1)
- The left kidney is usually clearly visible in the dorsal abdomen in the region of L_3–L_5. The right kidney may be less obvious and is situated cranially in the region of T_{13}–L_1. Renal length is approximately 1.25–1.75 times the length of the second lumbar vertebra (Hinton and Gibbs, 1982)
- The presence of intra-abdominal fat enhances the radiographic image of abdominal organs. The area cranial to the bladder is filled with fat deposited in the broad ligament in female rabbits and may be seen as a homogeneous grey area, especially in obese individuals
- The uterus is not normally visible in the non-pregnant doe but may be seen if it is enlarged by pregnancy or disease
- Nipples can be seen superimposed on the abdominal contents of some female rabbits. Nipples are rudimentary in males
- Sometimes mineralization of ovaries, uterine tumours or intra-abdominal abscesses may be seen
- Areas of calcification may be seen in association with soft tissue mineralization chronic abscesses or in areas of fat necrosis. Hard areas of necrotic fat in the mesometrium can be a sequel to ovarohysterectomy.

thought that the trichobezoar caused a pyloric obstruction. Anorexia, weight loss, reduced faecal output, depression and death due to starvation were attributed to the presence of a trichobezoar. Many theories were put forward about the cause of trichobezoar formation. Handbooks and leaflets on rabbit care suggest that regular grooming is

Box 10.2 Factors that affect gut motility

- **Phase of faecal excretion**: the nature and direction of the peristaltic waves alters with the excretion of hard or soft faeces. The *fusus coli* is a specially adapted area of the colon that acts as a differential pacemaker for the initiation of peristaltic waves in the proximal and distal colon. The *fusus coli* is under autonomic control. It is highly innervated and is influenced by hormones such as aldosterone and prostaglandins. Prostaglandin stimulates the excretion of soft faeces
- **Indigestible fibre**: the passage of large particles of indigestible fibre through the colon stimulates intestinal motility as a result of intestinal distension
- **Volatile fatty acids in the caecum**: an increase in caecal butyrate inhibits normal peristalsis of the gut. Low fibre diets result in decreased acetates and increased proprionates and butyrates
- **Motilin**: this is a polypeptide hormone secreted by enterochromaffin cells of the duodenum and jejunum. Motilin stimulates gastrointestinal smooth muscle. Fat stimulates and carbohydrate inhibits its release. In the small intestine, motilin activity is decreased aborally. It disappears in the caecum and reappears in the colon and rectum
- **Pain and stress**: cause adrenergic stimulation and inhibit gut motility
- **Disease**: e.g. dysautonomia, coccidiosis, *E. coli*, rotavirus, enterotoxins, plant toxins can affect gut motility in different ways. For example, in rabbits with diarrhoea experimentally induced by coccidiosis, the motility of the caecum is increased and the motility of the ileum and jejunum is reduced (Fiaramonti *et al.*, 1981)
- **Pharmacological agents**: e.g prokinetics, opioids, NSAIDS.

required to prevent excessive amounts of hair being swallowed and becoming impacted in the stomach. Some breeders still recommend one day a week without food for rabbits in order to 'clear the system' of ingested hair. Boredom, magnesium or copper deficiency, inadequate protein, individual caging and the presence of air filtration barriers have all been put forward as potential causes of trichobezoar formation (Ojerio and Ladiges, 1981). The rabbit's inability to vomit has also been cited as a contributory factor (Gillett *et al.*, 1983). Treatment was usually unsuccessful. The administration of liquid paraffin to lubricate the gastric contents or pineapple juice to dissolve the hair enzymatically with bromelain were suggested as therapies. Surgical removal of the trichobezoar was a last resort and carried a poor prognosis. The association between trichobezoars and fatty liver was noted by many authors (Ojerio and Ladiges, 1981; Gillett *et al.*, 1983). An association with pregnancy toxaemia was made by Patton *et al.* (1983). It is only in recent years that trichobezoars have been recognized as the result of anorexia rather than the cause. On *post-mortem* examination, the rabbit's stomach is never found to be empty (Okerman, 1988) and the presence of a small amount of fibrous food is normal. The presence of hair entangled in the food is also a normal finding because rabbits are continually grooming and ingesting large amounts of hair.

In 1984, Leary *et al.* attempted to induce the clinical syndrome associated with the presence of trichobezoars by the orogastric infusion of latex to reproduce a gastric foreign body. Monthly radiographs were taken and the rabbits monitored closely for food intake and faecal output for 24 weeks after infusion. Gastrotomies were then performed to remove the foreign material and the rabbits monitored closely for a further 4 weeks prior to euthanasia and *post-mortem* examination. The presence of a latex bezoar did not have any adverse effect on appetite and weight gain of any of the 12 rabbits that were infused. In the same study, the stomach contents of 208 clinically healthy commercial rabbits were examined after slaughter and well-defined trichobezoars were found in 23% of them. This study cast doubt on the concept that trichobezoars cause anorexia. In 1986, Fekete and Bokori found elevated cortisol levels in rabbits with trichobezoars, although they concluded that the elevation was associated with the stress of having a trichobezoar rather than the trichobezoar being the result of stress. In 1987, Buckwell described the successful medical treatment of

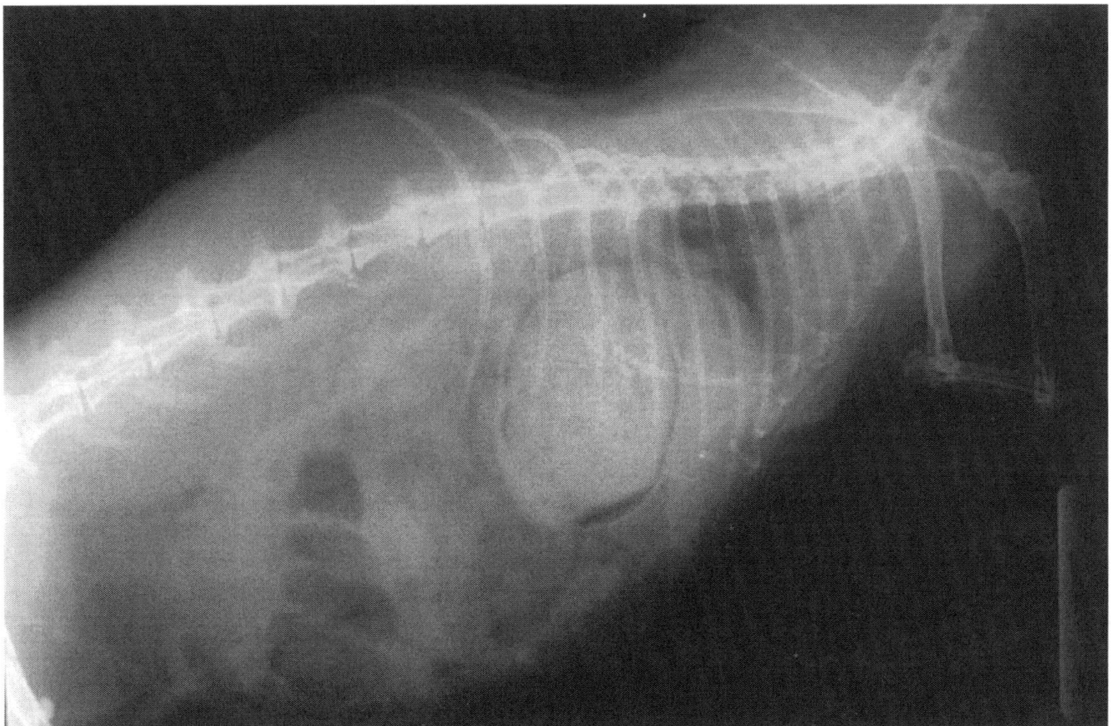

Figure 10.4. Lateral view of a rabbit with gastrointestinal hypomotility showing presence of a trichobezoar (hairball). Figure is an oblique view of a 3-year-old, obese female rabbit with gastrointestinal hypomotility. Gas shadows are evident in the stagnant caecum and stomach. The stomach contains a mass of impacted food and hair that has resulted from a decrease in gastrointestinal motility (see Section 10.3.1). The initiating cause was unknown, the rabbit was presented in a moribund state and subsequently died. Post-mortem examination confirmed the presence of hepatic lipidosis. There was also fatty degeneration of the kidneys.

'gut stasis' in rabbits exhibiting anorexia, reduced water intake, depression, weight loss and absence of faecal pellets. He described the presence of a palpable impacted mass in the region of the stomach. Treatment consisted of the administration of a motility stimulant, corticosteroid, oral fluid and the provision of hay. Since that time, trichobezoars have increasingly become recognized as the result, rather than the cause, of reduced gastrointestinal motility and are secondary to many other conditions.

Pain, stress and fright can all reduce gastrointestinal motility and lead to the accumulation of hair in the stomach and the formation of trichobezoars. In one study by Jackson (1991), intestinal stasis occurred more frequently in a group of laboratory rabbits that were restrained without the use of a towel. Once towel wrapping was introduced for the restraint of all rabbits, the incidence of the trichobezoars fell dramatically and the author concluded that stress played a significant role in the cause of the disease. Stimulation of the sympathetic nervous system causes adrenal hormones to be released into the circulation. One of the effects of adrenaline and noradrenaline is the inhibition of gastrointestinal motility. If gastrointestinal motility is reduced, water secretion into the stomach is also reduced and hair and ingesta accumulate and become impacted. The rabbit appears to be particularly susceptible to the effects of catecholamines on gut motility. In healthy rabbits with an uninterrupted daily routine, the passage of soft and hard faeces follows a circadian rhythm with an average day-to-day variation of approximately 30 minutes. Stress or even alterations in routine can have a significant effect on the caecotrophic rhythm. Simply switching a light on during the normal period of darkness caused one rabbit to stop producing faeces for 10 days in a study of caecotrophic rhythm by Jilge (1980). Thunderstorms, bonfire night, predator attacks, pain and surgery can all slow gut motility and, if left untreated, result in impacted stomach contents and trichobezoar formation.

Gut motility is affected by the indigestible fibre component of the diet. The provision of a high fibre diet has long been recognized as a preventative measure for the formation of hairballs (Sandford, 1996). Rabbits fed on a low fibre diet are at greater risk of developing gastric stasis and trichobezoar formation. Rabbits with slow gut motility crave fibre and will often eat hay or grass in preference to other foods. The provision of palatable indigestible fibre for rabbits that are at risk of gut stasis, e.g. postoperatively, is important. Fresh grass is the most acceptable form of fibre for rabbits, although good quality hay is acceptable.

Slow gut motility not only results in the development of trichobezoars. Gas accumulates in the stagnant stomach and caecum. Visceral distension causes pain that stimulates catecholamine release and exacerbates inhibition of gut motility. Gastric ulceration can occur. Alterations in the secretion and absorption of water and electrolytes cause dehydration and electrolyte imbalances. Reduced food intake leads to an energy deficit that stimulates mobilization of free fatty acids from adipose tissue and fatty infiltration of the liver. Ketoacidosis and hepatic lipidosis are the result. Liver failure from hepatic lipidosis is the usual end-point of untreated gastrointestinal stasis.

Reduced food intake and hypomotility of the proximal colon also reduce the amount of ingesta that is available as substrate for caecal microflora. Alterations in the caecal fermentation patterns can lead to changes in caecal pH and volatile fatty acid production. The balance of caecal microflora changes with the possibility of the proliferation of pathogenic bacteria such as *Clostridia* spp.

10.3.2 Anorexia and development of hepatic lipidosis

Anorexia, whatever the cause, can trigger a chain of events that can result in death of a rabbit from hepatic lipidosis and liver failure. Rabbits are obligate herbivores and their carbohydrate metabolism differs from carnivorous species such as the dog or cat. The endocrine control of the storage and mobilization of food are not as important in herbivorous species as in carnivores that eat periodically and need to regulate a fluctuating supply of nutrients from the digestive tract. Herbivorous animals withstand the absence of insulin far more readily than carnivorous ones (Bentley, 1998).

In rabbits, glucose and lactates are produced in the caecotrophs during the period of fermentation in the stomach and are absorbed during digestion of caecotrophs in the small intestine. Amylase is synthesized by the caecal flora and is present in caecotrophs to act on the carbohydrates that are present. Volatile fatty acids are a major energy source and represent about 40% of the maintenance energy requirement of rabbits (Marty and Vernay, 1984). They are absorbed from the digestive tract during digestion of caecotrophs and from the caecum where volatile fatty acids are produced by bacterial fermentation. Concentrations of volatile fatty acids in arterial blood are kept constant by the liver, despite fluctuations in absorption from the digestive tract. Volatile fatty acid absorption from the gut varies with the hard or soft phase of faecal excretion (Vernay, 1987) and is affected by gut motility. Lipids are absorbed from the diet or are derived from endogenous synthesis of free fatty acids in the liver (Madry *et al.*, 1976).

During periods of anorexia, glucose absorption from the gut falls and there is a reduction in volatile fatty acid production by the caecal microflora. The resultant drop in glucose and glucogenic volatile fatty acid absorption results in hypoglycaemia that stimulates lipolysis and the mobilization of free fatty acids from adipose tissue. The free fatty acids are transported to the liver to be metabolized as an energy source. The major pathway for their degradation is that of β-oxidation and ketone body production. Ketoacidosis occurs when ketone body production exceeds tissue metabolism. Rabbits do not have effective metabolic pathways for correcting acidosis (see Section 1.6.5) and are particularly susceptible to the effects of ketoacidosis. Also, during periods of increased mobilization of free fatty acids, a 'bottleneck' develops in the liver, which impairs the metabolic pathways that result in lipid transport to other tissues. Fat accumulates in the hepatocytes causing cholestasis and eventual liver failure and death. Hepatic lipidosis occurs most readily in obese rabbits because they have already accumulated triglycerides in the hepatocytes.

10.3.3 Obesity, pregnancy toxaemia and hepatic lipidosis

Any condition that causes prolonged anorexia in rabbits can result in fatty infiltration of the liver. Stress alone alters the fat metabolism of rabbits, especially in those that are already overweight. In a study by Lafontan and Agid (1979), minor stressful stimuli such as saline injections or venepuncture induced a prompt increase in plasma free fatty acid and glycerol concentrations in naturally obese rabbits. This increase did not occur in younger, lighter rabbits. Alpha-adrenergic responsiveness is increased in the large fat cells of obese rabbits in comparison with the small fat cells of underfed rabbits (Lafontan, 1981). High fat diets greatly increase the risk of hepatic lipidosis. In a study by Jean-Blain and Durix (1985), rabbits that were fed on a high fat diet showed a two-fold increase in ketonaemia during a period of fasting and were more hypoglycaemic than rabbits that were fed on a low fat diet. Obesity is a major problem in pet rabbits and animals that already have fatty livers can rapidly develop hepatic lipidosis if they become anorexic. Any surgical procedure in an obese rabbit carries a risk of hepatic lipidosis associated with pain, stress and withholding food.

It is well known among the rabbit breeders that female rabbits should not be too fat if they are to breed successfully. Rabbits with fatty livers readily develop ketosis (pregnancy toxaemia) in late pregnancy or during early lactation when glucose requirements are high. Healthy pregnant rabbits show a period of insulin resistance between days 24 and 30 of gestation during which high levels of insulin do not stimulate muscle glucose uptake (McLaughlin and Fish, 1994). Hepatic uptake of glucose and free fatty acids is also reduced in pregnant rabbits and brings about an arterial hyperglycaemia so more glucose is available to the uterus (Pere *et al.*, 1992). Insulin resistance results in increased hormone sensitive lipase (HSL) activity with increased amounts of triglyceride being hydrolysed from adipose tissue and transported to the liver.

Pregnant does are susceptible to the effects of anorexia and a drop in blood glucose rapidly stimulates fatty acid mobilization from adipose tissue to a liver that is already being compromised by fatty infiltration. An association between hairballs and pregnancy toxaemia was made by Patton *et al.* in 1983 illustrating the complex inter-relationship between anorexia, fibre, gastrointestinal motility, energy demand and fatty infiltration of the liver. Treatment of pregnancy toxaemia is unlikely to be successful, but follows the same principles as the treatment of hepatic lipidosis, apart from the complication of the fetuses. Pregnancy toxaemia can be prevented keeping breeding does slim and feeding them a high fibre diet.

10.3.4 Diagnosis and treatment of gastrointestinal hypomotility and prevention of hepatic lipidosis

Hepatic lipidosis can be prevented in anorexic rabbits by maintaining a positive energy balance with nutritional support and prompt treatment. It is important that rabbit owners are made aware that anorexia, in conjunction with lack of faecal output, is a potentially fatal condition and that rabbits that are not eating must be treated promptly. Hospitalization and intensive nursing are often required.

There are many differential diagnoses for the underlying causes of anorexia and gastrointestinal hypomotility, including dental disease and recent surgery (see Table 3.2). Recognition and treatment of the underlying cause is an essential part of treatment. The onset of gastrointestinal hypomotility can

Table 10.2 Therapeutic agents used in the treatment of enteric disorders

Enteric disorder	*Prokinetics*	*Narcotic analgesics*	*NSAIDs*	*Anti-ulcer drugs*	*Anti-biotics*	*Choles-tyramine*	*Liquid paraffin*	*Probiotics*	*Fluid therapy*	*Nutritional support*
Gastrointestinal hypomotility 'hairballs'	✓ Essential	✓ Except in mild cases	✓	In long-standing cases	X	X	In advanced cases to lubricate impacted stomach contents	Maybe useful adjunct to treatment	Oral fluids to soften stomach contents and to provide water and electrolytes Intravenous fluids in later stages	Provide indigestible fibre Provide tempting foods Syringe feed if necessary: carbohydrate to supply energy and prevent hepatic lipidosis Nasogastric tube as a last resort
Uneaten caecotrophs	X	May need sedation to clean perineum	If perineal skin is inflamed	X	If perineal skin is inflamed	X	X	Maybe useful adjunct to treatment	X	Increase indigestible fibre i.e lots hay/grass
Intestinal obstruction/ gastric dilatation	X **Contra-indicated**	✓ **Essential**	✓ Postop	✓	✓ Postop	✓ Postop	X	Maybe useful adjunct to treatment	✓ Intravenous (or intraosseous) fluids are essential	Tempting foods required post-operatively
Caecal impaction	✓	✓ Bupre-norphine	Use carprofen if NSAID is required. Less likely to interfere with caecotroph production	✓	X	X	✓	Maybe useful adjunct to treatment	✓	Tempting foods Easily digested foods e.g baby foods. No small fibre particles that cannot easily be digested by caecal bacterai.
Enteritis	X	✓	?	?	✓	✓	X	Maybe useful adjunct to treatment	Essential. Oral or subcut. in early stages Intravenous in later stages	Hay/grass Excel
Enterotoxaemia	X	✓	✓	X	Metro-nidazole	✓	X	Maybe useful adjunct to treatment	Essential Intravenous or intraosseous	Hay/grass Excel
Mucoid enteropathy	✓	✓	✓	✓	✓	✓	✓	Maybe useful adjunct to treatment	✓	Hay/grass Tempting foods

Table 10.3 Properties and dosages of therapeutic agents used in the treatment of enteric disorders of rabbits

Agent	*Dose*	*Comments*
Prokinetics		
Metaclopramide	0.5 mg/kg SC bid	Stimulates gastric emptying and GI motility
Cisapride	0.5 mg/kg Oral bid	Very effective product in rabbits. Unfortunately, the product has been withdrawn due to adverse drug interactions in humans. Contact manufacturers for more information
Narcotic analgesics		
Fentanyl/fluanisone	0.2–0.3 ml/kg IM (single dose)	Provides analgesia to treat abdominal pain that accompanies digestive disorders and gas distension of the viscera. Fentanyl/fluanisone is a good sedative to clean uneaten caecotrophs from the perineum
Buprenorphine	0.03 mg/kg SC bid	Buprenorphine provides analgesia without marked sedation. It is less potent but longer acting than fentanyl/fluanisone
NSAIDs		
Carprofen	3 mg/kg	NSAIDs are used to treat abdominal pain.Carprofen is a weak cyclo-oxygenase inhibitor and does not interfere with prostaglandin synthesis as much as other NSAIDs. Prostaglandins stimulate soft faeces production
Meloxicam (ketoprofen or flunixin can also be used)	100 µg (1 drop)/kg sid	
Anti-ulcer drugs		
Ranitidene	2 mg/kg IV or 5 mg/kg PO	In rabbits, gastric ulceration occurs in conjunction with stress and GI hypomotility In other species gastric ulceration can be associated with NSAID therapy
Antibiotics		
Trimethoprim/sulpha	40 mg/kg Oral bid	Safe antibiotic orally. It can be used against enteric pathogens such as *E. coli*. Also effective against coccidia
Metronidazole	40 mg/kg Oral bid	Metronidazole is effective against *Clostridia* spp. and has been cited as a treatment of choice for enterotoxaemia
Cholestyramine 'Questran'	0.5 g/kg bid	Binds with enterotoxins Can be used to treat enterotoxaemia Can be used prophylactically in situations where enterotoxaemia may develop
Liquid paraffin	1–2 ml/kg bid	Softens impacted gastric or caecal contents
Probiotics	As directed	May be useful either prophylactically or therapeutically to encourage a healthy gut flora Inactivated by concurrent oral antibiotic therapy
Fluid therapy		
Oral (Lectade)	Approximately 10 ml/kg every 2–3 h	Oral fluids help to soften impacted stomach contents in addition to providing water and electrolytes
Subcutaneous (5% glucose or Hartmann's solution)	10 ml/kg	Subcutaneous fluids can be used in animals that are not dehydrated although intravenous therapy is preferable for dehydrated patients with poor tissue perfusion
Intravenous	10–15 ml/kg/h	Immediate PCV, glucose, urea and electrolyte assay is advantageous. An I-stat analyser (Heska) is a very useful piece of equipment Stress can cause oliguria in rabbits 0.2–0.3 ml/kg i.m. fentanyl/fluanisone (Hypnorm, Jannsen) provides sedation and analgesia that reduce stress levels and facilitates intravenous fluid therapy
Nutritional support • Hay • Grass • Tempting food	Good quality hay, fresh grass and palatable foods should be available *ad lib.*	Hay/grass provides indigestible fibre that stimulates gut motility Dandelions, curly kale, spring greens and grated carrot will tempt most rabbits

continued

• Baby foods	10 ml/kg liquidized food every 2–3 h	Liquidized or cereal baby foods supply carbohydrates that are absorbed from the small intestine as an instant energy source that prevents mobilization of free fatty acids from adipose tissue and development of hepatic lipidosis
• Extruded complete food (Burgess Suparabbit Excel)	Can be ground up or mashed *Ad lib*	Ground up fibre (i.e. small enough to go through a syringe) provides substrate for caecal bacteria but does not affect gut motility
Vitamin C	50–100 mg/kg	Vitamin C reserves are depleted in times of stress
Anabolic steroids	2 mg/kg (nandrolone)	Anabolic steroids may stimulate appetite
Corticosteroids		
Prednisolone	0.5–2 mg/kg PO, IM, SC	Long-term use may be indicated in chronic diarrhoea (**not** uneaten caecotrophs) that could be immune mediated
Dexamethasone	1–3 mg/kg IM, IV	Single injections may be of use to counteract shock in cases of acute enterotoxaemia
Betamethasone	0.1 mg/kg IV	

Abbreviations: sid: once daily; bid: twice daily; IM: intramuscular injection; IV: intravenous injection; PO: orally; SC: subcutaneous injection.

be insidious and anorexic rabbits are often reasonably alert in the early stages. A reduced appetite and a reduction in faecal output are the early warning signs (Table 3.1). As the disease progresses, the rabbit becomes totally inappetant and depressed. It adopts a hunched appearance and may sit for hours, immobile in the corner of the cage or hutch. Affected rabbits do not groom and appear to be oblivious to their surroundings. They are no longer inquisitive and do not respond to being spoken to or the offer of an interesting titbit. The rabbit becomes clinically dehydrated. There are no specific clinical signs associated with the development of hepatic lipidosis but affected animals are depressed and unresponsive. In the terminal stages, they become totally inappetant and are often disorientated and ataxic. Hyperglycaemia occurs. Death is due to liver and kidney failure.

Diagnosis of gastrointestinal hypomotility can be made on clinical history and examination. It can be confirmed by radiography (see Box 10.1 and Figures 10.3 and 10.5). Faecal output ceases completely and the impacted stomach can often be palpated as a hard mass behind the ribs, especially in the later stages of the disease. A blood sample can aid differential diagnosis, assist with choice of fluid therapy and offer prognostic indicators. A lipaemic sample or the presence of hyperglycaemia in conjunction with ataxia is a poor prognostic sign. In the early stages, hypoglycaemia may be found. This is treated by oral, subcutaneous or intravenous glucose therapy. In contrast, some rabbits show hyperglycaemia in the early stages of the disease associated with stress or pain. A blood glucose value within the normal reference range is reassuring. A PCV in excess of 40–45% indicates dehydration. Prerenal azotaemia is common in rabbits with gastrointestinal stasis. It is found in conjunction with dehydration. Blood urea and creatinine levels can be markedly elevated. If the analytical equipment is available, electrolyte status is invaluable. Once hepatic lipidosis is established, fatty infiltration of the kidneys occurs and the rabbit goes into liver and kidney failure. There can be a range of bizarre biochemistry results at this stage.

Treatment of gastrointestinal hypomotility is aimed at restoring appetite, correcting electrolyte imbalances, correcting dehydration, stimulating gastric emptying, promoting normal gastrointestinal motility and softening and lubricating impacted food and hair. The medical treatment of gastrointestinal hypomotility and the properties of therapeutic agents are summarized in Tables 10.2 and 10.3. The general treatment of digestive disorders is given in Box 10.3. Nutritional support is important to prevent the development of hepatic lipidosis. Analgesics are always indicated, as gas accumulates in stagnant sections of the gastrointestinal tract, causing distension and pain, which compound the situation further.

Diet is a key part of the treatment of gastrointestinal hypomotility and nutritional support will prevent the development of hepatic lipidosis. All anorexic rabbits must be

Box 10.3 General principles of treatment of digestive disorders in rabbits

Treatment of digestive disease in rabbits is aimed at treating and removing the underlying cause, preventing dehydration and electrolyte imbalances, maintaining or restoring gut motility, protecting normal gut flora and preventing hepatic lipidosis. The dosages and properties of therapeutic agents are summarized in Table 10.3.

- Hospitalization is often necessary to permit observation of appetite and faecal output. Many rabbits with digestive disorders require fluid therapy, syringe feeding and medication by injection
- A healthy rabbit passes copious quantities of hard faecal pellets. Up to 180 pellets a day can be passed by a rabbit that is eating well and on a high fibrous diet. Hard faeces are always passed overnight by a healthy rabbit. The absence of hard faeces is a significant finding
- Small faeces, diarrhoea, uneaten or abnormal caecotrophs are easier to monitor in the hospitalized rabbit
- Rabbits with diarrhoea should not be fasted like a dog or cat
- Indigestible fibre is always required by all rabbits at all times and can be provided by a bed of good quality, palatable hay
- Fresh grass will tempt many rabbits to eat and is a good source of both indigestible and digestible (fermentable) fibre
- Tempting fibrous vegetables can be offered to rabbits with diarrhoea, although dandelions, fruit, lettuce and other salad items should be avoided
- Anorexic rabbits can be offered a selection of fresh, appetizing leafy green foods. Even rabbits that do not normally eat greens can safely be offered freshly picked grass, dandelions, spring greens, cabbage, kale, carrots or apple
- Syringe feeding is necessary for rabbits that have not eaten for more than 24 h
- Fluid therapy is an essential part of treatment for anorexic or diarrhoeic patients. Oral or subcutaneous fluids can be given to rabbits that are not dehydrated but intravenous or intraosseous therapy is essential in advances cases. Fluid therapy is described in Chapter 4. The safest choice of fluid for most conditions in rabbits is lactated Ringer's or Hartmann's solution
- Oral, subcutaneous or intravenous glucose is indicated in rabbits that are known to be hypoglycaemic from blood glucose measurements
- Analgesia is essential to treat the pain that is associated with colic or gas distension of the bowel
- There is a risk of gastric ulceration in anorexic rabbits and anti-ulcer therapy is indicated, especially in rabbits that have been anorexic for more than 48 h
- Motility stimulants are indicated in the treatment of motility disorders. They are an essential part of treatment for gastric stasis and can also be used to treat caecal impaction and mucoid enteropathy
- Antibiotics may be indicated for the treatment of enterotoxaemia and in some types of diarrhoea. Enrofloxacin, trimethoprim preparations or metronidazole are the least likely to cause disturbances in the gut flora. Metronidazole has been cited as a treatment of choice for enterotoxaemia caused by *Clostridium spiriforme* (Carman, 1994). Trimethoprim combinations can be used to treat coccidiosis
- Some rabbits may be malnourished due to poor diet or dental disease and the inclusion of a vitamin supplement in the treatment protocol can be beneficial. Although rabbits synthesize vitamin C, there is evidence that vitamin C requirements of rabbits increase during periods of stress when plasma ascorbic acid has been shown to decrease significantly (Verde and Piquer, 1986)
- Anabolic steroids can be effective as an appetite stimulant for rabbits and have some beneficial effect in the retention of electrolytes. There appear to be no adverse effects at low doses
- A probiotic can be used to introduce beneficial bacteria to the hindgut. There are many anecdotal reports of the efficacy of commercial probiotic preparations although they contain lactobacillus that is not a normal inhabitant of the rabbit gut. Alternatively, caecotrophs collected from a healthy rabbit can be used to introduce normal bacterial flora
- Rabbits with digestive disorders are at risk of developing enterotoxaemia. Cholestyramine (Questran), an ion exchange resin, can be given to absorb enterotoxins.

encouraged to eat. Hepatic lipidosis can develop in any rabbit that becomes anorexic, although the risk is greater in obese, pregnant or lactating animals. Tempting foods such as fresh grass, dandelions and appetizing vegetables such as curly kale, spring greens, carrots and apples should be offered. Good quality hay is important, both to stimulate appetite and to provide a sense of security to reduce stress levels. A bed of hay smells familiar. Grass and hay provide long particles of indigestible fibre that are important to stimulate gut motility. A quiet environment away from predators and barking dogs is important. In the initial stages (less than 24 h), analgesia and the provision of palatable fibre can be sufficient to stimulate gut motility and prevent progression of the disease. In the later stages (more than 24 h without food), syringe feeding is required to provide calories and fluid to soften and lubricate impacted stomach contents and provide water and electrolytes. Pureed vegetables or baby foods provide an easily assimilated digestible energy source that can be given through a syringe. A source of fermentable fibre is important to provide nutrients for caecal bacteria. Indigestible fibre cannot be administered through a syringe because the large particles clog the nozzle. There is no point in attempting to grind indigestible fibre down for syringe feeding in an attempt to stimulate gut motility. Grinding fibre to a particle size where it no longer clogs a syringe means that the particles are small enough to be moved into the caecum instead of the colon and the stimulatory action on the gut is lost. Nasogastric tube feeding may be necessary as a last resort for intractable cases, but nasogastric tubes can be counterproductive. They clog up easily and an Elizabethan collar is required. Elizabethan collars have been proven to be stressful to rabbits (Knudtzon, 1988).

Pineapple juice or proteolytic enzymes have been recommended as remedies for hairballs because they are reputed to dissolve hair. Gillett *et al.* (1983) conducted an experiment in which they incubated rabbit hair for up to 3 days either in papaya, proteolytic enzymes or pineapple juice. The pH of the solution was adjusted to 2 with hydrochloric acid to mimic conditions in the rabbit stomach. They found no difference between the treated and untreated control samples and the authors concluded that none of the enzyme treatments exhibited any ability to dissolve hair. The success of pineapple juice as a remedy for gastric stasis might be due to the introduction of liquid into the stomach that softens the hairball and aids its passage out of the stomach. Liquid paraffin can be used to soften and lubricate impacted stomach contents.

Motility stimulants are effective in promoting gastrointestinal motility. Cisapride is a very effective remedy for gastrointestinal hypomotility but, at the time of writing (October, 2000) adverse drug interactions in humans have led to its withdrawal and the agent is difficult to obtain (see Section 4.7.1). Metoclopramide is an alternative therapy but appears to be less effective than cisapride. Atropine and opioid analgesics can antagonize the effects of metoclopramide. There is *in vitro* evidence that metoclopramide is only effective in adult rabbits (see Section 4.7).

Fluid therapy is always indicated in rabbits in the later stages of gastrointestinal hypomotility. Oral or subcutaneous fluids might be sufficient if the rabbit is not clinically dehydrated but intravenous therapy or intraosseous fluid therapy is essential once dehydration becomes evident.

10.4 Gastric ulceration

Gastric ulcers are a common *post-mortem* finding in rabbits, especially in those that have been anorexic prior to death. In a survey of 1000 *post-mortem* examinations by Hinton (1980), 7.3% were found to have ulceration of the gastric mucosa. The majority of the ulcers were found in the fundic area of the stomach and did not exhibit significant tissue reaction suggesting that the lesions had developed rapidly and were associated with the stress of the associated illness. In 2% of the rabbits, the ulcers were in the pyloric area and the majority of these had perforated the mucosa. Many of the pyloric ulcers were found in female rabbits that had died in the perinatal period. Experimental stress ulcers can be induced in the gastric mucosa of laboratory rabbits by administering intraperitoneal injections of adrenaline (Behara *et al.*, 1980).

Rabbits are unable to vomit and therefore gastritis is more difficult to recognize than in the dog or cat. There are no specific clinical

Key points 10.2

- For many years, the presence of impacted food material and hair within the stomach was believed to be a cause of anorexia and weight loss. Now, it is recognized that gastrointestinal hypomotility is the cause of impacted stomach contents (trichobezoars or 'hairballs') and anorexia and weight loss are the result
- Stimulation of the sympathetic nervous system inhibits intestinal motility. Gastrointestinal hypomotility is associated with any stressful situation or condition that stimulates the sympathetic nervous system including pain, surgery, stress or fright
- A diet high in indigestible fibre stimulates gut motility and reduces the risk of gastrointestinal hypomotility
- Gastrointestinal hypomotility results in gas formation in stagnant organs such as the stomach or caecum. Gas distension of the viscera is painful and abdominal pain stimulates the sympathetic nervous system and compounds the situation
- Gastrointestinal hypomotility results in anorexia and a fall in glucose absorption from the stomach and small intestine. Volatile fatty acid production from the caecum is also reduced
- Hypoglycaemia stimulates lipolysis and mobilization of free fatty acids from adipose tissue. Free fatty acids are metabolized as an energy source. Oxidation of free fatty acids releases ketone bodies that can cause ketoacidosis
- Accumulation of free fatty acids in the liver results in the development of hepatic lipidosis. Fatty infiltration of other organs, such as the kidney, occurs and, ultimately, liver and kidney failure result in death of the rabbit
- Obese rabbits that already have a fatty liver are especially prone to the development of hepatic lipidosis
- Increased glucose demand during pregnancy and lactation increases susceptibility to hepatic lipidosis during periods of anorexia
- Stimulating gut motility and maintaining a positive energy balance to prevent oxidation of fatty acids, ketoacidosis and hepatic lipidosis are essential parts of the treatment protocol for many digestive disorders in rabbits
- Gastric ulceration is a common *post-mortem* finding in anorexic rabbits. Anti-ulcer treatment, such as ranitidine, can be used in rabbits.

signs associated with gastric ulceration and inappetant rabbits are often already in pain from other causes. Anthropomorphically, it seems likely that gastric ulceration would add to the pain that is already being experienced. The clinical role of anti-ulcer preparations in the treatment of anorexic rabbits has not been evaluated but the possibility of gastric ulceration is a consideration when treating anorexic rabbits, especially when non-steroidal preparations have been administered. Several human preparations may be of use. Rabbits secrete high levels of gastric acid and pepsin in comparison with dogs, cats, rats and guinea pigs and the effects of anti-ulcer medications on gastric pH have been investigated (Redfern *et al.*, 1991). Although omeprazole (Losec, Astra) is theoretically more effective than ranitidene (Zantac, GlaxoWellcome) in decreasing acid secretion and increasing postprandial pH, both preparations have a significant effect and appear safe as an adjunct to treatment of anorexia. Omeprazole is only available in capsule form for humans, which makes it difficult to administer a small dose to rabbits. Ranitidene is available as an oral syrup.

10.5 Gastric dilatation and intestinal obstruction

In pet rabbits, gastric dilatation is caused by some type of gastrointestinal obstruction. Rabbits continually secrete saliva and cannot vomit so fluid collects in the stomach, which distends rapidly with fluid if ingesta cannot pass through and down the digestive tract. Gas is produced which causes further distension. The stomach and intestine proximal to the obstruction becomes dilated with fluid and gas, giving a typical radiological picture (see Figure 10.5). Typical foreign bodies include pellets of impacted 'felts' of hair, whole dried pulses, pieces of carpet fibre or other small objects. The small intestine is the usual site of obstruction although pyloric obstructions can occur. Rabbits normally ingest large amounts of hair during grooming, which passes through the digestive tract with no problem. It is felts of impacted, matted hair that cause obstructions. During moulting, large felts of hair can accumulate, especially on the plantar aspect of the

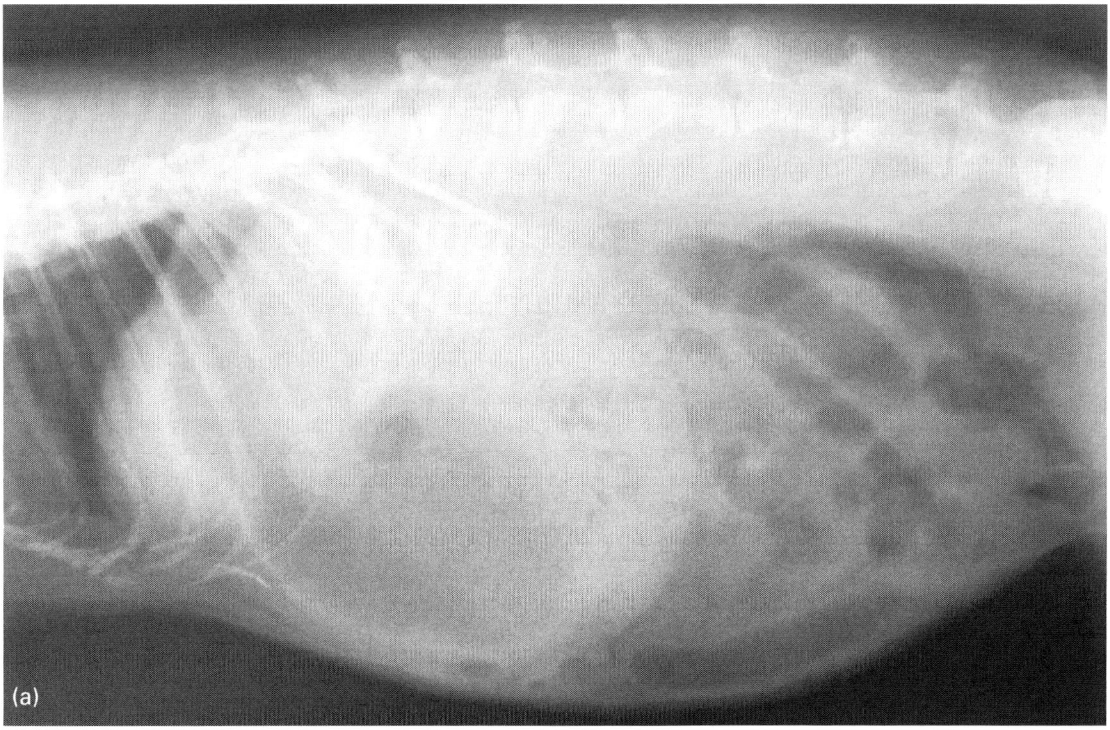

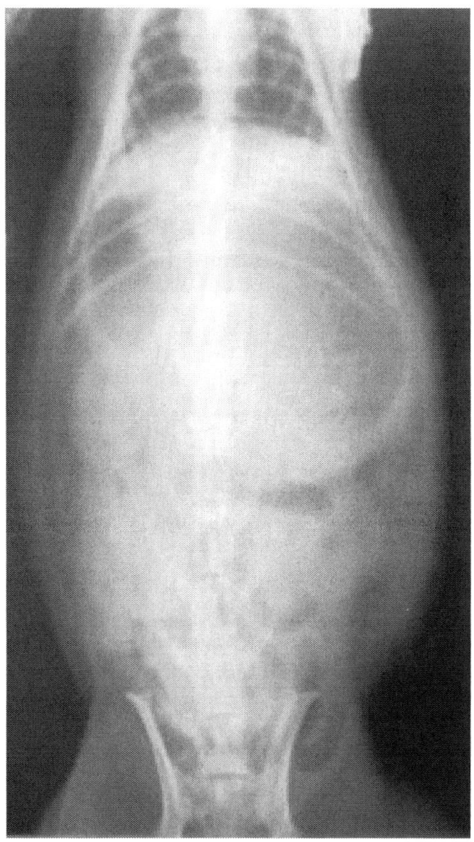

(b)

Figure 10.5. Lateral view of a rabbit with an intestinal obstruction.
Figure 10.5(a) shows a lateral view of a two-year-old Dwarf Lop male rabbit with an acute intestinal obstruction caused by a felt of ingested hair. The radiograph shows a grossly distended stomach containing fluid and gas. There is gas distension of the small intestine proximal to the site of obstruction that was in the ileum. This is a characteristic radiograph. The foreign body was surgically removed promptly (see Section 10.5.1) and the rabbit made an uneventful recovery. A differential diagnosis of intestinal obstruction is mucoid enteropathy, in which gastric dilatation may be seen in the terminal stages. An impacted caecum that can be palpated or seen radiographically is generally associated with mucoid enteropathy (see Figure 10.9).
Figure 10.5b. Dorsoventral view of a rabbit with an intestinal obstruction. Figure 10.4 shows the same rabbit as Figure 10.5. Knowledge of the topographical anatomy of the intestines aids diagnosis and location of a foreign body (see Figure 10.2). The radiographs in Figures 10.5a and 10.5b were taken after sedating the rabbit with 0.2 mls/kg fentanyl/fluanisone (see Box 5.5). It is possible to obtain a diagnostic radiograph by placing a conscious rabbit in ventral recumbency on an X-ray plate although positioning will be poor because the hind legs cannot be extended. Hypnosis and non-manual restraint with sandbags can be used to obtain a lateral view. A quiet room, gentle handling and patience are needed. The rabbit can be kept calm by covering its head with a towel.

metatarsus, and can be ingested by the rabbit during grooming. These felts of hair are found more frequently on Angora rabbits and fluffy Dwarf lops, although any breed can be affected. Rabbits with dental problems appear to be especially prone to intestinal obstruction. Rabbits with incisor problems cannot pull hair out effectively and large mats can build up before the rabbit can remove them. Owners of rabbits with grooming difficulties should be advised to watch for these felts and remove them promptly.

Dried pulses such as locust bean seeds or dried peas or sweet corn can also be exactly the right diameter to occlude the small intestine. This type of ingredient should not be included in rabbit food. Again, rabbits with dental problems appear to be prone to swallowing such ingredients whole (Harcourt-Brown and Friggens, 1999).

Inflammatory lesions or tumours in the wall of the intestine can cause obstructive disease at any site along the digestive tract, including the colon. Extramural lesions such as tumours, adhesions, abscesses and tapeworm cysts in the omentum can cause an obstruction (see Plate 36). A cystic calculus has been reported as a cause of intestinal blockage (Talbot and Ireton, 1975). The severity of symptoms and the course of the disease are related to the site of the obstruction. Complete occlusion of the small intestine is rapid in onset and fatal unless the obstruction is removed promptly. Sometimes the foreign body can move through the small intestine, intermittently obstructing the intestine causing abdominal pain and anorexia that passes off when the object passes through into the colon. The progress of the obstruction can be monitored radiographically from the gas shadows in the small intestine. The ileocaecal valve is a potential site of intestinal obstruction. Intestinal lymphoma has been found at this site in two cases (Harcourt-Brown, unpublished data), one of which developed an intussusception of the colon into the caecum. Occlusion of the colon shows a more protracted course that lasts for days rather than hours. Obstructions of the large intestine are not caused by ingested foreign bodies, as the lumen of the small intestine is much smaller than that of the colon. Instead tumours, adhesions and impacted caecal contents can obstruct the colon.

The typical history of a rabbit with an acute proximal intestinal obstruction is that the rabbit was well one minute and moribund the next (see Box 3.3). A feature of the condition is severe gastric dilatation with fluid and gas, which gives the rabbit a bloated appearance. Affected rabbits are totally inappetant, depressed and often collapsed. Dehydration and an unusual feeling abdomen are evident. A distended stomach may be palpable in the cranial abdomen, especially on the left side. Alternatively, the abdomen may be distended and tympanic, or feel doughy if intestinal rupture has occurred. Electrolyte imbalances cause a variety of symptoms. Twitching, blindness and convulsions can occur in the terminal stages. Abdominal radiography is usually diagnostic. The hugely distended stomach can be seen occupying the anterior half of the abdomen compromising respiratory and circulatory function. Gas shadows can be seen in the small intestine proximal to the obstruction (see Figure 10.2).

Prompt treatment is required for this painful and stressful condition. Analgesia and prompt decompression of the stomach are essential. The stomach can be decompressed

Key points 10.3

- In pet rabbits, gastric dilatation is usually associated with an intestinal obstruction. Mucoid enteropathy can also cause gastric dilatation
- Rabbits with intestinal obstruction are depressed, inappetant and shocked. The onset is sudden and the severity of symptoms depends on the site of the obstruction
- Felts of hair, carpet fibre, dried pulses, such as peas or beans, tumours, tapeworm cysts, abdominal abscesses, intussusceptions and adhesions are among the causes of intestinal obstruction
- Motility stimulants are contraindicated in cases of gastric dilatation
- Intestinal obstruction usually requires surgery that can be successful if performed promptly
- Occasionally, moving foreign bodies will pass through the ileocolic valve into the large intestine. Radiography can be used to monitor the progress of moving foreign bodies by the gas shadows in the intestines.

by passing a stomach tube to release the gas and liquid. Frequently the stomach tube blocks with hair and has to be emptied and repositioned. In most cases, the intestinal condition is rapidly fatal with death occurring within 12 h. There is a small chance of a moving foreign body passing through the small intestine and into the colon. Motility stimulants may aid this process but can also cause intestinal rupture if the gut is completely obstructed. Surgery is straightforward and successful if the case is presented early and surgery is performed rapidly. However, there are many potential life-threatening problems associated with enterotomy in rabbits; high risk anaesthesia, narrow intestinal lumen, soft friable tissue, small omentum, propensity to develop adhesions, water and electrolyte imbalances, postoperative ileus, infection and risk of recurrence due to stenosis of gut. Long-haired rabbits or those with dental problems will still have the predisposing cause even if they survive the surgery. Therefore, euthanasia is the most humane option unless the owners are keen for surgery, and accept all the risks and expense that are incurred.

Gastric dilatation is also a feature of mucoid enteropathy. The onset is usually more gradual than dilatation due to an intestinal obstruction. A palpably, impacted caecum in association with gastric dilatation is suggestive of mucoid enteropathy. Radiology can be used to differentiate the two conditions (see Figures 10.4 and 10.9), although exploratory laparotomy may be indicated to confirm the diagnosis.

10.5.1 Surgical removal of intestinal foreign bodies

Basic surgical principles in rabbits are described in Chapter 15. If the rabbit has been premedicated with low dose (0.2 ml/kg) fentanyl/fluanisone to obtain the abdominal radiographs, it can subsequently be masked down with isoflurane to induce anaesthesia (see Box 5.5). Prior to surgery, blood samples should be taken to assess PCV, glucose and electrolyte status before commencing fluid therapy. The passage of a stomach tube is required to decompress the stomach and remove as much fluid and gas as possible. The stomach tube can remain in place throughout surgery. Endotracheal intubation is advisable. If the anaesthetic induction agent does not contain an analgesic such as fentanyl/fluanisone, pre-emptive analgesia with butorphanol or buprenorphine is also required.

The abdomen is opened with a midline incision in the region of the umbilicus. In many cases, the small intestine lies just beneath the incision and is easily recognized. It is visibly distended with gas and fluid cranial to the obstruction. The topographical anatomy of the small intestine and its relationship to other abdominal organs is illustrated in Figure 10.5. Once the obstruction is located, the intestinal loop can be exteriorized and the surrounding tissues protected by sterile absorbent material. The intestinal contents are milked away from the obstruction before applying bowel clamps or asking an assistant to occlude the intestine with digital pressure. The enterotomy incision is made along the antimesenteric edge of the intestine distal to the foreign body to avoid placing sutures in devitalized tissue. The foreign body is removed and any everted mucosa trimmed off before suturing the wound with a single layer of appositional interrupted sutures making sure that they include the submucosa (see Figure 15.1). A fine inert, absorbable monofilament suture material with a high tensile strength is required, such as 5/0 poliglecaprone (Monocryl) or polydioxanone (PDS II, Ethicon). The repair of an intestinal incision is difficult due to the small diameter of the organ and the friability of the tissue. It is important to avoid stenosis as much as possible as it increases the possibility of re-obstruction at a later date. If enterectomy is indicated, the intestine should be sectioned at a slight angle to preserve its antimesenteric vascularity. Although techniques such as side-to-side or side-to-end anastomosis can be performed, they have no advantage over an end-to-end anastomosis, which is technically simpler (Bouvy and Dupré, 1997). A good seal to prevent leakage of intestinal contents is necessary as omentalization is difficult in rabbits due to the small omentum. Post-surgical adhesions to other organs form readily.

Withholding food postoperatively is not an option in rabbits. Small meals of soft

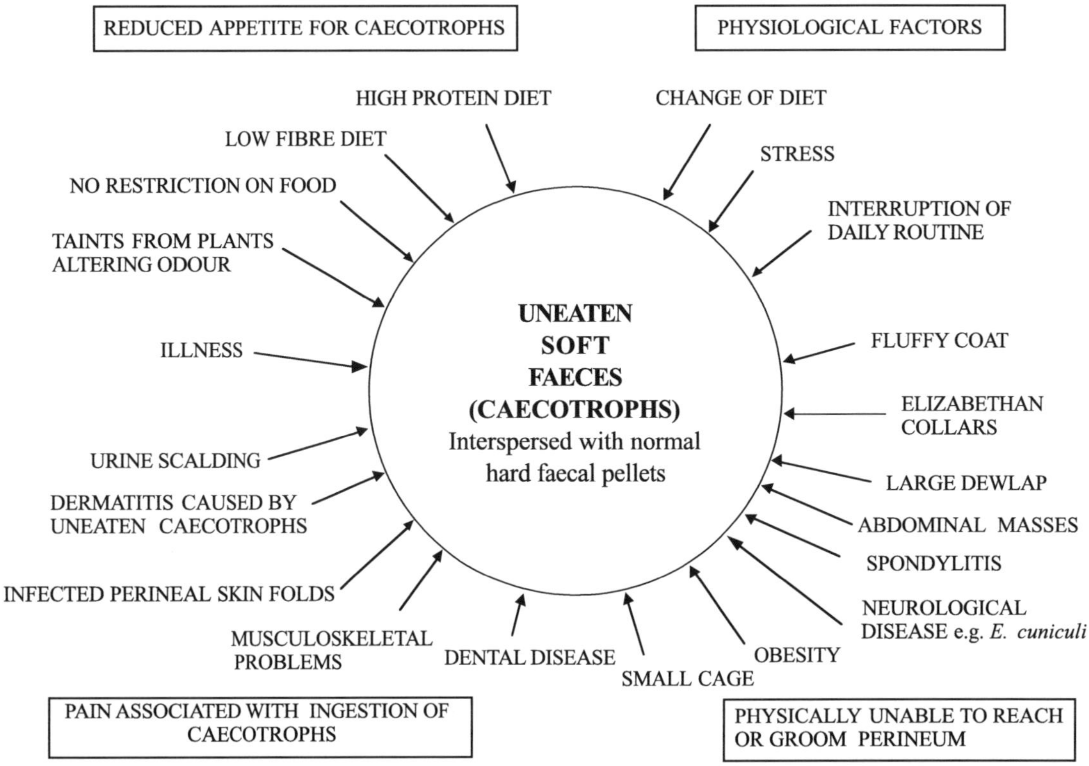

Figure 10.6. Causes of uneaten caecotrophs that may adhere to fur around anus.

digestable food can be fed for the first few days postoperatively to allow the intestine to heal. Postoperative analgesia and motility stimulants are essential.

10.6 Disorders of caecotrophy

10.6.1 Normal caecotrophy

Caecotrophy refers to the ingestion of soft faeces (caecotrophs) that are clusters of mucus encapsulated pellets of pasty, odorous material that originates from the caecum. Caecotrophs contain bacteria, protozoa, yeasts and their fermentation products, which are amino acids, volatile fatty acids, vitamins and enzymes such as amylase and lysozyme. Caecotrophs are a valuable source of nutrients to the rabbit. Caecotrophy starts at about 3 weeks of age and is established by 6 weeks (Lang, 1981).

Caecotrophs are produced approximately 4 h after the last meal during quiet periods of the day or night when the rabbits are at rest. A period without disturbance is required for ingestion (Lang, 1981). Many pet rabbits produce caecotrophs during the morning and if their routine is disturbed, they may deposit a pile of caecotrophs that are left uneaten. This phenomenon is sometimes observed in rabbits that have been admitted for an anaesthetic or some other procedure. Soft faeces may be found in the bottom of their cage or carrier and are not necessarily a cause for concern.

The ingestion of caecotrophs from the anus is triggered by stimulation of rectal mechanoreceptors and the perception of the specific odour of the soft faeces. The odour of the caecotrophs is influenced by the volatile fatty acids they contain. Germ-free rabbits do not eat their caecotrophs (Lang, 1981). Metabolites and hormones affect the rabbit's appetite for caecotrophs (Fekete, 1989). When food is scarce, all caecotrophs are consumed. When food is available *ad libitum*, the amount of caecotrophs consumed is influenced by the protein and fibre content of the diet. Increased levels of fibre increase caecotrophy whereas high protein levels reduce it. Increasing the indigestible fibre component of the diet not only stimulates the rabbit to eat the caecotrophs but also makes the pellets firmer and less sticky. Healthy rabbits that eat a high fibre diet will consume all their caecotroph whereas rabbits that are fed *ad libitum* on low fibre cereal diets will often leave caecotrophs uneaten. On some diets, particularly where certain herbs or legumes are included, the soft faeces appear less attractive than usual and are not ingested (Lang, 1981). Many diseases alter normal caecotrophic function, either by altering the consistency and composition of the caecotrophs or by interfering with the ingestion of caecotrophs from the anus (see Figure 10.6).

Rabbits that do not eat their caecotrophs are deprived of certain vitamins and amino acids that are synthesized by the caecal microflora. The effect of caecotrophy on protein and amino acid metabolism is greater in rabbits on a poor diet that is deficient in amino acids than on a diet with a higher protein content (Jécsai *et al.*, 1985).

10.6.2 Differentiation between uneaten caecotrophs and diarrhoea

A healthy rabbit on a balanced diet ingests caecotrophs straight from the anus without the owner ever seeing the caecotrophs or being aware of their existence. Many conditions interfere with the ingestion of caecotrophs (see Figure 10.6). Abnormalities in caecotrophy result in quantities of uneaten faecal material being deposited on the floor of the hutch or becoming entangled in the fur around the anus. The strong characteristic odour of uneaten caecotrophs and their soft, pasty consistency often misleads owners into believing their rabbit has diarrhoea. So, at the outset of the consultation, it is important to differentiate between uneaten soft faeces and true diarrhoea. Uneaten soft faeces is an unpleasant condition for both the owners and the rabbit but is not life threatening. Diarrhoea results in major disturbances in water and electrolyte metabolism and can be rapidly fatal. Caecotrophs are produced intermittently, usually once or twice every 24 h, when the animal is at rest. Copious amounts of hard faecal pellets are produced between episodes of soft faeces production and can be seen interspersed with any uneaten soft faeces in the bedding or on the floor of the hutch. Rabbits with enteritis and true diarrhoea do not produce hard faecal pellets. Instead, they produce soft faecal material that may be mixed with mucus. Rabbits suffering from caecotrophic disorders continue to eat well and produce large numbers of hard faecal pellets. Rabbits with diarrhoea are usually anorexic and depressed.

Although uneaten caecotrophs are not directly life threatening, the implications for the welfare of the individual rabbit are far reaching. The condition is difficult to treat successfully in the short term and tends to recur. Owners become disillusioned and are deterred by the smell and inconvenience of bathing and cleaning their pet's perineum. The constant smell and presence of the faecal mass can result in owners abandoning their pet, either by releasing it into the wild or by leaving it permanently confined to its hutch. The strong smell of uneaten caecotrophs attracts bluebottles during the summer months and affected rabbits are high-risk candidates for fly strike.

10.6.3 Physical conditions that interfere with caecotrophy

Many conditions can stop a rabbit consuming caecotrophs. Any skin condition that makes the perineal area sore and painful has the potential to prevent caecotrophy. The volatile fatty acid content of caecotrophs not only gives the characteristic odour but also scalds the skin under the mass of caked faecal material. The perineum of a rabbit is a very sensitive area and if the skin is sore, the rabbit may be reluctant to groom the area and ingest caecotrophs as they arrive at the anus. A vicious circle is formed, which results in sore, inflamed infected perineal skin (see Figure 9.1). Rabbits with fast growing, soft, fluffy coats can develop large mats of fur around the anus and under the tail. This fluffy coat texture is impossible for these rabbits to groom themselves. Soft faeces become entangled in the fur and can provide a physical barrier to the anus.

In order to reach the anus and ingest caecotrophs, the rabbit has to position itself correctly. Any condition that reduces flexibility or causes immobility can result in uneaten caecotrophs. This includes restriction in a small cage or carrier. Obese rabbits are often too fat to turn round and reach their perineum, both to groom or to ingest caecotrophs. Loose-skinned individuals often develop large perineal skin folds, especially if they are overweight. These skin folds can become infected and sore, which makes grooming painful. Faecal material can become entrapped in the folds of skin and exacerbate the problem. Some obese females or even castrated males develop huge dewlaps that pose an additional physical barrier to the perineum. Rabbits that are fed *ad libitum* on low fibre diets are not only more likely to leave caecotrophs uneaten but are also likely to become fat and lazy. Musculoskeletal conditions that either affect the rabbit's flexibility or cause pain when it turns round to reach its anus also interfere with caecotrophy. Spinal deformities such as kyphosis or vertebral spondylitis are a common radiological finding. Arthritic joints or painful infected hocks can make a rabbit reluctant to change position to clean and groom properly. Affected rabbits may not eat caecotrophs from the anus but will deposit them in the bedding and consume them later or not eat them at all.

Dental disease is a common reason for rabbits to leave caecotrophs uneaten and not to groom their perineal area. Sometimes caecotrophy abruptly ceases when sharp hooks develop on the cheek teeth and lacerate the tongue as the rabbit attempts to lick and groom. In other cases, incisor malocclusion prevents the rabbit from picking up and consuming caecotrophs.

Any condition that reduces appetite also reduces the appetite for caecotrophs, so almost any condition that makes a rabbit unwell can result in uneaten caecotrophs. Neurological diseases, that affect either the sense of smell or the neural pathways that supply the rectal mechanoreceptors, may interfere with caecotrophy. Degenerative disc disease, lumbosacral dislocations or fractures, and granulomatous lesions in the central nervous system caused by *E. cuniculi* are possible causes of such deficits.

10.6.4 Consistency of caecotrophs

Although softer than hard faeces, caecotrophs should have a firm pasty consistency. Uneaten caecotrophs that are soft in consis-

Key points 10.4

- Caecotrophs have a soft pasty consistency and a strong odour. Many owners mistake uneaten caecotrophs for diarrhoea, especially when they adhere to the fur around the anus
- It is important to make the distinction between uneaten caecotrophs and diarrhoea. Diarrhoea is a life-threatening condition in rabbits due to its effects on water and electrolyte metabolism. Uneaten caecotrophs are not life threatening
- Rabbits that are not ingesting caecotrophs do not have a reduced appetite and pass normal hard faeces in addition to uneaten caecotrophs
- Rabbits with enteritis do not pass hard faecal pellets. They are usually unwell and inappetant
- The consistency of caecotrophs can be soft or liquid and can mimic diarrhoea. Change in routine or dietary change such as the introduction of salad items or soft fruit can result in production of soft caecotrophs
- Several clinical conditions can either reduce a rabbit's appetite for caecotrophs, or prevent a rabbit from consuming caecotrophs from the anus
- Uneaten caecotrophs can become entangled in the fur around the anus and cause a superficial pyoderma in the skin beneath
- Treatment of uneaten caecotrophs is aimed at identifying and treating the underlying cause, clearing up any skin infection, improving the rabbit's appetite for caecotrophs and improving their consistency so they are not so sticky
- Decreasing dietary protein and increasing dietary fibre increase the rabbit's appetite for caecotrophs
- Increasing dietary fibre also results in caecotrophs of a firmer consistency.

Box 10.4 Treatment of uneaten caecotrophs and perineal soiling

Rabbits with 'sticky bottoms' can be a challenge to treat successfully. The first step is to clean and treat the soiled perineum. The next step is to identify and treat the underlying cause (see Figure 10.6).

In the short term

- Soiled fur should be carefully clipped away from the perineum. Simply bathing the area can be counterproductive as it leaves the fur soiled and damp and leads to infection of the underlying skin
- If the skin is inflamed, analgesia is indicated. Analgesics can also bring about a temporary respite from caecotroph production that is beneficial. Non-steroidal analgesics reduce caecotroph production by inhibiting endogenous prostaglandin synthesis (Pairet *et al.*, 1986). Meloxicam or ketoprofen have a greater influence on prostaglandin production than carprofen. Soft faeces production also appears to be temporarily reduced after sedation with narcotic analgesics, especially fentanyl/fluanisone (Hypnorm, Janssen)
- Analgesics also alleviate pain from spinal problems or arthritis, which may be preventing a rabbit from grooming and cleaning the perineal region
- Systemic antibiotics do not improve the consistency or reduce the production of soft faeces, although they may be beneficial in treating the perineal dermatitis. A 'safe' antibiotic such as enrofloxacin or trimethoprim that is unlikely to cause antibiotic-associated diarrhoea should be selected
- In the early stages, plenty of good quality hay or grass is required. Grass is ideal as it contains a mixture of fermentable and indigestible fibre and is palatable to most rabbits. A gradual dietary change will be required in the long term
- Probiotics may play a part in establishing a healthy caecal microflora.

In the long term

- Dietary modification is of paramount importance in altering the consistency of the caecotrophs and stimulating the rabbit's appetite for them
- Increasing the amount of fibre in the diet and reducing the amount of high calorie treats and cereals increases the rabbit's appetite for caecotrophs and makes them more fibrous and less sticky
- Cereal mixtures should be reduced or withdrawn and substituted with small amounts of complete rations. Treat foods such as chocolate should be cut out altogether. Vegetables, but not fruit may be offered, introducing one new item every few days starting with the more fibrous varieties such as spring cabbage or broccoli. Apples, carrots and garden weeds such as dandelions can be introduced later. Soft fruit and salad items such us cucumber, lettuce and tomatoes are not necessary and should be avoided altogether in rabbits that have a tendency to not to eat soft caecotrophs
- The introduction of fibrous green foods and vegetables is beneficial in increasing the fibre content and reducing the calorie content of the diet. In the short term, the introduction of new foods can unbalance the caecal flora, alter the consistency of the soft faeces, and compound the problem. Therefore, dietary modification should take place gradually
- Obesity is one of the main causes of perineal soiling and weight reduction is an essential part of the treatment (see Chapter 2). Exercise is also important
- Weight reduction and dietary modification may only be partially effective in resolving the problem in rabbits that have deep perineal folds. In obese animals, the skin folds often persist after the rabbit has lost weight. Surgical removal of the skin folds is a simple and effective remedy.

Long-term management of incurable cases of perineal soiling

In some cases of perineal soiling, the underlying cause cannot be removed and the owner will have to manage the problem for the lifetime of the rabbit. Other steps may be needed, in addition to modifying the diet to alter the consistency of caecotrophs.

- Fluffy coated breeds require constant grooming and clipping in the area around the tail and genitalia to prevent the hair becoming long and forming mats. Rabbits with maloccluded or no incisors require regular grooming in that area
- Enough space is required for the rabbit to move away from soiled bedding and decrease the likelihood of caecotrophs sticking to the fur
- Caecotroph production follows a circadian rhythm. Caecotrophs are usually produced during the morning. Observation of the individual rabbit's excretion pattern and changing the bedding accordingly can minimize soiling of the fur
- Long-term NSAID analgesic therapy may be helpful in the treatment of underlying spondylitic or arthritic conditions.

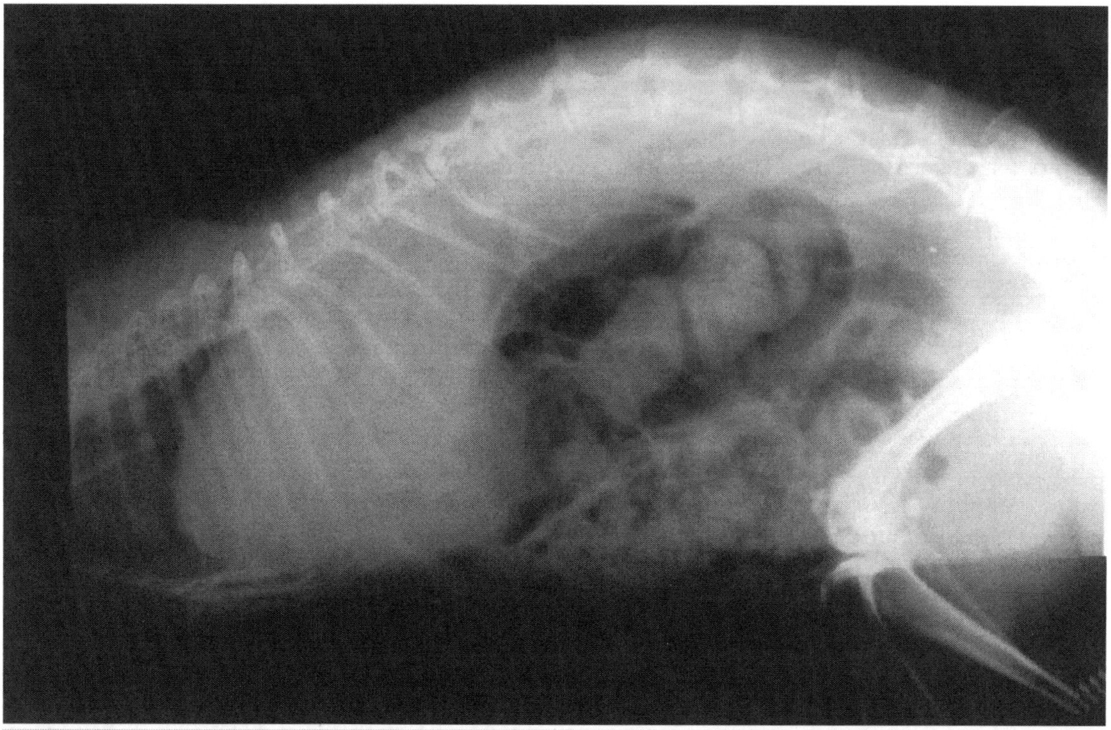

Figure 10.7. Lateral view of the abdomen of a rabbit with an impacted caecum. This radiograph was taken with the rabbit conscious. Gas has collected within the caecum and outlines several large pieces of impacted caecal material. Further impacted material can be seen in the caudoventral abdomen. In some cases, hard pieces of impacted material (caecoliths) can obstruct the colon as they are moved into the large intestine (see Figure 10.8). Like gastric impaction, impaction of the caecum can be the result of stress. The rabbit had recently been abandoned and, as a result, was subjected to the additional stresses of transport and rehoming. In this case, treatment was successful (see Section 10.7).

tency are more likely to become entangled in the fur under the tail, rather than drop into the bedding. Therefore changing the texture of the caecotrophs so that they are firmer is beneficial for both the rabbit and its owner.

Caecotrophs have a higher protein and water content and lower fibre content than hard faecal pellets. The amount and consistency of caecotrophs is affected by the fibre content of the diet. The type of fibre is important. Increasing the amount of indigestible fibre in the diet does not affect the volume or consistency of soft faeces because long fibre particles do not enter the caecum (Fraga *et al.*, 1991; Garcia *et al.*, 1995). Increasing the fermentable fibre content of the diet does have an effect on caecotroph consistency because small fibre particles are moved into the caecum. Most sources of fibre are a mixture of fermentable and indigestible fibre so increasing the overall fibre content of the diet is likely to increase the amount of fermentable fibre that reaches the caecum. Increasing dietary fibre also increases appetite for caecotrophs and the amount of soft faeces that are produced (Carabaõ and Piquer, 1998).

The consistency of soft faeces is also influenced by the water content. Water is absorbed from soft faeces during their passage through the colon and variations in transit time can lead to changes in consistency in soft faeces. The introduction of novel foods, especially succulent items such as lettuce or fruit can alter the consistency of caecotrophs so they are more liquid. This transitory change could be due to alterations in the transit time or changes in the caecal microflora. Dietary starch levels have no effect on the chemical composition of caecal contents or on the composition of hard or soft faeces (Carabaõ *et al.*, 1988).

The approach to treatment of uneaten caecotrophs is summarized in Box 10.4. In the short term, treatment is directed at clipping and cleaning the perineum and identifying the cause of uneaten caecotrophs. In the long term, dietary modification and weight reduction are required.

10.7 Caecal impaction

The cause of caecal impaction in rabbits is not always clear. Dry, impacted caecal contents in conjunction with mucus production in the colon is a feature of mucoid enteropathy, which is more often encountered in the juvenile rabbit than the adult. In the adult pet rabbit, caecal impaction occurs sporadically. Like gastric stasis, there is often a history of a stressful situation (see Figure 10.7). Dehydration may play a part in the aetiopathogenesis. It is known that feeding small fibre particles that absorb water can cause caecal impaction. Bulk laxatives, such as methylcellulose or psyllium are examples. Ground up lignified material can have a similar effect. Small particles, such as clay cat litter can also become impacted as they are moved into the caecum during mixing and separation of ingesta in the proximal colon.

The onset of caecal impaction can be insidious. In the initial stages, the rabbit may not look particularly unwell, but is inappetant and loses weight. The condition may be mistaken for dental disease as the rabbits may pick at food, eat a little and then drop it uneaten. Affected rabbits adopt a hunched stance. Faecal output is reduced or absent. There is often mucus production. The impacted organ can usually be palpated as a hard sausage-shaped structure in the ventral abdomen that can be seen on abdominal radiographs. On *post-mortem* examination, the caecal contents are solid and dry. Occasionally, a large lump of hard dry caecal contents can move into the colon and cause an obstruction. Caecal dilatation may be the result (see Figure 10.8).

Caecal impaction is difficult to treat. Surgery is unlikely to be successful. Medical treatment is directed at providing nutrition, relieving pain, promoting gastrointestinal motility, softening the caecal contents and promoting caecal evacuation. Fluid therapy by all routes, intravenous, subcutaneous and oral is indicated, plus liquid paraffin. All those foods that are reputed to cause 'diarrhoea' such as lettuce or fruit may tempt an inappetant rabbit to eat and provide additional fluid in addition to stimulating intestinal motility. As in all gastroenteric conditions in rabbits, good quality hay or fresh grass must be constantly available as a source of indigestible fibre. Motility stimulants such as cisapride and metaclopramide can be useful in stimulating motility, although their effect on caecal motility in rabbits is not clear. Sometimes, motility stimulants appear to cause stomach cramps perhaps due to their effects on the impacted organ. Analgesics are indicated although, theoretically, interference with prostaglandin production by non-steroidal analgesics could have an inhibitory effect on the *fusus coli*. Carprofen is a weak cyclo-oxygenase inhibitor and therefore has less effect on prostaglandin production than some other NSAIDs. Non-steroidal analgesic therapy could contribute to gastric ulceration, which is often a *post-mortem* feature of anorexic rabbits, and anti-ulcer treatment with ranitidene or omeprazole is indicated.

Experimentally, prostaglandin administration is followed by the passage of soft faeces (Pairet *et al.*, 1986). The author has used prostaglandin therapy (0.2 mg/kg dinoprost) as a last resort on a small number (3) of rabbits with impacted caeca. The caecal contents had been softened by orally administered liquid paraffin for 24–36 h prior to prostaglandin treatment. In all cases, the impacted caecal contents were evacuated 24–48 h after prostaglandin administration. All the rabbits went on to make a full recovery although they appeared to be in some abdominal discomfort for a few hours after the injection. However, prostaglandins have a number of systemic effects and the decision to use them should not be taken lightly. Concurrent oral and parenteral fluid therapy and analgesia are necessary. There might be adverse effects associated with the use of prostaglandins in rabbits.

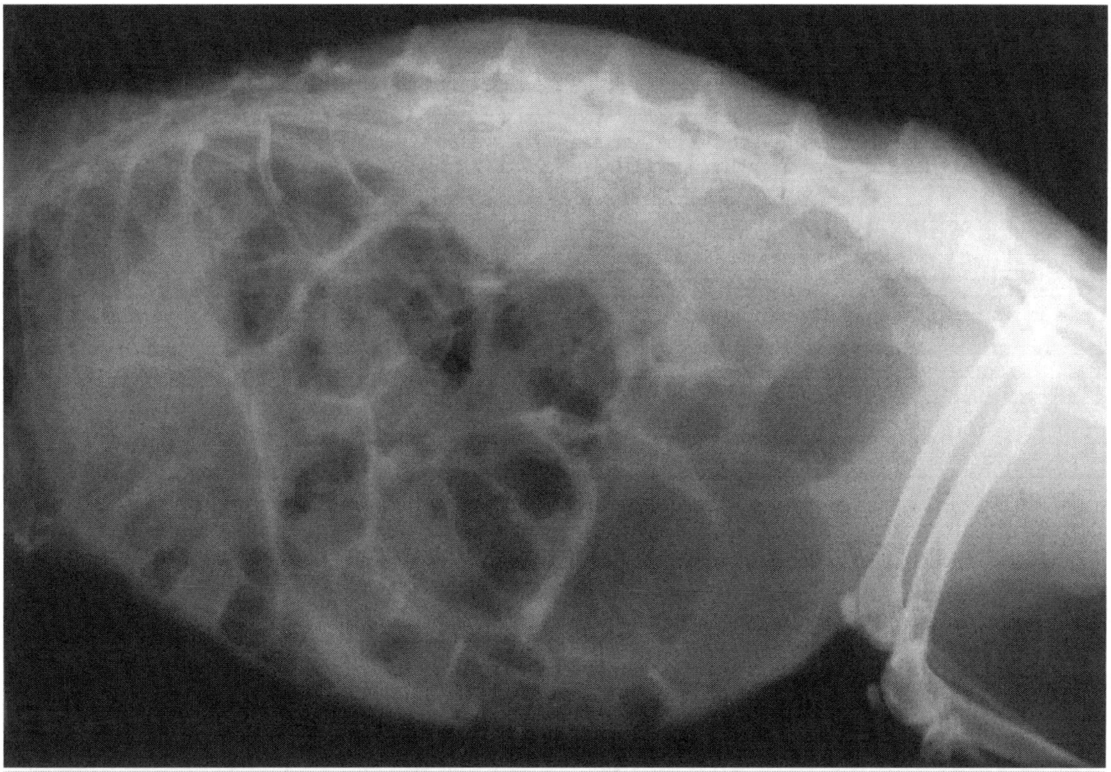

Figure 10.8. Lateral radiograph of a rabbit with caecal and intestinal tympany in association with chronic diarrhoea. The figure shows a lateral view of the abdomen of a 4-year-old neutered male rabbit that suffered from periodic bouts of anorexia and abdominal distension. In the interim, the rabbit had a good appetite but suffered from chronic diarrhoea. The stools were voluminous and contained a mixture of indigestible fibre particles and bacteria. Hard and soft faeces were indistinguishable. The rabbit was fed on a high fibre diet consisting of mainly grass hay with a small amount of good quality mixed ration. Vegetables appeared to exacerbate the problem. Blood samples showed a mild anaemia and hypoproteinaemia. Bouts of tympany responded to treatment with analgesics and oral trimethoprim/sulpha combinations. The rabbit was eventually euthanased. *Post-mortem* examination revealed a large (2–3 times normal size) flaccid caecum. Histopathological examination of the caecum and intestines showed lymphoplasmacytic enterotyphlocolitis suggestive of an immune-mediated aetiology. The author has seen several similar cases in which dietary modification and oral prednisolone has been prescribed, in addition to other treatment, with a limited degree of success.

A similar radiological picture can be seen in cases of caecal obstruction, which results in gas distension of the caecum. The cause of the obstruction is usually a large impacted lump of caecal material (caecolith) or a neoplasm such as a lymphoma. The cause of the obstruction can sometimes be seen radiographically or ultrasonagraphically. In cases of caecal obstruction, there is not the history of large loose voluminous faeces in association with a good appetite.

10.8 Dysautonomia

Dysautonomia is a dysfunction of the autonomic nervous system that results in loss of sympathetic and parasympathetic function. Dysautonomias have been described in dogs, hares, horses (grass sickness) and cats (Key-Gaskell syndrome). The disease mainly affects the digestive tract and is characterized by reduced gut motility, although other signs associated with loss of autonomic function, such as mydriasis, urine retention or dry mucous membranes, may also be evident. Histopathological changes are seen in the autonomic ganglia. Chromatolysis-like degenerative changes take place in the neurons. Dysautonomic disease is well documented in the dog, cat and horse in which loss of autonomic function carries a poor prognosis although the occasional mild case can survive with careful nursing. In recent years, dysautonomia has been described in rabbits suffering from mucoid enteropathy.

Cheeke (1987) observed that a strain of non-albino white rabbits with pigmented eyes were particularly susceptible to diarrhoea and that evidence of 'insufficient nerve ganglia in the intestine' was seen. An analogy with grass sickness in the horse was made. The discovery of degenerative changes in ganglionic neurons in rabbits suffering from mucoid enteritis had been made as early as 1967, but was not investigated further, although a syndrome of caecal impaction in conjunction with pulmonary oedema and urine retention was described by several authors (Van der Hage and Dorrestein, 1996). In 1991, *post-mortem* examination of two sick hares found on an English estate where horses had died from grass sickness revealed changes in the ganglia and alimentary tract that were remarkably similar to those seen in grass sickness (Whitwell, 1991; Griffiths and Whitwell, 1993). In 1996, Van der Hage and Dorrestein described the clinical findings, pathological lesions and microscopic and transmission electron microscopic features of the coeliac ganglia of 19 rabbits with mucoid enteropathy. Typical cases were selected that had died following a disease characterized by emaciation, respiratory distress, distended abdomen with a palpable obstipated caecum or a distended bladder. Degenerative changes, manifested as chromatolysis, were found in the coeliac ganglia. No viruses, infectious agents, aflatoxins or other causative agents were discovered on food analysis or on extensive examination of the liver and intestinal contents of affected animals. An analogy was again made with grass sickness in horses, which is thought to be caused by a neurotoxin.

Dysautonomia was first confirmed in rabbits in the UK in 1996 in a colony of Belgian Hares (which are actually rabbits) suffering from mucoid enteropathy (Whitwell and Needham, 1996). Histology of the ganglia showed chromatolysis-like degenerative changes in many neurons and some neuronal vacuolation. In 1997, Boucher and Nouvelle, in an outbreak of mucoid enteropathy, described clinical signs which were similar to dysautonomic disease in horses and cats, i.e. mydriasis, dry mucous membranes, reduced tear production, bradycardia (less than 100 bpm), urine retention and intestinal impaction. They described an age predisposition of 6–8 weeks and the presence of opportunistic pathogens such as coccidia, *Clostridium spiriforme* and *Clostridium perfringens*. Histological examination of the coeliac and mesenteric ganglia revealed characteristic lesions similar to dysautonomia in other species.

The incidence of dysautonomia or its importance in the syndrome of mucoid enteropathy is not clear at the present time. Mucoid enteropathy is not invariably linked with chromatolysis-like degenerative changes in the neurons. Detailed *post-mortem* examination is required to confirm the diagnosis of dysautonomia, which can be expensive. Most cases of mucoid enteropathy are not presented to veterinary surgeons for treatment and there is a great deal of confusion among rabbit breeders about the condition. 'Mucoid enteropathy' is a term that is used in a non-specific manner to describe a number of interrelated enteric diseases that occur in rabbits, especially around the time of weaning. Rabbit breeders will often cull and dispose of ill animals themselves. Caecal impaction in connection with pneumonia, and perhaps other autonomic signs such as bradycardia, dilated pupils or urine retention, is suggestive of dysautonomic disease. A feature of confirmed cases in the UK has been the presence of an inhalation pneumonia as affected rabbits have problems swallowing and may have uneaten food in the mouth and pharynx (Whitwell, personal communication).

Treatment for rabbits with dysautonomia follows the same principles as the treatment of mucoid enteropathy or an impacted caecum. In horses, some mild cases of grass sickness can survive with careful nursing and supportive care (Milne, 1997).

The diagnosis of dysautonomia can be confirmed at *post-mortem* examination, including histopathology of the autonomic ganglia and gut wall. The site of the mesenteric ganglia is illustrated in Figure 16.1 and a technique for removing autonomic ganglia is described in Section 17.3.

10.9 Mucoid enteropathy

Mucoid enteropathy is a confusing condition both in its terminology and in its aetiopathogenesis. Many lay people and rabbit breeders use the terms 'mucoid enteropathy', 'ME', 'mucoid enteritis', 'mucoid enteritis complex' interchangeably to describe any enteric condition of rabbits characterized by diarrhoea, mucus production, constipation or death. These signs are non-specific and can be caused by several diseases. 'Mucoid enteritis' has been the cause of significant losses in commercial breeding units with reported mortality rates of approximately 5–10% but rising to over 60% (McLeod and Katz, 1986). Colibacillosis, enterotoxaemia, Tyzzer's disease, coccidiosis and viral enteritis can all be included in the syndrome that often affects young rabbits especially around the time of weaning. 'Mucoid enteropathy' is characterized by the presence of large amounts of mucus in the colon and is usually associated with impaction of the caecum (see Figure 10.9). Inflammatory changes are minimal. The terms 'constipative mucoid enteropathy' or CME can also be used to describe this syndrome. At *post-mortem* examination, the caecum is often impacted with dried contents and gas (see Plate 23). The colon is distended with gelatinous mucus. The stomach and small intestine may be distended with fluid and gas.

The aetiopathogenesis of mucoid enteropathy is far from clear. It is not known what role diet, stress, pathogens, caecal microflora or dysautonomia have in the disease, although it seems likely that all these factors could have a part to play. Mucoid enteropathy is a disease of intensively reared domestic rabbits rather than wild ones (Lelkes and Chang, 1987). The disease is occasionally encountered in adult pet rabbits, especially after a stressful incident such as transport or parturition. It is known that increasing the amount of indigestible fibre in the diet of newly weaned rabbits significantly reduces the incidence of mucoid enteropathy. Stress appears to play a major role in the development of the disease. Enzyme deficiencies, infectious agents and enterotoxins have all been cited as other possible causes. Inflammation is not a feature of the disease and intestinal hypomotility or changes in the acidity of the caecum have been proposed as aetiological factors (Lelkes and Chang, 1987). Investigations are often hampered by the presence of concurrent

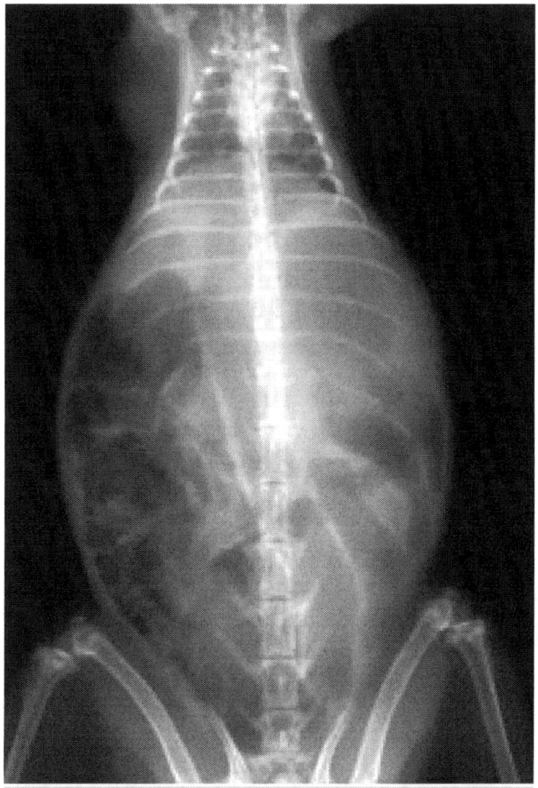

Figure 10.9. Ventrodorsal view of a rabbit with mucoid enteropathy. The figure shows a ventrodorsal view of a 4-month-old, mixed breed, male rabbit suffering from mucoid enteropathy. The stomach is dilated and filled with fluid. There is gas distension of the duodenum and jejunum. There is impacted material within the caecum that also contains gas. The rabbit died shortly after this radiograph was taken. Evidence of dysautonomia was not found on histopathological examination of the autonomic ganglia and other organs. Note the normal small volume of the thoracic cavity in comparison with the abdomen.

infections such as coccidiosis, Tyzzer's disease or opportunist pathogens such as *Clostridia* spp. or *E. coli*.

A feature of mucoid enteropathy is the presence of large amounts of mucus in the colon. At *post-mortem* examination, a large plug of mucus is often found obstructing the colon. In rabbits, mucus production is a response of the hindgut to untoward stimuli (Bergdall and Dysko, 1994) and is not necessarily specific to mucoid enteropathy. Experimentally, ligation of the caecum results in a mucoid enteropathy-like syndrome in some rabbits, with large amounts of mucus production in the colon. Incorporating the nerves and blood vessels in the ligature increases the likelihood of inducing a mucus hypersecretion 3–5 days after surgery (Hotchkiss and Merritt, 1996a). Surgical removal of the caecum does not result in mucus production whereas filtrates from the ligated caecum administered to *in vitro* sections of colon do stimulate mucus secretion. Injection of oxytetracycline into the ligated caecum prevents colonic mucus secretion suggesting that a bacterial secretory product is the stimulus for excessive goblet cell secretion characteristic of mucoid enteropathy. Mucus secretion is also stimulated in the respiratory tract. Injections of cholestyramine into the ligated caecum can prevent the development of mucoid enteropathy-like symptoms suggesting the presence of some type of toxin (Toofanian and Targowski, 1983).

The caecal microflora of rabbits with experimental mucoid enteropathy induced by caecal ligation is different from that of healthy rabbits. There is a decline in the number of gram-positive bacteria, protozoa and large anaerobic metachromatic bacilli and an increase in gram-negative organisms. The production of volatile fatty acids also alters after caecal ligation. In healthy rabbits, acetate predominates followed by butyrate and proprionate. In experimental mucoid enteropathy, caecal acetate and butyrate concentrations are reduced with an increase in proprionate, isobutyrate, valerate and isovalerate production (Toofanian and Hamar, 1986).

Typically, growing rabbits are affected by mucoid enteropathy but the disease is occasionally seen in adults, especially breeding does. Clinical signs include abdominal distension, subnormal body temperatures, depression, crouched stance and 'sloshy' sounding guts. There is a disruption of normal faeces production. Hard faecal pellets are not produced. Diarrhoea can be present in the early stages. In the later stages, large amounts of mucus, either on its own or mixed with faecal material are excreted. Faecal production may cease completely. Appetite is reduced, sometimes to the point of complete anorexia. Some rabbits are polydypsic whereas others may have a reduced water intake. A feature of the disease is tooth grinding, presumably due to abdominal pain. A solid impacted caecum may be palpable and seen radiographically. Some acute cases present with gastric dilatation rather than caecal impaction. Gas shadows may be seen in the caecum and small intestine. In the terminal stages, there is gastric distension with large amounts of fluid and/or gas in the stomach. There may be lung changes. Some rabbits are presented with respiratory signs. The disease is progressive and usually fatal.

In the live animal, differential diagnosis includes hepatic coccidiosis and enteritis caused by the variety of diseases that affect weanling and juvenile rabbits. Intercurrent disease is common. Confirmation of the diagnosis is usually made at *post-mortem* by the presence of large amounts of mucus in the colon.

Most rabbit breeders do not present cases of mucoid enteropathy to veterinary surgeons for diagnosis and treatment. Affected animals are culled or treated with a variety of home remedies. As a result, there is much confusion about the disease and there are claims of success with many different treatments, including antibiotics. In most cases, it is not clear if the treatments were effective against other diseases, such as respiratory or enteric pathogens or coccidiosis rather than mucoid enteropathy. In commercial units, affected rabbits are often not treated, although antibiotic therapy can be instigated, either prophylactically or therapeutically. Mucoid enteropathy is not common in pet rabbits. It may be seen in the newly acquired baby rabbits from the pet shop or breeder, or in an adult stressed by parturition, transport or a change of home. In these circumstances, the individual rabbit is valuable to the new owner and treatment is often requested. However, the prognosis is poor and most cases die despite aggressive treatment. Treat-

Key points 10.5

- Caecal impaction occurs in rabbits, either as a clinical entity or as part of the syndrome of mucoid enteropathy or dysautonomia. Stress appears to play a role in the aetiopathogenesis
- Feeding small fibre particles that absorb water, e.g. bulk laxatives, can cause caecal impaction
- Ingestion of clay litter material can cause caecal impaction
- The onset of caecal impaction is often insidious
- The impacted caecum can usually be palpated as a hard sausage-shaped structure in the ventral abdomen
- Analgesia is indicated. Narcotic analgesics such as buprenorphine or butorphanol may be preferable to NSAIDs that inhibit prostaglandin synthesis. Prostaglandins stimulate caecal emptying. Carprofen is a weak cyclo-oxygenase inhibitor and is preferable to other NSAIDs, if a NSAID is required
- Occasionally, large lumps of impacted caecal material can move into the colon and cause an obstruction. The caecum dilates with gas. Faecal output ceases and the rabbit becomes depressed and anorexic
- Dysautonomia has been identified in rabbits. Loss of sympathetic and parasympathetic function results in reduced gut motility, especially of the caecum. In the terminal stages, gastric dilatation and aspiration pneumonia can occur
- Dysautonomia can be confirmed at *post-mortem* examination by histopathological examination of the autonomic ganglia
- Enteric disease in rabbits is a complex inter-relationship of infectious and non-infectious diseases predisposed by poor diet, stress and intensive husbandry. Rabbit breeders tend to use the term 'mucoid enteropathy' to encompass any enteric condition that causes diarrhoea, mucus excretion, abdominal distension or death
- Strictly speaking, 'mucoid enteropathy' is a condition that is characterized by caecal impaction and the presence of large amounts of gelatinous mucus in the colon. Juvenile rabbits are most susceptible
- Clinical signs include abdominal distension, depression, crouched stance and 'sloshy' sounding guts. Tooth grinding is common
- Disruption of normal faecal output is one of the first signs of mucoid enteropathy. Diarrhoea and/or mucus may be seen in the early stages, followed by cessation of faecal output and abdominal distension
- Despite many investigations, the aetiology of mucoid enteropathy is still not clear. The syndrome can be reproduced in laboratory rabbits by ligation of the caecum
- The prognosis for rabbits with mucoid enteropathy is poor.

ment is non-specific and follows the same principles as for other digestive disorders (see Tables 10.2, 10.3 and Box 10.3). Frequent enemas have been recommended (Breitweiser, 1997). The role of antibiotics is unclear, although many breeders believe that antibiotics are effective. In advanced cases, euthanasia is the most humane choice.

10.10 Enteric diseases caused by specific pathogens

10.10.1 Coccidiosis

Coccidiosis is a disease of animals kept in crowded conditions and occurs in many breeding establishments. Intensive, damp, dirty conditions predispose to coccidiosis and the environment can become heavily contaminated. The disease is caused by a protozoan parasite with a complex life cycle. Wild rabbits can be affected and, theoretically, are a potential source of infection to pet rabbits that are fed on grass. Long grass picked by hand is less likely to be contaminated then short grass grazed by large numbers of wild rabbits.

The protozoan parasites that cause coccidiosis are Sporozoa belonging to the suborder Eimeriorina. *Eimeria* are parasites of epithelial cells. They invade the mucosa of the intestine, colon and caecum and the epithelium of various ducts. Infected rabbits void oocysts that require oxygen and a period of a several days to become infective. Ingestion of the oocyst releases sporozoites into the duodenum after the oocyst has been broken down by digestive enzymes. The sporozoites invade cells and cause tissue damage as they complete their complex life cycle ultimately to release oocysts into the lumen of the gut. *Eimeria* species are host and site specific. Oocysts can survive for many years in the environment but are susceptible to dry conditions. Recovered rabbits become immune to infection. As many as 14 species of *Eimeria* have been described in the rabbit. All but one species are found in the small intestine, caecum or colon and cause 'intestinal coccidiosis'. One species, *Eimeria steidae*, inhabits the epithelial cells of the bile ducts and causes 'hepatic coccidiosis'. There is no cross-immunity between the different *Eimeria* species.

10.10.1.1 Intestinal coccidiosis

Eimeria magna and *Eimeria irresidua* are the two most pathogenic coccidial species that affect the intestine of rabbits. Other less pathogenic intestinal species include *E. perforans, E. media, E. elongata, E. neoloporis, E. intestinalis, E. caecicola* and *E. piriformis*. The developmental stages are restricted to the ileum and jejunum but, in heavy infestations, overspill into the caecum has been observed (Owen, 1992). There are two asexual stages and oocysts appear in the faeces 7–8 days post-infection. Mixed infections can occur and coccidia are often found in conjunction with other pathogenic agents such as *E. coli*. It is not always clear how important intestinal coccidiosis is during an outbreak of enteritis, although the introduction of a pathogenic species into a susceptible population can prove fatal, especially in young rabbits around the time of weaning. Acute infection causes inappetance, weight loss, depression and diarrhoea that can be haemorrhagic. Intussusceptions may be associated with chronic infections. Subclinical coccidiosis results in reduced feed conversion.

On *post-mortem* examination, the parasite can be found on microscopic examination of intestinal scrapings. Lesions occur primarily in the ileum and jejunum and are immediately identifiable by inflammation and oedema at the site of infection. Mucosal ulcerations and haemorrhages may be seen. Characteristic changes can be seen histologically in the gut wall. During life, oocysts are found in the faeces. Sulpha drugs are used to treat coccidiosis. Groups of rabbits can be medicated in the food or drinking water. Oral trimethoprim preparations can be used to treat individual pets. Dose rates are given in Table 4.2.

10.10.1.2 Hepatic coccidiosis

Hepatic coccidiosis is a serious disease of rabbits caused by the species specific *Eimeria steidae*. Wild rabbits can be infected and transmission occurs by the ingestion of sporulated oocysts in food that has been contaminated by faeces. Sporulation of the oocysts is required for infectivity and requires at least 2 days outside the host. Oocysts are extremely resistant and can remain viable in soil, on vegetation and fomites for long periods of time (Harkness and Wagner, 1995). Recently voided faeces do not contain oocysts that are infective (Harkness, 1997) as a prepatent period in the presence of oxygen is required for development. *Eimeria steidae* has a slightly different life cycle to the intestinal *Eimeria* spp. Ingested oocysts hatch in the duodenum and sporozoites penetrate the intestinal mucosa before being transported to the liver, either in the blood stream, or in macrophages in the lymphatic system. Replication takes place in the mesenteric lymph nodes before transport via the hepatic portal circulation to the liver where they enter bile duct epithelial cells. Here the life cycle is completed with the ultimate release of oocysts into the bile duct. The prepatent period lasts for 15–16 days and oocysts are found in the faeces for at least 10–14 days after this (Owen, 1992).

Clinical symptoms of hepatic coccidiosis depend on the severity of infection and on the immune status of the individual. Signs are associated with the lesions in the liver and bile ducts, and include weight loss, ascites, jaundice, diarrhoea and hepatomegaly. Weanling rabbits are most commonly affected.

Post-mortem signs relate to the predilection of the parasite for the bile ducts. There are pale yellow foci or cords in the liver. The gall bladder and bile ducts may be thickened and distended. The liver is enlarged and fibrotic. The gall bladder is enlarged, distended, and packed with oocysts that can be seen in wet smears of the bile. Impression smears of the cut surface of the mesenteric lymph nodes or liver can reveal all stages of the parasite which is reputed to have nine different schizont stages (Owen, 1992). Remnants of the disease may be evident in the liver for life and can occasionally be discovered many years later, during *post-mortem* examination.

Newly weaned animals are most susceptible and those that recover have a solid lifelong immunity. The condition can be treated with sulpha drugs (Schmidt, 1995). Commercial pellets often contain a coccidiostat to prevent clinical disease in rabbit colonies while allowing an immunological response to confer immunity. Treatment of established disease can be problematical, as rabbits that are not eating well will not be receiving the medication in the feed. In a comparative study of the response of rabbits infected with *Eimeria steidae* to treatment with sulphaquinoxaline, robenidene, methyl benzoquate, clopidol and a mixture of methyl benzoquate and clopidol, only sulphaquinoxaline and the combination of methyl benzoquate and clopidol gave satisfactory control of the parasite (Joyner *et al.*, 1983). Toltrazuril (Baycox, Bayer) in the drinking water is highly effective in reducing oocyst output of intestinal and hepatic *Eimeria* species. A regimen of 2 days treatment repeated after 5 days reduces clinical signs and allows the development of immunity (Peeters and Geeroms, 1986).

10.10.1.3 Coccidiosis in pet rabbits

In pet rabbits, coccidiosis is sometimes encountered in the newly acquired young rabbit. Intestinal coccidiosis causes inappetance, weight loss and chronic diarrhoea, which can be blood tinged. Animals affected with hepatic coccidiosis are often thin, pot-bellied and small for their age. Occasionally icterus is seen. Mixed infections occur. Raised bilirubin values in rabbits of this age are virtually pathognomonic for hepatic coccidiosis, especially in conjunction with other biochemical evidence of liver damage such as a raised AST, ALT, gamma GT and alkaline phosphatase values. Coccidial oocysts may be evident in the faeces. By the time the animals are presented for treatment they are often recovering from infection. If the rabbit is active and eating well, the prognosis is usually good with administration of sulpha drugs. Paediatric suspension of trimethoprim/sulfamethoxazole can be used to treat the individual patient (see Table 10.3). A well balanced diet is also required as the hepatic coccidiosis interferes with vitamin metabolism.

10.10.2 Clostridial enterotoxaemia

Enterotoxaemia occurs in rabbits kept in colonies and occasionally in the individual pet rabbit. The disease is caused by *Clostridia* spp. that are anaerobic gram-positive bacilli capable of producing powerful enterotoxins. The organisms can reside in the gut without causing disease but under certain conditions will rapidly proliferate and cause a severe enteritis. *Clostridium spiroforme* is a major pathogen in rabbit enterotoxaemia, although *Clostridium difficile* and *Clostridium perfringens* may also be involved (Perkins *et al.*, 1995). Pathogenic rabbit strains of *C. spiroforme* are different from non-pathogenic strains in other species. A similar pathogenic strain has been isolated from humans affected with diarrhoea (Carman, 1993). Rabbit isolates of *C. spiroforme* produce a toxin that is neutralized by antiserum to *C. perfringens* type E iota toxin. Virtually all rabbit isolates of *C. spiroforme* are toxigenic, although this is not the case in other species. *Clostridium difficile* produces two exotoxins, toxin A and B. Toxin A is a lethal enterotoxin that binds to specific enteroreceptors and induces fluid secretion, mucosal damage and intestinal inflammation. Toxin B is a potent cytotoxin that interacts synergistically with toxin A (Perkins *et al.*, 1995).

In intensive situations, the mortality rate from enterotoxaemia can be high due to the prevalence of pathogen in the environment. Low fibre, high carbohydrate diets are associated with enterotoxaemia in commercial units. Recently weaned rabbits are most susceptible. Young rabbits do not digest and absorb starch as efficiently as adults (De Blas and Gidenne, 1998) and carry a greater risk of unabsorbed carbohydrate reaching the caecum to act as a bacterial substrate. Substantial amounts of glucose are required by *C. spiriforme* for toxin production. There is a marked difference in starch digestibility between adult and growing rabbits. In adult rabbits, carbohydrate is hydrolysed and absorbed before it reaches the caecum. Enterotoxaemia in adult pet rabbits is not associated with a high carbohydrate diet but usually follows a disruption of the gut flora by antibiotics, other pathogens, toxins or stress. Experimentally, enterotoxaemia can be induced by oral administration of clindamycin. The accidental inclusion of lincomycin in the diet of commercial rabbits has resulted in clinical outbreaks.

Enterotoxaemia is manifested by brown, watery diarrhoea, collapse or sudden death. It is an acute disease although it is sometimes preceded by a short period of anorexia. In most cases, enterotoxaemia is rapidly fatal due to toxaemia, dehydration and electrolyte loss although the occasional case can recover. Peracute cases may be found dead with no prior evidence of disease. Others are found moribund, often with liquid tarry brown diarrhoea. Chronic cases are manifested by anorexia and weight loss and intermittent diarrhoea (Carman and Evans, 1984).

At *post-mortem* examination, the rabbits are often in good bodily condition but may have liquid faeces oozing from the anus and staining the perineum and hind legs. Typical *post-mortem* findings include inflammation and hypereamia of the caecum. The small intestine or proximal colon can also be affected. Extensive petechial or ecchymotic haemorrhages on the serosal surface of the caecum are characteristic of enterotoxaemia. The caecal contents are very liquid and may contain gas. Haemorrhages or ulcers may be seen on the mucosal surface of the caecum. The submucosa can be thickened and oedematous. To be certain that enterotoxaemia was the cause of death, prompt *post-mortem* examination is required to differentiate the lesions from *post-mortem* changes.

Sometimes, enterotoxaemia can be confirmed by detection of the organism in caecal contents. Comma shaped organisms may be seen on gram-stained caecal smears. Anaerobic culture for 24–48 h on blood agar is required to grow the organism. Anaerobic conditions can be preserved by tying off a section of caecum or small intestine at each end before it is removed and submitted to the laboratory. Alternatively a swab of intestinal contents can be immediately plunged to the bottom of the transport medium where conditions remain anaerobic. *Clostridia* spp. concentrate at the interface of the deposit and supernatant after centrifugation of caecal contents and may be seen on a gram stain from material taken from this area. Toxin is also present in the supernatant but requires specialized tests such as the guinea pig dermonecrosis or the mouse lethality assay for detection (Delong and Manning, 1994).

Treatment of enterotoxaemia is not usually successful. Most cases are presented dead or dying. Prompt, intravenous fluid therapy and supportive care are necessary. Antibiotics and short-acting corticosteroids might be of value. Metronidazole is indicated to kill anaerobic *Clostridia* spp. Antibiotics such as ampicillin, clindamycin, lincomycin, amoxycillin, penicillin or erythromycin that are known to precipitate enterotoxaemia should be avoided. There is evidence that the ion exchange resin cholestyramine absorbs the enterotoxin and improves survival rate if it is given in the early stages (see Section 4.9.2). This preparation is safe enough to give to rabbits in any situations where enterotoxaemia could develop. Probiotics can also be administered, although it is not known if they are effective.

Vaccination protects sheep from clostridial enterotoxaemia and there are anecdotal reports from breeders that vaccinating rabbits with sheep vaccine reduces mortality rates in colonies of rabbits that have experienced losses from clostridial infections. Clostridial enterotoxaemia in sheep is caused by *C. perfringens* not *C. spiriforme,* which is the usual pathogen involved in enterotoxaemia. Experimentally, the protective value of toxoids prepared from *Clostridium spiriforme* have been evaluated in laboratory and farm bred rabbits (Ellis *et al.*, 1991). The trials showed that a single vaccination at 4 weeks of age was protective especially if a second dose was administered 14 days later. Maternal immunity was not passed from vaccinated dams to their offspring.

10.10.3 Coliform enteritis

Pathogenic strains of *Escherichia coli* can be a major cause of enteritis and losses in colonies of commercial rabbits or laboratories. *E. coli* is normally absent from the intestinal flora of rabbits or is only present in small numbers. Under some circumstances pathogenic strains of the organism proliferate and cause diarrhoea. Concurrent coccidiosis or dietary factors predispose to disease. Strains of *E. coli* vary in pathogenicity and some produce endotoxins. Antibiotics can be effective in treating some of the less virulent strains. There appears to be age susceptibility associated with *E. coil* with suckling rabbits being most susceptible. At *post-mortem* examination, the small intestine may appear normal but there is inflammation of the caecum and large intestine. In neonates, gram-stained smears from the small intestine may show large numbers of gram-negative rods (Okerman, 1988). In older animals, differential diagnosis from coccidiosis, enterotoxaemia, Tyzzer's disease and viral enteropathies depends on gross and microscopic changes and isolation of the pathogen. There may be concurrent disease such as rotavirus infection or coccidiosis. Antibiotic therapy, poor husbandry, overcrowding and stress are among predisposing factors.

10.10.4 Tyzzer's disease

Tyzzer's disease is an inflammation of the caecum caused by a sporulating, obligate intracellular bacterium, which has recently been reclassified as *Clostridium piliforme* rather than *Bacillus piliformis* based on molecular studies of the genome (Besch-Williford, 1997). The disease usually occurs in weanling rabbits 6–8 weeks old and is predisposed by poor husbandry, overcrowding, immunosuppression and incorrect diet. Serological testing of pet rabbits by the University of Missouri, USA, reported an incidence of 47%, although the majority of rabbits were asymptomatic (Besch-Williford, 1997).

Spores from *Clostridium piliforme* are shed in the faeces and can remain viable in the environment for over a year. Oral ingestion of spores from contaminated material results in bacterial invasion of the epithelium of the lower small intestine and caecum. The presence of antibodies in apparently healthy animals suggests that the organism can reside latently in the gastrointestinal tract. Overt disease is precipitated by stress or immunosuppression. Experimentally, corticosteroid administration is required to reproduce the disease (Delong and Manning, 1994). The organism penetrates the intestinal mucosa and disseminates throughout the liver and eventually the myocardium via the lymphatics.

Tyzzer's disease causes necrosis of the caecum, intestine, liver and heart. Peracute cases may show intestinal lesions only. Myocardial lesions occur later in the course of the disease and lesions are principally found in the left ventricle and septum.

Clinical signs include diarrhoea, faecal soiling of the perineum, dehydration and death and are therefore non-specific. Weanling rabbits 6–12 weeks old are primarily affected, although the disease can affect rabbits of any age. In common with many of the infectious agents that cause diarrhoea in rabbits, Tyzzer's disease is predisposed by stress, low fibre diets, intensive husbandry and intercurrent disease.

Chronic infection can occur with intestinal stenosis and fibrosis occurring at the sites of necrosis. There is little information about the clinical syndromes associated with intestinal stenosis or myocardial necrosis. Diagnosis is usually made at *post-mortem* examination and is confirmed by histological examination of the liver where the organism can be seen in hepatocytes. It is not known if Tyzzer's disease is a significant cause of disease in adult pet rabbits in the UK. Serological and PCR tests may become available which would facilitate the screening of stock for carriers and aid diagnosis in the live animal.

10.10.5 Salmonellosis

In common with most animals, rabbits can suffer from salmonellosis although the disease is uncommon, especially in the individual pet. *Salmonella typhimurium* or *S. enteriditis* can cause diarrhoea, septicaemia and rapid death.

10.10.6 Viral causes of enteritis

10.10.6.1 Rotavirus

Rotavirus has been associated with outbreaks of enteritis, usually in rabbits under 6 weeks of age. In most cases, diarrhoea is mild (Thouless *et al.*, 1996). Rotavirus was originally isolated from weanling rabbits with diarrhoea, although it has also been recovered from unaffected animals (Bryden *et al.*, 1976). Serological tests have revealed that rotavirus infection is widespread in colonies of domestic rabbits. The disease has been reported in many parts of the world including Japan, Europe, Canada and the USA (DiGiacomo and Mare, 1994). In infected colonies, adult animals are seropositive and confer maternal immunity on their offspring. The young rabbits become infected when maternal immunity wears off which coincides with weaning. Infected rabbits shed virus in faeces, which is probably the main route of transmission, although there is evidence for airborne spread. Severity of clinical signs depends on virus strain, intercurrent disease, immune status and all the other factors that are involved in enteric disease in weanling rabbits. In a study by Thouless *et al.* (1996), it was found that concurrent infection with rotavirus and *E. coli* resulted in increased mortality and morbidity due to diarrhoeal disease compared with infection with *E. coli* alone.

10.10.6.2 Coronavirus

Rabbit enteric coronavirus (RECV) has been reported in association with enteritis in rabbits. The virus has also been associated with pleural effusion and cardiomyopathy and an analogy has been made with feline infectious peritonitis (Deeb *et al.*, 1993). RECV has been implicated in outbreaks of enteric disease in a barrier maintained rabbit colony (DiGiacomo and Mare, 1994). RECV is unlikely to be a cause of disease in the pet rabbit.

10.11 Poisoning

10.11.1 Plant toxicity

Plant toxicity is a cause of concern to owners who give their rabbits the freedom of the garden or pick plants to feed to their pets. Actual proven cases of plant toxicity in rabbits are rare in the veterinary literature although there are some anecdotal reports and an abundance of myths (see Section 2.17.2). Rabbits are known to be resistant to the toxic components of deadly nightshade and ragwort. However, it is wise to avoid exposure to plants that are known to be toxic in other species (see Table 2.4).

10.11.2 Lead poisoning

Rabbits are susceptible to lead poisoning by chewing wood covered in lead-based paint, pipes or vinyl floor covering. The primary presenting signs are lethargy and reduced appetite, which can progress to other symptoms (Swartout and Gerken, 1987). Typical haematological changes of anaemia and basophilic stippling may be seen in chronic cases. Reduced appetite appears to be linked with slow gut motility. Radiographically, radiopaque material may be seen in the stomach and unevacuated hard faeces may be seen the large intestine. Treatment with motility agents such as cisapride or metaclopramide in addition to a chelating agent, such as sodium calcium edetate or D-penicillamine, facilitates excretion of the lead from the gut. An advantage of the rabbit's rapid elimination of large particles is that flakes of lead paint will be quickly passed out in the hard faeces rather than moved into the caecum and retained in the body for longer periods before being re-ingested.

10.12 Approach to an outbreak of enteric disease in a breeding colony

Many rabbit breeders keep a small number of animals that they use as exhibition animals and sell young stock into the pet trade. In many cases, diseases are treated with home remedies or by culling affected stock. Half-truths, myths and legends abound, although some traditional remedies have a grain of truth or some sound common sense in them. Professional veterinary advice is seldom sought except when a disease threatens all the stock, a prize-winning bloodline or perhaps a particularly valuable individual. Expense is always an issue. Cases of enteritis can be

Key points 10.6

- There are several *Eimeria* species that cause coccidiosis in rabbits. Mixed infections usually occur. There is no cross-immunity between the species
- Most *Eimeria* species affect the intestine and heavy infestations cause inappetance, weight loss and diarrhoea. Blood may be seen in the faeces
- One species, *Eimeria steidae*, has a complex life cycle involving the bile ducts. Infection causes 'hepatic coccidiosis', characterized by impaired liver function. Heavy infestations result in jaundice and liver failure
- Newly weaned rabbits are most susceptible to coccidiosis. It is rare in the individual, adult pet
- Sulpha drugs are used to treat coccidiosis in rabbits. The disease is controlled in commercial rabbit colonies and breeding stock by including coccidiostats in the food
- Enterotoxaemia is a cause of diarrhoea and sudden death in rabbits. Clostridial species, notably *C. spiroforme*, are the most usual pathogens
- *Clostridia* spp. can be present in the gut flora of healthy rabbits. Disruption of the normal bacterial population allows clostridia to proliferate
- Stress, antibiotic therapy and dietary change are predisposing factors to enterotoxaemia. Juvenile rabbits are most susceptible
- Glucose is required as a substrate for enterotoxin formation by *Clostridium spiroforme*. Juvenile rabbits absorb carbohydrates less efficiently than adults. High carbohydrate diets are believed to be a predisposing cause of enterotoxaemia in growing rabbits in commercial colonies
- Adult rabbits digest and absorb starch efficiently from the small intestine and high carbohydrate diets do not appear to predispose enterotoxaemia in adults
- The prognosis for rabbits with enterotoxaemia is poor
- *Escherichia coli* can cause diarrhoea. Pathogenicity is affected by the strain of *E. coli* and predisposing factors. Suckling rabbits are most susceptible
- Other infectious causes of enteritis in rabbits include Tyzzer's disease (caused by *Clostridium piliformis*), salmonella and viral infections such as rotavirus
- Poisoning can be manifested by digestive disease. Heavy metal poisons such as lead or poisonous plants can be ingested by rabbits, especially house rabbits.

difficult and expensive to investigate and treat. Prompt, detailed *post-mortem* examinations and laboratory investigations are required. The causes are often multifactorial and home visits to examine the stock and assess the husbandry may be needed. Successful treatment of individual rabbits with enteric conditions is difficult and usually expensive. Intensive therapy, including intravenous fluids, hospitalization and nursing, is required despite the breeder's expectation that some 'wonder drug' will provide an instant cure. Therefore compromises have to be made and general principles applied to prevent further losses. *Post-mortem* examination is extremely valuable and *all* dead rabbits should be examined, not just one or two, as soon after death as possible. Microscopic examination of impression smears, gut contents and faeces can be a cheap way of obtaining information. A provisional diagnosis of mucoid enteropathy, coccidiosis or enterotoxaemia can be made from *post-mortem* examination, although concurrent infections can be present. Histology or specialized laboratory techniques are required to confirm the diagnosis or detect viral infections.

In general, it is often easier to prevent further losses than it is to treat existing outbreaks. It may be advisable for breeders to take a break in their breeding programme and reduce stocking density so they have no young susceptible rabbits on the premises for a few weeks. A break gives the opportunity to clean and disinfect the premises thoroughly, and reduce the number of pathogens in the environment. Simply washing cages and hutches thoroughly in hot water and detergent to remove organic debris is beneficial and can be followed by the use of a disinfectant that kills viruses and bacteria. Povidone-iodine compounds such as Tamodine (Vetark) or non-irritant Virkon can be used. Coccidial oocysts are particularly resistant to disinfection but are susceptible to desiccation. The use of a blowtorch to flame hutches is a simple method of killing oocysts or a 10% solution of ammonia is effective (Pakes and Gerrity, 1994). Ammonia is unpleasant and potentially hazardous to handle. Soil may need to be removed and replaced in outdoor enclosures. The introduction of a feed containing a coccidiostat can be required in the long term.

References

Bentley, P.J. (1998). *Comparative Vertebrate Endocrinology*, 3rd edn. Cambridge University Press.

Behara, N., Silveira, M., Man, W. *et al.* (1980). Catecholamines and experimental stress ulcer: morphological and biochemical changes in the gastric mucosa (Abstract). *Br J Surg.*, **67**, 624–628.

Bergdall, V., Dysko, R.C. (1994). Metabolic, traumatic, mycotic and miscellaneous diseases. In *The Biology of the Laboratory Rabbit*, 2nd edn. (P.J. Manning, D.H. Ringler, C.E. Newcomer, eds). pp 336–355. Academic Press.

Besch-Williford, C. (1997). Tyzzers disease in rabbits. In *Rabbit Medicine and Procedures for Practitioners, Program and Abstracts*. House Rabbit Society Veterinary Conference, USA.

Blood, D.C., Studdert, V.P. (1999). *Saunders Comprehensive Veterinary Dictionary*, 2nd edn. W.B. Saunders.

Boucher S., Nouvelle L. (1997). Mucoid enteropathy syndrome (English Translation. Article in French) *L'Eleveur de Lapins*, No 67.

Breitweiser, B. (1997). Mucoid enteropathy in rabbits. *Proc N Am Vet Conf.*, **11**, 782–783.

Bryden, A.S., Thouless, M.E., Flewett, T.H. (1976). Rotavirus and rabbits. *Vet Rec.*, **99**, 323.

Buckwell, A.C. (1987). Gut stasis in rabbits. *Vet Rec.*, **120**, 143.

Carabaõ, R., Fraga, M.J., Santoma, G., de Blas, J. (1988). Effect of diet on composition of cecal contents and on excretion and composition of soft and hard feces of rabbits. *J Anim Sci.*, **66**, 901–910.

Carabaõ, R., Piquer, J. (1998). The digestive system of the rabbit. In *The Nutrition of the Rabbit* (C. de Blas, J. Wiseman, eds). pp 1–16. CABI Publishing.

Carman, R.J. (1993). Antibiotic associated diarrhea of rabbits. *J Small Exotic Anim Med.*, **2**, 69–71.

Carman, R.J. (1994). Clostridial enteropathies of rabbits. *J Small Exotic Anim Med.*, **2**, 179–181.

Carman, R.J., Evans, R.H. (1984). Experimental and spontaneous clostridial enteropathies of laboratory and free living lagomorphs. *Lab Anim Sci.*, **34**, 443–450.

Charney, A.N., Arnold, M., Johnstone, N. (1983). Acute respiratory alkalosis and acidosis and rabbit intestinal ion transport in vivo (Abstract). *Am J Physiol.*, **244**, G145–150.

Cheeke, P.R. (1987). *Rabbit Feeding and Nutrition*. Academic Press.

Cheeke, P.R., Grobner, M.A., Patton, N.M. (1986). Fiber digestion and utilisation in rabbits. *J Appl Rabbit Res.*, **9**, 25–27.

Chiou, P.W., Yu, B., Lin, C. (1998). The effect of different fibre components on growth rate, nutrient digestibility, rate of digesta passage and hindgut fermentation in domestic rabbits. *Lab Anim.*, **32**, 276–283.

De Blas, E., Gidenne, T. (1998). Digestion of starch and sugars. In *The Nutrition of the Rabbit* (C. de Blas, J. Wiseman, eds). pp 17–38. CABI Publishing.

Deeb, B.J., DiGiacomo, R.F., Evermann, J.F., Thouless, M.E. (1993). Prevalence of coronavirus antibodies in rabbits. *Lab Anim Sci.*, **43**, 431–433.

Delong, D., Manning, P.J. (1994). Bacterial diseases. In *The Biology of the Laboratory Rabbit*, 2nd edn. (P.J. Manning, D.H. Ringler, C.E. Newcomer, eds). pp 131–170. Academic Press.

DiGiacomo, R.F., Mare, J. (1994). Viral diseases. In *The Biology of the Laboratory Rabbit*, 2nd edn. (P.J. Manning, D.H. Ringler, C.E. Newcomer, eds). pp 171–197. Academic Press.

Ellis, T.M., Gregory, A.R., Logue, G.D. (1991). Evaluation of a toxoid for protection of rabbits against enterotoxaemia experimentally induced by trypsin-activated supernatant of Clostridium spririforme (Abstract). *Vet Microbiol.*, **28**, 93–102.

Fekete, S. (1989). Recent findings and future perspectives of digestive physiology in rabbits: a review. *Acta Vet Hung.*, **37**, 265–279.

Fekete, S., Bokori, J. (1986). The effect of trichobezoars on the digestive coefficients and fattening indices of rabbits. *J Appl Rabbit Res.*, **9**, 54–55.

Fioramonti, J., Ruckesbuch, Y. (1976). Caecal motility in the rabbit. III Duality of faecal excretion (English Abstract, article in French). *Ann Rech Vet.*, **7**, 281–295.

Fioramonti, J., Sorraing, J.M., Licois, D., Bueno, L. (1981). Intestinal motor and transit disturbances associated with experimental coccidiosis (*Eimeria magna*) in the rabbit. *Ann Rech Vét.*, **12**, 413–420.

Fraga, M.J., Perez de Ayala, P., Carabaõ, R., de Blas, J.C. (1991). Effect of type of fiber on the rate of passage and on the contribution of soft feces to nutrient intake of finishing rabbits (Abstract). *J Anim Sci.*, **69**, 1566–1574.

Garcia, J., de Blas, J.C., Carabaõ, R., Garcia, P. (1995). Effect of type of lucerne hay on caecal fermentation and nitrogen contribution through caecotrophy in rabbits (Abstract). *Reprod Nutr Dev.*, **35**, 267–275.

Gillett, N.A., Brooks, D.L., Tillman, P.C. (1983). Medical and surgical management of gastric obstruction from a hairball in the rabbit. *J Am Vet Med Assoc.*, **183**, 1176–1178.

Griffiths, I.R., Whitwell, K.E. (1993). Leporine dysautonomia: further evidence that hares suffer from grass sickness. *Vet Rec.*, **132**, 376–377.

Harcourt-Brown, F.M., Friggens, M.T. (1999). Intestinal obstruction in rabbits by locust bean seeds. *Vet Rec.*, **145**, 203.

Harkness, J.E., Wagner, J.E. (1995). *The Biology and Medicine of Rabbits and Rodents*, 4th edn. Williams and Wilkins.

Harkness, J.E. (1997). Gastroenteric conditions in rabbits. In *Proceedings of the House Rabbit Society Veterinary Conference*. pp 19–25.

Hinton, M. (1980). Gastric ulceration in the rabbit. *J Comp Pathol.*, **90**, 475–481.

Hinton, M.H., Gibbs, C. (1982). Radiological examination of the rabbit. II The abdomen. *J Small Anim Pract.*, **23**, 687–696.

Hotchkiss, C.E., Merritt, A.M. (1996a). Mucus secretagogue activity in cecal contents of rabbits with mucoid enteropathy. *Lab Anim Sci.*, **46**, 179–186.

Hotchkiss, C.E., Merritt, A.M. (1996b). Evaluation of cecal ligation as a model of mucoid enteropathy in specific pathogen-free rabbits (Abstract). *Lab Anim Sci.*, **46**, 174–178.

Jackson, G. (1991). Intestinal stasis and rupture in rabbits. *Vet Rec.*, **129**, 287–289.

Jean-Blain, C., Durix, A. (1985). Effects of dietary lipid level on ketonaemia and other plasma parameters related to glucose and fatty acid metabolism in the rabbit during fasting. *Reprod Nutr Develop.*, **25**, 345–354.

Jécsai, J., Teleki, M., Juhász, B. (1985). Effect of caecotrophy on protein and amino acid metabolism of Angora rabbits. *Acta Vet Hung.*, **33**, 51–57.

Jilge, B. (1980). The response of the caecotrophy rhythm of the rabbit to single light signals. *Lab Anim.*, **14**, 3–5.

Joyner, L.P., Catchpole, J., Berret, S. (1983). Eimeria steidae in rabbits: the demonstration of different responses to chemotherapy (Abstract). *Res Vet Sci.*, **34**, 64–67.

Knudtzon, J. (1988). Plasma levels of glucagon, insulin, glucose and free fatty acids in rabbits during laboratory handling procedures. *Z Versuchstierk*, **26**, 123–133.

Lafontan, M., Agid, R. (1979). An extra-adrenal action of adrenocorticotrophin: physiological induction of lipolysis by secretion of adrenocorticotrophin in obese rabbits (Abstract). *J Endocrin.*, **81**, 281–290.

Lafontan, M. (1981). Alpha-adrenergic responses in rabbit white fat cells: the influence of obesity and food restriction (Abstract). *J Lipid Res.*, **22**, 1084–1093.

Lang, J. (1981). The nutrition of the commercial rabbit. Part 1. Physiology, digestibility and nutrient requirements. *Nutr Abstracts Rev-Series B*, **51**, 197–217.

Leary, S.L., Manning, P.J., Anderson, L.C. (1984). Experimental and naturally occurring foreign bodies in laboratory rabbits. *Lab Anim Sci.*, **34**, 58–61.

Lelkes, L., Chang, C.L. (1987). Microbial dysbiosis in rabbit mucoid enteropathy. *Lab Anim Sci.*, **36**, 757–764.

Licois, D., Mongin, P. (1980). An hypothesis of the pathogenesis of diarrhoea in the rabbit based on intestinal contents (Article in French, English Abstract). *Reprod Nutr Dev.*, **20**, 1209–1216.

Licois, D., Coudert, P., Mongin, P. (1978). Changes in hydromineral metabolism in diarrhoeic rabbits 2. Study of the modifications of electrolyte metabolism. *Ann Rech Vet.*, **9**, 453–464.

Licois, D., Guillot, J.F., Mouline, C., Reynaud, A. (1992). Susceptibility of the rabbit to an enteropathogenic strain of Escherichia coli 0103; effect of animals age (Abstract). *Ann Rech Vet.*, **23**, 225–232.

Lofqvist, J. Nilsson, E. (1981). Influence of acid-base changes on carbechol and potassium induced contractions of taenia coli of the rabbit (Abstract). *Acta Physiol Scand.*, **111**, 59–68.

Madry, K., Lut, W., Lepert, R. *et al.* (1976). Lipid composition of plasma obtained from various parts of the vascular system of the rabbit. *Acta Physiol Pol.*, **27**, 485–492.

Marty, J., Vernay, M. (1984). Absorption and metabolism of the volatile fatty acids in the hind-gut of the rabbit (Abstract). *Br J Nutr.*, **51**, 265–277.

McLaughlin, R.M., Fish, R.E. (1994). Clinical biochemistry and haematology. In *The Biology of the Laboratory Rabbit*, 2nd edn. (P.J. Manning, D.H. Ringler, C.E. Newcomer, eds). pp 111–124. Academic Press.

McLeod, C.G., Katz, W. (1986). Opportunist bacteria isolated from the caecum of rabbits with mucoid enteritis. *Br Vet J.*, **142**, 177–187.

Milne, E. (1997). Grass sickness: an update. *In Practice*, **19**, 128–133.

Ojerio, A.D., Ladiges, W.C. (1981). Diagnostic exercise. *Lab Anim Sci.*, **31**, 33–34.

Okerman, L. (1988). *Diseases of Domestic Rabbits*. Blackwell.

Owen, D.G. (1992). Parasites of laboratory animals. In *Laboratory Animal Handbooks No 12*. Royal Society of Medicine Services Ltd.

Padilha, M.T., Licois, D., Gidenne, T. *et al.* (1995). Relationships between microflora and caecal fermentation in rabbits before and after weaning (Abstract). *Reprod Nutr Dev.*, **35**, 375–386.

Pairet, M., Bouyssou, T., Ruckesbuch, Y. (1986). Colonic formation of soft feces in rabbits: a role for endogenous prostaglandins. (Abstract). *Am J Physiol.*, **250**, G302–G308.

Pakes, S.P., Gerrity, L.W. (1994). Protozoal diseases. In *The Biology of the Laboratory Rabbit*, 2nd edn. (P.J. Manning, D.H. Ringler, C.E. Newcomer, eds). pp 205–224. Academic Press.

Patton, N.M., Holmes, P.R., Cheeke, P.R. (1983). Hairballs and pregnancy toxaemia. *J Appl Rabbit Res.*, **6**, 98–99.

Peeters, J.E., Geeroms, R. (1986). Efficacy of toltrazuril against intestinal and heptic coccidiosis in rabbits (Abstract). *Vet Parasitol.*, **1**, 21–35.

Pere, M.C., Baudelin, A., Briggs, K., Gilbert, M. (1992). Hepatic metabolism during fasting-refeeding transition in conscious pregnant rabbits (Abstract). *Am J Physiol.*, **262**, E899–E905.

Perkins, S.E., Fox, J.G., Taylor, N.S. *et al.* (1995). Detection of clostridium difficile toxins from the small intestine and cecum of rabbits with naturally acquired enterotoxaemia. *Lab Anim Sci.*, **45**, 379–447.

Redfern, J.S., Lin, H.J., McArthur, K.E. *et al.* (1991). Gastric acid and pepsin secretion in conscious rabbits. *Am J Physiol.*, **261**, G295–G304.

Riley, J.H., Cornelius, L.M. (1989). Electrolytes, blood gases, and acid base balance. In *The Clinical Chemistry of Laboratory Animals* (W.F. Loeb, F.W. Quimby, eds). pp 345–407. Pergamon Press.

Sandford, J.C. (1996). *The Domestic Rabbit*, 5th edn. Blackwell Science.

Schmidt, R.E. (1995). Protozoal diseases of rabbits and rodents. *Sem Avian Exotic Pet Med.*, **4**, 126–130.

Straw, T.E. (1988). Bacteria of the rabbit gut and their role in the health of the rabbit. *J Appl Rabbit Res.*, **11**, 142–146.

Swartout, M.S., Gerken, D.F. (1987). Lead induced toxicosis in two domestic rabbits. *J Am Vet Med Assoc.*, **191**, 717–719.

Talbot, A.C., Ireton, V.J. (1975). Unusual cause of intestinal blockage in the female rabbit. *Vet Rec.*, **96**, 477.

Thouless, M.E., DiGiacomo, R.F., Deeb, B. (1996). The effect of combined rotavirus and *Escherichia coli* infections in rabbits. *Lab Anim Sci.*, **46**, 381–384.

Toofanian, F., Targowski, S. (1983). Experimental production of rabbit mucoid enteritis. *Am J Vet Res.*, **44**, 705–708.

Toofanian, F., Hamar, D.W. (1986). Cecal short-chain fatty acids in experimental rabbit mucoid enteropathy (Abstract). *Am J Vet Res.*, **47**, 2423–2425.

Van der Hage, M.H., Dorrestein, G.M. (1996). Caecal impaction in the rabbit: relationships with dysautonomia. *Proc 6th World Rabbit Congr.*, **3**, 77–80.

Verde, M.T., Piquer, J.G. (1986). Effect of stress on the cortisone and ascorbic acid content of the blood plasma of rabbits. *J Appl Rabbit Res.*, **9**, 181–182.

Vernay, M. (1987). Origin and utilisation of volatile fatty acids and lactate in the rabbit: influence of the faecal excretion pattern. *Br J Nutr.*, **57**, 371–381.

Whitwell, K.E. (1991). Do hares suffer from grass sickness? *Vet Rec.* **128**, 395–396.

Whitwell, K., Needham, J. (1996). Mucoid enteropathy in UK rabbits: dysautonomia confirmed. *Vet Rec.*, **139**, 323–324.

11

Ophthalmic diseases

11.1 Ocular anatomy and physiology

Rabbits have large, prominent eyes that are positioned on the side of the head with a cornea that occupies approximately 25% of the globe. These features give rabbits a visual field of nearly 360°. However, despite their wide vision, accommodation is poor. The lens is large and spherical and the ciliary body poorly developed (Bagley and Lavach, 1995). The retina has a horizontal area of high photoreceptor density, the visual streak, that allows the rabbit to concentrate on all points of the horizon at one time, enabling it to be aware of a predator coming from any direction (Williams, 1999). Rods are the predominant photoreceptor cells and rabbits have good nocturnal vision (Bagley and Lavach, 1995).

Rabbits are born with their eyelids closed. Separation of the eyelids occurs at about 10 days of age. The upper eyelid is shorter, thicker, and more mobile than the lower lid. Both eyelids consist of four main layers: skin, muscle, fibrous tissue and conjunctiva. The layer of fibrous tissue in the eyelids provides firmness and shape. The eyelids contain a row of 40–50 meibomian glands, which are modified sebaceous glands, arranged parallel to one another. They contain a fatty secretion derived from the breakdown of epithelial cells that originate from the *stratum germinativum* that lines the meibomian gland (Eglitis, 1964).

Rabbits blink approximately 10–12 times per hour (Peiffer *et al.*, 1994). A third eyelid is present that does not actively nictitate but passively covers the cornea as the globe is retracted. It does not move more than two-thirds of the way across the cornea. Some of the palpebral hairs are larger than others and have a different root structure that contains blood sinuses, which provide an erectile function. These 'sinus hairs' or vibrissae have a rich sensory nerve supply and are tactile.

11.1.1 The glands of the eye

The glands of the eye are illustrated in Figure 11.1. The nomenclature for the glands of the eye in rabbits can be confusing. There are two glands associated with the third eyelid that are often collectively referred to as the Harderian gland. To conform to official veterinary nomenclature, the terms *glandula palpebrae tertiae superficialis* (superficial gland of the third eyelid) and *glandula palpebrae tertiae profunda* (deep gland of the third eyelid) are preferable. The deep gland of the third eyelid has two lobes. The dorsal lobe is white and the larger ventral lobe is pink despite a similar histological appearance (Janssens *et al.*, 1999). The deep gland of the third eyelid can prolapse causing swelling and protrusion of the third eyelid. It is larger in males then in females, especially during the breeding season. Within the orbit, the deep gland of the third eyelid lies adjacent to the globe and follows its contours. It is enclosed in a thin connective tissue capsule and is almost completely surrounded by the venous sinus. A duct from the gland opens on to the internal surface of the third eyelid.

The lacrimal gland is situated in the caudodorsal sector of the orbit. There is also a large accessory lacrimal gland that lies in the lower part of the orbit (Eglitis, 1964). The

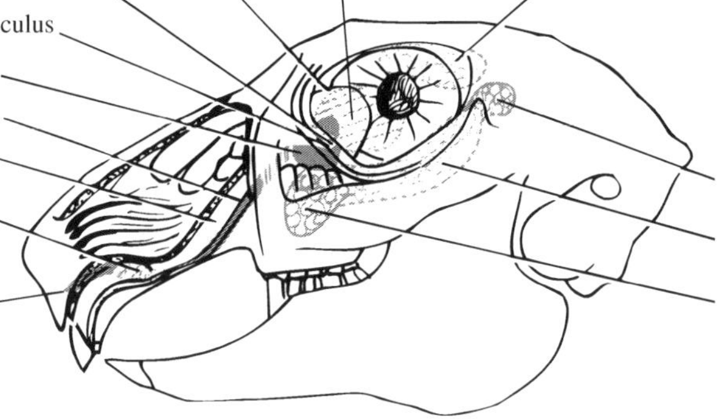

Figure 11.1. Nasolacrimal duct and glands of the eye. The figure shows the course of the nasolacrimal duct and its relationship with surrounding structures and was drawn from dissections using Barone *et al.* (1973), Burling (1991), Eglitis (1964) and Janssens *et al.* (1999) as reference sources. The aperture to the nasolacrimal duct, the *punctum lacrimale,* is situated in the anteromedial aspect of the lower eyelid. The punctum opens into a short (2 mm) canaliculus that opens into a dilation of the duct or lacrimal sac. The nasolacrimal duct leaves the lacrimal sac through a small aperture in the lacrimal bone (the lacrimal foramen, see Figure 11.3) into the maxilla where it is encased in the bony lacrimal canal. At the root of the primary maxillary incisor, the duct makes an abrupt mediodorsal bend and its diameter is reduced from approximately 2 mm to 1 mm. At this point, the duct is compressed between the alveolar bone surrounding the root of the primary maxillary incisor and the nasal cartilage. The duct then courses medially, alongside the incisor tooth root and emerges in the nasal cavity at the ventromedial aspect of the alar fold, a few millimetres inside the mucocutaneous junction.

There are three glands within the orbit: the lacrimal gland, the accessory lacrimal gland and the deep gland of the third eyelid. The lacrimal gland is situated in the caudodorsal sector of the orbit. The large accessory lacrimal gland lies in the lower part of the orbit and has three lobes: the orbital lobe, retro-orbital lobe and infraorbital lobe. The infraorbital lobe rests between the zygomatic bone, the superficial gland of the third eyelid and the globe. It is in close proximity with the alveolar bulla that contains the roots of the maxillary cheek teeth.

The deep gland of the third eyelid has two lobes. The white dorsal lobe and the larger, pink ventral lobe. Within the orbit, the deep gland of the third eyelid lies adjacent to the globe and follows its contours. It is enclosed in a thin connective tissue capsule and is almost completely surrounded by the venous sinus. A duct from the gland opens on to the internal surface of the third eyelid.

accessory lacrimal gland has three lobes: the orbital lobe, retro-orbital lobe and infraorbital lobe (Janssens *et al.*, 1999). The bulging infraorbital lobe rests between the zygomatic bone, the superficial gland of the third eyelid and the globe. This lobe has been confused with the zygomatic salivary gland. It is in close proximity with the alveolar bulla that contains the roots of the maxillary cheek teeth. Elongated roots of these teeth penetrate the infraorbital lobe of the accessory lacrimal gland. The glandular tissue of the lacrimal gland has marked regenerative properties. Thyroxine and testosterone stimulate growth of the lacrimal gland (Eglitis, 1964).

Secretions from the lacrimal glands and glands of the third eyelid moisten, lubricate and flush the surface of the eyeball. In rabbits, the secretion from the lacrimal gland is clear and the secretion from the glands of the third eyelid is milky (Eglitis, 1964). There are numerous goblet cells and intraepithelial cells within the fornix of the eye. The superficial epithelial cells are characterized by large osmiophilic granules (Peiffer *et al.*, 1994). The precorneal tear film is composed of glandular secretions in conjunction with secretions from the meibomian glands and goblet cells. Tears are drained from the conjunctival sac through the nasolacrimal system into the nose.

11.1.2 Nasolacrimal system

The mechanism of tear drainage through the nasolacrimal system has been studied extensively, especially in humans (Habin, 1993). The action of blinking propels tears medially into the lacrimal lake. During blinking, contraction of the orbicularis oris muscle causes occlusion of the *punctum lacrimale* and compression of the lacrimal canaliculus forces tears into the lacrimal sac and nasolacrimal duct. The lacrimal sac dilates during blinking and is compressed during relaxation of the eyelids. A valve mechanism is present within the lacrimal sac that prevents reflux, which aids the propulsion of tears from the eye into the nasolacrimal duct.

In rabbits, the aperture of the nasolacrimal duct, the *punctum lacrimale*, can be seen in the anteromedial aspect of the lower eyelid by gently pulling the lid away from the globe. Unlike the dog and cat, there is no *punctum* in the upper eyelid. The punctum opens into a short (2 mm) canaliculus that opens into a dilation of the duct or lacrimal sac. The nasolacrimal duct leaves the lacrimal sac through a small aperture in the lacrimal bone (the lacrimal foramen) into the maxilla where it is encased in the bony lacrimal canal (see Figure 11.1). This section of the nasolacrimal duct runs rostrally and medially until it reaches the root of the primary maxillary incisor. At this point, the duct makes an abrupt mediodorsal bend and the diameter is reduced from approximately 2 mm to 1 mm (Burling *et al.*, 1991). It is compressed between the alveolar bone surrounding the root of the primary maxillary incisor and the nasal cartilage. Elongation of the root of the incisor can easily occlude the duct at this point. The duct then courses medially, alongside the incisor tooth root and emerges in the nasal cavity at the ventromedial aspect of the alar fold, a few millimetres inside the mucocutaneous junction.

The nasolacrimal duct is lined with stratified or pseudostratified columnar epithelium richly supplied with goblet cells. In some areas, the epithelium is folded (Burling *et al.*, 1991).

11.2 Conjunctival flora

Swabs taken from the conjunctival sac of healthy rabbits can yield a variety of organisms. *Bacillus subtilis* and *Staphylococcus aureus*, *Pseudomonas*, *Neisseria*, *Bordetella*, *Moraxella* and *Pasteurella* spp. are among the organisms that have been isolated from healthy laboratory rabbits (Marini *et al.*, 1996). A survey of the conjunctival flora of healthy pet rabbits showed a predominance of DNase negative *Staphylococcus* spp. followed by *Micrococcus*, *Bacillus*, *Stomatococcus*, *Neisseria*, *Corynebacterium* and *Streptococcus* spp. (Cooper *et al.*, 2001).

11.3 Examination of the eye

Examination of the eyes begins with a comparison of the size and shape to look for evidence of exophthalmus or glaucoma. Fear can cause a bilateral exophthalmus. The eyelids open wide and the globe appears protuberant due to engorgement of the orbital vascular sinus (Eglitis, 1964). The condition is bilaterally symmetrical and no other abnormality is detected. The rabbit appears to be frightened, usually adopting a frozen, crouched stance. The bulging appearance of the eyes wears off after a few minutes. The eyes of entire males can also appear protuberant, especially during the breeding season, due to enlargement of the deep gland of the third eyelid. A unilateral bulging eye indicates the presence of a retrobulbar lesion, such as an abscess or tumour. A *Coenurus serialis* cyst has been reported in the orbit of a pet rabbit exhibiting unilateral exophthalmus (Wills, 2001). Ocular enlargement is due to glaucoma. In most cases, exophthalmus is advanced by the time the rabbit is presented for treatment and it easy to see whether a globe is enlarged or not. Placing a finger over the globe to estimate how hard an enlarged eye feels can be helpful but is often unreliable. Tonometry can be used. The normal intraocular pressure of rabbits is 15–23 mmHg (Williams, 1999).

Next, the eyelids should be examined for abnormalities. Eversion of the upper eyelid reveals the beige coloured rectus dorsalis muscle attached to the sclera. The normal position and structure of the eyelids can be altered by entropion, ectropion or acquired deformities. Progressive hyperaemia, oedema and thickening of the eyelids are caused by myxomatosis. Severe swelling of the eyelids prevents the eye opening and secondary bacterial infections and purulent discharges develop in the later stages.

The skin surrounding the eyes should be examined for evidence of ocular discharge or epiphora. Chronic epiphora results in matted, damp fur on the skin of the nose beneath the medial canthus of the eye. Secondary bacterial infection can cause inflammation and alopecia. Lack of grooming around the eye is often the result of underlying dental disease. Sharp spurs on the maxillary cheek teeth grow into the soft tissue of the cheek and cause pain if pressure is applied to the overlying skin. Epiphora is either due to excessive tear production or impaired tear drainage through the nasolacrimal system. Excessive tear production or blepharitis can be due to conjunctivitis, keratitis, corneal ulceration or ocular foreign bodies. Impaired tear drainage is often due to elongation of the root of the upper primary incisor.

The Schirmer tear test has been evaluated in rabbits and theoretically might be of value in the investigation of epiphora. The test paper is inserted into the lower conjunctival fold in the lateral third of the eyelid and is held in place for 1 minute. The amount of wetness is measured in millimetres. Topical anaesthesia is not used. Normal values for rabbits range from 0 to 11.22 mm/min with a mean of 5.30 + 2.96. High values indicate excessive tear production or impaired drainage but low values are of doubtful significance (Abrams *et al.*, 1990). Keratoconjunctivitis sicca has not been recognized in rabbits.

Good illumination is required for examination of external structures of the globe and the uveal tract. Instillation of local anaesthetic drops and fluorescein facilitates examination of the cornea and conjunctival sac for foreign bodies and areas of inflammation or ulceration. Fluorescein can be seen at the nostrils of rabbits that have patent nasolacrimal ducts. A prominent third eyelid may signify retrobulbar disease and exophthalmus. Samples for cytological or bacteriological examination can be taken from the fornix using a swab moistened with a few drops of sterile saline.

Mydriasis may be required for ophthalmoscopic examination of the fundus. Approximately 40% of rabbits produce atropinesterases that inactivate atropine. Tropicamide (0.5% or 1%) should be used as an alternative. The optic nerve is situated above the horizontal midline. It is necessary to look upward into the eye with an ophthalmoscope to view the optic disc, which has a deep natural depression or cup that can be mistaken for a coloboma. Two broad white bands of myelinated nerve fibres, the medullary rays, extend horizontally from the optic disc (Peiffer *et al.*, 1994). The retina is merangiotic or partially vascularized. There is an area of high photoreceptor density, the visual streak, which is inferior and parallel to the medullary rays. In non-pigmented rabbits, the choroidal vessels are easily seen.

11.4 Relationship between dental disease and ophthalmic conditions of pet rabbits

Dental examination of the teeth is a vital part of the investigation of ophthalmic disease in pet rabbits. There is a close anatomical relationship between the roots of the maxillary teeth and the structures of the eye and nasolacrimal duct (see Figure 11.1). Root elongation and periapical infections are part of the syndrome of acquired dental disease that is so common in pet rabbits (see Box 7.1) and dental disease is often manifested by ocular symptoms. Radiology is nearly always indicated to assess the position, shape and structure of the tooth roots and their association with the structures of the eye and nasolacrimal duct.

Elongated tooth roots, especially of the upper primary incisors, can block the nasolacrimal duct and interfere with drainage of tears from the conjunctival sac. Epiphora is often the first indication of acquired dental disease (see Section 7.6.5). Examination of the teeth and surrounding structures may reveal other signs of dental disease, such as horizontal ribbing of the enamel on the incisors, or palpable swellings along the ventral border of the mandible. Blockage of the nasolacrimal duct and impaired drainage of tears from the conjunctival sac allows bacteria and debris to accumulate. Secondary bacterial infection can ensue, causing conjunctivitis and/or infection and inflammation of the lacrimal sac (dacryocystitis). Dacryocystitis is characterized by a profuse mucopurulent ocular discharge that is most marked at the medial canthus. Digital pressure on the skin just below the medial canthus expresses purulent material from the lacrimal sac through the *punctum lacrimale* into the conjunctival sac.

Root elongation and periapical infections of the upper cheek teeth are sometimes manifested by epiphora, conjunctivitis, dacryocystitis or exophthalmos. Elongated, distorted premolar roots penetrate the maxilla and/or the lacrimal bone and can obstruct the nasolacrimal duct. They can also grow into the orbit causing ocular pain or infection of the periorbital structures. Retrobulbar abscesses or osteomyelitis are usually the result of periapical infection.

11.5 Congenital ocular conditions

11.5.1 Buphthalmia

Buphthalmia is an autosomal recessive trait in rabbits that causes unilateral or bilateral enlargement of the eyeball with secondary changes in the cornea. It can occur in rabbits of any breed. The age of onset is variable. Changes have been observed in baby rabbits as early as 2–3 weeks of age (Lindsey and Fox, 1994). The disease is due to a decrease in drainage of aqueous humour from the anterior chamber and a rise in intraocular pressure. Corneal oedema, conjunctivitis and increased prominence of the eyeball occur and, in severe cases, corneal ulceration can result in rupture and collapse of the eye with subsequent scarring and healing. The condition can be unilateral or bilateral. Protrusion of the anterior chamber gives rise to the term 'moon eye' that is sometimes used by breeders to describe the condition (Bauck, 1989). At one time, it was hypothesized that vitamin A deficiency was involved in hereditary buphthalmos. The theory was tested on rabbits of the hereditary buphthalmic strain with various levels of vitamin A. However, no correlation between intraocular pressure and serum vitamin A levels could be found (Fox *et al.*, 1982).

11.5.2 Congenital eyelid disorders

Entropion and ectropion occur in rabbits, especially in loose-skinned breeds such as the French lop. Short nosed breeds, such as the Netherland Dwarf, are prone to inadequate tear drainage and epiphora due to the conformation of the lower eyelid. Taut eyelids, a shallow medial canthal lake or mild medial lower lid entropion compromise drainage of tears through the *punctum lacrimale*. The natural bend in the nasolacrimal duct at the lacrimal foramen and at the base of the upper incisor can be enhanced in flat-faced individuals with a short, distorted nasolacrimal duct.

11.5.3 Conjunctival hyperplasia

Hyperplasia of the bulbar conjunctiva results in a circular flap of tissue that grows over the cornea. The condition can be unilateral or bilateral and the term 'precorneal membranous occlusion' has been used to describe it. The aetiology is unknown (Wagner *et al.*, 1998).

The flap is not adherent to the cornea and often does not affect vision. Treatment is not always necessary. Surgical excision is straightforward but the membrane tends to grow back within weeks. Extending the excision to a few millimetres posterior to the limbus was successful in a case described by Dupont *et al.* (1995). Alternatively, postoperative topical cyclosporin therapy can be used in an attempt to prevent regrowth.

11.6 Diseases of the eyelids and conjunctiva

11.6.1 Prolapse of the deep gland of the third eyelid

Occasionally, rabbits are presented with a mass protruding from under the third eyelid

Key points 11.1

- Although rabbits have a wide visual field, their accommodation is poor. The retina has an area of high photoreceptor density that allows the rabbit to concentrate on all parts of the horizon at one time. Nocturnal vision is good
- Tears are produced by the lacrimal glands and the glands of the third eyelid which have small ducts that open on to the inner surfaces of the eyelids
- The deep gland of the third eyelid is attached to the base of the nictitating membrane. This gland is influenced by testosterone and is larger in entire males
- Rabbits do not have an opening into the nasolacrimal duct on the upper eyelid
- A single *punctum lacrimale* is found on the lower eyelid near the fornix at the medial canthus. It opens into a short canaliculus that, in turn, opens into a relatively large lacrimal sac
- The lacrimal sac opens into the nasolacrimal duct that passes through a small foramen in the lacrimal bone before running though the bony nasolacrimal canal into the maxilla
- There is a close anatomical relationship between the maxillary teeth and the structures of the orbit and nasolacrimal system
- There is a natural bend in the nasolacrimal duct at the apex of the primary maxillary incisor. Blockage of the duct often occurs at this point, especially if the tooth root is elongated
- There are several congenital ocular disorders that are well documented in laboratory rabbits and are occasionally encountered in pets
- Buphthalmia is a congenital disorder caused by impaired drainage from the anterior chamber. The anterior chamber protrudes from the globe. Secondary corneal oedema and ulceration can occur. The term 'moon eye' is used by breeders to describe the condition
- Entropion and ectropion are seen in rabbits
- In some rabbits, hyperplasia of the conjunctiva results in a circular flap of tissue that grows across the cornea. The flap often regrows after surgical removal. Postoperative topical cyclosporin can prevent regrowth.

in the medial aspect of the eye. Sometimes the term 'cherry eye' is used to describe the condition. The protuberant tissue is composed of the deep gland of the third eyelid. Although the prolapsed glandular tissue can be removed, replacing it is preferable, as it will preserve its secretory function. A similar technique for replacing the gland of the third eyelid in dogs can be used.

11.6.2 Conjunctivitis

Inflammation of the conjunctiva is characterized by hyperaemia and oedema, lacrimation and/or an ocular discharge. There are some pathogens that cause primary conjunctivitis in rabbits, notably myxomatosis or, rarely, *Treponema cuniculi*, but these are uncommon in pets. Conjunctivitis may be seen in association with *Pasteurella multocida*, which can be a primary or secondary pathogen. However, most cases of conjunctivitis in pet rabbits are secondary to some other inciting cause. There is a wide range of bacteria present in the conjunctival sac, many of which can become opportunist pathogens. *Staphylococcus aureus* is frequently isolated from clinical cases of conjunctivitis (Hinton, 1977; Millichamp and Collins, 1986; Cobb *et al.*, 1999). *Chlamydia* has been found in conjunctival smears from laboratory rabbits (Krishna and Kulshrestha, 1985; Marini *et al.*, 1996).

Predisposing factors to conjunctivitis include mechanical irritation, eyelid abnormalities and, most importantly, dental disease. Poor ventilation and urine soaked bedding leads to high environmental ammonia levels that irritate the conjunctiva and predispose to secondary bacterial conjunctivitis. In intensive conditions, high protein diets increase nitrogen excretion and elevate ammonia levels. Hay dust irritates the eyes. Seeds or small pieces of hay can become lodged in the conjunctival sac, usually beneath the third eyelid. Using good quality dust-free hay and placing it on the floor or in hoppers rather than in overhead hayracks reduces the risk of mechanical irritation (Buckley and Lowman, 1979). Congenital or acquired entropion results in eyelashes irritating and inflaming the conjunctiva. Fight wounds, predator attacks and other types of trauma can cause bruising or lacerations of the conjunctiva and/or eyelids which can scar and distort as they heal. The large ears of some lop eared breeds hang over the eyes and mechanically irritate the eyelids.

The precorneal tear film is an important defence against bacterial infection. Inadequate drainage of tears from the conjunctiva compromises the function of the precorneal tear film and predisposes to conjunctivitis. Elongated tooth roots blocking the nasolacrimal duct is the most common cause of inadequate drainage of tears, although other conditions such as ectropion or conformational abnormalities can occlude the *punctum lacrimale*.

11.6.2.1 Treatment of conjunctivitis

Topical antibiotic eye ointments are indicated for the treatment of conjunctivitis. Bacterial culture may be required to identify pathogenic bacteria and as a basis for antibiotic selection. In the UK, there are two preparations licensed for use in rabbits at the present time (February, 2001). One contains fusidic acid (Fucithalmic Vet, Leo Laboratories Ltd.) and the other contains gentamicin (Tiacil, Virbac). The underlying reason for conjunctivitis should be identified and, if possible, treated. For example, eyelid abnormalities, such as entropion, require surgical correction. Conjunctival foreign bodies need to be removed. Improving the husbandry by providing ventilation and improving air quality, in addition to providing clean dry bedding and dust-free hay is an important part of the treatment of conjunctivitis. The treatment of conjunctivitis and epiphora have much in common (see Section 11.6.3).

11.6.3 Epiphora

Epiphora is defined as 'an abnormal flow of tears down the face' (Blood and Studdert, 1999). The lacrimal glands are innervated by the facial and trigeminal nerves and sympathetic fibres from the superior cervical ganglion. Stimulation of these nerves increases secretion of tears. Epiphora can be the result of excessive tear production or impairment of tear flow through the nasolacrimal apparatus. In pet rabbits, most cases of epiphora are caused by inadequate tear drainage due to dental disease. Increased tear production can be the result of irritating or painful ocular conditions such as conjunctivitis, keratitis, keratoconjunctivitis, uveitis, or glaucoma. In other species, disease of the paranasal sinuses and mechanical or olfactory

Box 11.1 Treatment of epiphora and dacryocystitis

- Radiography is indicated to confirm or negate the presence of underlying dental disease
- Dacryocystography using an iodinated contrast medium can be used to outline the nasolacrimal duct
- General anaesthesia is required for effective irrigation of the nasolacrimal duct. It is a procedure that can be distressing for the rabbit
- Irrigation of the nasolacrimal duct should be done gently. It is possible to cause soft tissue damage, especially with metal catheters. Rupture of the duct or lacrimal sac can occur if excessive pressure is applied
- It is sometimes necessary to pass a cannula through the lacrimal foramen to flush purulent material from the maxillary section of the nasolacrimal duct. The lacrimal foramen is illustrated in Figure 11.3
- Bacteriological culture of material flushed from the nasolacrimal duct aids antibiotic selection
- After flushing, antibiotic eye drops or ointment can be introduced into the duct through the catheter
- Systemic antibiotics are indicated in severe infections. Parenteral cephalexin is a useful antibiotic for the treatment of dacryocystitis, especially in combination with cefalonium eye ointment
- Long-term topical eye ointment is often indicated
- Manual expression of pus from the lacrimal sac two or three times a day can be helpful. Owners can be shown how to do this
- A bonded rabbit companion can be very effective in keeping the lacrimal sac empty and cleaning fur around the eye. Licking and cleaning the face is a part of normal mutual grooming behaviour
- Underlying dental disease needs to be treated. Diet and husbandry changes are often necessary.

stimulation of the nasal mucosa increase lacrimation (Habin, 1993). In rabbits, facial dermatitis is often seen in conjunction with chronic epiphora. The fur becomes matted and crusts with residues from the tears as they dry out and allows secondary bacterial infection of the underlying skin.

Treatment of epiphora depends on the underlying cause (see Box 11.1). Epiphora in association with root elongation of the maxillary incisors is difficult to cure. A clean, dry, ammonia-free, well-ventilated environment will reduce tear production and topical eye ointments can be used to control secondary infection. The eye ointment, or alternatively an antiseptic cream, can also be applied to the skin beneath the eye if it becomes infected. Soiled, matted fur requires regular clipping and cleansing to remove the crusty deposits that result from tear overflow. The most effective method of cleansing the skin in this area is a bonded companion who will spend time diligently licking and grooming the face of its mate.

Removal of the incisors has been advocated as a cure for epiphora and can be considered. However, surgical removal of the incisors is not without risk. Preoperative radiography is essential to show any abnormalities of the incisor roots that will make extraction difficult. If incisor malocclusion has occurred, then removal is indicated. If the incisors are in occlusion, then it is preferable to leave them alone. Most cases of epiphora cause more concern to the owner than to the rabbit and many cases spontaneously resolve as dental disease progresses and the teeth stop growing. Rupture of the nasolacrimal duct into the nasal passages provides an alternative route for the drainage of tears.

11.6.4 Dacryocystitis

Dacryocystitis is characterized by a mucopurulent discharge, which can be profuse and malodorous and is most marked at the medial canthus of the eye. Pressure on the skin beneath the medial canthus expresses a string of purulent material through the *punctum lacrimale* into the conjunctival sac. In some cases, the lacrimal sac is visually and palpably distended with pus. Secondary conjunctivitis is present and keratitis and corneal oedema may be found in association with the purulent material that is constantly discharging on to the cornea. In severe cases corneal ulceration develops. These cases are presented with blepharospasm, pain on palpation of the area around the medial canthus and a purulent ocular discharge. Sedation or anaesthesia is required for detailed examination.

Although primary bacterial dacryocystitis can occur in rabbits as a manifestation of pasteurellosis (Petersen-Jones and Carrington, 1988), most cases in pet rabbits are secondary to underlying dental disease and blockage of the nasolacrimal system. There are two sections of the nasolacrimal duct where the diameter narrows. The first section is at the start of the duct as it passes through the lacrimal foramen. The second section is at the base of the maxillary incisor where the duct curves round between the tooth root and palatine bone (see Figure 11.1). It is at this point that blockage usually occurs. Inflammation of the duct results in alteration in consistency of the tears, which can become viscid and gritty and can occlude the flexure at the incisor root, especially if the root is elongated (see Figure 11.1). The maxillary section of duct, proximal to the obstruction, becomes dilated and fills with mucopurulent material (see Figure 11.2). Secondary bacterial infection occurs. A range of bacteria can be cultured from affected cases. Focal epithelial erosions and submucosal infiltration of lymphocytes, macrophages and heterophils have been described in the nasolacrimal duct of rabbits affected with dacryocystitis (Marini *et al.*, 1996).

Dacryocystitis can be also be associated with changes in the cheek teeth. In cases of advanced dental disease, elongated roots of the upper premolars can distort and penetrate the maxillary bones, especially on the zygomatic prominence (see Plate 16 and Figure 11.1). In some cases, the bony reaction that occurs around the ectopic roots of these teeth impinges on the nasolacrimal duct as it passes through the nasolacrimal bone. Abscesses can occur around these roots and can block the duct completely. Elongated roots of the maxillary molars often grow through the alveolar bone into the lacrimal gland that is situated in the base of the orbit. Subsequent alteration in the position of the eye can interfere with drainage of tears through the *punctum lacrimale,* which predisposes to dacryocysti-

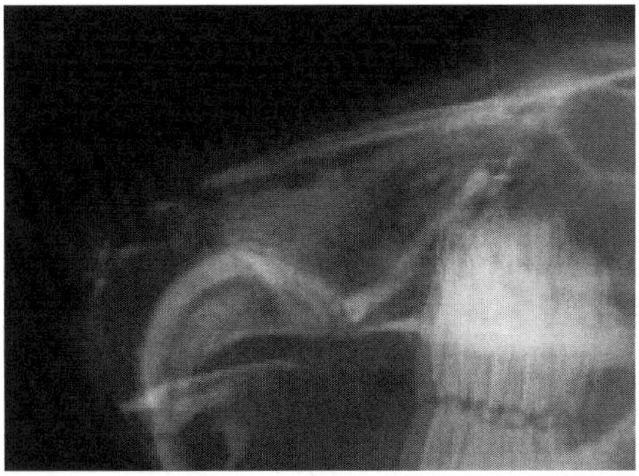

(a)

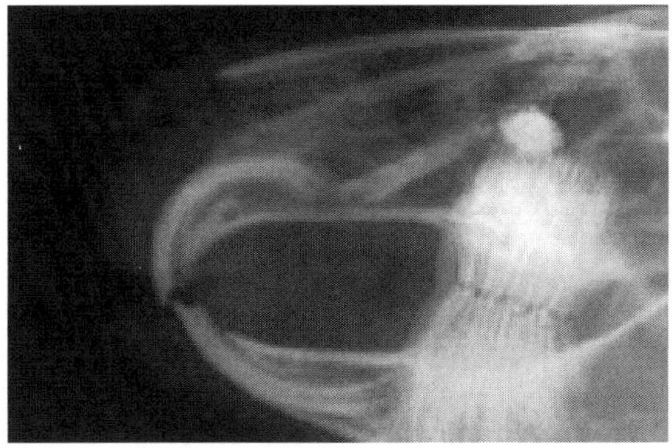

(b)

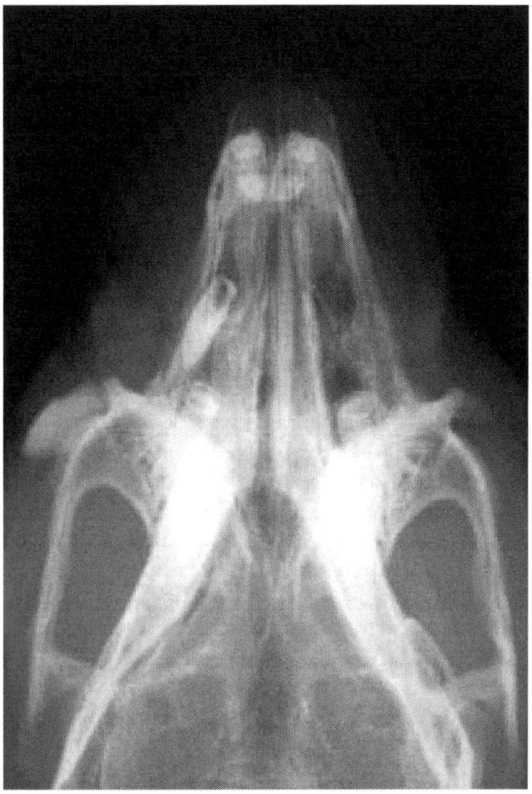

(c)

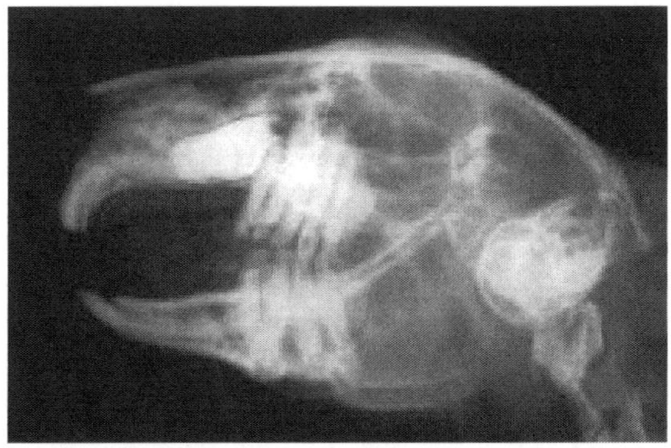

(d)

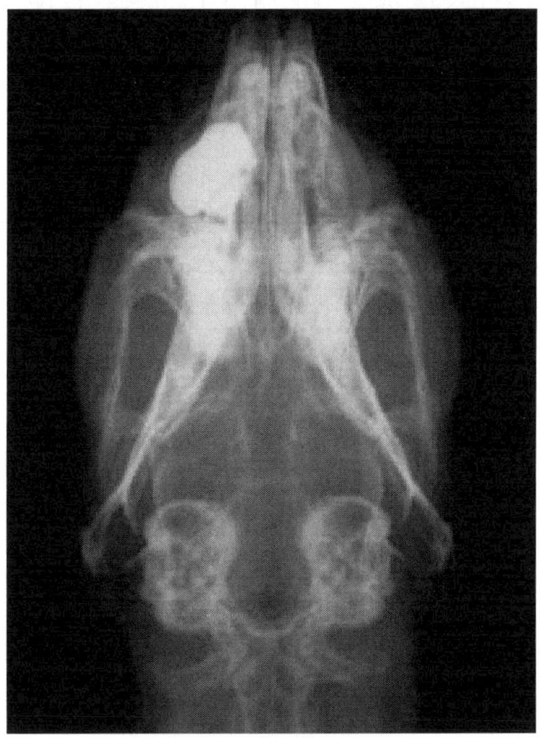

(e)

Figure 11.2.

Figure 11.2. Radiographic progression of dacryocystitis.
(a) Partial occlusion of the nasolacrimal duct by elongated incisor roots. Figure 11.2a is a lateral radiograph of an anaesthetised one-year-old Miniature Lop male rabbit. The rabbit is showing signs of acquired dental disease. There is marked elongation of the roots of the primary maxillary incisors. Contrast medium, sodium/meglumine iothalamate (Conray, 280) has been introduced into the lacrimal sac using a small plastic irrigating cannula. The cannula can be seen passing through the lacrimal foramen. The incisor tooth root is partially obstructing the duct at the mesiodorsal bend. The contrast material has passed through the duct into the nose. Some contrast material has been inhaled and is outlining the ventral nasal concha. There is also leaked contrast medium in the oral cavity.

(b) **Obstruction of the nasolacrimal duct by elongated incisor roots (lateral view).** Figure 11.2b shows a lateral view of the maxilla of a rabbit in the early stages of acquired dental disease. There is elongation of the root of the upper primary incisor that has completely occluded the duct. The rabbit was suffering from unilateral epiphora. Contrast medium, sodium/meglumine iothalamate (Conray, 280) has been introduced into the lacrimal sac using a small plastic irrigating cannula. The lacrimal sac can be seen filled with contrast medium. The blocked duct has become dilated. No contrast medium is passing through into the nasal cavity.

(c) **Obstruction of the nasolacrimal duct by elongated incisor roots (dorsoventral view).** Figure 11.2c shows a dorsoventral view of the same rabbit as in Figure 11.2c. The left lacrimal sac, filled with contrast medium is outlined. The dilated, contrast-filled, nasolacrimal duct is blocked by the elongated root of the maxillary incisor that is curving medially. The air-filled right maxillary sinus can also be seen.

(d) **Gross dilation of the nasolacrimal duct of a rabbit with advanced dental disease (lateral view).** Figure 11.2d shows a lateral view of the skull of an aged neutered male rabbit with advanced dental disease. Contrast medium, sodium/meglumine iothalamate (Conray, 280) has been introduced into the lacrimal sac using a small plastic irrigating cannula. Copious quantities of pus were flushed out through the *punctum lacrimale* and out through the nostril prior to instillation of the contrast medium. The nasolacrimal duct is grossly distended.

(e) **Gross dilation of the nasolacrimal duct of a rabbit with advanced dental disease (dorsoventral view).** Figure 11.2e shows a dorsoventral view of the same rabbit as shown in (d). The nasolacrimal duct has dilated to form a bony swelling that is bulging from the lateral aspect of the maxilla. The skull from a similar case is shown in Plate 17. The changes are bilateral. Although the rabbit suffered from epiphora in the early stages of dental disease, tears are no longer seen overflowing down his face. Between flare-ups of dacryocystitis the rabbit shows no external evidence of ocular disease. Infection has eroded a passage for the tears to flow into the nasal cavity in the area of the lacrimal foramen.

tis. In cases of advanced dental disease, there may be changes at the roots of all the maxillary teeth and obstruction, distortion and dilation of the nasolacrimal duct can be present at several sites. As the disease progresses, the maxillary section of the nasolacrimal duct can become grossly dilated causing a lateral bulge in the cribriform side of the maxilla. The blocked, dilated duct fills with mucopurulent material and debris (see Figure 11.2) that spills into the lacrimal and conjunctival sacs. Occasionally, the discharge from the *punctum lacrimale* ceases as infection of nasolacrimal duct eventually erodes through the nasolacrimal canal into the nasal cavity. There may also be a concomitant reduction in tear production from the lacrimal gland as it is often penetrated and infected by diseased roots of the maxillary molars.

Although clinical examination and bacteriology are valuable parts of the diagnostic workup of cases of dacryocystitis, radiography and detailed examination of the teeth are also required. General anaesthesia is necessary for irrigation of the nasolacrimal duct and to obtain a diagnostic set of radiographs.

11.6.4.1 Irrigation of the nasolacrimal duct

Treatment of dacryocystitis is summarized in Box 11.1. Cannulation and flushing the nasolacrimal duct with sterile water or saline is often cited as the treatment of dacryocystitis. Many authors suggest performing the procedure repetitively in the conscious animal. However, the nasal mucosa of the rabbit is sensitive and nasolacrimal duct flushing can be intensely stimulating, especially if the duct has ruptured and fluid is forced into the nasal passages. Some rabbits respond by screaming, even under general anaesthesia. General anaesthesia is always indicated for the initial investigation and irrigation of the nasolacrimal duct and is, in general, preferable for subsequent nasolacrimal duct flushing. Radiology prior to irrigation of the nasolacrimal duct is extremely informative and gives an idea of how difficult the procedure will be and whether it is likely to effect a cure. Most rabbits with dacryocystitis have major dental problems (see Box 7.1, Figure 11.2).

Flushing purulent debris through the nasolacrimal duct improves tear drainage and removes infected debris. The procedure is generally successful in curing primary bacterial nasolacrimal duct infections and improves secondary infections caused by underlying dental disease. Infected material that has been flushed from the duct can be collected and cultured for bacteriology and sensitivity. After the procedure, antibiotics can be instilled into the duct nasolacrimal duct through the catheter. A few drops of eye ointment can be expressed into a syringe for instillation through the catheter.

Changes of the nasolacrimal duct can be seen radiographically by instilling 1–2 ml of a contrast medium. Dilute preparations such as sodium/meglumine iothalamate (Conray 280) have the advantage of being cheap and easy to inject in comparison with more concentrated formulations that are more viscous and are more difficult to inject. Concentrated solutions give a clearer image and are retained in the duct for longer. It is more difficult to obtain a clear image of a patent duct than one that is blocked. Contrast material flows through a patent duct to the nose and is easily inhaled into the nasal passages causing superimposition.

Good illumination is required for irrigation of the nasolacrimal duct. The *punctum lacrimale* is identified in the medial canthus by gently everting the lower lid. Forceps can be used to hold the eyelid away from the cornea. A small plastic irrigating cannula is introduced through the *punctum lacrimale* into the canaliculus into the lacrimal sac. There is no punctum on the upper eyelid. In large rabbits, a cat catheter can be used. Metal irrigating cannulae are available and may be used in some cases, especially if the canaliculus is dilated. However, the risk of iatrogenic damage to the lacrimal sac and nasolacrimal duct is greater if metal catheters are used. Trauma can result in the formation of scar tissue and stenosis. Once a cannula has been introduced into the lacrimal sac, sterile water or saline can be used gently to flush out purulent material. In some cases, the pus can be flushed through the duct and out through the nostril. In other cases, although it is relatively simple to insert a cannula and flush material from the lacrimal sac, purulent material is left in the maxillary section of the nasolacrimal duct, especially if it is blocked and dilated. Applying gentle digital pressure to the *punctum lacrimale* during flushing forces fluid down the duct and can unblock it. Alternatively, the maxillary section of duct can be flushed by passing the cannula through the lacrimal foramen (see Figure 11.3). This is not possible in the conscious animal. A plastic, rather than metal, catheter is used and needs to be gently manipulated

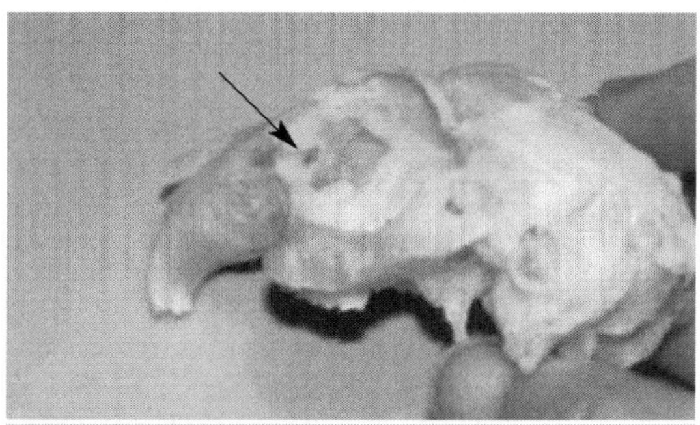

Figure 11.3. Lacrimal foramen. The nasolacrimal duct runs through the lacrimal bone via the lacrimal foramen. The direction of the duct is rostroventral and medial as it runs through the bony canal. In some cases of dacryocystitis, it is important to pass the irrigating cannula through this foramen to flush purulent material out of the nasal section of the nasal lacrimal duct. Flushing the nasolacrimal system can be extremely stimulating to rabbits, even if they are anaesthetized (see Section 11.6.4.1). General anaesthesia is essential.

Key points 11.2

- Although conjunctivitis can be caused by primary infections such as myxomatosis or pasteurellosis, in pet rabbits conjunctivitis is usually secondary to some underlying factor
- Dirty bedding and ammonia build-up in the environment causes conjunctival irritation and secondary bacterial infection
- Dusty hay can irritate the eyes. Stems or seeds can make their way into the conjunctival sac
- Dental disease can impair tear drainage through the nasolacrimal system so bacteria accumulate in the conjunctival sac which subsequently becomes inflamed and infected
- Blockage of the nasolacrimal duct results in epiphora, which is one of the first signs of acquired dental disease
- Epiphora caused by root elongation of the maxillary incisors is difficult to treat successfully. Surgical removal of the incisors can be considered but may not be curative
- Secondary infection of a blocked nasolacrimal duct results in dacryocystitis and accumulation of a purulent exudate in the lacrimal sac
- Pus can be expressed from the *punctum lacrimale* by gentle digital pressure below the medial canthus
- In cases of advanced dental disease, in addition to root elongation of the incisors, lesions at the apex of the premolars can interfere with drainage of tears through the nasolacrimal duct
- Radiography is essential for the assessment of recurrent dacryocystitis. The radiographic changes of underlying dental disease can be shown to owners who can then appreciate the difficulty in treating the condition
- The nasolacrimal duct can be irrigated to flush out purulent exudate. A cannula is introduced through the *punctum lacrimale*
- Flushing fluid through the nasolacrimal duct into the nose can be intensely stimulating and distressing for some rabbits. General anaesthesia is generally indicated
- It is almost impossible to cannulate the nasolacrimal duct from the nasal end
- Repetitively squeezing purulent material out of the lacrimal sac is beneficial in the treatment of chronic dacryocystitis
- Licking and grooming one another's face is part of rabbits' social behaviour. A bonded companion to keep the face and eyes clean is a definite advantage for rabbits suffering from chronic epiphora or dacryocystitis.

and directed through the lacrimal foramen. Only gentle pressure should be applied during irrigation of the nasolacrimal duct. There is a risk of rupturing the lacrimal sac, especially if the duct is blocked. If this happens, irrigation fluid is forced into the periorbital tissue.

It is difficult to cannulate the nasolacrimal duct from the nasal opening. The aperture is narrow and hard to locate.

11.7 Diseases of the globe

11.7.1 Keratitis, keratoconjunctivitis and corneal ulceration

Corneal inflammation in pet rabbits can be caused by infection, trauma, precorneal tear film abnormalities (often due to dental disease) and systemic or nutritional disorders. Vitamin A deficiency has induced keratitis in laboratory rabbits (Phillips and Bohstedt, 1937; Hunt and Harrington, 1974).

In pet rabbits, corneal oedema and/or ulceration are often associated with keratitis. The precorneal tear film plays an important role in protecting the cornea from infection and injury and any condition that affects it can result in keratitis. Inadequate tear drainage in rabbits with dacryocystitis can lead to keratitis, especially in the medial canthus where the cornea is in contact with purulent material from the *punctum lacrimale*. Trauma or scratches on the cornea from other rabbits or pieces of hay can become infected and result in a deep corneal ulceration. Affected rabbits are often presented with a large yellow necrotic ulcer in the centre of an inflamed opaque cornea surrounded with a scarlet inflamed conjunctiva. Pain, blepharospasm and lacrimation can be severe.

There is a temptation to enucleate these eyes as it can difficult to envisage healing but most cases respond well to medical treatment. Systemic cephalexin and topical cephalonium are an effective combination in rabbits. Cephalexin appears promptly in the aqueous humour of the non-inflamed eye of rabbits, in concentrations of 15–20% of serum levels (Gager *et al.*, 1969). Topical application of fusidic acid also penetrates the cornea and aqueous humour of rabbits (see Section 4.2.1.5). Minimum inhibitory concentrations against gram-positive infections persist for up to 24 h in the cornea (Taylor *et al.*, 1987). A topical eye ointment containing fusidic acid (Fucithalmic Vet, Leo Laboratories Limited) holds a product licence for use in rabbits and has sustained-release properties. The carbomer base significantly increases the concentration of fusidic acid in the tear film. Gentamicin is poorly absorbed into the inflamed eye and not at all in the normal eye of rabbits (Behrens-Baumann, 1996). Gentamicin ophthalmic solution (Tiacil, Virbac) is another licensed preparation that is available for rabbits.

11.7.2 Corneal opacities

In rabbits, the list of differential diagnoses for corneal opacities is similar to other species. Scars can result from deep corneal ulceration. Corneal dystrophies have been described in laboratory rabbits. For example, a dietary lipid keratopathy has been associated with high fat diets. Lipid degeneration of subepithelial stroma has been seen as a non-specific change following intraocular surgical procedures (Peiffer *et al.*, 1994).

11.7.3 Uveitis

Uveitis in rabbits is usually ascribed to *Pasteurella multocida* infection caused by haematogenous spread. Large iridal abscesses and panophthalmitis can develop. Uveitis can also be secondary to severe keratitis or caused by trauma or penetrating foreign bodies. Secondary uveitis and bacterial infection also occur in association with *Encephalitozoon cuniculi* infection.

11.7.3.1 *Encephalitozoon cuniculi* uveitis

Encephalitozoon cuniculi is a protozoan parasite that affects rabbits and other animals. Most cases are asymptomatic although neurological symptoms such as torticollis or renal disease can occur (See Sections 12.4, 14.5.1 and 16.4.2). Encephalitozoonosis is also a cause of ocular disease. Lens rupture, uveitis and cataract formation are the clinical signs that are found in young rabbits (Wolfer *et al.*, 1993; Stiles *et al.*, 1997). The anterior lens capsule spontaneously ruptures and causes a zonal granulomatous lens induced uveitis (Pieffer *et al.*, 1994). The condition is usually unilateral. Histologically, inflammation is centred around the break in the lens capsule. Neutrophils are present deep within the lens cortex surrounded by a ring of fibrous tissue containing lymphocytes and plasma cells (Wolfer *et al.*, 1993). *Encephalitozoon cuniculi* organisms may be seen within the liquefied lens cortex. It is believed that vertical transmission results in *E. cuniculi* organisms invading the developing lens of rabbits *in utero* when the lens capsule is very thin or absent (Wolfer *et al.*, 1993). At a later date, the parasite causes the lens to rupture at its thinnest point on the anterior surface, releasing lens material into the anterior chamber and causing phacoclastic uveitis.

Intraorbital changes such as iridal abscesses, hypopyon and acute uveitis are often seen in pet rabbits and it is probable that they are suffering from encephalitozoonosis and that *Pasteurella multocida* is a secondary opportunist infection. Serological testing will confirm or negate exposure to the *E. cuniculi*. Confirmation of the diagnosis can only be made by histological examination of the lens and surrounding structures.

Treatment of uveitis depends on the severity of signs and response to therapy. Most cases of phacoclastic uveitis due to *E. cuniculi* will respond to medical treatment and time. Occasionally, enucleation is necessary. Some cases settle down without any treatment. It is not unusual to find evidence of unilateral cataract and opaque remnants of lens tissue in the anterior chamber during routine clinical examination of pet rabbits. In a German survey, 10 out of 125 seropositive pet rabbits showed evidence of phacoclastic uveitis

(Ewringmann and Göbel, 1999). The authors describe treatment of these animals with systemic dexamethasone and oxytetracycline in conjunction with topical preparations containing the same drugs.

Treatment of encephalitozoonosis with corticosteroids is discussed in Section 16.4.2.5. Other authors have reported poor response to topical therapy and have resorted to enucleation (Wolfer *et al.*, 1993) or phacoemulsification (Stiles *et al.*, 1997). Lens extraction has also been suggested (Peiffer *et al.*, 1994).

Treatment with albendazole or fenbendazole is indicated to kill the parasite but it will not treat the inflammatory response that *E. cuniculi* has evoked.

11.7.4 Cataracts

Congenital cataracts have been described in laboratory rabbits (Peiffer *et al.*, 1994). Cataracts may also be seen in pet rabbits without an obvious cause. Cataracts are not a sign of diabetes mellitus in rabbits.

Rupture of the lens as a result of *E. cuniculi* infection results in cataract formation (see Plate 24). Opaque remnants of lens material may be seen in the anterior chamber. The condition is usually unilateral and asymptomatic. The rabbit does not appear to be visually impaired or in discomfort and there is no evidence of inflammation. Treatment is symptomatic. Serology will confirm exposure to *E. cuniculi* and a precautionary course of albendazole or fenbendazole can be prescribed for both the patient and in contact rabbits.

11.8 Lymphoma

Neoplastic disorders of lymphoid tissue are among the more common tumours that occur in pet rabbits. The condition can be encountered in relatively young animals. Although any organ may be infiltrated by neoplastic tissue, the internal structures of the eye, particularly the choroid, ciliary body, iris and anterior chamber, are one of the more common sites (Weisbroth, 1994). Rabbits are presented with a bilateral uveitis and visible tissue aggregates in the eye (see Plate 25). The spleen, liver and other organs can be affected.

Key points 11.3

- Fight wounds and scratches can damage the cornea and result in ulceration and keratitis or keratoconjunctivitis
- Keratitis or keratoconjunctivitis can also be associated with blockage of the nasolacrimal duct and dacryocystitis. *Pasteurella multocida* can invade as a secondary infection
- Most cases of corneal ulceration, keratitis and keratoconjunctivitis respond to topical and systemic antibiotic therapy. Severe changes can respond well to medical therapy without the need for enucleation
- Uveitis in rabbits can be associated with *Encephalitozoon cuniculi* infection. Infection *in utero* results in the parasite invading the lens. After birth, the lens ruptures releasing lens material into the anterior chamber
- Evidence of lens rupture and cataract formation can be seen in asymptomatic rabbits during routine clinical examination
- Phacoemulsification has been described in rabbits but is not usually required
- Albendazole can be used to kill *E. cuniculi* but does not treat the uveitis. Topical antibiotics and corticosteroids can be used
- Diabetes mellitus is not a cause of cataracts in rabbits
- Lymphoma can be a cause of ocular disease in rabbits.

11.9 Enucleation of the eye of a rabbit

Enucleation is indicated for conditions that cause a blind, painful eye such as intractable glaucoma or endophthalmitis. In rabbits, retrobulbar disease and exophthalmos are the most common indication because enucleation is required to investigate the orbit. Periapical abscessation of the upper cheek teeth causes retrobulbar swelling and protrusion of the globe. Endophthalmitis in rabbits can respond well to medical treatment and enucleation is a last resort. The surgical procedure is similar to other species, except for the presence of a large venous sinus (see Figure 3.7) that is closely associated with the glands of the orbit. Careful dissection, keeping close to the globe minimizes the risk of haemorrhage. If the venous sinus is punctured, haemorrhage can usually be controlled by applying pressure. Rabbit blood clots quickly.

References

Abrams, K.L., Brooks, D.E., Funk, R.S., Theran, P. (1990). Evaluation of the Schirmer tear test in clinically normal rabbits. *Am J Vet Res.*, **51**, 1912–1913.

Bagley, L.H., Lavach, D. (1995). Ophthalmic diseases of rabbits. *Californian Veterinarian*, **49**, 7–9.

Bauck, L. (1989). Ophthalmic conditions in pet rabbits and rodents. *Compendium of Continuing Education*, **11**, 258–266.

Behrens-Baumann, W. (1996). Absorption of topically administered ciprofloxacin, ofloxacin, and gentamicin in the inflamed rabbit eye (Abstract). *Ophthalmologica*, **210**, 119–122.

Blood, D.C., Studdert, V.P. (1999). *Saunders Comprehensive Veterinary Dictionary*, 2nd edn. W.B. Saunders.

Buckley, P., Lowman, M.R. (1979). Chronic non-infective conjunctivitis in rabbits. *Lab Anim.*, **13**, 69–73.

Burling, K., Murphy, C.J., Da Siva Curiel, J., Koblik, P., Bellhorn, R.W. (1991). Anatomy of rabbit nasolacrimal duct and its clinical implications. *Progr Vet Comp Ophthalmol.*, **1**, 33–40.

Cobb, M.A., Payne, B., Allen, W.M., Potts, J.M. (1999) A survey of the conjunctival flora in rabbits with clinical signs of superficial ocular infection. *BSAVA Congress Synopses*.

Cooper, S.C., McLellan, G.J., Ryecroft, A.N. (2001). Conjunctival flora observed in 70 healthy domestic rabbits (*Oryctolagus cuniculus*). *Veterinary Record* **149**, 232–235.

Dupont, C., Carrier, M., Gauvin, J. (1995). Bilateral precorneal membranous occlusion in a dwarf rabbit. *J Small Exotic Anim Med.*, **3**, 41–44.

Eglitis, I. (1964). The glands. In *The Rabbit in Eye Research* (J.H. Prince, ed.) pp 38–56, Charles C. Thomas.

Ewringmann, A., Göbel, T. (1999). Untersuchungen zur Klinik und Therapie der Encephalitozoonose beim Heimtierkaninchen (Article in German, English Abstract). *Kleintierpraxis*, **44**, 357–372.

Fox, R.R., Eaton, H.D., Crary, D.D. (1982). Vitamin A, beta carotene, and hereditary buphthalmus in the rabbit. *J Heredity*, **73**, 370–374.

Gager, W.E., Elsasa, F.J., Smith, J.L. (1969). Ocular penetration of cephalexin in the rabbit. *Br J Ophthalmol.*, **53**, 403–406.

Habin, D. (1993). The nasolacrimal system. In *BSAVA Manual of Small Animal Ophthalmology* (S.M. Petersen-Jones, S.M. Crispin, eds). pp 91–102. British Small Animal Veterinary Association.

Hinton, M. (1977). Treatment of purulent staphylococcal conjunctivitis in rabbits with autogenous vaccine. *Lab Anim.*, **11**, 163–164.

Hunt, C.E., Harrington, D.D. (1974). Nutrition and nutritional diseases of the rabbit. In *The Biology of the Laboratory Rabbit*. (S.H. Weisbroth, R.E. Flatt, A.L. Kraus eds). pp 403–428. Academic Press.

Janssens, G., Simoens, P., Muylle, S., Lauwers, H. (1999). Bilateral prolapse of the deep gland of the third eyelid in a rabbit: diagnosis and treatment. *Lab Anim Sci.*, **49**, 105–109.

Krishna, L, Kulshrestha, S.B. (1985). Spontaneous cases of chlamydial conjunctivitis in rabbits. *J Appl Rabbit Res.*, **8**, 75.

Lindsay, J.R., Fox, R.R. (1994). Inherited diseases and variations. In *The Biology of the Laboratory Rabbit*, 2nd edn. (P.J. Manning, D.H. Ringler, C.E. Newcomer, eds). pp 293–313. Academic Press.

Marini, R.P., Foltz, C.J., Kersten, D. *et al.* (1996). Microbiologic, radiographic and anatomic study of the nasolacrimal duct apparatus in the rabbit (*Oryctolagus cuniculus*). *Lab Anim Sci.*, **46**, 656–662.

Millichamp, N.J., Collins, B.R. (1986). Blepharoconjunctivitis associated with *Staphylococcus aureus* in a rabbit. *J Am Vet Med Assoc.*, **189**, 1153–1154.

Peiffer, R.L., Pohm-Thorsen, L., Corcoran, K. (1994). Models in ophthalmology and vision research. In *The Biology of the Laboratory Rabbit*, 2nd edn. (P.J. Manning, D.H. Ringler, C.E. Newcomer, eds). pp 410–434. Academic Press.

Petersen-Jones, S.M., Carrington, S.D. (1988). Pasteurella dacryocystitis in rabbits. *Vet Rec.*, **122**, 514–515.

Phillips, P.H., Bohstedt, G. (1937). Studies on the effects of a bovine blindness-producing ration upon rabbits. *J Nutr.*, **15**, 309–319.

Stiles, J., Didier E., Ritchie B., Greenacre C., Willis M., Martin C. (1997) Encephalitozoon cuniculi in the lens of a rabbit with phacoclastic uveitis: confirmation and treatment. *Vet Comp Ophthalmol.*, **7**, 233–238.

Taylor, P.B., Burd, E.M., Tabbara, K.F. (1987). Corneal and intraocular penetration of topical and subconjunctival fusidic acid (Abstract). *Br J Ophthalmol.*, **71**, 598–601.

Wagner, F., Brügmann, M., Heider, H.J. *et al.* (1998). Präkorneale membranöse Okklusion bei Zwergkaninchen-ein Fallbericht mit Literaturübersicht (Article in German, English summary) *Der praktische Tierarzt*, **79**, 404–409.

Weisbroth, S.H. (1994). Neoplastic diseases. In *The Biology of the Laboratory Rabbit*, 2nd edn. (P.J. Manning, D.H. Ringler, C.E. Newcomer, eds). pp 259–292. Academic Press.

Williams, D.L. (1999). Laboratory animal ophthalmology. In *Veterinary Ophthalmology*, 3rd edn. (K.N. Gelatt, ed.) pp 1209–1236. Lippincott, Williams and Wilkins.

Wills, J. (2001). Coenurosis in a pet rabbit. *Vet Rec.*, **148**, 188.

Wolfer, J., Grahn, B., Wilcock, B., Percy, D. (1993). Phacoclastic uveitis in the rabbit. *Prog. Vet Comp Ophthalmol.*, **3**, 92–97.

Neurological and locomotor disorders

12

12.1 Investigation of neurological and locomotor disorders

Neurological signs are common in rabbits. They may be caused by primary diseases of the central nervous system such as encephalitozoonosis or they may be secondary to some systemic problem such as ketoacidosis or hypokalaemia. Many diseases cause neurological signs, such as ataxia or seizures, in their terminal stages. Spinal deformities and associated neurological problems are also common in pet rabbits. Diseases of the central nervous system or locomotor system may be manifested by skin disease, digestive disorders or urinary tract problems. Therefore, a detailed clinical history and thorough examination are vital in determining the cause of neurological and locomotor disorders.

12.2 Lameness

Observation of a rabbit's gait can be very informative. Owners are often unaware that their pet has difficulty moving. They may not be familiar with normal rabbit locomotion or may not actually see their rabbit hopping about because it spends most of its life confined to a hutch. The rabbit can be placed on the floor to observe its gait. Obviously, the owner and the vet have to be confident that the rabbit can be caught again if it is allowed to have the freedom of the consulting room. Many rabbits dislike smooth flooring and benefit from a towel placed on the floor for them to hop over. Severe abnormalities of gait may be detected. Inspection and palpation of the limbs may reveal bony enlargements, swollen joints, abscesses or even fractures that have not been detected by the owner. Some causes of lameness in rabbits are listed in Box 12.1. Treatment of abscesses is described in Section 8.3.

Box 12.1 Differential diagnosis of lameness in rabbits

- Fracture
- Dislocation
- Ulcerative pododermatitis
- Spinal disease
- Septic arthritis
- Osteoarthritis
- Abscesses on plantar aspect of feet
- Osteomyelitis or abscesses in the bone
- Neoplasia (primary or metastatic)
- Hypertrophic osteopathy

Ulcerative pododermatitis is a common cause of lameness and interferes with normal stance and gait (see Section 9.10). In advanced cases, the superficial flexor tendon becomes displaced giving a 'dropped hock' appearance that can be mistaken for spinal cord disease (see Plate 9).

A case of hypertrophic osteopathy has been reported in a rabbit (DeSanto, 1997). The rabbit was presented with swollen hind legs that were painful on examination. Radiological examination revealed periosteal proliferation of the distal half of the tibia and tarsometatarsus. The hypertrophic osteopathy was secondary to a thoracic tumour that was a metastasized uterine adenocarcinoma.

12.2.1 Orthopaedic surgery

It is beyond the scope of this book to describe every orthopaedic procedure that may be necessary for pet rabbits. The same basic principles apply to rabbits as to cats. For fractured limbs, the aim of orthopaedic intervention is to restore anatomical alignment and immobilize the fracture site to permit rapid healing. Although splinting the limb may appear to be the simplest option, the shape of rabbits' legs does not lend itself to the easy application of satisfactory splints, slings or bandages so, in many cases, surgery is indicated. Internal fixation usually involves pinning rather than plating due to the small bones and thin cortices. Rabbit bones are brittle and fractures are often complex with multiple fragments. On the positive side, rabbit bone heals quickly. External fixation is often the solution for fracture repair in rabbits. The effects of external fixation on bone have been studied in laboratory rabbits. In an investigation of bone loss due to immobilization with an external fixator, no significant changes in bone strength, stiffness or mineral content were found after 6 weeks but bone strength was reduced by 87% and mineral content by 90% after 12 weeks. These effects were less pronounced using an external fixator rather than using metal plates (Terjesen and Benum, 1983).

12.2.2 Amputation

Amputation of a fractured limb offers an economic solution for a complex fracture and may be the only option for an intractable condition such as septic arthritis or neoplasia. Rabbits tolerate amputation well, especially of a forelimb. The procedure is similar to other species. The bone should be sectioned with a saw, rather than bone cutters, as it is liable to shatter. The main drawback of amputation, especially of a hindlimb, is the effect on the contralateral leg. There is a risk of avascular necrosis of the skin on the plantar aspect of the metatarsus (ulcerative pododermatitis, sore hocks) due to increased pressure (see Section 9.10). The risk can be reduced by preventing obesity, encouraging activity and housing the rabbit on clean, dry, compliant bedding.

Key points 12.1

- Neurological signs are common in pet rabbits. They may be caused by primary diseases of the central nervous system, such as *E. cuniculi*, or secondary to systemic diseases such as viral haemorrhagic disease or hepatic lipidosis
- Observation of the patient's gait is an important part of clinical examination. A towel can be placed on the consulting room floor for the rabbit to hop over. Both the owner and the vet must be confident they can catch the rabbit again
- Ulcerative pododermatitis is a common cause of lameness. Displacement of the superficial flexor tendon in advanced cases can result in a drooped hock that can be mistaken for neurological disease
- External fixation is often the method of choice to repair limb fractures in rabbits. The bones are brittle and liable to shatter
- External splints are difficult to apply and are usually unsatisfactory
- Rabbits manage well without an amputated limb, especially a forelimb. Amputation of a hind limb increases the pressure on the contralateral hock and can result in ulcerative pododermatitis. Amputees must be kept slim, encouraged to exercise and housed on dry, compliant bedding.

12.3 Neurological diseases

A detailed neurological examination is difficult in rabbits but proprioreceptive deficits, paresis or paralysis are easily detectable. The coat and perineum may show evidence of lack of grooming or perineal dermatitis that are indicative of spinal disease or other neurological problems. Cheyletiellosis and matted fur suggest reduced flexibility. There may be pain associated with palpation of the spine or there may be a history of aggression.

Laboratory investigations are helpful. Haematology may show evidence of chronic infection in the form of leucocytosis, neutrophilia or monocytosis, although absence of these changes does not negate the possibility of an abscess or chronic inflammation (see Section 6.2). Biochemical assays, especially serum potassium and glucose are informative. Liver and kidney function tests can show evidence of metabolic causes of neurological symptoms. Cisternal puncture for cerebrospinal fluid collection and myelography is feasible and follows the same principles as for a dog or cat. As in the dog, cisternal puncture is easier than lumbar puncture.

Radiography is essential for cases of paresis or paralysis. Bony abnormalities of the spinal column, such as fractures, subluxations or spondylosis may be seen. There may be evidence of underlying osteopaenia. Incidental findings such as urolithiasis or evidence of gastrointestinal hypomotility are significant. Skull radiography can be used to investigate vestibular disease and the tympanic bullae can clearly be seen on a dorsoventral view (see Figure 13.2).

Box 12.2 Clinical manifestations of *Encephalitozoon cuniculi* infection

Neurological symptoms

Acute

The onset of neurological signs associated with *E. cuniculi* can be sudden. Severe cases may be found dead.

- Vestibular disease
- Head tilt
- Seizures
- Ataxia
- Posterior paresis

Chronic

- 'Swaying' or 'nodding' at rest
- Stargazing
- Aggression
- Deafness
- Blindness
- Incontinence
- Loss of balance
- Uneaten caecotrophs

Kidney disease

- Polydypsia/polyuria
- Urinary incontinence
- Mild renal insufficiency
- Chronic renal failure

Ocular disease

- Lens rupture
- Uveitis
- Secondary hypopyon
- Cataracts
- Loss of vision

12.4 *Encephalitozoon cuniculi*

Encephalitozoon cuniculi is a microsporidian parasite that affects a wide range of species. A detailed description of the disease and its treatment is given in Section 16.4.2.5 and the clinical manifestations are summarized in Box 12.2. Encephalitozoonosis is widespread in rabbits, in which it causes granulomatous lesions in the brain and kidney. Focal necrosis gives the kidney a characteristic pitted appearance (see Section 14.5.1 and Plate 31). *E. cuniculi* can also cause phacoclastic uveitis (see Section 11.7.3.1). Clinical manifestations of *E. cuniculi* range from neurological disaster to mild renal insufficiency or infection can be latent. The parasite is endemic in many rabbit colonies. Commercial laboratories serologically screen their stock for *E. cuniculi* and cull affected animals. The most commonly recognized clinical manifestation is vestibular disease. Transmission of the parasite takes place via urine infected with spores. The spores invade the cells of the intestinal mucosa where they multiply and invade the reticuloendothelial system, which distributes the parasite throughout the body. The organism eventually localizes in the brain and kidney, and occasionally the myocardium. In the kidney, *E. cuniculi* can be found in the tubular epithelial cells and spores are flushed out in the urine. Cross-infection can take place between rabbits and rodents.

12.4.1 Central nervous system (CNS) signs of *Encephalitozoon cuniculi*

CNS signs relate to granulomatous encephalitis and include sudden death, seizures, ataxia, torticollis, paresis or paralysis. Signs develop rapidly when brain cells rupture to release parasites into surrounding tissues. Milder neurological symptoms also occur which may be noticed by observant owners. Some rabbits have nystagmus or sway slightly when they are at rest. Others are ataxic or appear clumsy. Deafness and strange behaviour have been recognized in seropositive animals. Incontinence, polydypsia and polyuria can also be associated with *Encephalitozoon cuniculi* infection, although it is not clear

Key points 12.2

- *Encephalitozoon cuniculi* is a common cause of neurological disease in pet rabbits
- Granulomatous encephalitis can cause a number of neurological syndromes ranging from acute neurological disaster and death to mild behavioural changes. Latent infections are common
- Vestibular disease (torticollis) is a common manifestation of *E. cuniculi* in pet rabbits
- *E. cuniculi* in rabbits can be treated with albendazole although there are no data available at the present time about its efficacy. Dosage and duration of treatment is empirical
- Oxytetracycline has also been used to treat symptoms of encephalitozoonosis in rabbits with anecdotal reports of success
- Corticosteroids may suppress the inflammatory response associated with cell rupture. Long-term treatment is immunosuppressive and therefore contraindicated
- Some rabbits will recover from neurological symptoms of *E. cuniculi* with no treatment at all
- In most cases, vestibular disease (wryneck, torticollis, head tilt) in rabbits is caused either by *E. cuniculi* or ascending *Pasteurella multocida* infection from the nasal cavity
- Other causes of torticollis include visceral larva migrans from *Baylisascaris* transmitted from raccoons (in the USA), neoplasia, trauma and other infections such as toxoplasmosis
- Dwarf rabbits appear particularly susceptible to encephalitozoonosis
- Pasteurellosis can cause abscesses along the vestibular tract
- If the rabbit is anorexic, the prognosis for vestibular disease is poor, whatever the cause
- Some mild cases of vestibular disease can survive to lead a relatively normal life although they may be left with a head tilt
- The prognosis for encephalitozoonosis is better than pasteurellosis which tends to be progressive
- Short-acting corticosteroids, oxytetracycline, albendazole and supportive care can be used as first aid blanket treatment for vestibular disease
- Serology can be used to prove exposure to *E. cuniculi*. In the USA, serological and PCR tests are available for diagnosis of *Pasteurella multocida*
- It is possible for rabbits to have been exposed to both *E. cuniculi* and *P. multocida*, which makes serological diagnosis difficult
- Neurological examination, radiology and blood samples can aid differential diagnosis.

whether this is a behavioural consequence of central lesions or due to mild renal insufficiency. The most commonly recognized neurological sign is vestibular disease that can range in severity from a minor head tilt to an animal that is unable to right itself and is rolling and hemiparetic.

Lesions do not develop in the central nervous system until at least 30 days after infection. Changes are those of a focal non-suppurative granulomatous meningoencephalomyelitis, with astrogliosis and perivascular lymphocytic infiltration (Percy and Barthold, 1993). Granulomas are characterized by a central area of necrosis surrounded by lymphocytes, plasma cells, microglia, epitheloid cells and sometimes giant cells (see Plate 26). In other instances, only dense accumulations of glial cells are noted. In the brain, there appears to be no predilection sites and granulomas are randomly distributed throughout all areas. Lesions can be found in the cerebellum and spinal cord. In many instances the organism cannot be identified in chronic lesions but is seen in large numbers in distended cells with no detectable inflammatory response (Pakes and Gerrity, 1994).

12.4.2 Vestibular disease

Vestibular disease is the most frequently recognized manifestation of *E. cuniculi* in pet rabbits. There are other causes of vestibular disease, such as pasteurellosis, which is the main differential diagnosis. The vestibular system is responsible for maintaining posture in relation to gravity, and for the movements of the eyes in relation to the position of the head. The peripheral vestibular system is composed of the labyrinth, the vestibular ganglion and the vestibular branch of the VIIIth cranial nerve. The labyrinth is situated in the inner ear surrounded by the petrous temporal bone. The vestibular nerve runs through the internal acoustic meatus into the cranial cavity and enters the rostral medulla at the cerebromedullary angle. Axons of the vestibular nerve terminate in the vestibular nuclei in the medulla or the cerebellum. Central vestibular disease results from lesions in the brainstem whereas peripheral vestibular disease is due to lesions in the cochlea and vestibular apparatus in the inner ear or along the vestibular nerve.

Vestibular disease in rabbits may be referred to as wryneck, torticollis, otitis media or interna, labyrinthitis or head tilt. A list of differential diagnoses includes neoplasia, abscesses, trauma, vascular disease, toxoplasmosis and other non-specific causes of neurological disease (see Table 3.2). In the USA, cerebral larval migrans by the larva of the ascarid *Baylisascaris* can cause torticollis. The parasite is ingested with food that has been contaminated by raccoon faeces. It is a problem associated with feeding hay. *Baylisascaris* does not occur in the UK. In pet rabbits in the UK, the two main causes of vestibular disease are pasteurellosis and *Encephalitozoon cuniculi* infection. Ascending *Pasteurella multocida* infection can spread from the nasal cavity to the middle ear along the eustachian tube to the inner ear and vestibular tract. In some cases, brain abscesses are found along the vestibular tract.

Kunstyr and Naumann (1983) compared the incidence of encephalitozoonosis and pasteurellosis as a cause of head tilt in dwarf and non-dwarf breeds of rabbits. The dwarf rabbits were pet animals and the non-dwarf group consisted of laboratory rabbits. All cases were euthanased when they developed torticollis. Outer and middle ears were examined for the presence of pus or ear mites, and inner organs and the brain were examined histologically. The non-dwarf laboratory rabbits had otitis interna and empyaemia. *Pasteurella multocida* was isolated from the pus and mucous membranes. With one exception, none of the group of pet rabbits showed signs of otitis, but they all had kidney and brain lesions characteristic of encephalitozoonosis. This study reflects the situation in pet rabbits in the UK.

12.4.3 Differentiation between pasteurellosis and encephalitozoonosis

In the UK, the main differential diagnosis of torticollis in pet rabbits is between pasteurellosis and *E. cuniculi* infection. Other diseases can cause vestibular symptoms, such as toxoplasmosis or brain tumours, but they are infrequent. A definitive diagnosis can only be made at *post-mortem* examination when the inner ear and brain tissue can be examined grossly and histologically. *P. multocida* is associated with purulent infection of the inner ear and abscesses along the vestibular tract. The abscesses are inaccessible and the only hope of therapy is to help wall off infection and prevent further spread with antibiotics. The disease tends to be progressive. *Encephalitozoon cuniculi* causes granulomatous lesions throughout the brain and spinal cord. Symptoms are associated with rupture of the brain cells. The condition does not appear to be progressive and the prognosis depends on the severity of the symptoms. If the initial episode is not life threatening, the rabbit can survive and make a partial or full recovery.

In most cases pasteurellosis causes peripheral vestibular disease and encephalitozoonosis causes central vestibular disease. Clinical examination can differentiate peripheral from central vestibular disease (see Table 12.1). Neurological examination of rabbits is difficult, especially if they are panicking and rolling and cannot be kept still. Serological testing may be a method of ruling out *Encephalitozoon cuniculi* as a cause of vestibular disease as, in experimental infections, antibodies are detected in the blood soon after infection and before lesions develop in the kidney and brain (Cox and Gallichio 1978). However, the significance of serology in relation to clinical signs in pet rabbits has yet to be established. It is also conceivable that a rabbit that has been exposed to *E. cuniculi* has developed pasteurellosis. Therefore a positive serological test does not give a definitive diagnosis but is strongly suggestive of encephalitozoonosis as a cause of vestibu-

Table 12.1 Differential diagnosis of signs of central and peripheral vestibular disease in rabbits

Clinical sign	*Central vestibular disease*	*Peripheral vestibular disease*
Loss of balance	Yes	Yes
Head tilt	Yes	Yes
Falling	Yes	Yes
Rolling	Yes	No
Nystagmus:	Yes	Yes
Horizontal	Yes	Yes
Rotatory	Yes	Yes
Vertical	Yes	No
Positional	Yes	No
Ventrolateral strabismus	Yes	Yes
Mental status	Possibly depressed	Probably not depressed
Cerebellar signs (intention tremor)	Possible	No
Hemiparesis with ipsilateral postural reaction deficits	Possible	No
Possible diagnosis		
Encephalitozoonosis cuniculi	Possible	No
Ascending *Pasteurella multocida* infection	Central lesions can occur in association with abscess formation along vestibular tract	Peripheral vestibular disease can result from otitis media
Other	*Bayliscararis* infection (USA) Neoplasia Trauma Toxoplasma	Neoplasia

lar disease. False negative results are unlikely in an animal showing acute signs of disease. Experimentally, no correlation has been found between antibody titre and the presence of *Encephalitozoon cuniculi* antigen in the brain (Kunstyr *et al.*, 1986). Haematology can show a leucocytosis or neutrophilia that suggests bacterial infection and pasteurellosis. Rabbits that are suffering from encephalitozoonosis can show mild renal insufficiency.

Examination of the external ear canal is unlikely to be diagnostic. Many rabbits, especially lop eared breeds, have purulent material along the horizontal canal. It can be difficult to remove this material to visualize the tympanic membrane with either an auriscope or endoscope. The presence of pus in the external ear canal does not mean that purulent infection is the cause of vestibular symptoms. Radiology can show lesions in the tympanic bullae that indicate the presence of infection which would suggest that pasteurellosis is the cause of any vestibular signs (see Figure 13.2).

12.4.4 Prognosis and treatment of rabbits with vestibular disease

Vestibular symptoms develop rapidly and treatment is usually required before serology results are available. The differential diagnosis between encephalitozoonosis and pasteurellosis based on clinical examination is difficult. Therefore, in severe cases, a blanket approach is necessary, working on the principle that the prognosis is poor and there is nothing to be lost by aggressive treatment. Conversely, mild cases of vestibular disease due to encephalitozoonosis often resolve with no treatment at all. Albendazole or fenbendazole should be included in the treatment protocol to eliminate *E. cuniculi* and to prevent spread to in-contact rabbits.

Both encephalitozoonosis and pasteurellosis carry a poor prognosis once vestibular signs have developed and the prognosis deteriorates in proportion to the severity of clinical signs. However, some individuals recover and many rabbits with a mild head tilt learn to cope with their disability and lead a relatively normal life. The nervous system is able to compensate for vestibular disorders if the lesion is stable or changing slowly. Enforced activity that appropriately challenges the vestibular system enhances the rate of compensation. Conversely, a period of immobilization after an acute vestibular lesion not only slows recovery but also actually limits the recovery of vestibular function (Thomas, 2000). Therefore, although cage confinement of an animal with acute vestibular disease may be necessary to prevent injury, normal activity should be encouraged as soon as possible. Rabbits with torticollis will eat if they can maintain an upright position. Appetite can be used as a prognostic indicator. Those rabbits with vestibular disease that cannot or do not eat voluntarily are unlikely to recover. The prognosis is better for rabbits that are still eating.

12.4.4.1 Corticosteroids

The use of corticosteroids in the treatment of neurological signs associated with *E. cuniculi* is controversial. On one hand, there is the argument that the neurological symptoms associated with *E. cuniculi* are due to the inflammatory reaction caused by rupture of brain cells by multiplying organisms rather than the organisms themselves (Feaga, 1997). Prompt treatment with a high dose of corticosteroid may suppress this inflammatory response. Experimentally, systemic glucocorticoid administration (dexamethasone) decreases the frequency of nystagmus and head deviation in surgically hemilabyrinthectomized rabbits (Yamanaka *et al.*, 1995). Corticosteroids are also used successfully to treat granulomatous encephalomeningitis in other species.

Conversely, it can be argued that corticosteroids are contraindicated in rabbits with encephalitozoonosis due to their immunosuppressive effects. In humans, clinical disease associated with encephalitozoonosis only occurs in immunosuppressed patients. Experimentally, encephalitozoonosis is fatal in rabbits that have been immunosuppressed with cyclophosphamide (Horvath *et al.*, 1999).

As a compromise, short courses of anti-inflammatory, rather than immunosuppressive doses, of corticosteroid are indicated for the initial treatment of vestibular signs, especially if they are severe. A dose of 0.2 mg/kg dexamethasone is suggested by Ewringmann and Göbel (1999).

12.4.4.2 Antibiotics

The selection of an antibiotic to treat vestibular disease in rabbits is empirical. Antibiotic therapy is indicated in the initial stages before a diagnosis is made. Occasionally, it is possible to culture purulent material that has burst through the tympanic membrane.

Oxytetracycline was the antibiotic selected by Ewringmann and Göbel (1999) to treat 23 seropositive rabbits with CNS signs. The selection was based on an *in vitro* study of the sensitivity of *E. cuniculi* to antibiotics (Waller, 1979). Oxytetracycline is also effective against *P. multocida*, although it is difficult to achieve sufficient tissue concentrations of any antibiotic to eliminate infection from the middle ear. In order to maintain minimum inhibitory concentrations of enrofloxacin for *P. multocida*, 12-hourly dosing of 5 mg/kg is required either orally or parenterally (Broome *et al.*, 1991).

12.4.4.3 Symptomatic treatment

Many types of drugs including anticholinergics, antihistamines and benzodiazepines are used to treat vestibular problems in humans. This type of medication may be helpful in the treatment of rabbits with vestibular symptoms. Prochlorperazine is a phenothiazine derivative with an alpha-adrenergic blocking activity that is used in man to treat vertigo and labyrinthine disorders. It acts on the neural pathways that arise in the vestibular apparatus. A palatable syrup is available that can be used as symptomatic treatment for rabbits with torticollis. Benzodiazepines such as diazepam or midazolam may be helpful in suppressing acute neurological signs associated with acute vestibular lesions. Long-term use of these drugs is not indicated because they suppress the sensory imbalance in the vestibular system that is an essential stimulus to recovery (Thomas, 2000). The differential diagnosis and treatment of encephalitozoonosis and pasteurellosis as a cause of vestibular disease is summarized in Table 12.2.

Table 12.2 Differential diagnosis and treatment of encephalitozoonosis and pasteurellosis as a causes of vestibular disease

	Encephalitozoonosis	*Pasteurellosis*
Radiography	*E. cuniculi* does not cause radiographic changes of the tympanic bullae	Radiographic changes may be seen in tympanic bullae associated with chronic otitis media
Bacteriology	Not applicable	There is a possibility of collecting material to culture from middle ear through ruptured tympanic membrane. Purulent material in horizontal ear canal is *not* diagnostic of pasteurella infection in the vestibular system
Serology	Serological tests are available for *E. cuniculi* in the UK Positive result indicates exposure to infection Negative result rules out encephalitozoonosis	Serological test for *P. multocida* is available in the USA Paired samples are required to show rising titre Positive result indicates exposure to infection. (Most rabbits have been exposed to *P. multocida*)
Haematology and biochemistry	No haematological changes associated with *E. cuniculi* Biochemistry may show mild renal insufficiency in association with *E. cuniculi*	Neutrophilia and shift to left is suggestive of pasteurellosis
Treatment	• Euthanasia for anorexic, severe cases • Consider short-term corticosteroids in acute severe cases of *E. cuniculi* • Albendazole or fenbendazole • Antibiotics: oxytetracycline has some effect against *E. cuniculi* • Some cases of *E. cuniculi* resolve with no treatment • Symptomatic treatment with human motion sickness remedies	• Euthanasia for anorexic, severe cases • Long-term corticosteroids contraindicated • Antibiotics unlikely to be curative but may be beneficial effects in early cases • Symptomatic treatment with human motion sickness remedies • Surgery. Bulla osteotomy or aural resection to remove pus from tympanic bulla is an option
Prognosis	Good for mild cases of *E. cuniculi.* Poor for severe cases, especially those that are unable to eat	Moderate for mild cases of pasteurellosis Head tilt is unlikely to resolve Prognosis grave for anorexic patients

NB. It is possible that *Encephalitozoon cuniculi* and *Pasteurella multocida* are present in the same animal. Either infection can be latent.

12.4.4.4 Bulla osteotomy

In other species, bulla osteotomy is used to remove purulent material from the tympanic bulla and to provide drainage and a route for topical therapy in the treatment of otitis media. Bulla osteotomy has been described in rabbits (Swindle and Shealy, 1996). It is a suggested treatment for otitis media associated with head tilt, opisthotonus, horizontal nystagmus and anorexia in association with bacterial or fungal infection (Redrobe, 2000). Theoretically, bulla osteotomy provides a means of draining pus from the middle ear of rabbits suffering from vestibular symptoms due to pasteurellosis. However, despite detailed descriptions of the surgical procedure, there are no follow-up data on the success of this operation. Anecdotally, the success rate is not good.

12.5 Seizures

Seizures occur in rabbits as in other species. *Encephalitozoon cuniculi* can cause seizures associated with the inflammatory response to rupture of brain cells. The seizures are sudden in onset and affected rabbits are sometimes left blind or comatose. Others make a complete recovery. Seizures are seen in the terminal stages of diseases such as hepatic lipidosis or viral haemorrhagic disease. Space occupying lesions such as tumours or abscesses can also cause seizures. Arteriosclerosis and mineralization of meningeal blood vessels has been associated with seizures in laboratory rabbits. Epilepsy has been reported, especially in blue-eyed white rabbits. Symptomatic treatment is similar to other species. Diazepam or midazolam can be given intravenously. Midazolam can be given intramuscularly or subcutaneously. If this is not possible, midazolam can be administered intranasally as it is absorbed across the nasal mucosa.

12.6 Generalized muscular weakness in rabbits

A syndrome of generalized muscular weakness has been recognized in the UK. The condition is colloquially known as 'floppy rabbit syndrome'. Affected rabbits suffer from a flaccid paralysis and are unable to move although they are able to eat and drink if food and water are placed within reach (see Figure 12.1). Many cases will recover with supportive care. There are many theories about the cause of this syndrome including hypokalaemia and plant toxicity. The condition warrants further investigation. It is important to recognize the good prognosis associated with the syndrome and not euthanase the rabbits in the initial stages. Recovery usually takes place within 2–3 days, whatever treatment is prescribed. Supportive care, especially assisted feeding is required.

Several conditions cause generalized muscular weakness in rabbits. The differential diagnoses include neurological, metabolic or muscular causes, which could be infectious, metabolic, congenital or nutritional in origin. Neurological conditions include *Encephalitozoon cuniculi*, compressive spinal lesions or cerebrovascular incidents. Metabolic diseases such as hepatic lipidosis or hypokalaemia can be manifested by ataxia or muscular weakness. Plant toxicity is another potential cause although it is difficult to prove, especially if the rabbit recovers. Myasthenia gravis has also been suggested as a possible cause of generalized muscular weakness (Boydell, 2000). A list of differential diagnoses is given in Table 12.3.

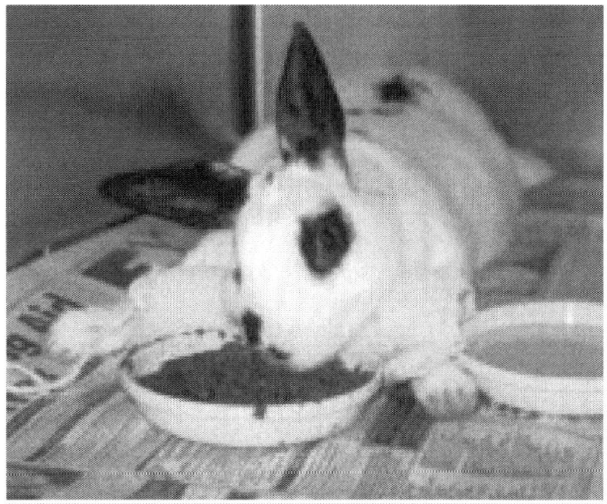

Figure 12.1. Floppy rabbit syndrome. 'Floppy rabbit syndrome' is the colloquial term for an idiopathic condition that affects pet rabbits causing generalized muscular weakness. The cause is not known although several possibilities exist (see Section 12.6). A feature of the condition is the recovery that can take place with supportive care, although not all rabbits survive. This 2.5-year-old, English, male rabbit was presented in the collapsed state that is typical of 'floppy rabbit syndrome'. He could not raise his head or move his limbs. The muscles were flaccid. The rabbit was one of a pair that were kept in a small yard during the day and placed in a hutch overnight. He was fed on *ad lib* mixed cereal rations, hay and vegetables. Rectal temperature, heart rate, heart sounds, respiratory sounds, capillary refill time and colour of the mucous membranes were considered normal. Radiographic examination, including myelography, revealed no abnormalities. Serology was negative for *Encephalitozoon cuniculi.* Culture of cerebrospinal fluid yielded no bacterial growth. An initial blood sample was taken without sedation or anaesthesia. Haematology showed mild anaemia and lymphopaenia. These findings are not unusual in pet rabbits (see Section 6.2.2). Biochemistry showed a hypoproteinaemia (51.2 g/l), slightly raised alkaline phosphatase (89.4 IU/l) and low serum potassium (2.75 mmol/l (reference range 3.5–7 mmol/l; Gillett, 1994)). He was treated with supportive care including intravenous fluid therapy (Hartmann's solution). The rabbit appeared hungry and could eat and drink if food and water was placed within reach. He made a complete recovery over a period of 3 days.

Table 12.3 Major differential diagnoses of neurological disease in pet rabbits

Symptom	*Possible causes*	*Diagnosis*
Seizures (fits, convulsions)	*Encephalitozoon cuniculi*	Serology Confirmed by histopathology of brain tissue
	Cerebral haemorrhage due to viral haemorrhagic disease	Terminal event Confirmed by *post-mortem* examination and histopathology of liver
	Epilepsy (idiopathic, previous trauma)	Diagnosis not easily confirmed
	Space occupying lesions (abscesses, tumours)	Neurological examination ?CSF analysis Haematology Brain scanning Confirmed by *post-mortem* examination
	Metabolic disease (end stage hepatic lipidosis)	History of inappetance Terminal event Confirmed by *post-mortem* examination
	Hypoxia	Terminal event Cause of hypoxia found at *post-mortem* examination
	Cardiovascular disease, e.g. arteriosclerosis	Radiology, ECG Confirmed by *post-mortem* examination
	Ingestion of toxic substances	History Diagnosis not easily confirmed during life Radiopaque material may be visible in GI tract Toxic principal may be found in digestive tract during *post-mortem* examination
Generalized muscular weakness ('floppy rabbit syndrome')	*Encephalitozoon cuniculi*	Serological testing will confirm exposure to organism
	Hypokalaemia	Serum potassium values < 3.0 mmol/l (NB Anaesthesia will depress serum potassium values) ECG changes associated with hypokalaemia include supraventricular or ventricular ectopic beats, depressed T-wave amplitude, depressed S–T segment, prolonged Q–T interval and prominent U waves
	Terminal disease, e.g VHD, septicaemia, liver failure due to hepatic lipidosis, renal failure, lymphoma, intestinal obstruction, predator attack, starvation	Diagnosis made at *post-mortem* examination
	Plant toxins (thiazines)	Diagnosis not easily confirmed
	Splay leg	Clinical examination. Caused by failure to adduct limbs. Can affect all the limbs
	Nutritional muscular dystrophy	Raised creatine kinase and AST blood levels. Confirmed at *post-mortem* examination and histopathology of muscle
	Spinal cord disease (fracture, subluxation, disc disease)	Radiology, myelography. Confirmed by *post-mortem* examination of spinal cord and related structures
	Myasthenia gravis	Response to intravenous edrophonium
	Cardiovascular disease	Clinical examination Thoracic radiography Electrocardiography
	Toxoplasma, neospora	Serology Muscle biopsy
	Idiopathic	
Ataxia	*Encephalitozoon cuniculi*	Serology

continued

Table 12.3 *continued*

Symptom	*Possible causes*	*Diagnosis*
	Spinal cord compression (fracture, subluxation, disc, abscess, tumour)	Neurological examination Radiology Myelography ?CSF analysis MRI scanning
	Space occupying lesions in brain, e.g. tumours, abscesses, haemorrhage due to recent trauma	Neurological examination Haematology ?Brain scanning
	Ketoacidosis (pregnancy toxaemia, hepatic lipidosis)	Clinical examination History of anorexia Blood/urine sampling
	Starvation	Clinical history Blood glucose
	Limb deformities (especially bilateral) e.g. septic arthritis, splay leg Terminal disease, e.g VHD, septicaemia, renal failure, lymphoma, intestinal obstruction, predator attack	Clinical examination Radiography
Posterior paresis or paralysis **NB**. The vertebrae of many pet rabbits are osteopaenic Metabolic bone disease due to calcium/vitamin D deficiency and/or disuse atrophy due to inactivity and confinement in a small cage or hutch predispose spinal fractures and deformities	Spinal fracture or subluxation	Clinical and neurological examination History of trauma Radiography: lumbar vertebrae commonly affected Myelography
	Degenerative disc disease	Clinical and neurological examination Maybe history of trauma Radiography Myelography
	Spondylosis, kyphosis, lordosis (**NB** very common in pet rabbits) Limb deformities e.g. bilateral fractures, splayleg, septic arthritis	Clinical findings (see Box 12.2) Radiography Clinical examination Radiography
	Ulcerative pododermatitis	Reluctance to walk In advanced cases, the superficial digital flexor tendon becomes displaced giving a 'dropped hock' appearance that can be mistaken for sciatic nerve paralysis (see Plate 12)
	CNS disease, e.g. *E. cuniculi,* brain abscess or tumour, VHD, trauma Terminal disease, e.g. VHD, septicaemia, renal failure, cardiovascular disease, intestinal obstruction, predator attack	Clinical and neurological examination Serology, haematology Diagnosis made at *post-mortem* examination

12.6.1 Possible causes of generalized muscular weakness in rabbits

12.6.1.1 Hypokalaemia

Hypokalaemia has been found in some cases of 'floppy rabbit syndrome' where serum electrolytes have been measured (Harcourt-Brown, unpublished data). Experimental potassium deficiency in rabbits has been investigated. Hove and Herndon (1954) fed a potassium-deficient diet to adult rabbits. Affected animals exhibited behavioural disorders such as restlessness before developing muscular dystrophy. Paralysis progressed from the hindquarters to the forequarters and neck muscles. Eventually the rabbits were unable to move. The paralysis was flaccid and every part of the body was limp. The authors noted that paralysis occurred at dietary levels of 0.3% potassium which is adequate for growth in the rat and pig. The dietary requirement of potassium for rabbits has been determined at a level of 0.6–0.9% (Hunt and Harrington, 1974). As herbivores, rabbits normally consume a potassium rich diet, so primary dietary deficiency is unlikely but could occur as a result of anorexia.

In healthy animals, about 95% of the total body potassium is intracellular. Insulin, aldosterone and catecholamines play a role in potassium balance and have a hypokalaemic effect. Dietary intake and absorption of potassium from the intestinal tract is variable and the kidneys regulate total body potassium by altering renal excretion rates. Aldosterone modifies renal excretion of potassium by its effects on the ion exchange mechanism in tubular epithelium. In the rabbit, variations in serum aldosterone concentrations are related to the excretion of hard or soft faeces. Potassium secretion into the colon also varies according to the type of faeces that are passing through. In other species, hypokalaemia is caused by excessive potassium loss, either by renal excretion or via the gastrointestinal tract. In cattle, hypokalaemia often follows a protracted illness and is associated with abnormal position of the head and neck, severe weakness, rumenal atony or hypomotility, abnormal faeces, anorexia and tachycardia (Sattler *et al.*, 1998).

In rabbits, the passage of electrolytes across the gut wall is complex and it is conceivable that digestive and motility disorders interfere with potassium exchange. Hypokalaemia could be the result of excessive loss into the digestive tract, especially if dietary intake is restricted due to anorexia. Soft faeces have a higher potassium content (1.8%) than hard faeces (0.57%) (Lang, 1981). Mucus is rich in potassium (Riley and Cornelius, 1989) and diarrhoea, especially mucoid diarrhoea, can induce hypokalaemia. Experimental diarrhoea induced by coccidiosis inoculation results in a marked hypokalaemia in rabbits. (Licois *et al.*, 1978).

In other species, massive catecholamine release can cause hypokalaemia. It is seen in post-resuscitation patients and human freshwater near-drownings (Willard, 1989). In rabbits, experimental intravenous adrenaline infusion causes a significant decrease in plasma potassium levels (Reverte *et al.*, 1993). In a catecholamine-susceptible species such as the rabbit it is also possible that hypokalaemia could result from stress, fright or hypothermia.

In the absence of specific information about rabbits, guidelines for potassium supplementation can only be given by following the basic principles that apply to other species. In most cases, providing a nutritional source of potassium is all that is required. In other species, intravenous supplementation is indicated if plasma potassium concentrations fall below 2.5 mmol/l (Bishop, 1998). In rabbits, serum potassium concentrations can fall during anaesthesia (Robson *et al.*, 1981) but low values in the unanaesthetized rabbit are a significant finding.

12.6.1.2 Toxins

Toxicity has been suggested as a cause of generalized muscular weakness or 'floppy rabbit syndrome' in rabbits. A condition known as 'head down disease', caused by ingestion of hay containing woolly pod milkweed (*Asclepias eriocarpa*) has been reported in the USA. Affected animals develop paralysis of the neck muscles and loss of coordination. Drooling, rough hair coat, subnormal temperature and tar-like faeces may occur. Recovery is possible if the rabbit has not consumed too much of the weed and food and water are placed within reach and the rabbit held so that it can eat and drink. Focal haemorrhages are observed on many organs at *post-mortem*. The toxic principal is a resinoid. Woolly milkweed does not grow in the UK.

Some herbicides can cause muscular weakness and therefore might be implicated in 'floppy rabbit syndrome'. Triazines are widely used in the UK. Not only is there a risk of poisoning by ingestion of the product but there is a small risk of poisoning by ingestion of the treated plants (Lorgue *et al.*, 1996). The repeated use of triazines in areas of monoculture, such as maize, results in the emergence of plants or weeds that are resistant to the chemical. Hay can be contaminated with treated triazine-resistant plants that are toxic. Muscle atonia, weakness and paraplegia are among reported clinical signs. In other species, the prognosis is good, and the condition is rarely fatal. Treatment is with symptomatic care. Although rabbits are not listed as animals most affected by this group of poisons, the LD_{50} for rabbits is considerably less than for rats. *Post-mortem*, lesions include cardiac haemorrhage, renal haemorrhage and pulmonary and renal congestion. Fresh stomach contents are required for analysis

12.6.1.3 Splayleg

Splayleg is a non-specific term that is used to describe any condition affecting the limbs that prevents standing. Several congenital abnormalities of rabbits affect the skeletal system and result in subluxations or limb deformities that prevent normal locomotion. Usually, the condition is due to an inability to adduct the limbs. The hind limbs are most frequently affected although splayleg can also be seen in the forelimbs. Treatment is not feasible for most cases. Each case should be considered on its own merit. Some rabbits cope well with disability.

12.6.1.4 Nutritional muscular dystrophy

In other species, muscular dystrophy caused by vitamin E or selenium deficiency causes generalized muscular weakness. Both vitamin E and selenium are antioxidants. Selenium is a constituent of the enzyme glutathione peroxidase that catalyses the detoxification of peroxides formed during tissue metabolism. Vitamin E is an antioxidant that prevents the development of peroxides and has a mutually sparing effect on selenium. In other species, such as rats, fed a selenium/vitamin E deficient diet, liver necrosis develops that can be prevented by the addition of either selenium or vitamin E. Rabbits fed on this diet develop muscular dystrophy, which can only be prevented by the addition of vitamin E. Selenium has no effect. Rabbit tissues have a high content of non-selenium glutathione peroxidase which could explain this phenomenon (Cheeke, 1987). Vitamin E deficiency has been described in commercial units as a cause of muscular dystrophy in young rabbits. Affected animals are unable to right themselves when placed on their backs and progress to posterior paralysis and death. Myocardial dysfunction can occur (Lowe, 1998). Hepatic coccidiosis caused by *Eimeria steidae* interferes with metabolism of fat soluble vitamins and increases the requirement for dietary vitamin E. Unsaturated fatty acids or vegetable oils also increase the requirement of vitamin E. Leafy green vegetables and cereals are good sources of vitamin E although activity can decline with storage.

12.7 Spinal disorders

12.7.1 Anatomy of the spinal cord

In the rabbit, the numbers of vertebrae in each sector of the spinal column are C8, T12, L7, S4, C6. The dura mater is not firmly attached to the spinal cord so there is an epidural space surrounding the spinal cord. The brachial plexus originates from C_4, C_5, C_6, C_7, C_8, T_1 and the lumbosacral plexus originates from L_4, L_5, L_6, L_7, S_1, S_2, S_3. The spinal cord tapers to a filament at about S_2–S_3 which runs alongside the posterior spinal nerves in the spinal canal as the *cauda equina*.

12.7.2 Clinical signs associated with spinal disease in pet rabbits

Clinical signs associated with spinal disease are summarized in Box 12.3. Vertebral spondylosis, kyphosis (see Figure 12.2), scoliosis and lordosis are common in pet rabbits and are often observed as incidental findings on radiographs. Abnormalities of gait are often overlooked by owners who never see their rabbit hopping around if it spends most of its life confined to a hutch. The uncomplaining nature of rabbits means that painful conditions of the spine are often not recognized. Rabbits do not cry out in pain like a dog or cat. Instead, they are quiet and immobile although they can become unaccountably aggressive towards their companions or owners. A common presentation of spinal disease is a reluctance or inability to reach the perineum and area at the base of the tail resulting in an unkempt coat or failure to ingest caecotrophs and perineal soiling. Some rabbits with spinal problems cannot or will not adopt the correct position to urinate away from the body and become

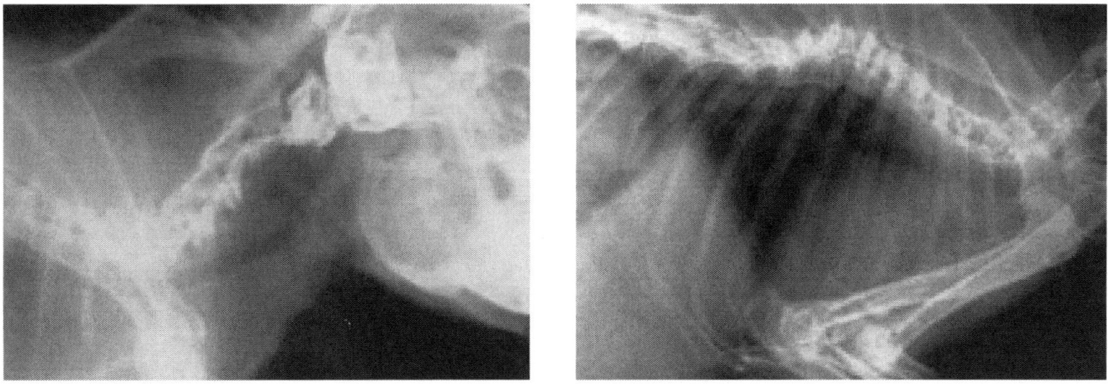

(a) (b)

Figure 12.2. Spinal defects.
(a) **Spondylosis of cervical vertebrae.** Degenerative changes of the spine are frequently seen on radiographs of pet rabbits. In dogs, spondylosis causes pain and reluctance to exercise. In rabbits, the condition is often overlooked because pain is not recognized. Rabbits in pain are quiet and immobile although they can become unaccountably aggressive towards their companions or owners. The figure is a lateral radiograph of the cervical vertebrae of an aged male rabbit showing spondylitic changes and collapse of the intervertebral spaces from C_1 to C_6. The rabbit was presented because he had become ataxic and was unable to groom. His perineal area was constantly soiled with urine and faeces. His condition had deteriorated to the point where he was unable to stand. The rabbit was euthanased. Myelography would have been necessary to make an accurate assessment of the compressive nature of the spinal lesions.

(b) **Kyphosis of thoracic vertebrae.** Like spondylosis, spinal defects such as kyphosis, scoliosis and lordosis are frequently seen on radiographs of pet rabbits. Spinal defects are significant in rabbits, not only because they are a potential source of pain, but also because they affect flexibility and interfere with the rabbit's ability to reach its perineum. A common presentation of spinal disease is a reluctance or inability to groom the area at the base or to ingest caecotrophs. Perineal soiling by uneaten soft faeces or urine can be the result. This figure is a lateral view of a 2-year-old female Dwarf lop rabbit that was radiographed because she was anorexic. Gastrointestinal hypomotility was suspected and the rabbit responded to analgesia, prokinetic therapy and nutritional support. The kyphotic changes were believed to be an incidental finding although, on questioning the owner, it materialized that the rabbit would ingest caecotrophs from its bedding rather than its anus. It is not known if spinal pain contributed to the gastrointestinal hypomotility.

Rabbits are also prone to spinal fractures. In commercial rabbits, spinal deformities have been linked to small cage size and to periods of high calcium demand such as pregnancy and lactation. Metabolic bone disease could also be a contributory factor in spinal deformities in the pet rabbit population.

saturated in urine in a result. The urine scalds the skin between the back legs (see Section 14.4.3). Fly strike can be the sequel to spinal disease. Rabbits with flexibility problems cannot groom the area at the base of the tail or on the scruff of the neck effectively. Skin debris accumulates and mites proliferate resulting in clinical skin disease. A reluctance to move around and exercise predisposes to obesity which exacerbates the problems with grooming and cleaning the perineal area and the base of the tail (see Section 9.7.3). Ataxia, posterior paresis or paralysis may also be the result of spinal cord disease.

12.7.3 Causes of spinal disease

There are several causes of spinal disorders in rabbits. Congenital defects occur, such as hemivertebrae, that can be asymptomatic (Hoogstraten-Miller, 1994; Boydell, 2000).

Box 12.3 Clinical signs associated with spinal disease

Many pet rabbits have spinal deformities such as spondylosis, kyphosis, lordosis, hemivertebrae. Clinical signs may not be evident or may be manifested by symptoms of skin, urogenital or digestive disease.

Impaired flexibility results in:

- Abnormal gait
- Grooming difficulties. The rabbit is unable to reach many parts of the body, especially the area around the tail and along the dorsum. Dead hair and skin debris accumulate
- Cheyletiellosis. The rabbit is unable to remove skin parasites and scale allowing build up of mites in the fur
- Uneaten caecotrophs. The rabbit cannot reach the anus to ingest caecotrophs as they are excreted
- Perineal dermatitis. The rabbit cannot reach the area around the anus and genitalia which becomes soiled and infected
- Facial dermatitis and/or tear staining. The rabbit is unable to sit on its haunches to groom the face and ears with its front legs.

Spinal pain can result in:

- Aggression towards companions or owners
- Reduced gut motility
- Quiet, unresponsive demeanour
- Reluctance to exercise

Compression of spinal cord can cause neurological deficits such as:

- Ataxia
- Lack of proprioreception
- Paresis
- Paralysis
- Urinary incontinence
- Faecal incontinence

Low calcium diets cause a decrease in vertebral bone density (Gilsanz *et al.*, 1991) and calcium deficient rabbits are used as laboratory models of osteoporosis in humans. Rabbits have 20% less vertebral bone after only 14 weeks of a calcium deficient diet (Wu *et al.*, 1990). Metabolic bone disease caused by calcium and/or vitamin D deficiency is a cause of spinal deformities in pet rabbits. Young rabbits that are growing are more susceptible to nutritional osteodystrophy although its effects may not be evident until later in life. The selection of calcium deficient cereal and legumes from mixed cereal rations can result in a calcium deficient diet (Harcourt-Brown, 1996) and pet rabbits that are housed indoors can have undetectable vitamin D concentrations, especially in the spring (Fairham and Harcourt-Brown, 1999). Many young rabbits are reared indoors on mixed cereal rations. Nutritional secondary hyperparathyroidism is associated with generalized demineralization of the skeleton (Rübel *et al.*, 1991).

Spinal deformities are also associated with inactivity and small cage size. Rothfritz *et al.* (1992) compared the vertebral columns of caged and group-housed rabbits. They found no changes in the vertebrae of the group-housed rabbits but lumbar fractures were common among the caged group. Drescher and Loeffler (1996) studied kyphosis, scoliosis and lordosis in rabbits. They found a sex predilection towards females and that the degree of deformity was dependent on cage size. The authors concluded that lack of exercise and alterations in posture, in addition to a high calcium requirement due to pregnancy and lactation, resulted in spinal deformities. Conrad (1997) investigated the bone mineral density of female rabbits and compared group-housed and single-housed does. The author concluded that pregnancy and lactation had a considerable influence on bone density.

Degenerative disc disease occurs in rabbits. Disc protrusion and nuclear extrusion has been confirmed, by *post-mortem* examination, as a cause of hind leg paralysis in rabbits (Smith Baxter, 1975). The author suggests that forceful movement produces hyperflexion of the spine that causes disc damage, dislocations and fractures. He emphasized the importance of supporting the rear end of rabbits and avoiding sudden noises and fear provoking stimuli that may send *'any member of this rather nervous species into self destructive impulsive behaviour'*.

Spontaneous degenerative spinal disease has been studied in laboratory rabbits. Green *et al.* (1984) described three spontaneous degenerative changes that take place in the vertebral column: chondroid metaplasia of the nucleus pulposus, calcification of the nucleus pulposus and spondylosis. The spinal columns of 35 rabbits ranging in age from 3 months to 8.5 years were examined in detail. Spondylitic lesions were found on the vertebral bodies especially in the cervicothoracic region although lesions were found in lumbar vertebrae too. In the thoracolumbar region, osteophytosis of the apophyseal joints was more prevalent than spondylitic changes. Degenerative changes were found in the nucleus pulposus as early as 3 months of age although the frequency and severity of lesions did not increase after 9 months of age. Calcification of the discs was observed in the lumbar region in older rabbits. The study confirmed the findings of previous workers that rabbit vertebral epiphyses do not close until about 3 years of age.

Key points 12.3

- Seizures in rabbits can be caused by *E. cuniculi*
- Many terminal diseases (viral haemorrhagic disease, hepatic lipidosis) can present as seizures in their final stages
- Epilepsy can occur. Treatment is similar to the dog or cat
- Midazolam or diazepam can be used to control seizures
- There are several conditions that can cause general muscular weakness in rabbits, e.g. encephalitozoonosis, hypokalaemia, toxins, muscular dystrophy, quadriplegia
- There is a syndrome of generalized muscular weakness in rabbits that can respond to supportive care. This syndrome is colloquially known as 'floppy rabbit syndrome'. Affected rabbits continue to eat and drink if food and water are placed within reach
- Splayleg is a non-specific term used to describe a number of congenital defects that prevent normal locomotion. In most cases, the rabbit is unable to adduct one or more limbs. Symptoms are evident from an early age
- Spinal disorders are common in pet rabbits and underly many other diseases. Problems with flexibility can interfere with grooming, urination and caecotrophy
- Congenital defects, metabolic bone disease, inactivity due to small cage size and degenerative disc disease can all result in spinal disorders
- Meloxicam is a useful NSAID for long-term therapy of arthritic conditions in rabbits
- Myelography, CSF collection and spinal surgery are feasible in rabbits although few cases have been described in the literature
- Spinal fractures and subluxations are common sequels to trauma
- The prognosis for rabbits with spinal fracture, subluxations and compressive lesions is poor.

12.7.4 Treatment of spinal disease in rabbits

Treatment of spinal disease follows the same principles as the dog or cat. Treatment depends on the severity of the condition and the quality of the rabbit's life. NSAIDs can be used as long-term anti-inflammatory and analgesic treatment. Meloxicam (Metacam, Boehringer) is a useful product for long-term therapy.

The prognosis for rabbits with spinal fractures, subluxations and other compressive lesions is poor. Although spinal surgery is a possibility, it is still in its infancy in rabbits in comparison with dogs and cats. There are few reported cases in the literature and no follow-up studies. Euthanasia is the sensible option for paralysed rabbits but some owners are reluctant to agree and will diligently nurse paraplegic rabbits despite problems with incontinence. Boydell (2000) even illustrates a paraplegic rabbit in a cart.

References

Boydell, P. (2000). Nervous system and disorders. In *Manual of Rabbit Medicine and Surgery* (P.A. Flecknell, ed.) pp 57–62. British Small Animal Veterinary Association.

Broome, R.L., Brooks, D.L., Babish, J.G. *et al.* (1991). Pharmacokinetic properties of enrofloxacin in rabbits. *Am. J. Vet. Res.*, **52**, 1835–1841.

Cheeke, P.R. (1987). *Rabbit Feeding and Nutrition.* Academic Press.

Conrad, J. (1997). *Untersuchungen zur Knochendichte bei weiblichen ZIKA-Zuchtkaninchen an calcaneus sowie am distalen Tibiaende über einen Zeitram von mehreren Reproduktionszylen mittels peripherer Qunatitativ Computertomogrpahie (pQCTtm).* Doctoral Thesis. English Abstract.

Cox, J.C., Gallichio, H.A. (1978). Serological and histological studies on adult rabbits with recent naturally acquired encephalitozoonosis. *Res Vet Sci.*, **24**, 260–261.

DeSanto, J. (1997). Hypertrophic osteopathy associated with an intrathoracic neoplasm in a rabbit. *J Am Vet Med Assoc.*, **210**, 1322–1323.

Drescher, B., Loeffler, K. (1996). Scoliosis, lordosis and kyphosis in breeding rabbits. *Tierarztl Prax*, **24**, 292–300.

Ewringmann, A., Göbel, T. (1999). Untersuchungen zur Klinik und Therapie der Encephalitozoonose beim Heimtierkaninchen (Article in German, English summary). *Klientierpraxis*, **44**, 357–372.

Fairham, J., Harcourt-Brown, F.M. (1999). Preliminary investigation of the vitamin D status of pet rabbits. *Vet Rec.*, **145**, 452–454.

Feaga, W.P. (1997). Wry neck in rabbits. *J Am Vet Med Assoc.*, **210**, 480.

Gilsanz, V., Roe, T.F., Antunes, J. *et al.* (1991). Effect of dietary calcium on bone density in growing rabbits. *Am J Physiol.*, **260**, E471–E476.

Green, P.W., Fox, R.R., Sokoloff, L. (1984). Spontaneous degenerative spinal disease in the laboratory rabbit. *J Orthop Res.*, **2**, 161–168.

Harcourt-Brown, F.M. (1996). Calcium deficiency, diet and dental disease in pet rabbits. *Vet Rec.*, **139**, 567–571.

Hoogstraten-Miller, S.L. (1994) 'What is your diagnosis'. *J Am Vet Med Assoc.*, **204**, 1566–1567.

Horvath, M., Leng, L., Stefkovic, M. *et al.* (1999). Lethal encephalitozoonosis in cyclophosphamide-treated rabbits (Abstract). *Acta Vet Hung.*, **47**, 85–93.

Hove, E.L., Herndon, J.F. (1954). Potassium deficiency in the rabbit as a cause of muscular dystrophy. *J Nutr.*, **55**, 363–374.

Hunt, C.E., Harrington, D.D. (1974). Nutrition and nutritional diseases of the rabbit. In *The Biology of the Laboratory Rabbit*, (S.H. Weisbroth, R.E. Flatt, A.L. Kraus eds). pp 403–428. Academic Press.

Kunstyr, I., Naumann, S. (1983). Head tilt in rabbits caused by Pasteurella and Encephalitozoonosis. *Lab Anim.*, **19**, 208–213.

Kunstyr, I., Lev, L., Naumann, S. (1986). Humoral antibody response to rabbits to experimental infection with *Encephalitozoon cuniculi*. *Vet Parasitol.*, **21**, 223–232.

Lang, J. (1981). The nutrition of the commercial rabbit. Part 1. Physiology, digestibility and nutrient requirements. *Nutr abstr rev -Series B*, **51**, 197–217.

Licois, D., Coudert, P., Mongin, P. (1978). Changes in hydromineral metabolism in diarrhoeic rabbits 2. Study of the modifications of electrolyte metabolism. *Ann Rech Vet.*, **9**, 453–464.

Lorgue, G., Lechenet, J., Rivière. (1996). *Clinical Veterinary Toxicology, English Edition.* (M.J. Chapman, ed.) Blackwell.

Lowe, J.A. (1998). Pet rabbit feeding and nutrition. In *The Nutrition of the Rabbit* (C. de Blas, J. Wiseman, eds). pp 309–332. CABI Publishing.

Pakes, S.P., Gerrity, L.W. (1994). Protozoal diseases. In *The Biology of the Laboratory Rabbit*, 2nd edn. (P.J. Manning, D.H. Ringler, C.E. Newcomer, eds). pp 205–224. Academic Press.

Percy, D.H., Barthold, S.W. (1993). Rabbit. In *Pathology of Laboratory Rodents and Rabbits*, pp 179–223. Iowa State University Press.

Redrobe, S. (2000). Surgical procedures and dental disorders. In *Manual of Rabbit Medicine and Surgery* (P.A. Flecknell, ed.) pp 117–134. British Small Animal Veterinary Association.

Reverte, M., Garcia-Barrado, M.J., Hernandez-Garcia, F.J., Moratinos, J. (1993). Coexistence of beta 2- and beta 3-adrenoreceptors in plasma potassium control in conscious rabbits (Abstract). *J Auton Pharmacol.*, **13**, 227–236.

Riley, J.H., Cornelius, L.M. (1989). Electrolytes, blood gases and acid base balance. In *The Clinical Chemistry of Laboratory Animals* (W.F. Loeb, F.W. Quimby, eds). pp 347–408. Pergamon Press.

Robson, W.L., Bayliss. C.E., Feldman, R. *et al.* (1981). Evaluation of the effect of pentobarbitone anaesthesia on the plasma potassium concentration of the rabbit and the dog. *Can Anaesth Soc J.*, **28**, 210–216.

Rothfritz, P., Loeffler, K., Drescher, B. (1992). Einflu-unterschiedlicher Haltungs-verfahren und Bewegungsmöglichkeiten auf die Spongiosastruktur der Rippen sowie Brust- und Lendenwirbel von Versuchs- und Fieischkaninchen (Article in German). *TierärztlUmschau*, **47**, 758–768.

Rübel, G.A., Isenbügel, E., Wolvekamp, P. (1991). Rabbit. In *Diagnostic Radiology of Exotic Pets*. Wolfe Publishing Ltd.

Sattler, N., Fecteau, G., Girard, C., Couture, Y. (1998). Description of 14 cases of bovine hypokalaemia syndrome. *Vet Rec.*, **14**, 503–507.

Smith Baxter, J. (1975). Posterior paralysis in the rabbit. *J Small Anim Pract.*, **16**, 267–271.

Swindle, M.M, Shealy, P.M. (1996). Common surgical procedures in rodents and rabbits. In *Handbook of Rodent and Rabbit Medicine* (K. Laber-Laird, M.M. Swindle, P. Flecknell, eds). pp 239–255. Pergamon Press.

Terjesen, T., Benum, P. (1983). Stress protection after external fixation on the intact rabbit tibia (Abstract). *Acta Orthop Scand.*, **54**, 648–654.

Thomas, W.B. (2000). Vestibular dysfunction. *Vet Clin N Am: Small Anim Pract.*, **30**, 227–249.

Waller, T. (1979). Sensitivity of *Encephalitozoon cuniculi* to various temperatures, disinfectants and drugs. *Lab Anim.*, **13**, 227–230.

Willard, M.D. (1989). Disorders of potassium homeostasis. *Vet Clin N Am: Small Anim Pract.*, **19**, 241–263.

Wu, D.D., Boyd, R.D., Fix, T.J., Burr, D.B. (1990). Regional patterns of bone loss and altered bone remodelling in response to calcium deprivation in laboratory rabbits. *Calcif Tissue Int.*, **47**, 18–23.

Yamanaka, T., Sasa, M., Amano, T. *et al.* (1995). Role of glucocorticoid in vestibular compensation in relation to activation of vestibular nucleus neurons (Abstract). *Acta Otolaryngol Suppl.*, **519**, 168–172.

13

Cardiorespiratory disease

13.1 Anatomy and physiology of the respiratory system

Rabbits have sensitive nostrils and a good sense of smell. There are 20–25 vibrissae in each upper lip. In healthy rabbits, the nostrils are constantly twitching at a rate of 2–120 times per minute, unless the rabbit is at rest (Brewer and Cruise, 1994) or is unwell. The nasal cavity is lined with a protective layer of mucus that entraps foreign particles and bacteria. The mucus also prevents water loss and enhances the sense of smell. The nasal glands secrete serous fluid into the nasal cavity. In the rabbit, there is glandular tissue along the nasal septum and a cluster of glands, collectively known as the lateral nasal gland, occupy the entire wall between the nasal cavity and maxillary sinus (Bojsen-Moller, 1964). The function of these nasal glands is to moisten inspired air, which has a role in thermoregulation. The position of the conchal and maxillary sinuses and the structures of the nasal cavity are illustrated in Figures 3.9 and 7.1. There is no frontal sinus.

The oropharynx is narrow and the base of the tongue is large in rabbits. The glottis is small. Breathing takes place through the nostrils. Mouth breathing only occurs during severe respiratory distress.

Each lung is divided into cranial, middle and caudal lobes and there is an accessory lobe on the right lung. Respiratory movement in rabbits is mainly diaphragmatic rather than due to the action of the intercostal muscles. The thoracic cavity is small and the thymus, which remains large throughout life, occupies the anterior ventral thoracic cavity (see Figure 13.3).

13.2 Respiratory diseases

13.2.1 Pasteurellosis

Pasteurella multocida is associated with a number of diseases of rabbits (see Section 16.5.1). Pasteurellosis is not a recognized problem in wild rabbits but is a serious disease in colonies of commercial or laboratory rabbits. In pet rabbits, although *P. multocida* is found as an opportunist pathogen in many secondary infections, primary pasteurellosis is uncommon. It is usually encountered in the newly acquired rabbit that has recently been bought from a breeder or pet shop. Respiratory disease is the most common manifestation. Acute infections and septicaemia occur, especially in young animals, but chronic, insidious recurrent infections are more common in the adult pet rabbit. Rhinitis, conjunctivitis, nasolacrimal duct infections, otitis media, tracheitis and bronchopneumonia can all be caused by *Pasteurella multocida.* The organism can spread to other sites from the nasal cavity where it can reside as a commensal organism. Infection often persists despite mucosal and humoral antibody responses in addition to effusive neutrophilic exudation. The deleterious effect of pasteurellosis on laboratory colonies of rabbits and interference with experimental procedures has resulted in the evolution of expensive 'pasteurella-free' rabbits for use in research. The epidemiology of pasteurellosis is discussed in Section 16.5.1. Many predisposing factors trigger disease.

13.2.2 Respiratory disease due to pasteurellosis

Pet rabbits are often already infected with *P. multocida* when they are purchased from a pet shop or breeder. The development of rhinitis and other respiratory tract problems in the newly acquired young rabbit is likely to be due to pasteurellosis. In the older animal, stress or poor husbandry can result in a flare up of a latent infection. Poor air quality, caused by high ammonia levels, or dusty hay irritate the respiratory tract and predisposes secondary infection. Many owners like to protect their rabbits from inclement weather by covering the hutch or placing them in a poorly ventilated damp shed during the winter months. Ventilation and good air quality is important in disease prevention. Pasteurellosis can be spread between animals and the disease is endemic in most breeding establishments. It often causes problems in premises, such as sanctuaries, where several animals are housed in close proximity. A distance of greater than 1.8 m (6 feet) or 'sneezing distance' is needed to control the spread of infection between individuals (Whittaker, 1989).

13.2.3 Rhinitis ('snuffles')

Repetitive sneezing and upper respiratory tract noise is a feature of rhinitis. Rhinitis and sinusitis can be manifestations of pasteurellosis, although other organisms such as staphylococci or *Bordetella* can also be involved. The differential diagnosis of upper respiratory tract disease in rabbits includes nasal foreign bodies and periapical abscesses of the maxillary incisors or premolars. Both these conditions are common in the pet rabbit so it cannot be assumed that all rabbits with a purulent nasal discharge are suffering from pasteurellosis or that all cases of 'snuffles' are due to infectious agents.

In the initial stages of pasteurellosis, the nasal discharge is serous and the condition is responsive to antibiotic therapy. In advanced cases, the nasal discharge is thick, yellow and viscid. Copious amounts of mucopurulent material can be discharged from the nostrils and form crusts on the surrounding skin. Affected rabbits wipe the purulent discharges from their nose with their forepaws, which become matted and discoloured. Coughing is not as common as sneezing and snortling. Respiratory noises may be audible to the owner who may think their rabbit is 'wheezing'. Anorexia can occur, perhaps due to a reduced sense of smell or because it is difficult to chew and breathe at the same time. Grooming difficulties occur because the rabbit finds it difficult to breathe and groom simultaneously. Response to antibiotic therapy is poor in advanced cases and relapse is common. *Post-mortem* examination of the sinuses and nasal passages of rabbits with chronic rhinitis shows why these cases are so difficult to treat. The nasal cavity is filled with pus, which can spread into the paranasal sinuses (see Figure 7.1 and Figure 13.1). The pus becomes thick and inspissated. There is ulceration of the mucous membranes and osteomyelitis of the turbinates causing severe atrophy and erosion (Deeb, 1997). The presence of pus in the nasal cavity impedes gas exchange and causes physical discomfort and irritation.

13.2.3.1 Differential diagnosis of rhinitis

The clinical history can be very suggestive of pasteurellosis. Young rabbits that have recently been stressed by weaning, change in routine and transport are often exposed to infection at the breeding establishment where they originated. Rabbits housed with several others in sheds and outhouses are susceptible. In older, individual pet rabbits, bacterial infection is less likely to be a cause of rhinitis than dental disease, which is common. Nasal foreign bodies can cause rhinitis (see Section 13.3). Myxomatosis is another possible cause of rhinitis. Myxomatosis in rabbit colonies can present as rhinitis in association with ocular discharge. Aerosol infection is more likely to give respiratory tract signs that insect spread (see Section 16.6.1). Myxomatosis is progressive and almost invariably fatal.

Bacteriology can be used to identify bacteria that are present in the nasal passages of rabbits with rhinitis and to ascertain antibiotic sensitivity. The rabbit's nose is sensitive and it can be difficult to insert the swab deep into the nasal passages in the conscious animal.

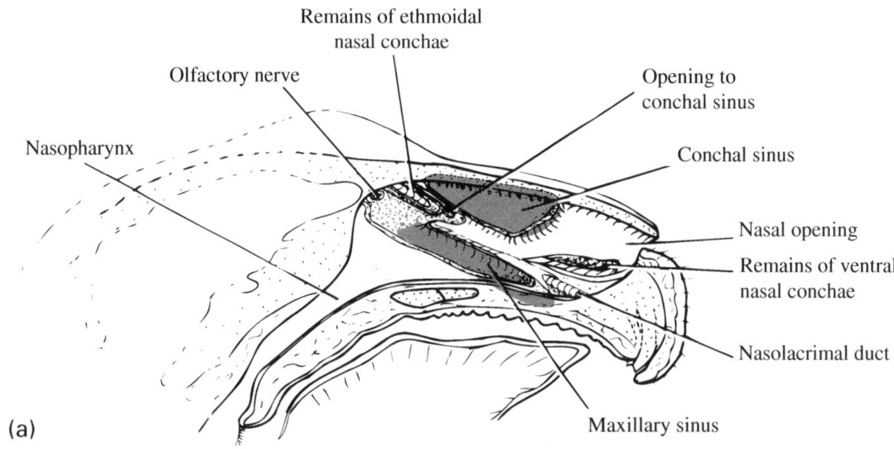

(a)

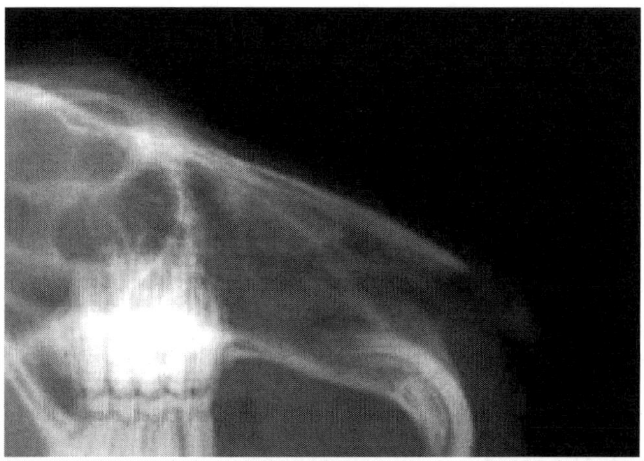

(b)

Figure 13.1. (a) **Sagittal section through the head to show the position of the paranasal sinuses.** This figure was drawn from a *post mortem* specimen of a sagittal section through a decalcified head. The nasal conchae have been removed. There are two paranasal sinuses in rabbits: the conchal sinus and the maxillary sinus. There is no frontal sinus. Both the conchal and the maxillary sinus form blind cavities. At the cranial end of each sinus there is a single opening into the nasal passage. The structures of the nasal cavity are illustrated in Figure 3.9. The position of the paranasal sinuses is also illustrated in Figure 7.1. (b) **Chronic infection of the conchal sinus.** This figure is a lateral view of the nasal cavity of an 18-month-old Dwarf Lop female rabbit with chronic rhinitis. The rabbit had started sneezing and developed a nasal discharge shortly after she was purchased at 10 weeks of age. Antibiotic therapy and mucolytic therapy failed to cure the condition although the symptoms were temporarily alleviated. Radiology shows increased radiopacity of the conchal sinus indicating the presence of infection. There is erosion of the turbinates. The conchae and ethmoturbinates are not visible on the radiograph. Rhinitis was due to infection and not related to dental disease.

Sedation or anaesthesia is usually required to take a deep nasal swab for culture.

Underlying dental problems can be diagnosed by visual examination and by radiography (see Section 7.6 and Figure 13.1a). The structures of the nose and teeth can be assessed on skull radiographs. The paranasal sinuses can be identified (see Figures 7.5 and 13.1) and abnormalities may be detected radiologically. Opacity of the

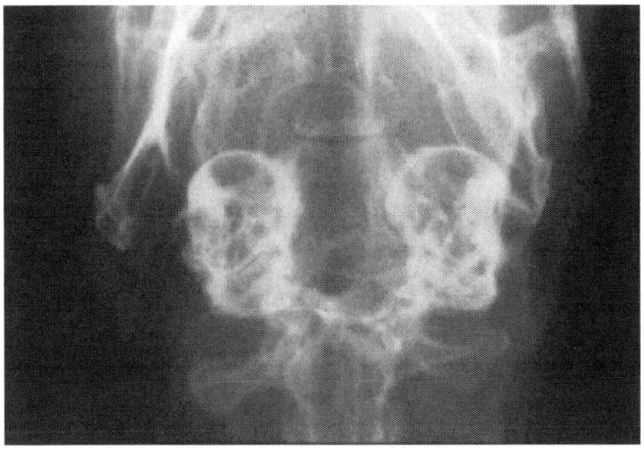

(a)

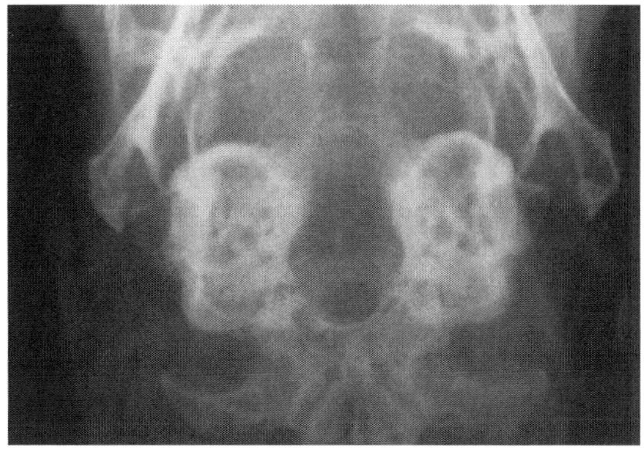

(b)

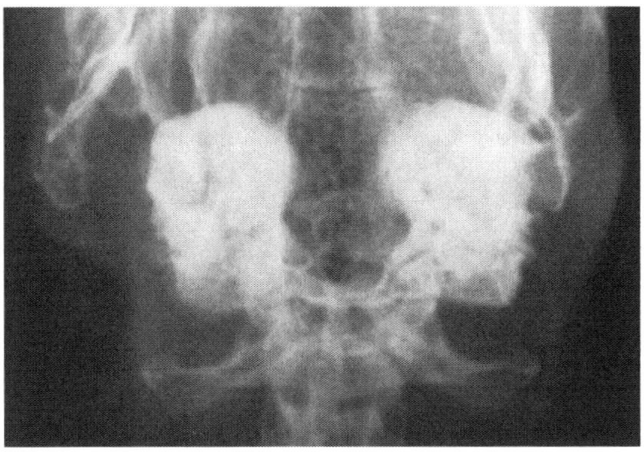

(c)

Figure 13.2. Radiographic changes of the tympanic bulla. (a)–(c) are dorso ventral views of the caudal area of the skull to show progressive changes of the tympanic bullae from normal (a) to severe (c); (b) was an incidental finding on a rabbit that was radiographed to investigate his dental disease.; and (c) was of a 3-year-old French Lop male that was rescued by the RSPCA from a small shed containing between 20–30 rabbits. Upper respiratory problems were endemic. The rabbit appeared totally deaf and was ataxic. He was quiet and subdued. He was euthanased due to dental problems. Post-mortem examination showed pus in both tympanic bullae.

conchal sinus indicates the presence of exudate (see Figure 13.1b). Erosion of the ethmoturbinates can be seen on a well-exposed radiograph. However, the presence of *P. multocida* or other bacterial infection and erosion of the turbinates does not rule out the possibility of an underlying foreign body or perapical abscess. Large abscesses or rhinoliths can form in the nasal passages because of tooth root infection (see Plate 17).

13.2.4 Otitis media

Pasteurella multocida primarily resides in the nasal cavity but can spread via the eustachian tube to the tympanic bulla and affect the middle ear (see Plate 27). Infection can spread further to affect the inner ear and vestibular apparatus or track through the acoustic meatus and along the vestibulocochlear nerve. On *post-mortem* examination abscesses can be found in the cranial cavity.

It is not easy to diagnose otitis media in the live rabbit. The presence of exudate in the external ear canal does not signify the presence of otitis media. In many pet rabbits, especially lop eared breeds, it is difficult to visualize the tympanic membrane due to the presence of waxy ear secretion. *Post-mortem* examination of the horizontal ear canal of pet rabbits often reveals the presence of inspissated pus that occludes the horizontal canal. The presence of purulent material in the external ear canal does not necessarily signify the presence of pus in the tympanic bulla. Neither does pus in the tympanic bulla always cause otitis interna and vestibular symptoms (see Section 12.4.3). Radiological changes can often be seen as an incidental finding on skull radiographs (see Figure 13.2). It seems likely that rabbits with pus in the external ear canal and/or the tympanic bulla will have impaired hearing although they may appear clinically normal. Some observant owners can detect hearing deficits in their pets and aggression in rabbits has been attributed to deafness when rabbits have been startled by the unheard approach of their owners.

In a study by Flatt *et al.* (1977), otitis media was found in 4% of 2001 young rabbits and 32% of adults slaughtered for human consumption. The animals were clinically healthy on *ante-mortem* inspection. Gross lesions included the presence of white tenacious exudate filling the tympanic bulla. The mucous membrane lining the bulla was thickened, translucent and discoloured. The eustachian tube was dilated and filled with pus. Microscopic lesions consisted of an accumulation of heterophils in the lumen of the tympanic bulla and in the mucosa and underlying periosteum. In some of the affected ears, the simple squamous epithelium over the tympanic membrane and auditory ossicles had undergone squamous metaplasia with necrosis of the mucosa in severe cases. In the rabbits with periosteal changes, the thickened periosteum was infiltrated by a variable number of heterophils, plasma cells and lymphocytes. Occasionally granulation tissue was present. In some cases, the tympanic membrane was ruptured and a suppurative exudate was present in the tympanic cavity and the external auditory canal.

13.2.5 Pneumonia

Septicaemia and acute suppurative pneumonia can be caused by *Pasteurella multocida*. Infection can be peracute and cause rapid death (see Plate 28). Chronic pneumonia and abscesses in the thoracic cavity also occur. Poor exercise tolerance and increased respiratory rate may not be obvious to owners of pet rabbits that are confined to hutches or small runs with no opportunity to exercise. These individuals pose a poor anaesthetic risk due to poor gas exchange in consolidated lungs.

13.2.6 Treatment of pasteurellosis

Pasteurellosis is a difficult condition to cure. Acute upper or lower respiratory infections can be responsive to prompt antibiotic and non-steroidal anti-inflammatory medication. An antibiotic that is unlikely to cause diarrhoea but is effective against *Pasteurella multocida* should be selected. Examples include enrofloxacin, trimethoprim sulpha combinations, tetracyclines, parenteral cephalexin or penicillin. *In vitro*, most rabbit isolates of *P. multocida* are susceptible to penicillin, chloramphenicol, tetracycline, erythromycin, novobiocin and nitrofurans with a variable susceptibility to streptomycin, kanamycin, neomycin and sulphonamides. *P. multocida* is usually resistant to clindamycin and lincomycin (Manning *et al.*, 1989). Penicillin has been used widely to treat rhinitis in laboratory rabbits (Gaertner, 1991). Concurrent infection with other pathogens such as *Bordetella bronchiseptica* can affect the response to therapy. Tilmicosin is an effective antibiotic in the treatment of acute pasteurellosis in sheep and has been used to treat rabbits despite the possibility of a fatal adverse reaction to the drug (see Section 4.2.1.11).

Long-term or periodic courses of antibiotic can be given to control long-standing infections although they are unlikely to be curative. Antibiotics can also be introduced directly into the nose. Some rabbits will tolerate this procedure. Gentamicin is available as an ophthalmic preparation (Tiacil, Virbac) that can be used as nose drops. Purulent exudate needs to be removed before the drops are instlled.

Chronic pasteurellosis is manifested by the presence of copious quantities of thick, viscid, mucopurulent material that presents a physical barrier to medication. The pus is often in inaccessible sites such as the nasal passages, paranasal sinuses, tympanic bullae or even the brain. Surgery, such as trephination, to remove the pus, provide drainage and create a route for local medication, is theoretically possible. Bulla osteotomy has been suggested as a treatment for rabbits with severe, refractory, chronic otitis media in association with vestibular signs such as head tilt and anorexia (Redrobe, 2000). The surgical technique has been described (Swindle and Shealy, 1996; Redrobe, 2000), but there are no follow-up reports of the success of the procedure. Anecdotally, the results of bulla osteotomy are disappointing. Anorexic rabbits are not good surgical subjects. Trephination of sinuses has not been described in rabbits but rarely provides freedom from clinical signs of chronic sinusitis in cats.

The chances of successful treatment of pasteurellosis are greater in sites where the pus can be removed, e.g. by flushing an infected nasolacrimal duct or removing an abscess or infected organ such as a uterus or testicle. Dacryocystitis, facial abscesses or purulent nasal discharges are often associated with underlying dental disease that needs to be addressed if there is to be any hope of success in treating the secondary pasteurella infection (see Section 7.5.5 and 8.1).

In cases of rhinitis, it is important to establish adequate systemic hydration by ensuring adequate fluid intake. Dry airways result in increased viscosity of secretions, decreased ciliary function, inflammation, and degeneration of the mucosa. The inclusion of fresh leafy vegetables in the diet can increase a rabbit's fluid intake. Water can be added to inspired gases by the use of humidifiers or placing the rabbit in a steamed-up room such as a bathroom. Nebulization is sometimes used as a method of introducing antibiotic, decongestants and other agents directly into the respiratory tract and to loosen secretions and bring relief. Nebulization introduces charged particles into the respiratory tract as an aerosol. In other species, nebulization is used to treat lower respiratory tract disease. Medication introduced by nebulization is unlikely to reach the tympanic bullae or paranasal sinuses or to penetrate thick mucopurulent exudate in rabbits. Mucolytic agents such as bromexine or *N*-acetyl-cysteine have been recommended for nebulization in rabbits with rhinitis (Meredith, 2000). In other species, *N*-acetyl-cysteine is irritating to mucosal surfaces and can inactivate certain antibiotics when it is mixed with them (McKiernan, 1983). Systemic bromhexine (Bisolvon, Boehringer Ingelheim) can be used as a mucolytic in rabbits. In cattle and pigs, when bromhexine is administered simultaneously with oxytetracycline, the antibiotic in the bronchial mucus is considerably increased (product datasheet).

Occasionally, zealous owners administer human decongestants to their rabbits. There is no proven efficacy in the use of such products in the treatment of 'snuffles'.

Key points 13.1

- Healthy rabbits can twitch their nose at a rate of 2–120 times per minute
- The nasal gland of the rabbit is well developed and humidifies inspired air, which is part of temperature regulation
- Mouth breathing only occurs during severe respiratory distress
- *P. multocida* is a significant cause of acute and chronic respiratory disease in rabbits
- Rhinitis ('snuffles') can be caused by dental disease or nasal foreign bodies as well as pasteurellosis. Other bacterial and fungal agents can also be involved
- In the initial stages, when the nasal discharge is serous, antibiotics can be effective in the treatment of pasteurellosis. As the disease progresses, the discharge becomes a thick, viscid, mucopurulent exudate that is refractory to treatment
- Osteomyelitis and erosion of the nasal turbinates occurs in long-standing infections. Pus can be present in the sinuses or tympanic bullae. Abscesses may develop in the brain
- Treatment of advanced cases of rhinitis is unlikely to be successful. Antibiotics may be effective in controlling the disease. Long-term or intermittent periodic antibiotic therapy may be indicated
- Antibiotics can be introduced into the nose using nose drops
- Hydration of the nasal mucosa is important. The inclusion of fresh vegetables in the diet will increase water intake. Steam therapy by placing the rabbit in a steam filled room may be helpful
- Nebulization can be used to introduce antibiotics and/or mucolytics into the respiratory tract and to loosen secretions. Nebulization is more likely to be effective in the treatment of lower respiratory tract disease than in cases of rhinitis, sinusitis or otitis media where mucopurulent exudates form an effective barrier
- The mucolytic agent, bromhexine (Bisolvon, Boehringer Ingelheim) can be given orally or by nebulization
- Human decongestants are unlikely to be effective.

Oxymetazoline is a common topical nasal decongestant that has been investigated in

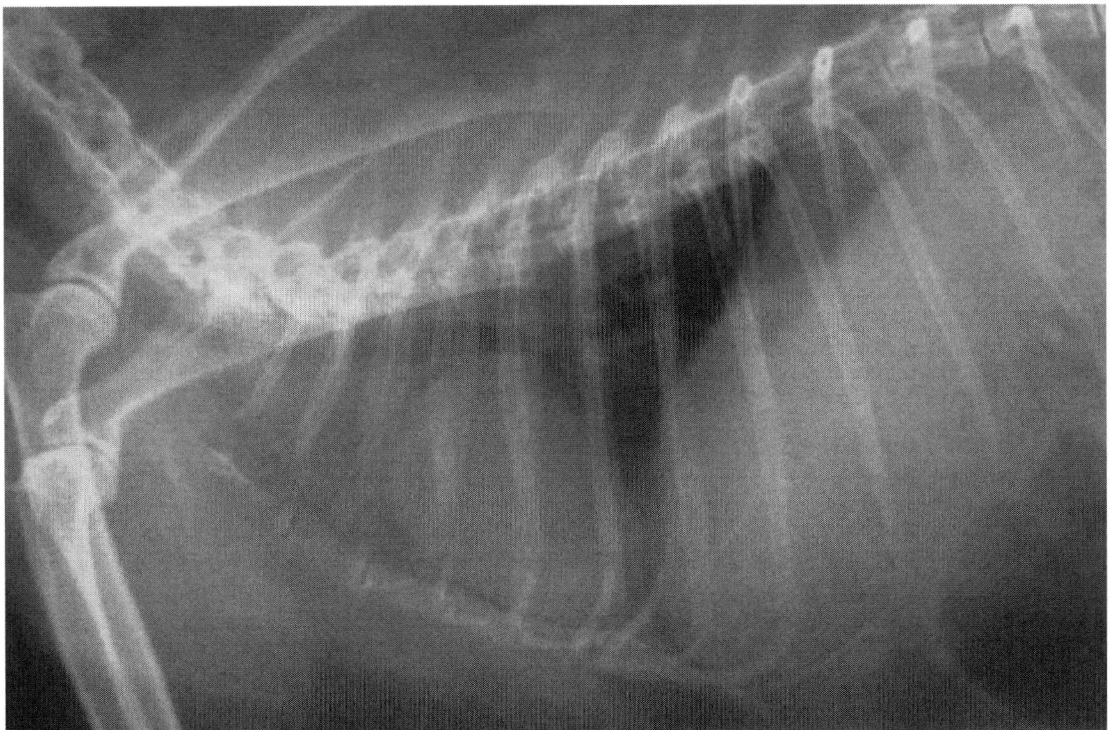

(a)

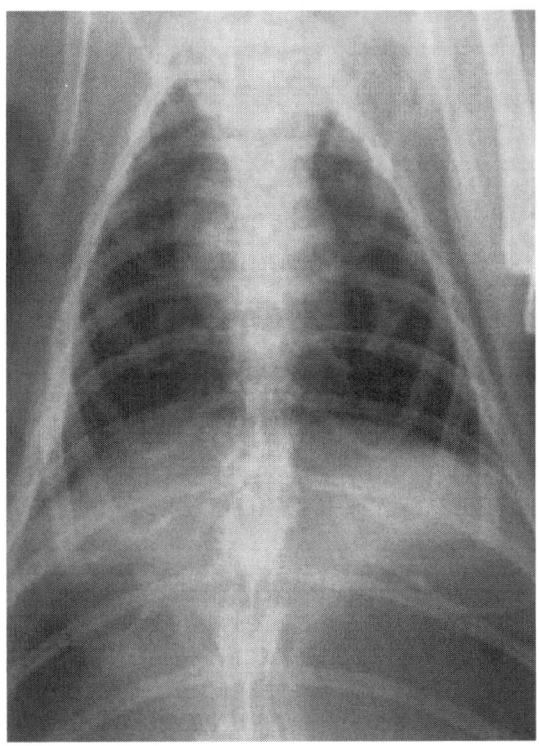

(b)

Figure 13.3. Radiographic anatomy of the thoracic cavity. Sedation or general anaesthesia is required to position a rabbit for thoracic radiography. The forelegs need to be retracted cranially to prevent superimposition of the scapulae on the cranial portion of the thoracic cavity.

Normal findings:

- The thoracic cavity is small in comparison with the abdominal cavity.
- The heart occupies a relatively large volume of the thoracic cavity.
- The small cranial lung lobes are not as seen in as much detail as the caudal lobes.
- The thymus remains large throughout life.
- The aorta and caudal vena cava should be visible.
- In obese animals, intrathoracic fat deposits can sometimes be seen (Rübel *et al.*,1991).
- Cartilage rings are often visible within the tracheal wall.
- The carina lies at the 4th or 5th intercostal space.
- The pulmonary vessels can be seen within the lungs.

(a) Shows a normal lateral view of the thoracic cavity, and (b) shows the dorsoventral view.

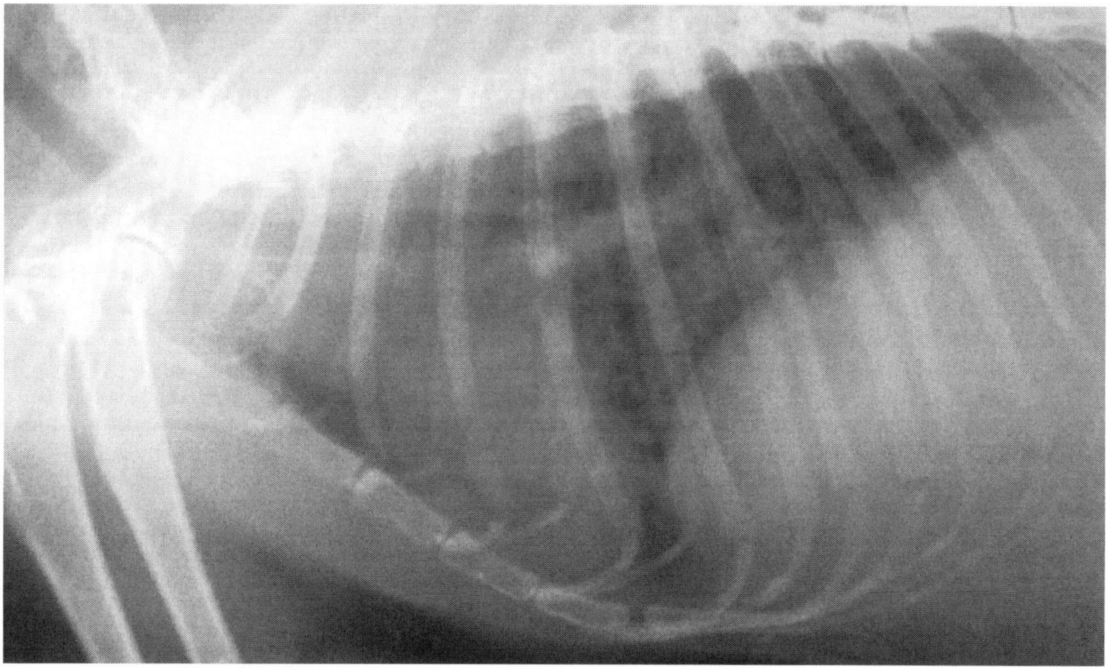

(a)

Figure 13.4: Pneumonia
Figures 13.4a and 13.4b show a lateral and dorsoventral view of a four-year-old Himalayan neutered male rabbit that was thin, anorexic and dyspnoeic. An alveolar pattern can be seen on both views. At *post mortem* examination, pneumonic changes were found throughout the lung tissue.

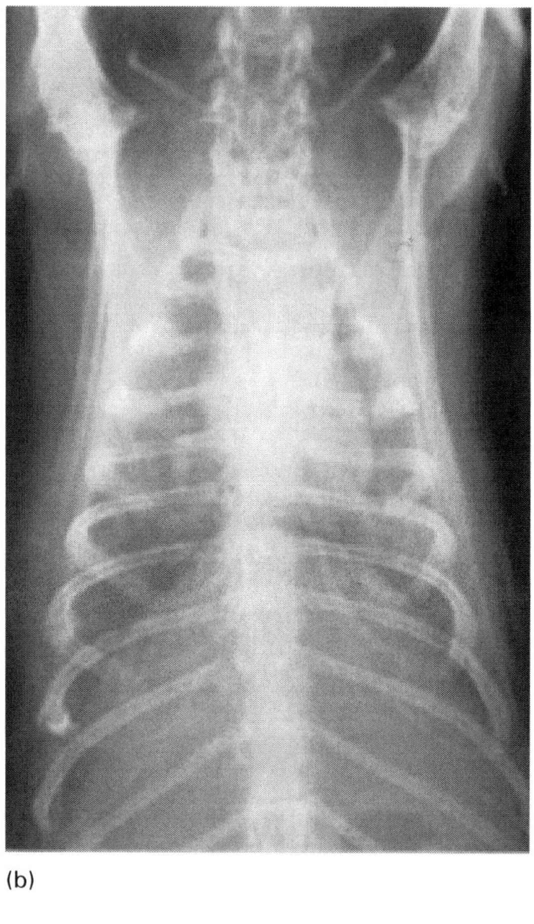

(b)

experimentally induced infections of the maxillary sinus in rabbits (Bende *et al.*, 1996). Paradoxically, a higher degree of inflammation was found in the oxymetazoline treated sinuses. The authors concluded that oxymetazoline nose drops interfere with the normal defence mechanisms possibly by a decrease in mucosal blood flow.

13.3 Nasal foreign bodies

Pieces of hay, grass seeds or shafts of hair can enter and become lodged in the nasal cavity. Repetitive sneezing, nose rubbing and a unilateral discharge are indicative of a nasal foreign body. If the foreign material has penetrated deep into the nasopharynx, snortling and dyspnoea can occur which can be mistaken for pneumonia. The patency of the nasal passages can be assessed by occluding each nostril in turn and listening to the respiratory noises. Sometimes the end of a blade of hay or hair shaft can be seen protruding from the nostril (see Plate 29). The foreign body can be gently pulled out. In other cases, endoscopy is required. Dislodging or removing a nasal foreign body often results in a complete recovery.

13.3.1 Endoscopic examination of the nasal passages

The nasal passages can be examined endoscopically. They require flushing to clear away discharges and exudate prior to endoscopic examination. Foreign material can also be flushed out during the procedure. Nasal flushing in rabbits poses problems due to the small nasopharynx and inaccessible larynx. Great care is required to prevent purulent material entering the larynx and trachea. Endotracheal intubation is mandatory and the rabbit should be positioned so fluid drains out of the mouth. The nasal passages are examined using a rigid endoscope such as a 1.9 mm needlescope (Stortz) and irrigation sheath. The endoscope can go from the nostril to the nasopharynx via the ventral meatus and can also be used to explore the turbinate area.

13.4 Dyspnoea

The differential diagnoses for dyspnoea is given in Table 3.2 and includes acute pasteurellosis, viral haemorrhagic disease, heat stroke, cardiac disease and pleural effusions due to cardiac disease. Metastatic tumours can also cause dyspnoea. Uterine adenocarcinomas can metastasize to the lungs where they are seen as multiple spherical opacities (Rübel *et al.*, 1991). Some rabbits with upper respiratory tract disease are dyspnoeic because they cannot breathe through their nose. As in other species, external trauma can cause chest injuries and respiratory problems. Bite wounds from predators can penetrate the chest wall causing serious internal injury and introducing infection. A small external wound can easily be overlooked. Abscesses can develop within the thoracic cavity as result of haematogenous spread from other sites. Auscultation and radiology are useful adjuncts to clinical examination. Radiographic features of the normal chest are illustrated in Figure 13.3. Chronic pneumonia is illustrated in Figure 13.4.

13.5 Heat stroke

Rabbits are tolerant of low temperatures and can withstand sub-zero environmental temperatures without discomfort providing they are acclimatized and healthy, and have shelter with plenty of bedding. Their dense fur insulates them from the effects of cold weather but can be a liability in hot weather.

Rabbits do not sweat and cannot pant effectively. The ears play an important part in thermoregulation. Signs of heat stroke are similar to other species: anorexia, increased respiratory rate, prostration, pulmonary oedema, cyanosis and death. Some cases can have blood-tinged fluid from the nose and mouth. A high rectal temperature (in excess of 40°C) is suggestive of heat stroke. Treatment is aimed at reducing body temperature, e.g. bathing in cold water, wetting the ears and blowing them with a cold hair drier. The administration of a vasodilator such as acetylpromazine may be helpful.

13.6 Cardiovascular disease

Most recorded information about cardiac diseases relates to infectious, toxin-induced or diet-related diseases of laboratory rabbits. Heart disease also occurs in pet rabbits and hopefully, more information will become available as rabbits live longer and more diagnostic and therapeutic procedures are adopted for the individual animal. Congenital abnormalities such as ventricular septal defects do occur. Diagnosis and treatment follow the same lines as for dogs and cats with most cases being positively diagnosed by echocardiography. Electrocardiography is also feasible in rabbits. Some reference values for normal parameters determined in laboratory rabbits are give in Box 13.1

Box 13.1 Circulatory data

Electrocardiography (from Kozma *et al.*, 1974)

P wave:	0.1–0.15 mv and 0.03–0.04 s
	Low or negative in lead I
	Always positive in leads II–III
P–R:	0.05–0.1 s
QRS:	0.015–0.04 s

Arterial blood pressure

Systolic:	90–130 mmHg
Diastolic:	80–90 mmHg

Arterial blood pH

7.2–7.5

Key points 13.2

- Dyspnoea can be caused by upper respiratory disease, pasteurellosis, viral haemorrhagic disease, heat stroke, cardiac disease, trauma or pleural effusion. Pleural effusion can be secondary to primary or secondary neoplasia
- Heat stroke occurs readily in rabbits as they do not sweat or pant effectively. A rectal temperature in excess of 40°C is indicative of heat stroke
- Cardiac disease occurs in pet rabbits.
- Cardiomyopathy of unknown aetiology is associated with giant breeds
- Congenital abnormalities such as septal defects occur
- In laboratory rabbits, vitamin E deficiency, coronavirus, *E. cuniculi* and bacterial infections such as Tyzzer's disease have been shown to cause myocardial changes.

13.6.1 Cardiomyopathy

Cardiomyopathy occurs in pet rabbits. Giant breeds appear most susceptible (see Plate 30) but the aetiology is unknown at the present time. Histopathological findings indicate the presence of myocardial fibrosis.

The rabbit myocardium can be affected by several diseases. Vitamin E deficiency, coronavirus infection and some bacterial infections such as salmonellosis and pasteurellosis have been recorded as causes of cardiomyopathy in laboratory rabbits (Marini *et al.*, 1999). Tyzzer's disease not only causes intestinal and hepatic lesions but can also cause a myocarditis resulting in myocardial fibrosis in those animals that survive (Percy and Barthold, 1993). *Encephalitozoon cuniculi* has been reported as a cause of myocarditis in rabbits (Pakes and Gerrity, 1994). Stress and catecholamines are proven causes of cardiomyopathy and experimental models of the human disease can be provided by keeping rabbits in overcrowded conditions (Weber and Van der Walt, 1975). Myocardial necrosis and fibrosis have been recorded in rabbits anaesthetized with ketamine/xylazine combinations by continuous infusion. Marini *et al.* (1999) postulate that hypoxaemia and coronary vasoconstriction result in cell death and necrosis. The rabbit has limited collateral coronary circulation and is therefore predisposed to ischaemia induced by coronary vasoconstriction. The authors draw an analogy with rabbits used as models of catecholamine-induced cardiomyopathy in which alpha-adrenergic mediated coronary vasoconstriction occurs. Hypotension and hypoxaemia are further contributory factors.

13.6.2 Arteriosclerosis

Arteriosclerosis is a thickening and hardening of the arteriolar walls resulting from proliferative or degenerative changes. Aortic arteriosclerosis occurs in rabbits and can cause seizures or vague symptoms such as inactivity and weight loss. Mineralization of the aorta occurs in hypercalcaemic rabbits, usually in association with renal disease that impairs calcium excretion. Mineralization of the aorta is seen radiologically (Shell and Saunders, 1989) and on *post-mortem* examination. Calcification of the aorta is often associated with calcification of the kidney (see Section 14.4.2). Calcification of soft tissues can be caused by excessive intestinal absorption of calcium, such as in cases of vitamin D toxicity.

13.6.3 Coronavirus

Coronaviris infection in rabbits can result in cardiomyopathy and pleural effusion. Experimentally, coronavirus infected rabbits are used as laboratory models to study virus-induced cardiomyopathy. The disease was first discovered in Sweden in the 1960s in rabbits inoculated with emulsified testicular tissue containing *Treponema pallidum* (human syphilis). Coronavirus was found in the testicular tissue. An analogy has been made between rabbit coronavirus and feline infectious peritonitis. Clinical signs vary, but infected rabbits are generally pyrexic and many die within 5 days of infection. Pulmonary oedema, pleural effusion and dilation of the right ventricle are found at *post-mortem*. As in feline infectious peritonitis, hypergammaglobulinaemia is a feature of chronic infection that can be manifested by myocardial degeneration, ascites and uveitis. An enteric form has also been described. At the present time, coronavirus induced pleural effusion and cardiomyopathy have only been reported in experimentally inoculated rabbits (DiGiacomo and Mare, 1994). It has not been described in pet rabbits.

References

Bende, M., Fukami, M., Arfors, K.E. *et al.* (1996). Effect of oxymetazoline nose drops on acute sinusitis in the rabbit (Abstract). *Ann Otol Rhinol Laryngol.*, **105**, 222–225.

Bojsen-Moller, F. (1964). Topography of the nasal glands in rats and some other mammals. *Anat Rec.*, **150**, 11–24.

Brewer, N.R., Cruise, L.J. (1994). Physiology. In *The Biology of the Laboratory Rabbit*, 2nd edn. (P.J. Manning, D.H. Ringler, C.E. Newcomer, eds). pp 63–70. Academic Press.

Deeb, B.J. (1997). Respiratory disease and the pasteurella complex. In *Ferrets, Rabbits and Rodents, Clinical Medicine and Surgery* (E.V. Hillyer, K.E. Quesenberry, eds). pp 189–201. W.B. Saunders.

DiGiacomo, R.F., Mare, J. (1994). Viral diseases. In *The Biology of the Laboratory Rabbit*, 2nd edn. (P.J. Manning, D.H. Ringler, C.E. Newcomer, eds). pp 171–197. Academic Press.

Flatt, R.E., Deyoung, D.W., Hogle, R.M. (1977). Suppurative otitis media in the rabbit: prevalence, pathology and microbiology. *Lab Anim Sci.*, **27**, 343–347.

Gaertner, D.J. (1991). Comparison of penicillin and gentamycin for treatment of pasteurellosis in rabbits. *Lab Anim Sci.*, **41**, 78–79.

Kozma, C., Macklin, W., Cummins, L.M. Mauer, R. (1974). The anatomy, physiology and the biochemistry of the rabbit. In *The Biology of the Laboratory Rabbit* (S.H. Weisbroth, R.E. Flatt, A.L. Kraus, eds). pp 50–69. Academic Press.

Manning, P.J., Digiacomo, R.F., Delong, D. (1989). Pasteurellosis in laboratory animals. In *Pasteurella and Pasteurellosis* (C. Adlam, J.M. Rutter eds). pp 264–289. Academic Press.

Marini, R.P., Xiantung, L., Harpster, N.K., Dangler, C. (1999). Cardiovascular pathology possibly associated with ketamine/xylazine anesthesia in Dutch Belted rabbits. *Lab Anim Sci.*, **49**, 153–160.

McKiernan, B.C. (1983). Lower respiratory tract disease. In *Textbook of Veterinary Internal Medicine, Diseases of the Dog and Cat*, 2nd edn. (S.J. Ettinger, ed.) pp 760–828. W.B. Saunders.

Meredith, A. (2000). Respiratory system and disorders. In *Manual of Rabbit Medicine and Surgery* (P.A. Flecknell, ed.) pp 33–38. British Small Animal Veterinary Association.

Pakes, S.P., Gerrity, L.W. (1994). Protozoal diseases. In *The Biology of the Laboratory Rabbit*, 2nd edn. (P.J. Manning, D.H. Ringler, C.E. Newcomer, eds). pp 205–224. Academic Press.

Percy, D.H., Barthold S.W. (1993). Rabbit. In *Pathology of Laboratory Rodents and Rabbits.* pp 179–223. Iowa State University Press.

Redrobe, S. (2000). Surgical procedures and dental disorders. In *Manual of Rabbit Medicine and Surgery* (P.A. Flecknell, ed.) pp 117–134. British Small Animal Veterinary Association.

Rübel, G.A., Isenbügel, E., Wolvekamp, P. (1991). Rabbit. In *Diagnostic Radiology of Exotic Pets.* Wolfe Publishing Ltd.

Shell, L.G., Saunders, G. (1989). Arteriosclerosis in a rabbit. *J Am Vet Med Assoc.*, **194**, 679–680.

Swindle, M.M., Shealy, P.M. (1996). Common surgical procedures in rodents and rabbits. In *Handbook of Rodent and Rabbit Medicine* (K. Laber-Laird, M.M. Swindle, P. Flecknell, eds). pp 239–255. Pergamon Press.

Weber, H.W., Van der Walt, J.J. (1975). Cardiomyopathy in crowded rabbits (Abstract). *Recent Adv Stud Cardiac Struct Metab.*, **6**, 471–477.

Whittaker, D.(1989). Pasteurellosis in the laboratory rabbit: a review. *Vet Ann.*, **29**, 285–291.

Urinogenital diseases

14

14.1 Anatomy of the urogenital tract

The anatomy of the urogenital tract is illustrated by Barone *et al.* (1973). The rabbit kidney is unipapillate with extensive evaginations of the pelvis into the medullary tissue. The rabbit is the only known mammal in which the tubules can be separated from kidney slices with the tubular epithelium intact. Rabbit kidneys are therefore used for many *in vitro* studies of renal function. The right kidney can be palpated in the thoracolumbar region and is cranial to the left kidney. There may be substantial amounts of perirenal fat in some individuals, which displaces the kidneys ventrally. Both kidneys are usually visible on abdominal X-ray plates (see Box 10.2). The thin walled bladder occupies the ventrocaudal abdomen.

In the female the urethra opens into a vestibulum in the vagina called the urogenital sinus (Cruise and Brewer, 1994). A bulbourethral gland is situated in the dorsal wall of the urogenital sinus and the clitoris lies along the ventral surface. The external margins of the urogenital sinus form the vulva. The vaginal body is a flaccid structure which can retain urine. The uterus is bicornuate with a cervix on each horn.

The sexually mature male has two external testicles that lie on either side of the penis in two hairless scrotal sacs. The testicles descend at approximately 10–12 weeks. During periods of food deprivation or illness, the testicles can be withdrawn into the inguinal canal by the well-developed external cremaster muscle. The vas deferens enters a seminal vesicle that opens into the prostatic segment of the urethra. A vesicular gland lies with the prostate gland in the dorsal wall of the seminal vesicle. A small pair of bulbourethral glands forms a bilobed swelling in the dorsal wall of the urethra immediately posterior to the prostate (Cruise and Brewer, 1994).

Externally, immediately adjacent to the penis or the vulva lie two deep inguinal spaces which are closely associated with inguinal glands that secrete a thick brown or white waxy exudate into the space (see Figure 3.1). Immediately dorsal to the genital opening is the anus.

Key points 14.1

- Laboratory rabbits are used extensively for kidney research
- The right kidney is palpable in the thoracolumbar region and is cranial to the left kidney
- Perirenal fat can displace the kidneys ventrally
- Both kidneys are usually visible on abdominal X-ray plates
- The vagina of rabbits is a flaccid structure that can retain urine
- The bicornuate uterus has two cervices
- Testicles descend into scrotal sacs at 10–12 weeks of age
- The inguinal ring is open and testicles can be withdrawn into the inguinal canal during periods of stress
- Genuine cryptorchid males with abdominal testicles can occur although testicles that are absent from the scrotal sac may have been removed during attacks by other rabbits
- There are two deep skin folds adjacent to the external genitalia of both males and females. The folds normally contain a thick waxy, odorous secretion.

14.2 Renal function in rabbits

Rabbits are very susceptible to the effects of acid–base disturbances, pain, stress, anorexia and dehydration because of their renal responses. The role of the rabbit kidney in calcium homeostasis results in the excretion of large amounts of calcium that form a calcium carbonate precipitate in the alkaline urine, giving it a turbid appearance in healthy animals.

14.2.1 Renal response to acid–base disturbances

Rabbits excrete alkaline urine and have a limited ability to excrete hydrogen ions (see Section 1.6.5). As a result, they are susceptible to acid–base disturbances. Some of the renal compensatory mechanisms that are present in other species are absent from rabbits. Carbonic anhydrase, an enzyme which catalyses the reversible conversion of carbon dioxide to bicarbonate, is present in tubule epithelial cells in large amounts in species such as humans, monkeys and rats, in comparison with the rabbit (Dobyan *et al.*, 1982). In other mammals, ammonia is produced in the kidney by glutamine deamination in response to a fall in plasma pH, or a decreased concentration of bicarbonate. In rabbits glutamine deamination only takes place in response to reduced serum bicarbonate concentrations but not a drop in plasma pH. The alternative biochemical pathways that are present in other species and result in ammonia synthesis appear to be absent in the rabbit (Brewer and Cruise 1994). As a result of their limited ability to excrete hydrogen ions, rabbits are susceptible to metabolic acidosis. Rabbits are not as sensitive to the effects of loop diuretics as other species due to the insensitivity of the inner medullary collecting duct cells (Brewer and Cruise, 1994).

14.2.2 Stress and renal blood flow

In rabbits, pain and stress have a significant effect on renal blood flow. Experimental studies suggest that adrenaline is responsible for a marked and prolonged reduction in renal plasma flow and glomerular filtration (Brod and Sirota, 1949). In a study by Kaplan and Smith (1935) into the effects of diuresis and urine flow in rabbits, the forcible oral administration of large amounts of water (> 40 ml/kg every 30 minutes) was fatal in some rabbits. They became oliguric, convulsed and died. The experiment was repeated using a single dose of 50 ml/kg of water before subjecting the rabbits to unpleasant or painful stimuli. The rabbits were subjected to electric shocks, loud bangs or being tied in a supine position to an animal board for long periods of time. In all cases the disturbing stimuli were immediately followed by a marked decrease in urine flow, renal plasma flow and filtration rate. Oliguria was frequently severe, lasting from 30 to 120 minutes. Some rabbits that were infused with water at 0.3 ml/minute during this period died in convulsions. Rabbits that were not stimulated and remained undisturbed could withstand diuresis by increasing urine flow.

In a later study of the renal circulation in rabbits (Korner, 1963), the author found that it was '*particularly important to keep the animals in their experimental cages without restraint, to avoid handling the animals when collecting blood and urine samples, to avoid overhydration by the administration of excessive water loads and to prevent dehydration by the prolonged use of strong osmotic agents*'. These conclusions are relevant to the handling and treatment of the pet rabbit especially with regard to fluid therapy.

14.2.3 Calcium excretion

Calcium metabolism in rabbits is described in Section 1.6.5. Briefly, calcium is readily absorbed from the intestine in rabbits (Cheeke and Amberg, 1973). Calcium absorption from a diet with adequate calcium concentrations appears to be passive and vitamin D independent (Bourdeau *et al.*, 1986; Kamphues *et al.*, 1986). Blood calcium concentrations are higher and more variable in rabbits than in other species. Calcium homeostasis is mainly regulated by the kidney that responds rapidly to changes in calcium status. Responses are mediated by PTH and 1,25-dihydroxyvitamin D_3

(Bourdeau *et al.*, 1988) and result in excretion rates of calcium that are proportional to dietary intake (Kennedy, 1965). The kidney plays a vital role in calcium regulation in rabbits. During periods of calcium deprivation, tubular reabsorption of calcium by the kidney increases (Bourdeau and Lau, 1992). During periods of high calcium intake, the kidney can increase the excretion of calcium into the urine considerably (Whiting and Quamme, 1984). Urinary calcium excretion is also increased during periods of restricted phosphate intake (Depalo *et al.*, 1988; Bourdeau *et al.*, 1990). Calcium carbonate is formed in the alkaline urine of rabbits and forms a white precipitate.

14.3 Urine examination

There is a variety of ways in which urine can be collected from rabbits (see Section 3.12.3). Many rabbits will urinate in an empty litter tray or urine can be collected by cystocentesis. Normal rabbit urine varies in its visual appearance. The colour can vary from the pale yellow colour through a range of oranges and browns to a deep red colour that can be mistaken for blood. The colour depends on the diet and variations are the result of the excretion of plant pigments. Vegetable such as beetroot, cabbage, broccoli and dandelions often result in the excretion of red urine. There are also some clinical conditions, such as urolithiasis or uterine disorders, that can cause red urine due to haematuria. Examination of the urine with a dipstick (Hemostix, Ames) will differentiate between blood and plant pigments. Alternatively, a Wood's lamp can be used as urinary pigments fluoresce when exposed to ultraviolet light (Benson and Paul-Murphy, 1999). Normal rabbit urine is turbid due to the presence of calcium carbonate precipitates. The amount of precipitate varies with the calcium content of the diet and the health, age, reproductive and hydration status of the rabbit. Young rabbits and pregnant or lactating does usually produce clear urine. High calcium diets, dehydration and urine retention can result in large amounts of calcium carbonate precipitate that forms a thick sludge in the bladder and causes urethral irritation and dysfunction. It is sometimes

Key points 14.2

- As a herbivorous species, rabbits excrete alkaline urine (pH 8–8.2). Rabbits have limited ability to excrete hydrogen ions
- Some renal compensatory mechanisms that are present in other species are absent in rabbits, making them susceptible to acid–base disorders, especially metabolic acidosis
- Adrenaline can cause a marked and prolonged reduction in renal blood flow and temporary oliguria. This response can be fatal in rabbits that are stressed and overhydrated, e.g. during fluid therapy
- Calcium homeostasis in rabbits is mainly regulated by the kidney that responds rapidly to changes in calcium status
- During periods of calcium deprivation, tubular reabsorption of calcium by the kidney increases (Bourdeau and Lau, 1992)
- During periods of high calcium intake, the rabbit kidney is capable of increasing the fractional excretion of calcium into the urine considerably
- Dietary phosphate restriction increases urinary calcium excretion in rabbits
- Normal rabbit urine can vary in colour from yellow to orange, brown or red
- Plants such as dandelions and brassicas often result in the excretion of red urine that can be differentiated from haematuria by testing with a dipstick such as Hemostix (Ames)
- Calcium carbonate is formed in the alkaline urine of rabbits and forms a white precipitate
- Growing rabbits and pregnant or lactating females usually produce clear urine. The urine of anorexic rabbits may also be clear
- High calcium diets, dehydration and urine retention can result in large amounts of calcium carbonate precipitate that forms a thick sludge in the bladder and causes urethral irritation and dysfunction
- In addition to the presence of calcium carbonate crystals, ammonium magnesium phosphate (struvite) and oxalate crystals can also be found in normal rabbit urine
- In female rabbits, haematuria can be caused by uterine disease. Blood from the uterus can be mixed with urine in the vagina before it is voided.

difficult to differentiate between normal calcium carbonate deposits and abnormal amounts of sludge. Normal rabbit urine can be radiopaque on abdominal radiographs.

In addition to the presence of calcium carbonate crystals, ammonium magnesium phosphate crystals are also found in normal rabbit urine. The specific gravity of urine can be difficult to evaluate accurately due to the presence of mineral deposits (Goad *et al.*, 1989) but is approximately 1.003–1036. The urine is naturally alkaline with a pH of 8–8.2. Traces of glucose and protein can be present. Urine can be spun and the sediment examined microscopically for the present of crystals, red cells, inflammatory cells and bacteria. Urine cultures can confirm bacterial infection and aid antibiotic selection.

Haematuria may be caused by blood from the reproductive or urinary tract. The list of differential diagnoses is similar to other species (see Table 3.2). In entire female rabbits, uterine disease is often present. Uterine adenocarcinomas, polyps or endometrial venous aneurysms can rupture and bleed intermittently. In rabbits, blood from the uterus is often voided mixed with urine because the vaginal vestibule fills with urine during micturition. Blood clots may be present in the urine in association with uterine disease. Urolithiasis and/or cystitis can also cause haematuria. Chronic polypoid cystitis, renal infarcts and disseminated intravascular coagulopathy have all been described as causes of haematuria in laboratory rabbits (Garibaldi *et al.*, 1987).

14.4 Lower urinary tract disease

Like cats, pet rabbits are prone to a variety of interacting urinary tract disorders that can be grouped together. Feline lower urinary tract disease (FLUTD) or feline urological syndrome (FUS) is also called 'the fat lazy cat syndrome' (Blood and Studdert, 1999). An analogy can be made with the fat lazy pet rabbit, which is also prone to lower urinary tract disorders. The exact aetiology is unknown but there appear to be many predisposing factors. In rabbits, the syndrome includes urinary incontinence, 'sludgy urine' and cystic calculi. Ureteral calculi and nephrolithiasis are also seen and cause eventual renal failure.

Clinical signs of lower urinary tract disease in rabbits include inappropriate urination, depression, a hunched posture, teeth grinding, dysuria, perineal scalding, urinary incontinence, polyuria and polydypsia. Visual examination of the urine, urinanalysis, sediment examination and culture can be used to establish the presence of cystitis and bacterial infection. Examination of the perineum and consideration of the patient's mobility, husbandry and general state of health are important as there is an interrelationship between the predisposing causes. Abdominal radiography is nearly always indicated to evaluate the spine, kidneys, ureters, uterus and bladder. Further investigations such as examination of the oral cavity for the presence of molar spurs, or serological testing for *E. cuniculi* may be required. Ultrasound examination can also be helpful, especially if uterine disease is suspected. Evaluation of renal function is necessary in rabbits with urolithiasis, especially if there are stones in the kidney or ureters.

14.4.1 The role of hypercalcaemia and hypercalcuria in urinary tract disease in rabbits

The susceptibility of pet rabbits to urinary tract disorders is often attributed to excessive dietary intake of calcium. It is postulated that high dietary calcium results in hypercalcaemia, hypercalciuria and the accumulation of calcium deposits in the urine. This association between the rabbit's unusual calcium metabolism and the development of urinary tract disorders warrants further investigation as there are other factors, apart from high dietary calcium levels, that predispose to urinary tract disorders. The rabbit's kidney is adapted to the excretion of calcium and the presence of sediment in the urine is a normal finding in many rabbits. In a study of the haematological and biochemical parameters of pet rabbits with dental disease, a comparison was made with a group of free-range rabbits with access to natural vegetation. Total serum calcium concentrations as high as 4.28 mmol/l were recorded in the free-range group who showed no evidence of urinary tract disease other than turbid urine, which was considered to be normal (Harcourt-Brown and Baker, 2001). The free-range group lived out their natural life without evidence of any urinary tract disorders. At least two of the group are still alive at the time of writing (February, 2001), 6 years after the blood samples were taken.

Although high dietary calcium intake is not always associated with urinary tract disease, a low calcium intake does appear to prevent the development of sludgy urine and related disorders. The incidence of urinary tract disease is much higher in the USA than in the UK where most pet rabbits are kept in hutches and fed on mixed cereal rations. Selective feeding from mixed rations can result in a calcium deficient diet (Harcourt-Brown, 1996). Calcium deficiency and/or vitamin D deficiency results in metabolic bone disease that predisposes to dental disease (see Section 7.5.1.1). In the UK, dental disease is far more common than urinary tract disease in the pet rabbit population.

Dietary phosphorus levels are an important factor in the urinary excretion of calcium. Experimentally, dietary phosphorus restriction results in substantial hypercalciuria (Depalo *et al.*, 1988; Bourdeau *et al.*, 1990). Calcium and phosphorus are mobilized from bone in response to hypophosphataemia and excess calcium is excreted in the urine. Phosphorus is deficient in the soil of some parts of the world and hay and mature herbage are poor sources of the mineral in comparison with cereals. The availability of phosphorus in alfalfa is low in rabbits (Cheeke *et al.*, 1985).

Urine retention in association with large amounts of calcium deposits in the urine can result in urinary tract disease. There are many behavioural and physical reasons for pet rabbits to retain urine. Wild rabbits urinate frequently. They do not urinate in their burrow, but do so above ground over landmarks or other rabbits' terrain as part of their territory marking behaviour. Neutered rabbits do not void urine and territory mark as much as their entire counterparts. The stimulus to urinate and mark territory is absent from solitary rabbits with no neighbours to threaten to their territory. Sedentary pet rabbits are often forced to urinate in a hutch and may retain urine for as long as possible. Rabbits that are overweight or suffer from painful conditions such as spondylitis or sore hocks are reluctant or unable to adopt the correct position to urinate (see Plate 32) and can retain urine as a result. Urine retention in rabbits leads to the sedimentation of the urine within the bladder. During urination, the supernatant is voided and the

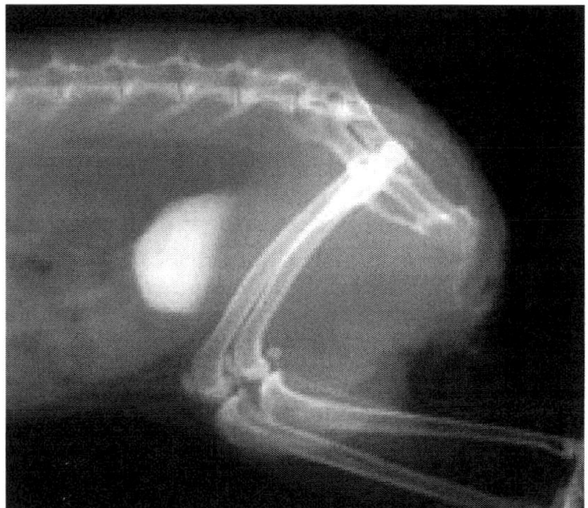

Figure 14.1. Lateral view of the caudal abdomen of a rabbit with 'sludgy urine'. Figure shows a lateral view of the caudal abdomen of a 3-year-old neutered male Dwarf Lop house rabbit. There is a quantity of radiodense sediment in the bladder. The rabbit was suffering from urine scalding of the perineum and inner thighs (see Plate 33). He was maintained on a diet of hay and vegetables with a small amount of complete extruded rabbit food each day. Total serum calcium concentration was 3.17 mmol/l, which is within the reference range for laboratory rabbits. Ionized blood calcium was 1.67 mmol/l. The bladder was enlarged and tense. Palpation of the bladder evoked straining that would produce a small amount of urine. The figure shows the bladder after the rabbit had urinated. The urine that remained within the bladder had formed a thick sediment that was impossible for the rabbit to void.

Under general anaesthesia, the bladder was emptied by gentle, manual compression. The urine that was expressed was thick and viscid (see Plate 34). Radiography also revealed a displaced 7th lumbar vertebra and a narrowed lumbosacral disc space. The rabbit could not adopt the correct position to urinate. He was euthanased. Sludgy urine is discussed in Section 14.4.2.

sediment is retained in the bladder. Eventually the sediment forms a thick, viscid sludge (see Figure 14.1). Secondary bacterial infection and urinary incontinence ensue.

14.4.2 'Sludgy urine'

Calcium carbonate deposits that build up in the bladder result in the accumulation of a thick paste or sludge. Cystitis develops and blood can be present in the urine. Affected rabbits are depressed and adopt a hunched position. Urination appears to be painful. The bladder feels enlarged and turgid. Palpation of the bladders appears to be uncomfortable for the rabbit and often evokes a straining response. Urine is passed in small quantities and may dribble from the urethra. Perineal scalding occurs (see Plate 33). Voided urine may appear only slightly turbid but radiographically the bladder is filled with radiodense sediment (see Figure 14.1). Under general anaesthesia, copious quantities of a viscid sludgy material can be expressed from the bladder (see Plate 34). There appears to be a difference in the urine from rabbits with 'sludge' and normal urine containing calcium carbonate deposits. The sediment in sludgy urine forms a dense precipitate whereas calcium carbonate deposits in normal urine can easily be shaken up to form a suspension. Sludgy urine is distressing for the rabbit. The sludge irritates the bladder, urethra and perineal skin causing pain and irritation. Secondary infection and cystitis is common. Superficial bacterial dermatitis, pain and a reluctance to urinate exacerbate the condition. Urethritis leads to urinary incontinence.

14.4.3 Urinary incontinence and urine scalding of the perineal skin

Any condition that affects normal urination can trigger a chain of events that results in urine scalding of the perineal skin. The main causes of urine scalding of the perineal skin are summarized in Box 14.1. A vicious circle of perineal pain, painful urination, urinary incontinence, urine scalding, perineal inflammation and perineal pain occurs (see Figure 14.2). Urinary incontinence may be due to loss of bladder control as a result of neurological conditions such as encephalitozoonosis or spinal problems. Incontinent rabbits dribble urine so the perineal area is constantly damp and inflamed. Diseases that cause polydypsia and polyuria increase the amount of urine that is produced to soak the bedding. Urine scalding can also be the result of anatomical conditions that affect the direction of the jet of urine so it lands on the skin causing chronic inflam-

Box 14.1 Causes of urine scalding of the perineal skin

- Primary incontinence due to neurological conditions such as encephalitozoonosis or compressive lesions of the spinal cord. Incontinent rabbits dribble urine so the perineal area is constantly damp and inflamed
- Many conditions can prevent a rabbit from adopting the correct stance to urinate. Examples include painful conditions such as pododermatitis or arthritis, or flexibility problems such as obesity, spondylitis or small cramped cages. Affected rabbits are unable to lift their hindquarters during urination to direct urine away from the skin and constantly sit in a pool of urine (see Plate 33)
- Several conditions can prevent normal grooming and allow the sensitive perineum to become inflamed and painful. Affected rabbits may be reluctant to adopt the correct stance to urinate or to groom the inflamed, infected painful perineal skin. Urethritis causes urine to dribble onto the perineal skin. Examples include dental disease, obesity, spondylitis or a fine fluffy coat
- Calcium carbonate deposits can form a sediment in immobile rabbits or those that retain urine for any length of time. The sediment can form a thick sludge that is mechanically irritating to the bladder, urethra and perineal skin. Cystitis and urethritis lead to urine dribbling and incontinence
- Anatomical conditions can affect the direction of the jet of urine so it lands on the skin. Fight wounds can lead to scarring of the prepuce so that urine is directed towards the surrounding skin during urination
- Poor husbandry and urine-soaked bedding will soak the fur and scald the perineal skin
- Reproductive disease or *Treponema cuniculi* can cause perineal infection and inflammation of the perineal area causing urethritis and urinary incontinence.

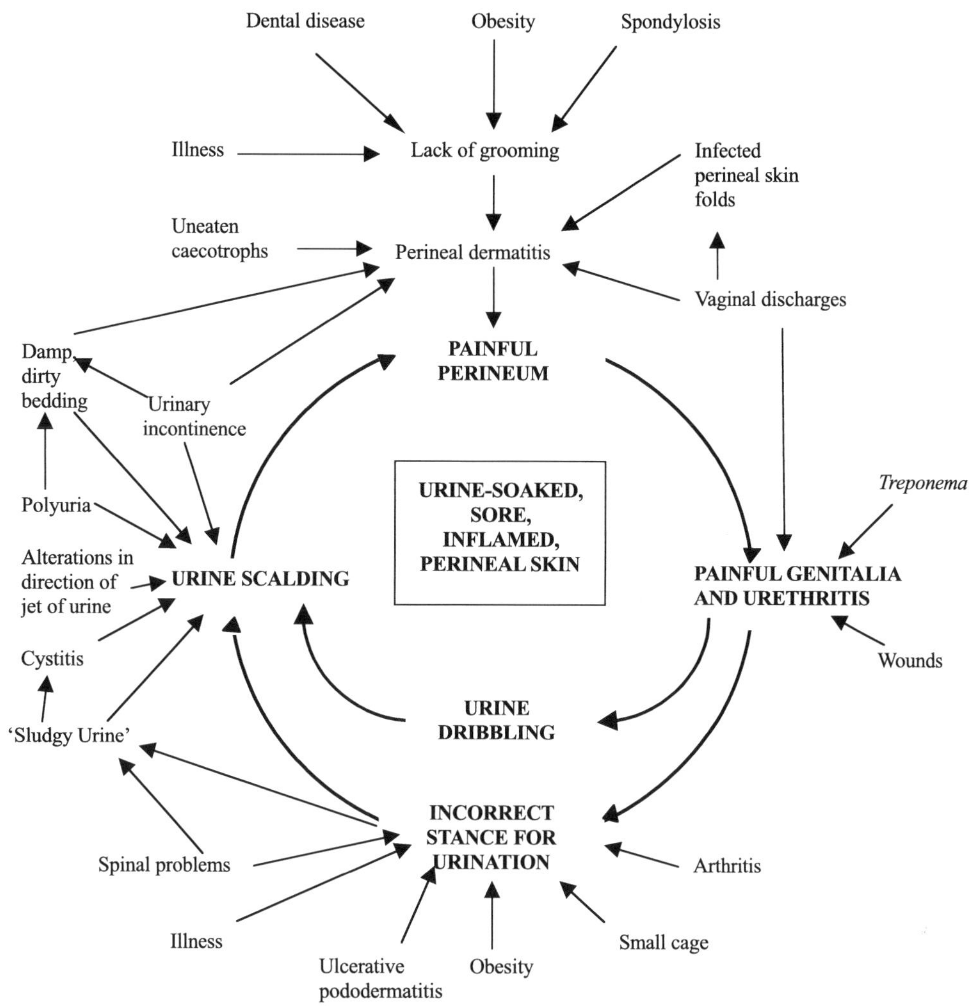

Figure 14.2. Inter-relationship of conditions that result in urine scalding of perineum.

mation and pain. Scarred preputial skin as a result of bite wounds or infection can alter the direction of urination.

Pain or mobility problems caused by paraplegia, obesity, ulcerative pododermatitis, spondylitis or small cramped cages can prevent a rabbit from adopting the correct stance for urination so that it constantly sits in a pool of urine (see Plates 32 and 33). Immobility allows urine to sediment in the bladder, which predisposes to sludgy urine, cystitis, urethritis and urine leakage. Pain or mobility problems also prevent a rabbit from grooming effectively so that the perineal skin becomes infected and inflamed. Matted fur soiled with uneaten caecotrophs can be the result of dental disease, obesity and flexibility problems. Reproductive disease or *Treponema cuniculi* can cause perineal infection and inflammation of the perineal skin. Hormone responsive incontinence has been described in two ovarohysterectomized does (Caslow, 1989).

Once the perineal area is inflamed, secondary bacterial dermatitis occurs, exacerbated by wet, soiled, matted fur covering the skin. Licking and grooming inflamed skin becomes painful so uneaten caecotrophs can become entangled in the matted fur, exacerbating the condition even further. Owners

Box 14.2 Treatment of urinary tract disease in rabbits

- Identify and, if possible, treat any underlying problems that interfere with normal urination. For example, spinal disorders, encephalitozoonosis, anatomical defects, ulcerative pododermatitis
- Clip away soiled matted fur and treat infected skin around the genitalia, perineum and thighs. Sedation may be necessary. Fentanyl/fluanisone (Hypnorm, Janssen) is satisfactory. Topical fusidic acid (Fuciderm, Leo Animal Health) can be applied to the infected skin
- Provide clean dry bedding
- Provide analgesia. Opioids (buprenorphine) or NSAIDS (carprofen or meloxicam) or a combination of the two can be used
- Give antibiotics, e.g. enrofloxacin or trimethoprim/sulpha, to treat cystitis, urethritis and secondary pyoderma. Urine culture and sensitivity is indicated. Long courses of antibiotics may be necessary to treat cystitis
- If possible, provide the opportunity to exercise and urinate away from the bedding.

For cases of 'sludgy urine' it may also be necessary to:

- Induce diuresis, taking care not to stress the rabbit. Stress can reduce renal blood flow and cause oliguria. Fentanyl/fluanisone (Hypnorm, Janssen) can be used as a sedative during intravenous fluid therapy or fluids may be given subcutaneously or orally
- Increase voluntary water intake. Plenty of leafy green vegetables and sweetening the water with sucrose or fruit juice may be effective. Some plants such as dandelions, goosegrass, plantain and yarrow are reputed to have diuretic properties
- Reduce the amount of calcium in the diet so less calcium is excreted by the kidneys. The calcium content of common ingredients of rabbit food is listed in Table 2.3.

Surgical treatments for urinary tract disease

- Cystic or urethral uroliths require surgical removal but they are often found in conjunction with nephrolithiasis that causes eventual renal failure. Abdominal radiography is required before embarking on surgery
- Perineal dermoplasty is necessary in rabbits with deep perineal skin folds. Obese female rabbits are most susceptible. The folds become chronically infected and sore, especially in rabbits with urine scalding of the perineal area
- Scars from fight wounds on the prepuce can alter the direction of the jet of urine so that it lands on the skin inside the thighs. Corrective surgery on the prepuce is indicated to cure the condition
- The direction of urine flow can be surgically altered in rabbits that are unable to lift their hindquarters to adopt the correct stance for urination. Removal of an area of skin dorsal to the genitalia pulls the urethral orifice dorsally. The tail needs to be amputated.

often attempt to bathe and clean the area without removing the soiled fur. Matted, damp contaminated fur in contact with inflamed skin makes the situation even worse. Inflammation and pain around the urethral entrance results in urine dribbling so a vicious circle is formed (see Figure 14.2). Treatment is directed at breaking this vicious circle.

14.4.4 Treatment of lower urinary tract disorders such as 'sludgy urine' and urine scalding

The treatment of lower urinary tract disorders is summarized in Box 14.2. If possible, the underlying cause of urinary tract disease should be identified and addressed. Sometimes, it is not possible to cure the initiating factor, e.g. encephalitozoonosis or spondylitis, in which case the owner can be informed of the long-term management implications and may opt for euthanasia.

In the short term, rabbits with urine scalding benefit greatly from clipping soiled matted hair from around the perineum and the inner aspects of the thighs. The procedure is time consuming but essential. Care is required to prevent iatrogenic skin damage (see Section 9.3). After the soiled, damp fur has been removed, the skin can be cleansed with an antiseptic such as chlorhexidene and dried before applying topical therapy.

Fuciderm (Leo Laboratories Ltd) is effective. Eliminating the superficial skin infection of the perineum and inner thighs makes urination less painful and breaks the vicious circle that occurs in rabbits with lower urinary tract disorders. It also makes the rabbit more comfortable and mobile. Sedation with 0.2–0.3 ml/kg fentanyl/fluanisone (Hypnorm) may be required for fractious patients and has the added advantage of providing analgesia for a few hours until other medications take effect. Clean dry bedding is essential.

Long-term analgesia is indicated for rabbits with lower urinary tract disease, both to treat the pain associated with a sore perineum and to treat any other underlying condition that is painful. The use of analgesics encourages mobility and the adoption of the correct stance for urination. NSAIDs can be given orally by the owner for long-term management if required.

Antibiotics are indicated for the treatment of cystitis, urethritis and superficial pyoderma. Enrofloxacin or trimethoprim combinations are safe and effective. Urine culture for bacteriology and sensitivity can identify pathogens and aid antibiotic selection. Long courses of antibiotics can be necessary to eliminate infection.

Sludgy urine can be removed by manual expression of the bladder under sedation or general anaesthesia. Catheterization may be necessary to flush the bladder with sterile saline or water. Analgesics are always required postoperatively.

An increase in the amount of fluid passing through the urinary tract aids the expulsion of calcium carbonate deposits and dilutes the urine. Diuresis can be induced with intravenous, subcutaneous or oral fluids. Sweetening the drinking water with sucrose or fruit juice such as Ribena may encourage the rabbit to drink more. Diuretic drugs can be used, although it is safer, cheaper and pleasanter for the rabbit to change its diet to include plenty of vegetables that contain water. Many wild plants such as dandelions, goosegrass, plantain and yarrow are reputed to have diuretic properties and are enjoyed by rabbits. Giving the rabbit the opportunity to graze grass and the freedom to exercise will improve its water intake and encourage it to exercise and urinate.

A balanced diet with sufficient, but not excessive, quantities of calcium and phosphorus is required. It is important not to feed a diet that is deficient in either calcium or phosphorus. Calcium deficiency can result in osteoporosis and dental problems. Phosphorus restriction increases urinary calcium excretion and exacerbates both hypercalciuria and bone loss.

All vitamin and mineral supplements should be excluded from the diet and mineral blocks taken away. Plenty of fibre in the form of good quality hay or grass is essential. A balanced concentrated ration can also be offered. High calcium vegetables such as kale, broccoli, turnip, chinese cabbage and watercress should be avoided although small quantities of dandelions are acceptable because of their diuretic properties. Vegetables with a moderate calcium content include cabbage, carrots, celery and lettuce. Alfalfa should be avoided.

14.4.4.1 Surgical procedures for rabbits with lower urinary tract disease

Some rabbits, especially obese rabbits or those that have lost weight, develop deep folds of skin that envelop the genitalia. These skin folds easily become infected, especially if the rabbit has problems urinating so the perineal skin is constantly damp. Infected, inflamed skin is painful and affected rabbits are reluctant or unable to groom effectively or adopt the correct stance for urination. Surgical removal of the skin fold is a simple and effective remedy. The technique is described in Section 9.7.3.1.

Chronic or recurrent cases of urine scalding warrant examination under anaesthetic. There are several conditions that can alter the direction of urine flow and corrective surgery can be curative. Fight wounds and scarring of the prepuce can alter the direction of urine flow so that urine is directed on to the skin inside the thighs.

Removal of an area of skin dorsal to the urethral orifice has been described as method of altering the direction of urine flow away from the perineal skin (Jenkins, 1997). Amputation of the tail is necessary. The operation is indicated for rabbits with incurable conditions that affect their ability to raise their hindquarters and adopt the correct stance for urination. Examples include rabbits with spondylosis or ulcerative pododermatitis. A crescent-shaped area of skin around the tail is removed with the tail so that the anus and urethral orifice is pulled dorsally. The tail is amputated at the third or fourth coccygeal vertebrae.

14.4.5 Urolithiasis

Urolithiasis is a separate condition from 'sludgy urine' in rabbits, although the two conditions may be related. Several factors predispose to urolithiasis in any species. Any factor that increases the urinary concentration of stone-forming ions, or promotes crystal formation can cause crystals to aggregate and form a stone. Analysis of the stone confirms its composition and can give an indication of possible causes. Rabbits differ from other species because their urine contains many crystals. Oxalate and struvite crystals can be found in normal rabbit urine. Uric acid (the final degradation product of purine metabolism) is handled differently by the kidney in different species of mammals. In the dog and the rat, more than 50% of the filtered load of urate is reabsorbed and less than 40% is secreted. In the rabbit, more than 100% of the filtered load is excreted, indicating that urate is secreted into the urine by the kidney. This high excretion rate of uric acid occurs because the urate–anion exchange mechanism that is present in other species is not present in rabbits (Brewer and Cruise, 1994).

Calcium carbonate deposits can be found in large quantities in normal rabbit urine. Urolithiasis occurs commonly in pet rabbits (see Figure 14.3) and calcium carbonate is the most likely constituent of uroliths. Documented cases of urolithiasis have been due to calcium carbonate stones (Garibaldi and Pecquet-Goad, 1988; Whary and Peper, 1994). The formation of calcium carbonate uroliths is usually attributed to excessive amounts of calcium carbonate in the urine due to high dietary calcium levels. This association between urolithiasis and high dietary calcium intake is not proven. Experimentally, forced excessive dietary intake of calcium results in calcification of the aorta and kidney (Kamphues *et al.*, 1986) and large amounts of calcium in the urine but not

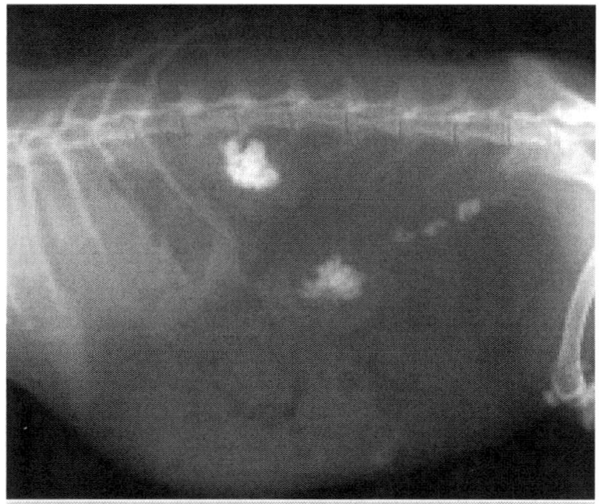

Figure 14.3. Lateral view of the abdomen of a rabbit with renal and ureteral uroliths. The figure shows an oblique lateral view of a 4-year-old, entire, female anorexic English rabbit. The radiograph shows extensive renal and ureteral urolithiasis. The rabbit was presented for treatment for anorexia. A blood sample showed a urea level of 49.8 mmol/l and creatinine of 813.2 µmol/l. Haematology was unremarkable despite the presence of pus around the uroliths, both in the kidney and in the ureters. The rabbit was euthanased.

urolith formation. Instead, urolithiasis can be induced in the rabbit by mechanical obstruction of the urinary tract. In a study by Itanani *et al.* (1979), temporary obstruction of the upper urinary tract of rabbits on a normal diet resulted in rapid formation of a renal urolith in 100% of cases. The stones were composed of calcium carbonate, calcium oxalate and calcium phosphate.

Mechanical obstruction of the urinary tract can be caused by adhesions, abscesses, tumours or sludgy urine. Other factors might also play a part in the development of uroliths in rabbits, such as high dietary oxalate, restricted water intake, changes in urine pH, urine retention and cystitis.

Bladder stones require surgical removal. In some cases, the stones obstruct the urethra and need to be pushed back into the bladder before they can be removed. Renal calculi are often present in conjunction with cystic calculi. Careful examination of abdominal radiographs for the presence of renal calculi is necessary before embarking on surgery.

Key points 14.3

- Rabbits suffer from a variety of interacting urinary tract disorders. The exact aetiology is complex and unclear but, like cats, fat, lazy, neutered indoor animals are most susceptible
- The susceptibility of pet rabbits to urinary tract disorders is often attributed to excessive dietary intake of calcium and the accumulation of calcium deposits in the urine. However, there are other causes and predisposing factors
- Urine retention leads to sedimentation of urine within the bladder. The sediment is retained in the bladder to form sludge that is irritant to the bladder, urethra and perineal skin and can cause cystitis, urethritis and urinary incontinence
- There are many reasons for urine retention in pet rabbits. Wild, entire rabbits continually spray urine to mark territory, this behaviour is absent in the neutered, litter trained house rabbit
- Obesity, illness, perineal dermatitis, ulcerative pododermatitis, arthritis, spinal problems are among the reasons for rabbits to retain urine. They can also prevent a rabbit from raising its hindquarters to urinate so that it constantly sits in a pool of urine
- Urine scalding of the skin around the genitalia is painful for the rabbit. It can cause urethritis and urinary incontinence which compund the situation and start a vicious circle
- Clipping the hair from the perineal skin and treating the perineal dermatitis can break the vicious circle. Fentanyl/fluanisone (Hypnorm, Janssen) is a useful sedative for rabbits that require clipping and cleaning of the perineum. It is also a potent analgesic
- Conditions that cause urinary incontinence, such as *E. cuniculi* or spinal problems can result in urine scalding of the perineum
- Abnormalities of the penis or prepuce can alter the direction of the jet of urine and cause urine scalding
- Bathing the perineum without clipping away soiled fur can be counterproductive as matted, wet, soiled fur encourages bacterial infection of the underlying skin
- Clean, dry bedding, analgesia and antibiotics are important in the treatment of urine scalding
- Urolithiasis can be induced by urinary tract obstruction. In rabbits, calcium carbonate uroliths are most common
- Experimentally, high dietary calcium or vitamin D levels are not associated with stone formation although they can result in large amounts of calcium carbonate in the urine. Forced intake of high levels of calcium results in mineralization of soft tissues such as the aorta or kidney, but not urolithiasis
- Uroliths are often found in the kidney of rabbits with cystic calculi. The prognosis for rabbits with nephrolithiasis is poor. Secondary calcification of the aorta can occur
- Cystic or urethral uroliths can be removed by cystotomy. The bladder should be repaired with a fine absorbable suture material of low reactivity to prevent calculus formation. 4/0 Poliglecaprone (Monocryl) is suitable
- The treatment of lower urinary tract disorders in rabbits is summarized in Box 14.2.

Renal calculi obstruct the renal pelvis and eventually cause renal failure.

It is advisable to empty the bladder by cystocentesis prior to cystotomy. Manual expression of the bladder can result in bladder rupture, especially if the neck is obstructed with a urolith. A midline abdominal incision is made between the umbilicus and the pubis. The bladder can then be exteriorized before incising it longitudinally. Stay sutures are used to hold the bladder out of the abdominal cavity while uroliths are removed. The bladder is repaired using a single layer of simple, interrupted sutures without penetrating the lumen of the bladder. The suture pattern should appose the edges of the bladder wall, including the submucosa, to ensure a watertight seal and rapid healing. A modified Gambee suture is suitable (see Figure 15.1). Rabbits are prone to developing calculi along a cystotomy suture line (Kaminski *et al.*, 1978). Calculus formation can be reversible and the persistence of calculi appears to be dependent on the longevity of the suture material that is used (Morris *et al.*, 1986). In rabbits, the bladder heals quickly;

epithelializiation of the suture line occurs after 3 days (Hanke *et al.*, 1994). A fine absorbable suture material of low reactivity will prevent calculus formation: 4/0 Poliglecaprone (Monocryl) is suitable. Although polyglactin (Vicryl, Ethicon) is not recommended for urinary tract surgery in other species because it undergoes rapid hydrolysis in an alkaline medium (Bouvy and Dupré, 1997), experimental studies have shown that it can be satisfactory for bladder repair in rabbits (Hanke *et al.*, 1994).

14.5 Renal disease

A variety of kidney diseases affect rabbits. Renal agenesis and asymptomatic congenital renal cysts have been recorded (Lindsey and Fox, 1994). Lesions associated with bacterial infections include renal abscesses, staphylococcal nephritis, pyelonephritis and pyelitis (Hinton, 1981). Malignant neoplasms such as lymphoma and renal carcinomas occur. A benign tumour, an embryonal nephroma, is a reportedly common tumour of laboratory rabbits (Weisbroth, 1994). The tumours can be an incidental *post-mortem* finding and do not affect renal function. They appear as whitish, sharply circumscribed nodules of tissue projecting above the cortical surface. Renal amyloidosis can be found in association with chronic inflammatory conditions such as abscesses. Renal fibrosis can occur in older rabbits or can be associated with encephalitozoonosis (Hinton, 1981). Obstruction of the flow of urine from the kidney can lead to hydronephrosis and impaired renal function in the short term and to nephrolithiasis in the long term.

14.5.1 *Encephalitozoon cuniculi*

The protozoan parasite *Encephalitozoon cuniculi* has a predeliction for nervous tissue and the kidney in rabbits. A detailed description of the parasite is given in Section 16.4.2. *E. cuniculi* causes areas of fibrosis of the kidney that can be seen on gross *post-mortem* examination (see Plate 31). It is often an incidental *post-mortem* finding. Focal, irregular, depressed areas can be seen on the surface of the kidney giving it a pitted appearance. Histologically, early lesions show focal to segmental granulomatous interstitial nephritis. Lesions may be present at all levels of the renal tubule and ovoid spores are sometimes evident within epithelial cells, in macrophages, in inflammatory foci or free within collecting tubules. The spores stain heavily with gram stain. In the later stages, interstitial fibrosis occurs and the parasite is not visible (Percy and Barthold, 1993). Significant renal impairment is not usually associated with encephalitozoonosis, although a recent survey of 125 seropositive pet rabbits 16 (31.4%) showed haematological and biochemical evidence of renal failure. A serological test is available that confirms exposure to *E. cuniculi* (see Section 16.4.2.4). Albendazole can be used to treat encephalitozoonosis. There is an individual case report of an HIV seropositive human who developed renal failure in association with *Encephalitozoon* infection. Treatment with albendazole resulted in disappearance of microsporidia from urine, clinical improvement and return of renal function almost to normal (Aarons *et al.*, 1994).

14.5.2 Calcification of the kidney

Calcification of the kidney is associated with any condition that results in blood calcium levels that exceed the kidney's ability to excrete calcium. Conditions that result in high blood calcium levels, such as forced intake of a high calcium diet and vitamin D toxicity result in calcification of soft tissues such as the kidney and aorta (Kamphues *et al.*, 1986; Zimmerman *et al.*, 1990). Impaired excretion of calcium due to poor renal function can also result in soft tissue calcification, especially of the aorta. Mineralization can include the kidney. Experimentally, surgical resection of part of the kidney or cautery of kidney tissue to induce chronic renal failure also results in dystrophic calcification (Eddy *et al.*, 1986; Tvedegaard, 1987).

14.5.3 Renal failure

14.5.3.1 Acute renal failure

Acute renal failure is the end stage of many fatal conditions of rabbits and can be prevented or treated with judicious fluid therapy (see Section 4.11). Fatty infiltration of the kidney occurs in conjunction with hepatic lipidosis (see Section 10.3.2) and causes acute kidney failure

Prerenal azotaemia can occur in rabbits in association with stress, fright, water deprivation, severe dehydration, heat stroke and toxic insults. The rabbit has a limited capacity to concentrate urea and a greater volume of urine is required when urea load increases (Brewer and Cruise, 1994). Dehydration can result in high urea and creatinine values that would indicate renal disease in other species. Therefore urea and creatinine levels should be checked on a second sample before making an absolute diagnosis of renal failure in rabbits, as high values can return to normal once the animal is rehydrated. Adrenaline can reduce renal blood flow and cause oliguria in rabbits (Brod and Sirota, 1949). Care must be taken not to overperfuse the circulation and rabbits should be kept as stress free as possible during rehydration.

14.5.3.2 Chronic renal failure

Chronic renal failure causes inappetance, polydypsia, polyuria, weight loss, anaemia and lethargy in rabbits. These symptoms are non-specific and may be confused with other conditions such as dental disease or gastrointestinal hypomotility. Many diseases can cause chronic renal failure (see Table 3.2). *Encephalitozoon cuniculi* is a cause of low grade kidney disease with mild elevations in blood urea. Most cases are subclinical. *E. cuniculi* infection causes granulomatous lesions in the kidneys that become pitted and scarred with fibrotic areas. Radiographs should be taken of any rabbit with raised urea and creatinine levels (see Figure 14.3). Nephrolithiasis is a cause of kidney disease in the rabbit and can be detected radiographically. Overmineralization of the skeleton and calcification of the aorta may also be seen.

In other species, such as dogs and cats, chronic renal disease affects conversion of 25-OH-D to 1,25 (OH_2)D in the kidney. Calcium absorption is impaired and demineralization of the bones occurs. In rabbits, renal failure compromises calcium excretion but not absorption. Passive absorption of calcium from the intestine continues in the absence of vitamin D. Hypercalcaemia occurs in conjunction with excretion of clear urine. This can lead to excessive mineralization of the bones. Calcification of the aorta is often seen in rabbits with chronic renal failure, especially in the area at the base of the heart. Mineralization of the kidneys can also occur, which impairs renal function further.

The prognosis for rabbits with clinical signs of chronic renal failure is poor, although symptomatic treatment may prolong life. Antibiotics are indicated, especially for infectious causes of kidney disease and are beneficial for rabbits with renal or ureteral calculi as they are usually embedded in purulent

Key points 14.4

- A number of renal diseases affect rabbits. Some are asymptomatic such as renal cysts and a benign tumour, embryonal nephroma
- Malignant neoplasms such as lymphoma and renal carcinoma occur
- *Encephalitozoon cuniculi* infection can result in areas of renal fibrosis. Focal, irregular, depressed areas can be seen on the surface of the kidney giving it a pitted appearance
- Calcification of the kidney and other soft tissue, such as the aorta, occurs when blood calcium levels exceed the ability of the kidney to excrete calcium. Very high dietary calcium intake, vitamin D toxicity or chronic renal disease are among possible causes
- Prerenal azotaemia can occur in rabbits in association with stress, fright, water deprivation, severe dehydration, heat stroke and toxic insults
- Blood urea and creatinine values can attain high levels during periods of dehydration. Similar values would indicate renal failure in dogs or cats
- Chronic renal failure in rabbits causes inappetance, polydypsia, polyuria, weight loss, anaemia and lethargy. These symptoms are non-specific and may be confused with other conditions such as dental disease or gastrointestinal hypomotility
- Nephrolithiasis is a common cause of kidney disease in the rabbit and abdominal radiographs should be taken of rabbits with raised urea and creatinine levels
- *E. cuniculi* can cause low grade kidney disease with mild elevations in blood urea. Most cases are subclinical.

material. Dietary calcium restriction but not deprivation is necessary. Maintaining hydration and providing electrolytes with oral fluid replacement therapy is helpful.

14.6 Reproductive disease

Reproductive physiology is described in Section 1.4.

14.6.1 Obstetrics

Obstetrical problems are rare in rabbits. Does are susceptible to pregnancy toxaemia during late gestation and it is important to ensure that they do not become stressed or anorexic (see Section 10.3.3). Complications of pregnancy can be treated in a similar manner to other species and a brief description of normal pregnancy and parturition is given so that an abnormal situation can be recognized.

The gestation period of the rabbits is normally 30–32 days with small litters being carried a day or two longer. Viable young may be born between 29 and 35 days (Cheeke *et al.*, 1982). Pregnancy can be diagnosed by abdominal palpation from 10 days *post-coitus*. The fetal units are felt as olive-sized masses in the ventral abdomen. At around 14 days, it becomes more difficult to distinguish fetal units from other abdominal organs. Radiographically, fetuses are seen after the 12th day of pregnancy. Resorption of the fetal units can take place before the 20th day of pregnancy (Adams, 1987). The process is very rapid. Abortion is uncommon and only occurs after the 24th day of pregnancy. In cases of prolonged gestation, the litter is often small and may contain one or two abnormally large kits that are usually born dead. After day 35 the fetuses will die *in utero* if they are not expelled. Mummification or maceration then occurs.

Parturition usually takes place in the morning and takes about 30 minutes. Anterior and posterior presentations are normal. Occasionally part of the litter is born some hours or even days after the first fetus and can still be viable. Some does will split the litter between two nest sites (Cheeke *et al.*, 1982). Each fetus is expelled with its placenta that is eaten immediately by the doe who continues to lick and clean the young. Newborn rabbits move to the teats to suckle while the remainder of the litter is born.

14.6.2 Caesarean section

Caesarean section is relatively straightforward in rabbits. The gravid uterus lies immediately beneath a midline laparotomy incision and can be swiftly exteriorized before incising it to deliver the fetuses. Alternatively, a lateral flank approach can be used that has the advantage of avoiding the mammary glands.

14.6.3 Pseudopregnancy

Rabbits are reflex ovulators. Mating stimulates ovulation approximately 10 hours *post-coitus*. Ovulation can also be induced by mechanical stimulation of the vagina or by the act of being mounted by another female, which can result in pseudopregnancy. Neutered or entire rabbits of either sex may mount each other to establish dominance or during periods of excitement. Pseudopregnancy can also be the result of sexual arousal from the close proximity or scent of a male. Reflex ovulation takes place and results in the formation of corpora lutea that secrete progesterone. Pseudopregnancy lasts for 16–18 days. The doe is not receptive to a buck during this time. At the end of the period, the doe may pull hair from her body and attempt to make a nest. She may become territorial and attack other rabbits or people that come near.

Although there are anecdotal reports of treating pseudopregnancy in rabbits with hormone preparations, in most circumstances, treatment is unnecessary as the condition is self-limiting. Repeated false pregnancies can be prevented by neutering or separating females that are stimulating each other. It may be necessary to house entire males and females in separate locations in multi-rabbit establishments.

14.6.4 Extrauterine pregnancy

Extrauterine pregnancy is relatively common in domestic rabbits (Bergdall and Dysko,

1994). It is due to the escape of a fertilized ovum into the abdominal cavity or rupture of a pregnant uterus (Harper and Ensley, 1982). Implantation usually occurs on the parietal peritoneum. The fetus becomes mummified and is palpated as an abdomenal mass. Radiology or ultrasound can be used in the differential diagnosis of this condition.

Arvidsson (1998) described a case of extrauterine pregnancy that was discovered during *post-mortem* examination. Three mummified fetuses were found in the abdominal cavity. The doe had give birth to three offspring 3 weeks previously. Beddow (1999) described a case of ectopic pregnancy in a young doe that was presented for sexing. Fetuses were palpated in the abdomen but parturition did not occur. The rabbit remained healthy with no symptoms of nest making. During subsequent laparotomy to perform an ovarohysterectomy, the ovaries and uterus appeared normal but six mummified fetal masses were found enveloped in omentum and loops of adherent gut. These were dissected free and removed and the rabbit made an uneventful recovery.

14.6.5 Bladder eversion

Transurethral, bladder eversion has been described in two does which had recently given birth (Greenacre *et al.*, 1999). Affected does were presented with a mass protruding from the vagina and were straining to urinate. One case was treated successfully with surgery.

14.6.6 Diseases of the uterus

The entire doe can suffer from a number of uterine disorders, even if they are not used for breeding. Uterine or ovarian tumours, abscesses, cysts, pyometra, hydrometra are discovered during clinical or *post-mortem* examination. Abdominal palpation, radiography, ultrasound examination, urinanalysis and inspection of the vulva are helpful in diagnosis. Many reproductive tract problems show no obvious clinical signs and exploratory surgery is required before a definitive diagnosis can be made. Pyometra can cause a purulent vaginal discharge and

Key points 14.5

- Obstetrical problems are rare in rabbits
- Pregnancy toxaemia can occur especially in does that become stressed or anorexic in late pregnancy
- The gestation period of the rabbits is normally 30–32 days with small litters being carried a day or two longer. Viable young may be born between 29 and 35 days
- Rapid resorption of the fetal units can take place before the 20th day of pregnancy
- Abortion is uncommon and only occurs after 24th day of pregnancy
- Parturition usually takes place in the morning and takes about 30 minutes. Anterior and posterior presentations are normal
- Pseudopregnancy can result from an infertile mating or from sexual activity that occurs between two does that are housed together
- Pseudopregnancy can also be the result of sexual arousal from the close proximity or scent of a male
- Pseudopregnancy lasts for 16–18 days. The doe is not receptive to a buck during this time. At the end of the period, the doe may pull hair from her body and attempt to make a nest. She may become territorial and attack other rabbits or people that come near
- Extrauterine pregnancy can occur in rabbits. It is due to the escape of a fertilized ovum into the abdominal cavity or rupture of a pregnant uterus. Implantation usually occurs on the parietal peritoneum. The fetus becomes mummified and can be palpated as an abdominal mass
- A number of uterine conditions affect female rabbits. Pyometra can cause a purulent vaginal discharge and can be a manifestation of *Pasteurella multocida* transmitted during coitus
- The most common tumour in female rabbits is the adenocarcinoma of the uterine endometrium. It is often encountered in adult entire does
- Uterine adenocarcinomas are often multicentric and involve both horns of the uterus appearing as globular polypoid structures that project into the uterus
- Metastasis of uterine adenocarcinomas occurs via local spread into the peritoneum and other abdominal organs such as the liver, or by haematogenous spread to distant sites such as the lung, brain, skin or bones.

can be a manifestation of *Pasteurella multocida* transmitted during coitus. Ovarohysterectomy is curative but surgery can be hazardous due to the presence of adhesions between the uterus and surrounding tissue. Endometrial venous aneurysms also occur in rabbits. They can rupture spontaneously and cause intrauterine haemorrhage. Hydrometra has been described in a laboratory rabbit (Bray *et al.*, 1991).

14.6.6.1 Uterine adenocarcinoma

The most common tumour in female rabbits is adenocarcinoma of the uterine endometrium. The incidence of this tumour increases with age and has been reported to reach 60% in animals over 4 years of age. A survey by Greene (1941) of 14 breeds of laboratory rabbits revealed 145 tumour-bearing animals among 849 females by 2 years of age. The Dutch type of rabbit was more susceptible to uterine adenocarcinoma than other breeds. The tumours were detected by abdominal palpation and confirmed by biopsy or autopsy. Statistical analysis of the results led the author to conclude that '*if a rabbit survived to the 5th year of life without the occurrence of a uterine tumour, which is contrary to probability, the chances are better than 3 to 1 that a tumour would develop by the 7th year*'. Uterine adenocarcinomas are often multicentric and involve both horns of the uterus appearing as globular polypoid structures that project into the uterus. As the condition advances, the tumours enlarge and coalesce so that large portions of the uterus are affected and become progressively more palpable. They may contain large areas of haemorrhage, necrosis or calcification. Uterine adenocarcinomas are often multicentric and involve both horns of the uterus appearing as globular polypoid structures that project into the uterus. Metastasis occurs via local spread into the peritoneum and other abdominal organs such as the liver, or by haematogenous spread to distant sites such as the lung, brain, skin or bones.

References

Aarons, E.J., Woodrow, D. *et al.* (1994). Reversible renal failure caused by a microsporidian infection (Abstract). *AIDS*, **8**, 1119–1121.

Adams, C.E. (1987). The laboratory rabbit. In *The UFAW Handbook on the Care and Management of Laboratory Animals*, 6th edn. pp 415–436, Longman Scientific and Technical.

Arvidsson, A. (1998). Extra-uterine pregnancy in a rabbit. *Vet Rec.*, 176.

Barone, R., Pavaux, C., Blin, P.C., Cuq, P. (1973). *Atlas d'anotomie du lapin*. Masson et Cie.

Beddow, B.A. (1999). Ectopic pregnancy in a rabbit. *Vet Rec.*, **144**, 624.

Benson, K.G., Paul-Murphy, J. (1999). Clinical pathology of the domestic rabbit. *Vet Clin N Am: Exotic Anim Pract.*, **2**, 539–552.

Bergdall, V., Dysko R.C. (1994). Metabolic, traumatic, mycotic and miscellaneous diseases. In *The Biology of the Laboratory Rabbit*, 2nd edn. (P.J. Manning, D.H.Ringler, C.E.Newcomer, eds). pp 336–355. Academic Press.

Blood, D.C., Studdert, V.P. (1999). *Saunders Comprehensive Veterinary Dictionary*, 2nd edn. W.B. Saunders.

Bourdeau, J.E., Lau, K., (1992). Regulation of cystosolic free calcium concentration in the rabbit connecting tubule: a calcium absorbing renal epithelium. *J Lab Clin Med.*, **119**, 650–662.

Bourdeau, J.E., Shwer-Dymerski, D.A., Stern, P.A., Langman, C.B. (1986). Calcium and phosphorous metabolism in chronically vitamin D-deficient laboratory rabbits. *Miner Electrolyte Metab.*, **12**, 176–185.

Bourdeau, J.E., Bouillon, R., Zikos, D., Langman, C.B. (1988). Renal responses to calcium deprivation in young rabbits. *Miner Electrolyte Metab.*, **14**, 150–157.

Bourdeau, J. E., DePalo, D., Barr, D.R., Hu, J. (1990). Effects of moderate dietary phosphorus restriction on intestinal absorption and external balances of phosphorus and calcium in growing female rabbits. *Miner Electrolyte Metab.*, **16**, 378–384.

Bouvy, B., Dupré, G. (1997). Surgical soft tissue suture techniques: current recommendations for the dog and cat. *Waltham Focus*, **7**, 7–15.

Bray, M.V., Gaertner, D.J., Brownstein, D.G., Moody, K.D. (1991). Hydrometra in a New Zealand White rabbit. *Lab Anim Sci.*, **41**, 628–629.

Brewer, N.R. and Cruise, L.J. (1994). Physiology. In *The Biology of the Laboratory Rabbit*, 2nd edn. (P.J. Manning, D.H. Ringler, C.E. Newcomer, eds). pp 63–70. Academic Press.

Brod, J., Sirota J.H.(1949) Effects of emotional disturbance on water diuresis and renal blood flow in the rabbit. *Am J Physiol.*, **157**, 31–39.

Caslow, D. (1989). Hormone responsive perineal urine soiling in two female ovariohysterectomised rabbits. *Companion Anim Pract.*, **19**, 32–33.

Cheeke, P.R. Amberg, J.W. (1973). Comparative calcium excretion by rats and rabbits. *J Anim Sci.*, **37**, 450.

Cheeke, P.R., Patton, N.M., Templeton, G.S. (1982). *Rabbit Production*, Interstate Publishers.

Cheeke, P.R., Bronson, J., Robinson, K.L., Patton N.M. (1985). Availability of calcium, phosphorus and magnesium in rabbit feeds and mineral supplements. *J Appl Rabbit Res.*, **8**, 72–74.

Cruise, L.J., Brewer, N.R. (1994). Anatomy. In *The Biology of the Laboratory Rabbit*, 2nd edn. (P.J. Manning, D.H. Ringler, C.E. Newcomer, eds). pp 47–61. Academic Press.

DePalo, D., Theisen, A.L., Langman, C.B. *et al.* (1988). Renal responses to calcium deprivation in young rabbits. *Miner Electrolyte Metab.*, **14**, 313–320.

Dobyan, D.C., Magill, L.S., Friedman, P.A. *et al.* (1982). Carbonic anhydrase histochemistry in rabbit and mouse kidneys (Abstract). *Anat Rec.*, **204**, 185–197.

Eddy, A.A., Falk, R.J., Sibley, R.K., Hostetter, T.H. (1986). Subtotal nephrectomy in the rabbit: a model of chronic hypercalcaemia, nephrolithiasis and obstructive nephropathy (Abstract). *J Lab Clin Med.*, **107**, 508–516.

Garibaldi, B.A., Fox, J.G., Otto, G. *et al.* (1987). Hematuria in rabbits. *Lab Anim Sci.*, **37**, 769–772.

Garibaldi, B.A., Pecquet Goad, M.E. (1988). Hypercalcaemia with secondary nephrolithiasis in a rabbit. *Lab Anim Sci.*, **38**, 331–332.

Goad, D.L., Pecquet, M.E., Warren, H.B. (1989). Total serum calcium concentrations in rabbits. *J Am Vet Med Assoc.*, **194**, 1520–1521.

Greene, H.S.N. (1941). Uterine adenomata in the rabbit. *J Exp Med.*, **73**, 273–292.

Greenacre, C.B., Allen, S.W., Ritchie, B.W. (1999). Urinary bladder eversion in rabbit does. *Compendium of Continuing Education*, **21**, 524–528.

Hanke, P.R., Timm, P., Falk, G., Kramer, W. (1994). Behaviour of different suture materials in the urinary bladder of the rabbit with special reference to wound healing, epithelization and crystallisation (Abstract). *Urol Int.* **52**, 26–33.

Harcourt-Brown, F.M. (1996). Calcium deficiency, diet and dental disease in pet rabbits. *Vet Rec.*, **139**, 567–571.

Harcourt-Brown, F.M., Baker, S.J. (2001). Parathyroid hormone, haematological and biochemical parameters in relation to dental disease and husbandry in pet rabbits. *J Small Anim Pract.*, **42**, 130–136.

Harper, P.A., Ensley, P.K. (1982). Mummified fetus associated with uterine rupture in a New Zealand White rabbit (*Oryctolagus cuniculus*) (Abstract). *Lab Anim Sci.*, **32**, 518–519.

Hinton, M.(1981). Kidney disease in the rabbit: a histological survey. *Lab Anim.*, **15**, 263–265.

Itatani, H., Yoshioka, T., Namiki, M. *et al.* (1979) Experimental model of calcium containing renal stone formation in a rabbit. *Invest Urol.*, **17**, 234–241.

Jenkins, J.R. (1997). Soft tissue surgery and dental procedures. In *Ferrets, Rabbits and Rodents. Clinical Medicine and Surgery* (E.V. Hillyer, K.E. Quesenberry, eds). pp 227–240. W.B. Saunders.

Kaminski, J.M., Katz, A.R., Woodward, S.C. (1978). Urinary bladder calculus formation on sutures in rabbits, cats and dogs (Abstract). *Surg Gynecol Obstet.*, **146**, 353–357.

Kamphues, V.J., Carstensen, P. Schroeder, D. *et al.* (1986). Effect of increasing calcium and vitamin D supply on calcium metabolism in rabbits (Article in German with an English Summary). *J Anim Physiol Nutr.*, **50**, 191–208.

Kaplan, B.L., Smith, H.W.(1935). Excretion of inulin, creatinine, xylose and urea in the normal rabbit. *Am J Physiol.*, **113**, 354–360.

Kennedy, A. (1965). The urinary excretion of calcium by normal rabbits. *J Comp Pathol.*, **75**, 69–74.

Korner, P.I. (1963). Renal blood flow, glomerular filtration rate, renal PAH extraction ratio and the role of renal vasomotor nerves in the unanesthetised rabbit. *Circ Res.*, **12**, 353–360.

Lindsey, J.R., Fox, R.R. (1994). Inherited diseases and variations. In *The Biology of the Laboratory Rabbit*, 2nd edn. (P.J. Manning, D.H. Ringler, C.E. Newcomer, eds). pp 293–313. Academic Press.

Morris, M.C., Baquero, A., Redovan, E. *et al.* (1986). Urolithiasis on absorbable and non-absorbable suture materials in the rabbit bladder. *J Urol.*, **135**, 602–603.

Percy, D.H., Barthold, S.W. (1993). Rabbit. In *Pathology of Laboratory Rodents and Rabbits.* pp 179–223. Iowa State University Press.

Tvedegaard, E. (1987). Arterial disease in chronic renal failure. An experimental study in the rabbit. *Acta Pathol Microbiol Immunol Scand Section A. Suppl 290*, **95**, 3–28.

Weisbroth, S.H. (1994). Neoplastic diseases. In *The Biology of the Laboratory Rabbit*, 2nd edn. (P.J. Manning, D.H. Ringler, C.E. Newcomer, eds). pp 259–292. Academic Press.

Whary, M.T., Peper, R.L. (1994). Calcium carbonate urolithiasis in a rabbit. *Lab Anim Sci.*, **44**, 534–536.

Whiting, S.J., Quamme, G.A. (1984). Effects of dietary calcium on renal calcium, magnesium and phosphate excretion by the rabbit. *Miner Electrolyte Metab.*, **10**, 217–221.

Zimmerman, T.E., Giddens, W.E., DiGiacomo, R.F., Ladiges, W.C. (1990). Soft tissue mineralization in rabbits fed a diet containing excess vitamin D. *Lab Anim Sci.*, **40**, 212–215.

15

General surgical principles and neutering

Anaesthesia and postoperative care are covered in Chapter 5. Endoscopy in rabbits is summarized in Table 15.1.

15.1 Skin preparation

Rabbit skin is thin and prone to injury. It contains many hair follicles with multiple shafts of fine dense hair. Removing the hair without damaging the skin or clogging the clipper blades can be difficult. A good quality, robust set of clippers is a sound investment. Rabbit hair is so fine that it quickly becomes trapped between fine clipper blades. Running the clipper blade slowly through the fur can prevent this. Depilatory creams can be used but tend to be messy and difficult to clean off satisfactorily. The application of excessive quantities of spirit to the operation site can cause heat loss especially in small, thin rabbits. Excessive scrubbing or iatrogenic skin damage from the clippers may cause postoperative irritation, pain and possibly self-mutilation especially around the perineum. Chlorhexidene in spirit (Vetasept, Animalcare) is suitable for preoperative skin sterilization as it can be applied as a single application and does not require skin scrubbing.

15.2 Surgical considerations

Good illumination is essential for rabbit surgery. The tissue is thin, delicate and friable in comparison with the dog or cat. Some surgeons prefer to operate using optical loupes or an operating microscope. Transparent, plastic drapes are an asset as they allow the anaesthetist to observe the respiratory movements during surgery. A set of fine surgical instruments is required. A kit has been put together especially for surgery on rabbits (Animalcare, York). It contains a selection of 5" (12.7 cm) straight and curved Criles and Halstead forceps, Martin splinter forceps, Debakey (2 mm) and Adson (1/2tm 5") dissecting forceps, an Olsen hegar scissor needle holder and 5" (12.7 cm) straight sharp/blunt and 4.5" (11.5 cm) Strabismus scissors. A no. 9 scalpel blade and a pair of 6" (15 cm) straight Metzenbaum scissors are also included.

The blood volume of rabbits is 55–65 ml/kg (Gillet, 1994). Up to 10% of this amount can be lost without untoward effect. Above 20–25% results in hypovolaemic shock.

Rabbits are prone to the development of adhesions after surgery. The omentum in rabbits is small and it is often not possible to omentalize viscera satisfactorily. Foreign material such as talc from gloves or lint from gauze swabs can induce adhesion formation. Gentle surgical technique with minimal tissue handling is important. Fat necrosis occurs readily, especially in the broad ligament. The fat decomposes into fatty acids and glycerol that combine with ions such as sodium, potassium and calcium. It is associated with trauma.

Rabbits are used extensively as experimental models of post-surgical adhesions in humans, especially after urogenital surgery. In laboratory rabbits, it has been discovered that calcium channel blockers are effective in preventing adhesions (Steinleitner *et al.*, 1990). Verapamil (200 μg/kg), given subcutaneously every 8 h for a total of nine doses, can be used in situations where adhesions are

Table 15.1 Endoscopy in rabbits

- As a general rule, the largest endoscope possible should be used. Large endoscopes give a better view with good illumination and are stronger and less liable to damage
- Rigid endoscopes are most suitable for most endoscopic procedures in rabbits. They require an irrigation sheath that is used for flushing, sucking and insufflation. A larger sheath can be used to provide an instrument channel
- General anaesthesia is required.

Site	*Type of endoscope*	*Indications*	*Comments*
Oropharynx	Rigid 2.7 mm 0° is OK 4 mm is preferable 30° can be useful	To view tongue and teeth	• Withhold food for 1–2 h prior to examination • Caecotrophs may still be found in the oral cavity and obscure the view
Larynx	Rigid 2.7 mm 0° or 4 mm 0°	Visual examination of larynx and surrounding structures Can be used for endotracheal intubation by placing tube over scope.	• Positioning is important • The larynx of the rabbit is small so a 2.7 mm scope is required to pass through it • The large base of the tongue is an obstacle
Rhinoscopy	1.2 mm 0° (microendoscope and sheath, Storz) A rigid 2.7 mm 0° endoscope plus sheath can be used in large rabbits	Examination of the nasal passages Removal of foreign bodies such as stems of hay	• Endotracheal intubation is vital. A tight-fitting, endotracheal tube is required to prevent inhalation of water or purulent material during flushing • Foreign material that cannot be grasped can be pushed into nasopharynx and oesophagus
Otoscopy	Rigid plus sheath 2.7 mm 0° or 1.2 mm 0° (microendoscope and sheath, Storz)	Examination of tympanic membrane	
Oesophagus and stomach	Possible with 7.9 mm flexible, paediatric gastroscope in average sized rabbit (2.5–3 kg) Alternative is 3 mm ureteroscope		• Unlike dogs and cats, the rabbit's stomach is never empty • Stomach contents impede view
Colon	Rigid 2.7 mm 0° or 4 mm 0°		Can only visualize distal portion of descending colon
Laparoscopy	Rigid 4 mm 0° or 5 mm 0° plus CO_2insufflation	Visualization and biopsy of abdominal viscera	• Requires careful anaesthesia. Intermittent positive pressure is preferable, which requires a tight fitting endotracheal tube • Distension of the abdominal cavity can compromise respiration • Must be done aseptically • Enter abdomen at umbilicus taking care not to damage thin-walled abdominal viscera • Abdominal fat can obscure the view • Light transmission can be a problem • Postoperative analgesia is required
Urogenital tract	Rigid plus sheath 2.7 mm 0° or 1.2 mm 0° (microendoscope and instrument sheath, Storz)	Examination of urogenital tract Retrieval of small uroliths from neck of bladder (Murray, 2000)	Only in female

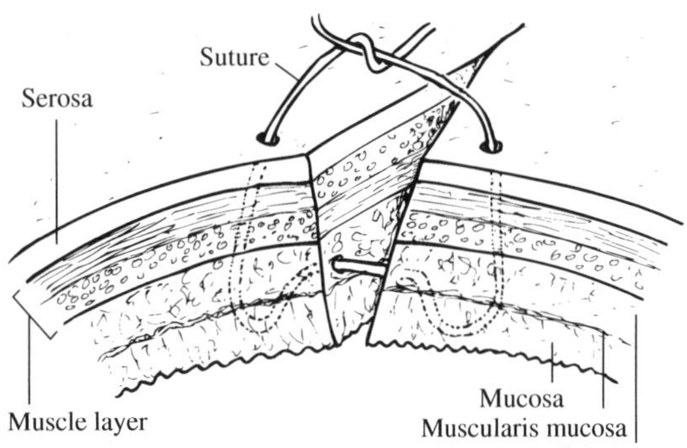

(a) Modified Gambee suture

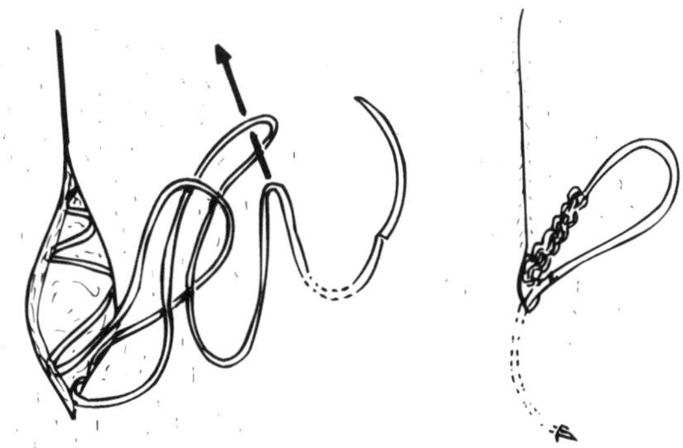

(b) Aberdeen knot

Figure 15.1. Recommended suture patterns. (a) **Modified Gambee suture pattern for edge-to-edge intestinal repair.** The submucosal layer is important during intestinal healing due to its abundance of collagen. During repair, it is essential to pass sutures through the submucosal layer and to bring it and the wound edges into direct apposition without crushing the tissue or everting the mucosa. Single layer enterotomy closures are preferable because double layer closures reduce the lumen diameter. Classic inverting sutures can induce stenosis, which is a major problem in rabbits that have a narrow intestinal lumen. Fine (5/0), absorbable, monofilament suture material such as poliglecaprone (Monocryl, Ethicon) or polydioxanone (PDS II, Ethicon) are suitable for the closure of intestinal incisions. A modified Gambee suture, using single interrupted sutures 2–3 mm apart and 2–3 mm from the cut edge, is satisfactory. With correct instrumentation, this suture pattern is surprisingly easy. (b) **Subcuticular skin closure using an Aberdeen knot.** Skin sutures can easily be removed by rabbits although, if the suture line is comfortable, most rabbits will leave a surgical incision alone. Elizabethan collars are unsatisfactory and stressful to rabbits and are not an alternative to good surgical technique. It is important that surgical incisions are repaired securely and without tension on the sutures. Skin closure with a continuous subcuticular suture with a buried Aberdeen knot is recommended (Flecknell, 1998). This method leaves no visible skin sutures for the rabbit to remove. Fine, absorbable, monofilament suture material such as poliglecaprone (4/0 Monocryl, Ethicon) or polydioxanone (4/0 PDS II, Ethicon) are suitable for subcuticular suturing.

likely to develop. Examples include surgery on the large intestine, ruptured pyometra or abdominal abscess removal.

15.3 Suture techniques and materials

Experimental studies have indicated that the size of the suture material is more important than tissue reactivity in adhesion formation (Holtz, 1982). Therefore, the choice of fine suture material in addition to good suture technique is important to minimize adhesion formation in rabbits. Small gauge (3/0, 4/0 or 5/0) modern suture materials swaged on needles are satisfactory. Polydioxanone (PDS 11) or poliglecaprone (Monocryl, Ethicon) can be used for most situations, although 3/0 or 4/0 catgut is suitable to tie off blood vessels or ligaments.

15.4 Abdominal incisions

A midline approach through the linea alba is suitable for most abdominal procedures in rabbits. A good choice for repairing the incision is 4/0 polydioxanone (PDS 11) as it has high tensile strength and is degraded slowly. An alternative is 4/0 poliglecaprone (Monocryl, Ethicon). The abdominal fascia is repaired in a single layer. Studies in rabbits have shown that a double layer abdominal closure has no advantage over a single layer technique (Nilsson, 1981). The knots at the ends of the suture must be made with particular care if a continuous suture is used. The first throw draws the edges of the fascia together without crushing. An additional four throws are required at the start of the suture and six at the end. (Bouvy and Dupré, 1997). Alternatively, a row of simple interrupted sutures can be used. Skin closure with a continuous subcuticular suture with a buried Aberdeen knot is recommended (see Figure 15.1) (Flecknell, 1998). Additional skin sutures or tissue adhesive can be used, if necessary. Owners appreciate skin sutures and worry that the patient has removed them if they cannot be seen. It is important that the abdominal incision is repaired securely and without tension on the sutures. Tight sutures and ischaemia of the peritoneum increase the risk of abdominal adhesions (Niles and Williams, 1999). If the suture line is comfortable, most rabbits will leave the incision alone, although some will remove the skin sutures. If the subcuticular suture is secure, this is not important.

Surgical staples can be used to close the skin wound as an alternative to subcuticular sutures. Staples have the advantage of being quick to place and difficult, although not impossible, for the patient to remove. Elizabethan collars are unsatisfactory and stressful to rabbits and should not be used as an alternative to good surgical technique.

15.5 Skin sutures

For operations where there is no skin tension, e.g. perineal dermoplasty, absorbable skin sutures that do not require removal can be used. Polyglactin 910 (Vicryl Rapide, Ethicon) is satisfactory for such procedures. The inflammatory response to polyglactic acid in rabbits is mild (Wainstein *et al.*, 1997).

It is sometimes necessary to suture contaminated wounds, notably after abscess removal or exploration. Closure of infected skin wounds is sometimes necessary after surgery on abscesses. Skin sutures are necessary after placement of antibiotic impregnated beads in order to retain them. The presence of buried suture material in wounds associated with abscesses in rabbits carries a high risk of secondary abscess formation. The risk can be minimized by using fine materials and small knots. Monofilament suture materials withstand contamination better than multifilament sutures so materials such as polydioxanone (PDS, Ethicon) or poliglecaprone (Monocryl, Ethicon) are preferable to braided or multifilament materials. Bacteria can persist within the interstices of the multifilament fibres where they are resistant to removal by macrophages (Niles and Williams, 1999). Alternatively, absorbable materials such as catgut can be used which are removed from the wound by macrophages together with any associated bacteria.

15.6 Repair of hollow abdominal organs

Fine, absorbable, monofilament suture material such as poliglecaprone (Monocryl, Ethicon) or polydioxanone (PDS II, Ethicon) are suitable for the closure of most abdominal organs in rabbits. Catgut is not suitable for closure of the stomach because of the acidic environment. Poliglecaprone elicits minimal inflammatory reaction and handles and knots well. A number of suture patterns are acceptable. Single interrupted sutures 2–3 mm apart and 2–3 mm from the cut edge can be used. The submucosal layer is most important in wound healing due to its abundance of collagen. During repair of the intestine, it is essential to pass sutures through the submucosal layer and to bring the wound edges into direct apposition without crushing the tissue or everting the mucosa. Penetration of the lumen is often required (Bouvy and Dupré, 1997). Single layer enterotomy closures are preferable because a double layer closure reduces the lumen diameter. A modified Gambee suture is suitable (see Figure 15.1). Classic inverting sutures induce stenosis, which is a major problem in a species with a narrow intestinal lumen, such as rabbits. During repair of the bladder, penetration of the lumen should be avoided because of the risk of subsequent calculus formation.

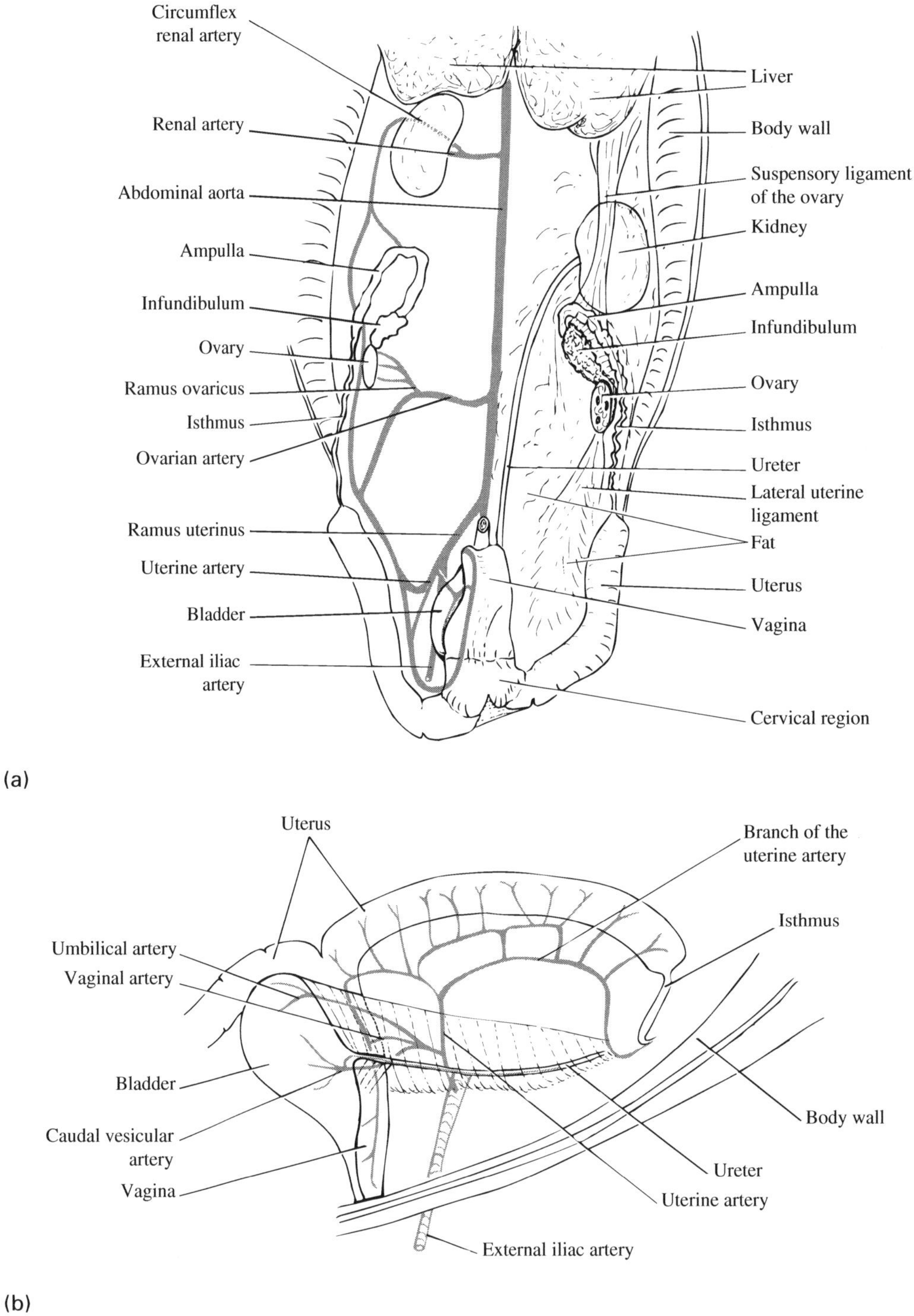
Circumflex renal artery
Renal artery
Abdominal aorta
Ampulla
Infundibulum
Ovary
Ramus ovaricus
Isthmus
Ovarian artery
Ramus uterinus
Uterine artery
Bladder
External iliac artery
Liver
Body wall
Suspensory ligament of the ovary
Kidney
Ampulla
Infundibulum
Ovary
Isthmus
Ureter
Lateral uterine ligament
Fat
Uterus
Vagina
Cervical region
(a)
Uterus
Branch of the uterine artery
Isthmus
Umbilical artery
Vaginal artery
Bladder
Caudal vesicular artery
Vagina
Body wall
Ureter
Uterine artery
External iliac artery
(b)

Figure 15.2.

Figure 15.2. Anatomy of female reproductive tract. (a) A view of dorsal abdomen with intestinal tract removed and uterus reflected caudally. (b) A caudolateral view of the urogenital tract with the uterus pulled cranioventrally. This figure illustrates the anatomy of the female reproductive tract of the rabbit, including the blood supply and peritoneal attachments. There are several anatomical features that are relevant during ovariohysterectomy:

- The vaginal body is long and flaccid. The cervix is easily exteriorized via a midline abdominal incision. The incision should be made closer to the ovaries, which are more difficult to exteriorize. The landmarks are the umbilicus and the pubis. A 1–2 cm incision is made midway between these points
- The Fallopian tube, that consists of the isthmus, ampulla and infundibulum, is long, convoluted and friable. The narrow isthmus separates the cranial end of the uterine horn from the long ampulla, infundibulum and ovary. The ampulla and infundibulum are a deep red colour resembling a blood vessel
- The ovaries are easily identifiable and are situated in the dorsal part of the mid abdomen. The left ovary is close to the kidney. Both ovaries must be identified and removed
- Substantial amounts of fat may be laid down in the broad ligament and suspensory ligament of the ovary
- The ovarian artery lies within the broad ligament caudal to the infundibulum
- The cervix is bicornuate
- The flaccid vaginal body fills with urine during micturition. A secure transfixing cervical ligature is required
- A branch of the uterine artery, the caudal vesicular artery, supplies the bladder. This branch can be inadvertently incorporated in a cervical ligature if it is placed incorrectly (see (a)). It is also possible to incorporate the ureter in an incorrectly placed ligature around the caudal vagina
- A ligature placed across the cervix is easier to place and to transfix than a ligature placed around the vagina, but carries a small risk of leaving sufficient uterine tissue to form a uterine adenocarcinoma.

15.7 Neutering

15.7.1 Ovariohysterectomy

Spaying female rabbits is indicated to prevent unwanted pregnancy and pseudopregnancy, modify sexually related behaviour such as territorial aggression and prevent or treat neoplasia of the uterus or pyometra and other uterine disorders. The procedure is now routine in many veterinary practices. Rabbits should be sexually mature, i.e. at least 5 months of age. Immature females have vestigial, thread-like uterine horns and tiny ovaries that can be very difficult to locate. Obese rabbits should lose weight prior to surgery. Apart from the practical considerations associated with large quantities of abdominal and subcutaneous fat, some rabbits are inappetant for 12–36 h after spaying, even with analgesia. Even a short period of fasting is dangerous in obese individuals with a fatty liver, as they are prone to developing hepatic lipidosis (see Section 10.3.3). Does can be spayed during early pregnancy without additional complications.

Some authorities advocate expressing the bladder prior to surgery. If the bladder is emptied manually, great care should be taken as the organ is thin walled and easily traumatized or even ruptured.

The uterus is easily accessible through a 1–2 cm midline incision approximately half way between the umbilicus and the pubic symphysis. Care must be taken when entering the abdominal cavity to avoid the thin-walled caecum and bladder that may be lying immediately beneath the incision. The body wall should be grasped with forceps and elevated prior to incising into the abdominal cavity.

The anatomy and blood supply to the uterus is illustrated in Figure 15.2. The Fallopian tubes are long and friable. The Fallopian tube has three sections: the isthmus, the ampulla and the infundibulum. Gentle traction is required to exteriorize the ovary and ovarian ligament. Ligatures are required to tie off the ovarian blood vessels and those in the broad ligament. A ligature placed just cranially to the cervices lies securely and avoids the ureters and common blood supply

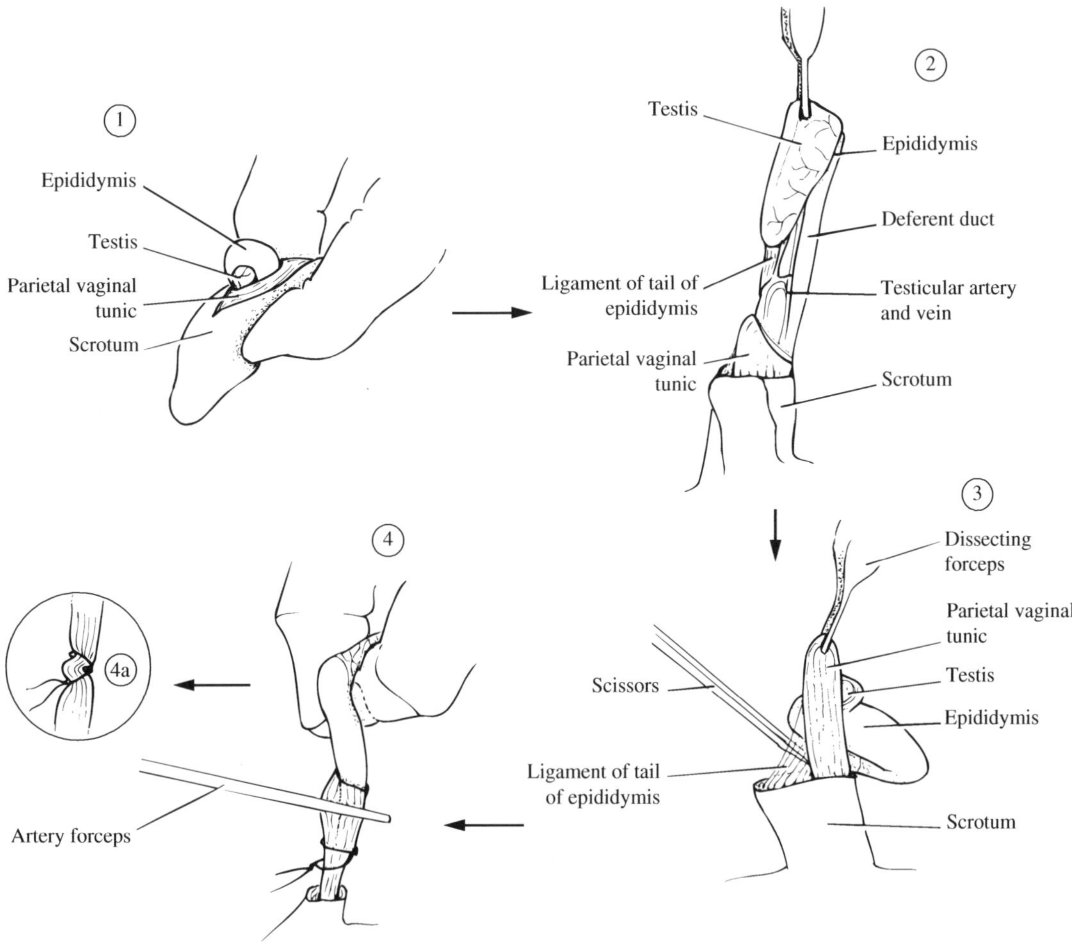

Figure 15.3. Recommended technique for castration. The inguinal ring of rabbits remains open throughout life. There is a risk of herniation of abdominal contents through the inguinal ring after castration unless the ring is satisfactorily closed. Herniation can be prevented by an inguinal ligature that incorporates the parietal vaginal tunic as well as the spermatic cord. This figure illustrates a simple, quick castration technique that closes the inguinal ring and requires no skin sutures.

1. The fur surrounding the scrotum is clipped and the skin prepared for surgery. The scrotal sac containing a testicle is grasped between finger and thumb and a 1 cm incision made through the skin at the cranial end. The parietal vaginal tunic is incised to expose the epididymis and testicle
2. The testicle is exteriorized and pulled out of the incision, which places tension on the parietal vaginal tunic that is attached to the testicle by the gubernaculum
3. The parietal vaginal tunic is grasped and the connective tissue that holds it to the scrotal skin is dissected with scissors
4. The testicle, surrounded by parietal vaginal tunic is pulled out of the incision and a secure ligature placed around the entire structure, close to the inguinal ring (using 3/0 absorbable suture material). The ligated remnant of the spermatic cord is returned to the scrotum and the skin pulled over it. No sutures are required in the scrotal skin.

Key points 15.1

- Rabbit skin is thin and prone to injury during skin preparation. A good set of clippers and fine clipper blades are a sound investment
- Good illumination and a fine set of surgical instruments are required for rabbit surgery. The tissue is thin and friable. Many surgeons prefer to use optical loupes
- The blood volume of rabbits is 55–65 ml/kg (Gillet, 1994). Up to 10% of this amount can be lost without untoward effect. Above 20–25% results in hypovolaemic shock
- Adhesions develop easily in rabbits. Gentle tissue handling and minimum contamination by haemorrhage, talc, lint from swabs and other foreign material will reduce risk of adhesion formation
- Fat necrosis occurs readily, especially in the broad ligament around ligatures placed during spaying
- The calcium channel blocker, Verapamil (200 μg/kg), can be given subcutaneously every 8 h for a total of nine doses, and may be used in situations where adhesions are likely to develop
- Rabbit blood clots quickly
- Small gauge (3/0, 4/0 or 5/0) modern suture materials, swaged on needles are ideal for rabbit surgery. 3/0 suture material is suitable for skin repair. 4/0 suture material is required for subcuticular repair of abdominal incisions and 5/0 suture material is required for intestinal surgery
- Polydioxanone (PDS 11) can be used for most situations as it has high tensile strength and is degraded slowly. An alternative is poliglecaprone (Monocryl, Ethicon). These suture materials can be used to repair abdominal organs and close abdominal incisions. Cat gut can be used to tie off blood vessels or ligaments
- A midline abdominal approach is suitable for most abdominal operations. The abdominal fascia is repaired in a single layer with continuous or simple interrupted sutures using PDS or Monocryl
- Rabbits have the reputation for removing skin sutures. Elizabethan collars are not recommended as they are stressful and prevent caecotrophy
- Sutures are less likely to be removed if the skin incision is comfortable and repaired without tension on the sutures. A subcuticular suture or skin staples reduce the risk or patient interference and subsequent wound breakdown
- Polyglactin 910 (Vicryl Rapide) (4/0) is a useful skin suture for plastic surgery such as perineal dermoplasty. It is soft and knots easily. Sutures do not require removal
- The submucosal layer of abdominal organs is most important in wound healing due to its abundance of collagen. During repair of organs such as intestine or bladder, it is essential to pass sutures through the submucosal layer and to bring the wound edges into direct apposition without crushing the tissue
- The cervical ligature can be placed above or below the cervix during ovariohysterectomy. A transfixing suture is recommended
- Placing the ligature above the cervix results in a secure ligature but carries a risk of leaving residual uterine tissue that, theoretically, could develop adenocarcinoma
- A ligature placed below the cervix is less secure due to the flaccid nature of vaginal tissue and carries a risk of urine leakage through the stump
- Ligatures placed low down the vagina carry a small risk of including the ureters or blood vessels to the bladder (see Figure 15.2)
- A closed castration technique with closure of the inguinal ring is required to prevent postoperative herniation of abdominal contents. A simple technique is illustrated in Figure 15.3.

to the bladder. A transfixing suture is advisable. 3/0 cat gut can be used without adverse effects (Millis and Walshaw, 1992). Placing the cervical ligature around the uterine side of the cervix results in a small amount of residual uterine tissue that could be a site for adenocarcinoma formation. However, the risk is small once the hormonal influence of the ovaries is removed. An alternative approach is to place the ligature around the vaginal side of the cervix. However, at this site, the tissue is flaccid and it is more difficult to place the ligature securely. There is also the possibility of contamination of the abdominal cavity from leaked urine through the vaginal stump. In rabbits, the vagina fills with urine when the bladder is emptied. There is a risk of including ureters and the blood vessels that supply the bladder if the ligature is placed too low.

15.7.2 Castration

Testicles descend into the scrotal sacs at 10–12 weeks of age. Rabbits are able to retract their testicles through the inguinal ring, which remains open throughout life. This response can also be evoked by handling the testicle even under light anaesthesia. Immature or debilitated rabbits have abdominal or inguinal testicles and genuine cryptorchid males also occur (Richardson, 1999). A testicle that has been retracted through the inguinal ring can be brought into the scrotal sac during surgery. Retracted testicles and cryptorchidism can also be confused with absent testicles. Rabbits often attack the scrotum during fighting and can remove one or both testicles. Remnants of the spermatic cord and surrounding structures are found in the inguinal region.

There are several methods of castration and the choice depends on the preference of the surgeon. Some authors describe removal of the testicles through a prescrotal or even abdominal incision (Millis and Walshaw, 1992). Surgery follows the same principles as castration in other species, except that the inguinal ring should be closed to prevent prolapse of abdominal contents after surgery. A traditional closed castration via the scrotum is often recommended (Redrobe, 2000). Alternatively, a simple technique that involves exteriorizing the testicle can be used. The testicle is pulled out of the incision so the tunic can easily be dissected away from the scrotum with scissors (see Figure 15.3). A ligature is placed around the spermatic cord encased in the tunic as close as possible to the inguinal ring. The testicle and surrounding tissue is cut off below the ligature. No skin sutures are required and there is no risk of herniation. This is effectively a closed castration although it is much simpler to perform.

References

Bouvy, B., Dupré, G. (1997). Surgical soft tissue suture techniques: current recommendations for the dog and cat. *Waltham Focus*, **7**, 7–15.

Flecknell, P.A. (1998). Developments in the veterinary care of rabbits and rodents. *In Practice*, **20**, 286–295.

Gillett, C.S. (1994). Selected drug dosages and clinical reference data. In *The Biology of the Laboratory Rabbit*, 2nd edn. (P.J. Manning, D.H Ringler, C.E. Newcomer, eds). pp 468–471. Academic Press.

Holtz, G. (1982). Adhesion induction by suture of varying tissue reactivity and caliber (Abstract). *Int J Fertil.*, **27**, 134–135.

Millis, D.L., Walshaw, R. (1992). Elective castrations and ovariohysterectomies in pet rabbits. *J Am Anim Hosp Assoc.*, **28**, 491–497.

Murray, M. J. (2000). Application of rigid endoscopy in small exotic mammals. *Exotic DVM*, **23**, 13–18.

Niles, J., Williams, J. (1999). Suture materials and patterns. *In Practice*, **21**, 308–320.

Nilsson, T. (1981) Closure of the abdominal wound with single-layer and double-layer technique. *Acta Chir Scand.*, **147**, 399–403.

Redrobe, S. (2000). Surgical procedures and dental disorders. In *Manual of Rabbit Medicine and Surgery*. pp 117–134. British Small Animal Veterinary Association.

Richardson, V. (2000). *Rabbits. Health Husbandry and Diseases*. Blackwell Sciences.

Steinleitner, A, Lambert, H, Kazensky, C. *et al.* (1990). Reduction of primary postoperative adhesion formation under calcium channel blockade in the rabbit. *J Surg Res.*, **48**, 42–45.

Wainstein, M., Anderson, J., Elder, J.S. (1997). Comparison of effects of suture materials on wound healing in a rabbit pyeloplasty model (Abstract). *Urology*, **49**, 261–264.

16

Infectious diseases of domestic rabbits

16.1 Parasites of rabbits

Wild rabbits are host to a variety of parasites that can be transmitted to domestic rabbits. The type and species of parasite varies throughout the world and it is beyond the scope of this book to describe them all. A detailed, illustrated description is given by Hofing and Kraus (1994). The parasites that affect domestic rabbits are described in detail by Owen (1992). This is the major reference source for the parasite section of this chapter.

16.2 Ectoparasites

16.2.1 Fleas

Spilopsyllus cuniculi is a common flea that infests wild rabbits in Europe. It does not occur in the USA (Kraus *et al.*, 1984). The fleas have a predilection for the ears where they can be found in clusters along the edges of the pinnae. The fleas are mobile and move between the environment and the host. Wild rabbit fleas are not usually found on pet rabbits. *Spilopsyllus cuniculi* is a small flea whose life cycle is influenced by the reproductive status of the host. Egg maturation is dependent on female reproductive hormones. Successful reproduction of the rabbit flea requires contact with a rabbit in late pregnancy or with a newborn nestling. Increased blood corticosteroid concentrations in late pregnancy attract fleas, which attach firmly to the doe to feed. Within a few hours of parturition, fleas move from the doe to the newborn babies to feed, copulate and lay eggs in the nest. The eggs hatch and the larvae feed on flea dirt deposited in the nest by the adult fleas feeding on the pregnant doe. In this way, fleas are spread from one generation to the next and are an important vector of disease, especially myxomatosis.

Ctenocephalides canis or *felis*, the common cat and dog flea, is the usual flea that is found on pet rabbits. Infestation results from rabbits living in a house inhabited by dogs and cats. Infestation causes intense pruritus and allergic dermatitis can develop. Fleas and flea dirt can be found on the rabbit by combing the coat with a fine-toothed comb.

16.2.2 Lice

Haemodipsus ventricosus is a sucking louse that affects wild rabbits and may act as a vector for myxomatosis. It is a large louse 1.5–2.5 mm in length. It is occasionally found on pet rabbits (Owen, 1992).

16.2.3 Mites

Psoroptes cuniculi is the common ear mite of rabbits that causes crusting and ulceration of the external ear canal. The mites are large and active and are just visible to the naked eye. They are surface dwellers that cause intense irritation when they are present in large numbers (see Figure 16.1). Occasionally they are found in other areas of the body such as the perineal skin folds (see Section 9.14.2.1).

Cheyletiella parasitovorax is a fur dwelling mite that can be found in large numbers in pet rabbits (see Section 9.14.2.3). Areas of dense, flaky, encrusted skin are found along the back especially above the tail base and on

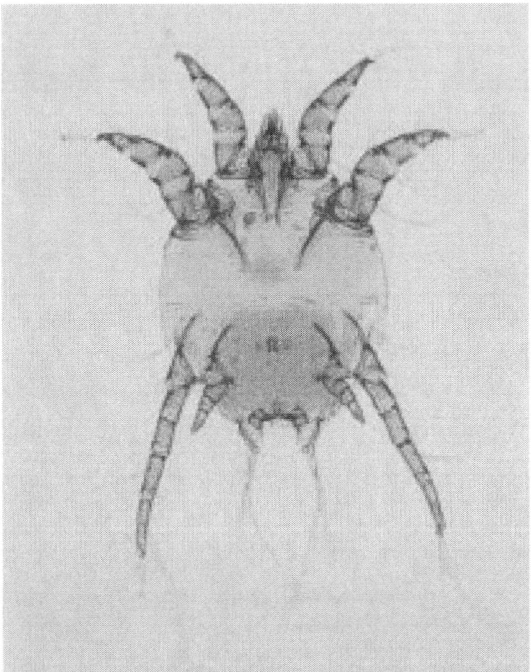

Figure 16.1. *Psoroptes cuniculi* (Image supplied by Dr Sheelagh Lloyd, Division of Animal Pathology, University of Cambridge). The rabbit ear mite, *Psoroptes cuniculi* causes crusting and inflammation of the external ear canal, which often extends up the pinna (see Plate 4). Lesions are sometimes found on other parts of the body such as the perineal skin folds. Mites can just be seen with the naked eye in exudate from the lesions. Large numbers of *Psoroptes cuniculi* are visible on microscopic examination of the exudate, which can be softened in liquid paraffin before placing on a glass slide.

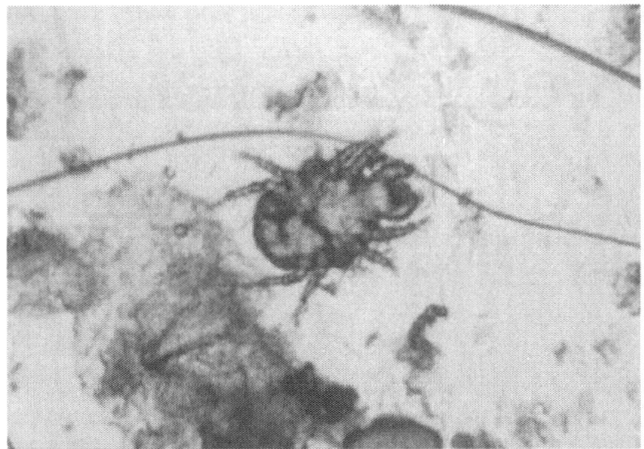

Figure 16.2. *Cheyletiella parasitovorax.* This mite can be found in the fur of healthy rabbits. It is not always associated with skin lesions. In large numbers, *Cheyletiella parasitovorax* mites cause pruritus and areas of white, flaky skin. Heavy infestation is usually linked to some underlying problem with grooming, such as dental disease, obesity or spinal disorders. Mites may be seen moving among skin flakes that are combed out and placed under a bright light. *Cheyletiella parasitovorax* can also be detected by combing out the flakes and applying acetate strips to the exposed underlying skin. The acetate strip is placed on a microscope slide and examined on low power. In heavy infestations a variety of nymphal stages, eggs and adult mites are seen.

the neck. The mites are easily identified by microscopic examination of skin brushings or pluckings (see Figure 16.2). Infestation with cheyletiella is often associated with obesity, spinal disorders or dental disease. *Cheyletiella parasitovorax* is zoonotic and can cause erythema and pruritus in man. Pruritic lesions are found on the forearm or neck of humans that have handled infested rabbits. The lesions regress over 24 h.

Leporacus gibbus (formerly known as *Listrophorus gibbus*) is the common fur mite of rabbits (see Section 9.14.2.4). Infestation is normally asymptomatic and is not significant, except that large numbers can indicate some underlying disease. The mite is usually found attached to the hair shaft where it feeds on sebaceous gland secretions (see Figure 16.3). The mites are just visible to the naked eye especially on light coloured rabbits when infestation gives the coat the appearance of being sprinkled with pepper. This effect is more obvious when the coat is wet.

Notoedres and *Sarcoptes* have been described as causes of mange in rabbits.

16.2.4 Warble flies

Cuterebra horripilum and *C. buccata* are warble flies that affect rabbits in the USA but do not occur in the UK.

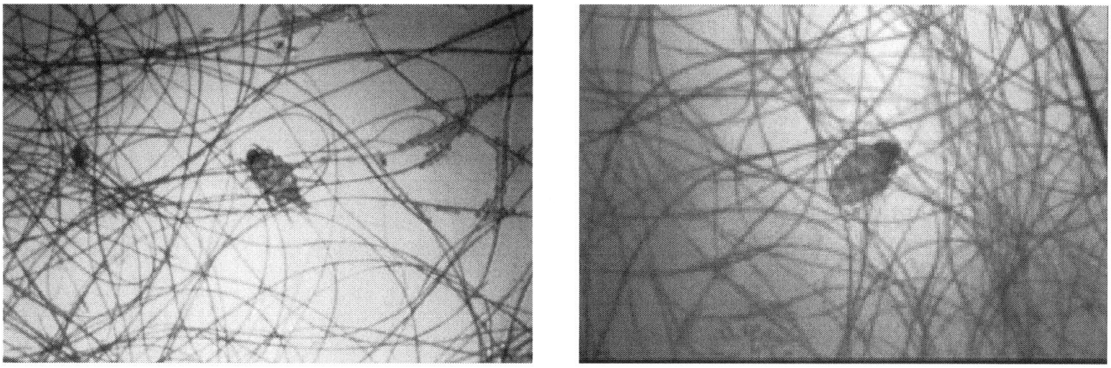

(a) (b)

Figure 16.3. *Leporacus gibbus* (formerly *Listrophorus gibbus*). *Leporacus gibbus* can be found in the fur of many pet rabbits. Infestation is usually asymptomatic. Like *Cheyletiella parasitovorax,* heavy infestation is linked to some underlying problem with grooming, such as dental disease, obesity or spinal disorders. The mite is just visible to the naked eye, especially in light-coloured rabbits. A simple method of detecting *Leporacus gibbus* is to comb through the fur with a fine-toothed flea comb and place the combings in a small, clear plastic bag. The contents of the bag are viewed microscopically under low power and the mites are seen moving along hair shafts. Eggs and empty egg cases can be seen attached to hair shafts. Immature and adult mites are visible. There are morphological differences between male (a) and female mites (b).

16.3 Endoparasites

16.3.1 Intestinal worms

There is a range of nematodes that affect wild rabbits in various parts of the world. With the exception of *Passalurus ambiguus,* infestations in domestic rabbits are rare, especially in pets and are unlikely to be encountered. *Passalurus ambiguus* is an oxyurid that is found in the caecum and large intestine. The adult worms measure 5–10 mm and are not pathogenic in the adult animal. Heavy infestations in young rabbits can be a contributory factor to the enteritis complex of diseases that occur around weaning (see Section 10.2).

The small, thread-like worm is seen in the faeces of affected animals. The life cycle is direct. *Passalurus ambiguus* is susceptible to most anthelmintics, e.g. piperazine and fenbendazole. Ivermectin is ineffective (Morrisey, 1996).

There are other helminth parasites that principally affect wild rabbits and are not found in the domestic pet. They include *Graphidium strigosum* and *Trichostrongylus retortaeformis* (Allan *et al.,* 1999). *Obeliscoides cuniculi* occurs in wild rabbits in various parts of the world and in domestic rabbits in the USA (Hofing and Kraus, 1994). *Obeliscoides cuniculi* has been used as a laboratory model of *Trichostrongylus* and *Ostertagia* species of ruminants. No species of trematode has been reported in rabbits (Kraus *et al.,* 1984).

16.3.2 Tapeworms

The rabbit is the intermediate host for several tapeworms that affect dogs and cats. Pet rabbits that graze in gardens inhabited by pet dogs or visited by foxes can become infected. The incidence of these parasites is not high as most pet owners now worm their dogs with preparations that are effective against tapeworms.

Cysticercus pisiformis is the larval stage of *Taenia pisiformis,* which is a tapeworm that affects dogs and foxes with rabbits acting as the intermediate host. Tapeworm segments packed with eggs are shed in faeces and contaminate pasture. Grazing rabbits ingest eggs that pass into the small intestine where the onchosphere emerges and migrates to the peritoneal cavity via the liver. Multiple oval cysts are found in the mesentery (see Plate 36). The cysts contain the inverted scolex of the tapeworm. Heavy infections cause abdominal discomfort and distension. In severe cases, they can cause intestinal obstruction. Migration through the liver results in the development of fibrous tracks and necrotic foci.

Coenurus serialis is the larval stage of *Taenia serialis*, which is a tapeworm that affects dogs and foxes. A variety of mammals can act as intermediate hosts, usually wild rabbits and hares, but primates and even man can host the intermediate stage. Onchospheres from this tapeworm migrate to the subcutaneous tissue where they form cysts that are palpated as soft swellings under the skin. The cyst contains fluid and inverted secondary buds, each containing a scolex. Occasionally a cyst may be found in the orbit where it causes a retrobulbar swelling (Wills, 2001).

Echinococcus granulosus affects dogs and foxes. Most mammalian species, including man and rabbits, can act as intermediate hosts. The adult tapeworm is small in comparison to other tapeworms. It measures 2–9 mm. Onchospheres from ingested eggs migrate to the liver or the lung via the mesenteric blood vessels. The onchosphere then develops into a huge cyst that is able to produce secondary buds, each with an inverted scolex that can produce daughter cysts. The daughter cysts can, in turn, produce daughter cysts with the result that a huge cyst full of smaller cysts develops. Rupture of the cyst seeds the surrounding tissues with smaller cysts, all of which are capable of developing.

The rabbit can also be a primary host for tapeworms. The cestode species varies in wild rabbits from different parts of the world. An example is *Cittotaenia ctenoides* that has a free-living mite as its intermediate host.

Key points 16.1

- There is a wide range of infectious diseases that affect rabbits throughout the world
- Infectious and parasitic diseases are common in wild rabbits and colonies of commercial or laboratory rabbits but relatively rare in the individual pet
- In pet rabbits, flea infestations are usually transmitted from other household pets such as dogs or cats
- The rabbit louse *Haemodipsus ventricosus* can be found in wild rabbits and is occasionally found in domestic rabbits
- Several mites affect rabbits. *Psoroptes cuniculi, Cheyletiella parasitovorax* and *Leporacus gibbus* are the most common in domestic rabbits
- The warble flies, *Cuterebra horripilum* and *C. buccata* that affect rabbits do not occur in the UK
- With the exception of cestodes and *Passalurus ambiguus*, endoparasite infestations in domestic rabbits are rare
- *Passalurus ambiguus* is a small, thread-like worm that can be seen in the faeces of affected animals. It inhabits the caecum and colon. It is not usually pathogenic. The life cycle is direct
- *Obeliscoides cuniculi* occurs in wild rabbits in various parts of the world and in domestic rabbits in the USA
- The rabbit is the intermediate host for several tapeworms that affect dogs and cats. Pet rabbits that graze in gardens inhabited by pet dogs or visited by foxes can become infected
- Multiple oval cysts of *Cysticercus pisiformis* may be found in the mesentery
- Onchospheres from *Coenurus serialis* migrate to the subcutaneous tissue where they form cysts that may be palpated as soft swellings under the skin
- Onchospheres from *Echinococcus granulosus* can develop into huge cysts in the liver that are able to produce secondary buds, each with an inverted scolex that can produce daughter cysts
- In some parts of the world rabbits are the primary hosts to some tapeworms. Infection is unlikely in domestic rabbits in the UK.

16.4 Protozoa

16.4.1 Coccidiosis

There are as many as 14 species of *Eimeria* which affect rabbits and vary in pathogenicity. Coccidiosis can be a serious problem of rabbit colonies. The disease is described in Section 10.10.1. *Eimeria magna* and *Eimeria irresidua* are the two most pathogenic species that affect the intestine. Other less pathogenic species include *E. perforans*, *E. media*, *E. elongata*, *E. neoloporis*, *E. intestinalis*, *E. caecicola* and *E. piriformis*.

Eimeria steidae causes hepatic coccidiosis and has a slightly different life cycle from the intestinal *Eimeria* species. Oocysts can survive for many years in the environment but are susceptible to dry conditions. Recovered rabbits become immune to infection.

16.4.2 *Encephalitozoon cuniculi*

Encephalitozoon is an obligate intracellular protozoan parasite. It belongs to the Microsporidia genus that is a member of the subphylum Sporozoa. Microsporidia are characterized by having small spores and one polar capsule. There are several *Encephalitozoon* species (e.g. *E. intestinalis*, *E. hellum*, *E. bieneusi*, *E. septata*) most of which are opportunist pathogens in immunocompromised humans. Diarrhoea, renal disease and keratoconjunctivitis are among the diseases that have been associated with encephalitozoonosis in humans. In animals, *Encephalitozoon cuniculi* is the most important member of the Microsporidia genus. *E. cuniculi* primarily affects rabbits but can be found in other species. Microsporidia are unusual in that they lack mitochondria, presumably gaining their nutrition from the host cells (Pakes and Gerrity, 1994). They are characterized by a firm capsule that is strongly gram-negative (Owen, 1992). A long polar filament is neatly coiled within it. The spore has a polar cap. Infection of the host usually occurs by oral ingestion of food contaminated with infected urine. Once in the alimentary tract, the spore comes in close contact with the mucosa and infects a host cell by extruding the polar filament. Sporoplasm is transferred through the polar filament into a vacuole in the host cell where multiplication takes place. Dividing organisms are lined up along the vacuolar membrane that is thought to be of host origin (Pakes and Gerrity, 1994). The cells of the reticuloendothelial system are among those that are invaded and they distribute the parasite around the body. Eventually the organisms develop into mature spores that are oval in shape and measure approximately 2.5×1.5 µm with a thick cell wall (Pakes and Gerrity, 1994). The vacuole becomes distended and the cell eventually ruptures releasing spores that invade new cells. Rupture of the cells is associated with an inflammatory response (Pattison *et al.*, 1971). Chronic inflammation results in the development of granulomatous lesions in target organs, primarily the kidney and brain, although the liver may be involved (see Plates 26 and 31). Myocarditis has also been reported (Pakes and Gerrity, 1994). Clinical signs are associated with granulomatous encephalitis or nephritis, notably vestibular disease and chronic renal failure. *E. cuniculi* can also cause lens rupture, pyogranulomatous uveitis and cataracts in rabbits (see Section 11.7.3.1 and Plate 24). *In utero* infection of the lens in the developing embryo occurs and causes the lens to rupture in later life (Stiles *et al.*, 1997).

Spores of *E. cuniculi* are shed in the urine of infected rabbits and transmit infection between individuals. The infection can be experimentally transmitted to rabbits by both the oral and tracheal route and young rabbits can be infected by their dam in the first few days of life. There appears to be maternal transfer of immunity to newborn rabbits (Bywater and Kellett, 1979; Lyngset, 1980). It has been suggested that ecto- and endoparasites also play a role in the transmission of *E. cuniculi* (Pakes and Gerrity, 1994).

Following ingestion or inhalation, spores pass via infected mononuclear cells into the systemic circulation. Initially, target organs are those of high blood flow, such as the lungs, liver and kidney (Percy and Barthold, 1993) with infection of nervous tissue taking place later on in the course of the disease. An antibody response is initiated soon after infection. Antibodies to *E. cuniculi* can be demonstrated at least 2 weeks before intracellular organisms are demonstrated and 4 weeks before histopathological changes are seen in the kidney or organisms in the urine. Histopathogical changes in the brain are observed over 8 weeks after seroconversion (Cox and Gallachio, 1978). *In vitro* studies of the effects of immune and non-immune rabbit serum on *E. cuniculi* suggest enhanced phagocytosis of the parasite by macrophages in immune animals (Niederkorn and Shaddock, 1980). Serum antibody levels become detectable 3–4 weeks after infection, reaching high titres 6–9 weeks post-infection. Spores can be seen in the urine 1 month after infection and are excreted in large numbers up to 2 months post-infection. Shedding of spores is essentially terminated by 3 months post-infection (Percy and Barthold, 1993). Spores of *E. cuniculi* survive for less than 1 week at 4°C but remain viable for at least 6 weeks at 22°C.

16.4.2.1 *E. cuniculi* in other species

E. cuniculi can infect a number of mammalian species with predilection sites and disease variation between hosts. Infections have been reported in rabbits, mice, guinea pigs, hamsters, dogs, cats, monkeys and man. There are no morphological or immunological differences between strains of *E. cuniculi* affecting laboratory animals.

A serological survey of stray dogs showed antibodies in 13.3% (Hollister *et al.*, 1989). Encephalitozoonosis has also been reported in birds (Poonacha and Stamper, 1985). Guinea pigs housed with infected rabbits were found to be at more risk than those housed separately in a survey by Gannon (1980). Nephritis was common but cerebral granulomas were not seen in the guinea pigs. *E. cuniculi* has been described in a wild rabbit in 1955 (Pakes and Gerrity, 1994) but more recent serological surveys have failed to find evidence of infection in wild rabbits, although they can be infected experimentally (Cox *et al.*, 1980; Cox and Ross, 1980). It has been suggested that the natural hygiene habits of wild rabbits significantly decrease post-natal infection.

16.4.2.2 Zoonotic potential of *E. cuniculi*

Although *E. cuniculi* can infect a range of hosts, severe systemic disease is rare in other species except in athymic or immunosuppressed mice and neonatal dogs or foxes. Athymic mice do not develop a cellular or humoral response to the parasite and masses of spores are found in the liver and other viscera (Gannon, 1980). *E. cuniculi* has been recognized as an opportunistic pathogen in human patients with acquired immunodeficiency syndrome (AIDS) in which it can cause interstitial pneumonitis, diarrhoea and wasting (Deplazes *et al.*, 1996; Joste *et al.*, 1996). Experimental infection of rabbits with *E. cuniculi* cultures administered into the rectum with a catheter after weeks of repeated colonic enemas resulted in *E. cuniculi* infection with hepatic lesions predominating rather than the typical brain and kidney changes (Fuentealba *et al.*, 1992).

16.4.2.3 Clinical signs associated with *E. cuniculi* infection in rabbits

E. cuniculi was first described in 1922 in rabbits exhibiting hind leg paralysis and other neurological signs. Kimman and Akkermans (1987) described an outbreak in a colony of laboratory rabbits that resulted in heavy losses. Affected animals showed muscular weakness, emaciation, polydypsia, polyuria and occasional neurological signs. Other texts describe encephalitozoonosis as a chronic, latent disease of rabbits that is significant because of its effects on experimental results. Infection with *E. cuniculi* in laboratory rabbits has caused many problems to scientific studies. Subclinical infection has vitiated experimental results and lesions caused by the parasite have been wrongly attributed to a number of other ailments (Wilson, 1979). Encephalitozoonosis can interfere with test results. Blood samples of rabbits with spontaneous encephalitozoonosis have been shown to have significantly lower levels of catecholamines than healthy rabbits (Levkut *et al.*, 1997). Nowadays, laboratory rabbits are screened for *E. cuniculi* and seropositive animals eliminated.

Encephalitozoonosis is widespread in pet rabbits. There is a range of manifestation signs from acute neurological disaster to latent infections that do not exhibit clinical signs of disease. In Germany, a serological survey of 277 pet rabbits showed that 41% were seropositive (Ewringmann and Göbel, 1999). Of the seropositive rabbits, 51 (40.8%) showed clinical signs of encephalitozoonosis. In the UK, a random survey of 30 pet rabbits revealed eight seropositive individuals (Carmichael, Idexx and Harcourt-Brown, unpublished data). After the animals had been found to be seropositive, the owners were questioned and four reported vague symptoms such as head nodding or swaying at rest, deafness or impaired mental ability.

When clinical signs occur, they are usually associated with granulomatous lesions in the brain, kidney or lens although the liver, heart and other organs can be affected. In the German survey of 277 rabbits, 51 (40% of the seropositive animals) showed signs relating to infection. Twenty-three rabbits suffered from CNS disorders, 16 from renal disease and seven with uveitis. Two rabbits had both CNS and renal disease and three animals had CNS symptoms, renal disease and uveitis (Ewringmann and Göbel, 1999). Renal disease associated with *E. cuniculi* is described in Section 14.5.1 and ocular disease in Section 11.7.3.1.

16.4.2.4 Diagnosis of *E. cuniculi*

The definitive diagnosis of *E. cuniculi* as a cause of disease can be problematical. In the live animal, evidence of uveitis can be seen in rabbits that have been infected *in utero*. At *post-mortem* examination, kidneys from infected rabbits show an obvious pitted appearance on gross examination due to areas of fibrosis (see Plate 31). There are no macroscopic lesions in the central nervous system, even on gross examination of the brain. Microscopic examination of tissues is required to confirm the diagnosis. Characteristic granulomatous lesions are seen in the brain, kidney and, occasionally, the liver. The microsporidial parasite may or may not be evident.

Many diagnostic tests have been developed to detect antibodies to *E. cuniculi* in the live animal, including intradermal and a range of serological tests. Serological screening is used by some laboratories to identify and cull potentially infected animals to reduce interference with experimental results (Pakes and Gerrity, 1994). In the pet rabbit, a humoral response to *E. cuniculi* infection cannot be relied upon for accurate diagnosis. In laboratory rabbits, serum antibodies develop after 3 weeks and excretion of the parasite occurs 6 weeks after experimental infection with *E. cuniculi* (Cox *et al.*, 1979). Passive immunity is transferred from infected dams to their offspring, which can have titres of 1:25 to 1:800 that last until they are about 4 weeks old. After a seronegative period, young rabbits seroconvert at 8–10 weeks of age in response to natural infection (Lyngset, 1980). Therefore the presence of antibodies only indicates exposure to the organism and does not confirm *E. cuniculi* as a cause of disease.

The antibody titre or type of immune response could be helpful in deciding whether a positive result is indicative of disease but these tests are not available in the UK at the present time. Experimentally, high antibody titres have been found in rabbits showing signs of chronic infection (Pye and Cox, 1977). IgG titres reached a level of 160–2560 after a latent phase of 13–28 days in a study of rabbits experimentally infected with *E. cuniculi* (Kunstyr *et al.*, 1986). Some of the rabbits showed an episodic humoral response and became seronegative after a few weeks. There was wide individual variability in antibody response but the authors suggested that differences in IgM and IgG could distinguish between recent and chronic infection. IgM seroconversion occurs at the beginning of the antibody response and simultaneous IgG and IgM detection suggest recent infection.

E. cuniculi organisms can be found in the urine of infected animals (Pye and Cox, 1977). The spores are evident as ovoid, gram-positive organisms approximately 1.5–2.5 μm in size. Staining procedures using carbol fuchsin will stain the organisms a distinct purple colour (Percy and Barthold, 1993). Theoretically, urine examination is a means of confirming the presence of antigen in the live animal, although it is impractical as a routine diagnostic technique in general practice. Organisms are intermittently excreted and urine collection can be difficult. Normal rabbit urine often contains sediment. In humans, microsporidia can be detected by centrifuging urine and resuspending the sediment in sterile non-bacteriostatic saline (De Groote *et al.*, 1995). The suspension is smeared on a slide and stained with Weber's chromotrope-based stain. A polymerase chain reaction (PCR) test has been used for detecting encephalitozoon DNA in human samples but is not available for veterinary use at the present time (De Groote *et al.*, 1995).

16.4.2.5 Treatment of encephalitozoonosis

Although the incidence and pathogenesis of *E. cuniculi* has been extensively reviewed in the scientific literature, there is a dearth of information about treatment. In colonies that screen for the disease, affected animals are culled and in colonies that do not screen, infection can be subclinical with no obvious sign of disease. It is for the individual pet rabbit that treatment is usually sought. Observant owners may notice clinical signs that would be overlooked in the colony situation and are reluctant to have their animals euthanased. Several treatment protocols have been suggested based either on basic principles of therapy for granulomatous encephalitis or on *in vitro* susceptibility of *E. cuniculi* organisms to various therapeutic agents. Some cases appear to improve spontaneously without treatment, presumably due to the host's immune response. In the absence of a simple diagnostic test for the presence of the antigen in the live animal, it is difficult to monitor the efficacy of therapeutic agents in eliminating the parasite. Antibody titres have been used as a guide to the progress of the disease but controlled studies are needed to evaluate their significance as prognostic indicators. Clinical signs are not only associated with the presence of the parasite but also the associated inflammatory response that persists after the organism is eliminated. Some data have been obtained from the treatment of AIDS patients who are able to describe their symptoms and can therefore be assessed more easily than pet rabbits. Parasite excretion has been monitored using PCR assays that are not generally available for pet rabbits. In general, *E. cuniculi* in pet rabbits is either treated with corticosteroids to suppress the inflammatory reaction or with albendazole or oxytetracycline, both of which kill the organism *in vitro*.

The effect of various antimicrobial agents on *E. cuniculi* has been studied in vitro. One technique involves incubating infected fibroblasts with various drugs for 3 days before counting the parasitic foci. Albendazole was found to inhibit 90% of microsporidial growth using this technique, which led to the use of albendazole to treat infected human AIDS patients. A wide range of other drugs was also tested, including some that are available in veterinary medicine. Metronidazole, doxycycline, sulphonamides and itraconazole could not be evaluated because of their toxic effects on the fibroblast tissue culture (Beauvais *et al.*, 1994). Fumigallin, an agent used to treat bees for nosematosis, was found to be effective against *E. cuniculi* as well as albendazole. Franssen *et al.* (1995) found that toltrazuril, metronidazole and itraconazole were ineffective in preventing spore formation in tissue cultures of *E. cuniculi* and confirmed the efficacy of albendazole and fumigallin. Thiabendazole and oxbendazole were also found to be effective against the organism *in vitro*.

Albendazole is a benzimidazole anthelmintic available as an oral preparation for cattle and sheep. It has been used to eliminate the *Encephalitozoon* spp. from human AIDS patients, sometimes with dramatic success (De Groote *et al.*, 1995). Elimination of the parasite is accompanied by relief of clinical symptoms in humans. Eradication of the parasite has been confirmed at autopsy (Sobottka *et al.*, 1995; Joste *et al.*, 1996). Albendazole has also been used to treat clinical cases of *E. cuniculi* in pet rabbits with no reports of adverse effects and apparent improvement in clinical symptoms. The pharmacokinetic effects of the agent have been tested on rabbits (Li *et al.*, 1995). An empirical course of 3–10 days treatment appears to be beneficial. In-contact rabbits should be treated as a precaution although albendazole is potentially teratogenic and is not advisable in breeding females. Oxytetracycline has also been used to treat clinical cases of encephalitozoonosis (Ewringmann and Göbel, 1999).

Fenbendazole is effective against *Encephalitozoon* species *in vitro*. Fenbendazole has been shown to be effective in preventing experimental infection of *E. cuniculi* in laboratory rabbits and for eliminating the spores from the central nervous system of naturally infected rabbits (Suter et al., 2001). Fenbendazole was given at a dose rate of 20 mg/kg daily for up to 4 weeks.

16.4.3 *Toxoplasma gondii*

In common with all mammals, rabbits can be infected with *Toxoplasma gondii* although infection is usually subclinical. Ingested sporulated oocysts hatch in the duodenum. Sporozoites invade neighbouring cells and are dispersed throughout the body via the

Key points 16.2

- Domestic rabbits are susceptible to a variety of protozoan diseases including coccidiosis, *Encephalitozoon cuniculi*, *Toxoplasma gondii*, *Cryptosporidia*, *Giardia* and *Sarcocystis*
- *E. cuniculi* is an intracellular protozoan parasite. It is spread through urine
- Sporoplasm from ingested spores is transferred to cells of intestinal mucosa. The parasite is then distributed throughout the body by the reticuloendothelial system
- The predilection sites for *E. cuniculi* are the brain and kidney. *In utero*, the lens is another predilection site
- Granulomatous encephalitis, chronic renal insufficiency and phacoclastic uveitis are among the clinical syndromes associated with encephalitozoonosis. Vestibular disease is the most commonly recognized manifestation
- Multiplication of spores within infected cells takes place until, eventually, the cell ruptures releasing spores that can invade neighbouring cells
- Cell rupture is associated with an inflammatory response and the development of granulomas
- In the kidney, spores are released into the urine to infect other animals
- *E. cuniculi* is uncommon in wild rabbits. It can affect other mammals and birds, especially if they are immunosuppressed. Serological studies have demonstrated antibodies to *E. cuniculi* in dogs
- *E. cuniculi* is potentially zoonotic although there are no reports of infections in healthy individuals. Immunosuppressed humans such as AIDS patients are susceptible
- An antibody response occurs in rabbits and infected animals become immune. Serological testing can be used to detect exposure to infection
- *E. cuniculi* is susceptible to a range of drugs *in vitro*. Albendazole has been used to treat human patients with success in eliminating the parasite
- Albendazole is available and safe for use in rabbits although there are no data available at the present time about its efficacy. Dosage and duration of treatment is empirical. It is indicated to limit spread of infection to other rabbits
- Oxytetracycline has been used to treat encephalitozoonosis in rabbits
- Toxoplasmosis is rare in rabbits, but does occasionally occur
- Although toxoplasmosis is potentially zoonotic, toxoplasma is only transmissable from rabbits to humans who handle or eat undercooked rabbit meat. Infection is not spread through rabbit faeces.

blood and lymphatics. Once the host immune responses are established, the organisms can be found as cysts in various tissues where they can remain for years (Owen, 1992). The source of infection for rabbits is feed contaminated by cat faeces and symptoms have been described in rabbits that grazed an area frequented by cats. Clinical signs are most common in the acute phase in young rabbits. Sudden anorexia, pyrexia and death are the usual signs, although CNS symptoms such as posterior paralysis or seizures can also occur (Leland *et al.*, 1992). Outbreaks have been described in commercial rabbits (Harcourt, 1967; Okerman, 1988). High antibody titres have been found in wild rabbits collected from sewerage farms in Australia (Cox *et al.*, 1981). Positive serology only indicates exposure to infection. Gustaffson *et al.* (1997) compared the difference in susceptibility to toxoplasmosis between two lagomorphs; the mountain hare (*Lepus timidus*) and the domestic rabbit (*Oryctolagus cuniculus*). Domestic rabbits were found to be resistant to toxoplasmosis in comparison with the mountain hare. In the mountain hare, toxoplasmosis is acutely fatal and characterized by necrosis and tissue damage in the small intestine, mesenteric lymph nodes and liver. In the domestic rabbit, lesions are mild consisting of focal accumulations of mononuclear cells, mainly in the liver and heart. Histopathology is diagnostic. Antibodies are detected early as 7–8 days post-infection (Gustaffson *et al.*, 1997).

Although toxoplasmosis is potentially zoonotic, toxoplasma is only transmissible from rabbits to humans who handle or eat undercooked rabbit meat. Infection is not spread through rabbit faeces.

16.4.4 Other protozoan parasites of rabbits

Cryptosporidia species have been described in rabbits but not as a major cause of disease. *Giardia duodenalis* has also been reported in rabbits, although it does not appear to be pathogenic. A single outbreak of catarrhal enteritis in rabbits has been attributed to giardiasis. There is no evidence of transmission to humans (Pakes and Gerrity, 1994). *Sarcocystis cuniculi* affects rabbits although it is rarely reported in the European rabbit (*Oryctolagus cuniculus*). It is more commonly encountered in the cottontail (*Sylvilagus floridanus*). Sarcocystis forms cysts in skeletal and cardiac muscle. The source of infection is believed to be cats.

16.5 Bacterial diseases

16.5.1 Pasteurellosis

Pasteurella multocida is a very small, non-motile, gram-negative, ovoid, coccoid or short rod that shows bipolar staining. It is aerobic and facultatively anaerobic. The organism forms circular, convex smooth colonies on blood agar after 24 h incubation. The colonies are generally 2–2.5 mm in diameter and slightly iridescent, although variations can occur. The colonies are mucoid in appearance.

There are multiple antigenic strains of *P. multocida* associated with different species of animal. The organism is potentially pathogenic to a variety of animals. It can also be found as a commensal organism, for example *P. multocida* has been isolated from the tonsils of healthy dogs and from the respiratory tract in humans. In rabbits, *P. multocida* can reside in the nasal cavity without causing disease. In pet rabbits that are kept individually or in small numbers, *P. multocida* seldom causes primary disease, although the bacterium is often found as a secondary pathogen in any purulent or suppurative condition. In colonies of rabbits kept for breeding, meat and fur production, or for laboratory purposes, pasteurellosis is a serious, infectious disease. Disease occurs when predisposing factors give the bacteria the opportunity to multiply uncontrollably and overwhelm the physiological and immunological defences of the respiratory tract. During these episodes, clones of virulent bacteria increase which are easily transmitted to neighbouring animals.

The protein pattern of the outer membrane of *P. multocida* shows a relationship between the protein type and the animal host. Bacterial capsular polysaccharides inhibit phagocytosis. Bacterial lipopolysaccharides confer resistance to complement and bactericidal activity of serum (Deeb, 1993). There are several capsular and somatic serotypes of *P. multocida* that are pathogenic for domestic livestock and poultry, but only a few are pathogenic for rabbits. Serotyping entails the identification of the capsular antigen and serotypes. In rabbits, serotypes 12:A, 3:A and 3:D are the usual types identified (Percy and Barthold, 1993). Snuffles is most frequently associated with 12:A, whereas 3:A and occasionally 3:D are more frequently associated with disease of the lower respiratory tract. Virulence of infection varies between serotypes. *Pasteurella multocida* produces an endotoxin that varies with serotype. The role of the endotoxin in clinical disease is unclear, although it may be significant in septicaemic cases. The bacteria also produce adhesins which adhere the bacteria to epithelial tissue. Filamentous appendages elaborated by the bacteria may help *P. multocida* colonize mucous membranes (Deeb, 1993). The adhesive properties vary with different serotypes of *P. multocida* and could be important in the pathogenesis of the disease (Manning *et al.*, 1989). Mucosal antibodies (IgA) inhibit growth of bacteria and are produced in response to exposure to *P. multocida*. High humoral (IgG) antibody levels are associated with chronic infection and have been used to identify infected rabbits in laboratory colonies (Deeb, 1993).

16.5.1.1 Epidemiology

When sufficient numbers of *P. multocida* bacteria are transmitted between rabbits, a subclinical infection is established in the upper respiratory tract. Bacteria become abundant in the mucous film covering the mucous membranes but are scarce in the sinuses (Whittaker, 1989). Clinical disease occurs when there is disruption of the balance between mucociliary clearance and bacterial proliferation. Pregnancy, parturition, lactation, poor husbandry, overcrowding, stress, nutritional deficiencies, genetic predisposition and bacterial serotype can affect the course of the disease which tends to be a greater problem in the colony rabbit than in the adult pet rabbit.

P. multocida is spread to newborn rabbits shortly after birth from infected does that harbour infection in their nasal cavity. There are many predisposing factors in young rabbits, including the age of weaning, the presence of vaginal infection and the prevalence of infection within the colony. There appears to be genetic susceptibility to pasteurellosis. For example, Chinchilla rabbits appear to be more susceptible than Blue Beverans (Manning *et al.*, 1989). The incidence of disease increases with age up to about 5 months of age. After colonization of the upper respiratory tract, infection extends to the rest of the respiratory tract and tympanic bulla and can cause clinical rhinitis, conjunctivitis, pneumonia, tracheitis, dacryocystitis or otitis media. Some rabbits remain asymptomatic despite the presence of *P. multocida* in the nares. Such individuals are carriers and infective to contact animals. Other animals are negative on nasal culture but harbour *P. multocida* in the tympanic bulla.

Transmission of disease can occur between rabbits by direct contact and by airborne spread. Uninfected rabbits in direct contact with infected rabbits contract pasteurellosis within 8 days to 3 weeks (Manning *et al.*, 1989). Physical separation of rabbits by a distance of a few feet will delay transmission of infection (Lelkes and Corbett, 1983). Fomite spread has been demonstrated and contaminated water supplies have been suggested as a source of infection (Whittaker, 1989).

16.5.1.2 Clinical signs of pasteurellosis

P. multocida infection can be acute, subacute or chronic. There are several clinical syndromes associated with pasteurellosis. Surveillance of rabbits for pasteurellosis at a laboratory animal facility revealed the following syndromes in a decreasing order of magnitude: rhinitis, conjunctivitis, abscesses and otitis media (DiGiacomo *et al.*, 1983)

16.5.1.3 Rhinitis ('snuffles')

The colloquial term 'snuffles' refers to upper respiratory tract infections manifested by a serous followed by purulent discharge from the nose. Affected rabbits sneeze and cough and may have an audible upper respiratory noise or 'snuffle'. 'Snuffles' is usually associated with *P. multocida* infection although other infectious agents such as *Staphylococcus aureus* can be involved. In pet rabbits, dental disease and nasal foreign bodies can cause similar signs (see Section 13.2.3). The thick sticky white discharge from the nose is wiped away with the forelegs leading to a yellow staining and matting of the fur. Poor husbandry, overcrowding, poor ventilation, dust conditions and ammonia buildup exacerbate the disease. Investigations of rhinitis in laboratory rabbits have shown that some rabbits can have rhinitis for up to 2 weeks before *P. multocida* is isolated from nasal swabs. Clinical signs wax and wane but symptoms often persist despite treatment.

16.5.1.4 Pneumonia

P. multocida is a cause of pneumonia in rabbits. The disease can be acute and rapidly fatal. Chronic or subacute infections also occur in rabbits with no clinical signs. It is not unusual to find incidental pneumonic lesions during *post-mortem* examination of apparently healthy rabbits. Large abscesses can be present in the thoracic cavity.

16.5.1.5 Genital infection

P. multocida can be recovered from the vagina in a relatively high percentage of carrier animals (Percy and Barthold, 1993) and the organ can act as a reservoir of infection. *P. multocida* can be spread during mating. Bucks may harbour infection in their genital tract. Orchitis, pyometra and genital infections can be manifestations of pasteurellosis.

16.5.1.6 Wound infections and abscesses

P. multocida is often isolated from abscesses and infected bite wounds. The organism is present in the nasal cavity of many rabbits and can contaminate tissues during licking and grooming. It can also be spread haematogenously. *P. multocida* may be isolated from post-surgical wound breakdowns and can cause osteomyelitis after orthopaedic surgery (Leibenberg and Badger, 1984). *P. multocida* can be isolated from facial abscesses that result from periapical infection or tissue damage caused by elongated crowns in rabbit with dental disease.

16.5.1.7 Dacryocystitis

P. multocida can cause dacryocystitis (Petersen-Jones and Carrington, 1988). The organism may be isolated from purulent infections of the nasolacrimal duct which can result from spread of infection from the nasal cavity or as secondary infections in ducts blocked by elongated tooth roots especially of the maxillary incisors.

16.5.1.8 Otitis media

P. multocida can spread from the nasal cavity to the tympanic bulla via the eustachian tube. A common *post-mortem* and radiographic finding is the presence of inspissated pus in the deeper structures of the ear (see Plate 27). Infection can spread along the vestibulocochlear nerve and cause vestibular disease resulting in neurological signs such as rolling and nystagmus.

16.5.1.9 Detection of pasteurellosis

Confirmation of pasteurellosis in rabbit colonies is required to limit the spread of disease. Clinical signs are indicative of infection but diagnostic tests are required to isolate the organism and detect subclinical carriers. A deep nasal swab is required for bacteriology. It can be difficult to obtain satisfactory swabs in the conscious animal and sedation or anaesthesia is required. Bacterial culture cannot always be relied upon. Infection can be deep within the nasal passages or in the paranasal sinuses and false negative results can occur. Some rabbits have already been treated with antibiotics. *Pasteurella multocida* does not survive well in transport media (Sanchez *et al.*, 2000). It survives for less than 24 h at room temperature. Some strains of *P. multocida* grow best at 34–35°C, which is lower than most routine cultures.

Serological tests and a polymerase chain reaction (PCR) test are available in the USA. A rising titre demonstrates exposure to infection. However, the presence of antibodies does not confirm the presence of active infection. Sanchez *et al.* (2000) conducted a study of a combination of bacterial culture, serology and PCR testing in rabbits with clinical signs suggestive of pasteurellosis. They found that the combination of PCR and serology was more useful than culture from nasal swabs. The authors concluded that there are other organisms, such as *Bordetella*, *Pseudomonas* and *Staphylococcus* spp. that cause clinical signs similar to those of pasteurellosis.

16.5.1.10 Control of pasteurellosis in rabbit colonies

Pasteurellosis is a major problem in breeding, laboratory or commercial colonies of rabbits. The disease also presents problems in multi-rabbit households or in sanctuaries and rescue centres that house several rabbits in a small space. Stress, intercurrent disease, overcrowding, and poor air quality can trigger the flare up of latent infection. As with any infectious disease in an intensive situation, good husbandry is important in the control of the disease. Affected animals should be isolated and treated promptly or even culled, as they are a source of infection to other stock. Keeping the numbers down and minimizing contact between batches of rabbits reduces transmission of disease.

In infected colonies, clinical disease can be minimized by separating newly weaned rabbits from adults and by carefully controlling the environment and reducing stress factors. A clean, dry, well-ventilated environment is required with no draughts. Rabbits can withstand cold but become stressed by high temperatures. Closed stuffy sheds increase the risk of disease especially if the air quality is poor due to ammonia buildup. Fluctuations of temperature should be avoided with an optimum temperature maintained at 16–20°C and humidity of 50–70% (Whittaker, 1989). Air quality should be good with around 20 air changes per hour and preferably a filter system.

16.5.1.11 Prevention of pasteurellosis

Over the years, several control strategies for pasteurellosis have been tried in rabbit colonies with varying degrees of success. Many laboratory colonies are now disease free and are vigilantly barrier-housed to prevent the introduction of infection. *Pasteurella*-free stock is selected by placing rabbits in isolation for 2–4 weeks and repeatedly culturing the nasal passages. Rabbits with positive cultures or signs of rhinitis are culled. Surviving rabbits are bred from and after 3 years, the colony is considered to be disease free. Other methods of producing disease-free rabbits involve caesarean derivation with hand-rearing (Manning *et al.*, 1989) or the transfer of fertilized ova to *Pasteurella*-free does. Early weaning and the use of antibiotics can increase the number of disease-free stock. To ensure an uninfected status, periodic serological testing for antibodies to pasteurella is necessary. Recently a polymerase chain reaction test has been developed that can be used to detect infection (Sanchez *et al.*, 2000).

Antibiotics have also been used prophylactically in an attempt to prevent pasteurellosis by administering them either in the feed or drinking water to pregnant does. There appears to be genetic resistance to pasteurella and attempts have been made to produce disease-free strains of rabbit.

Vaccines against *P. multocida* are used successfully in other species such as sheep and attempts have been made to produce an effective vaccine against pasteurellosis in rabbits. Both live and dead vaccines have been used and found to be effective in reducing mortality and clinical disease caused by a homologous strain of the bacteria. Most pathogenic strains from rabbits carry somatic antigens 3 and 12 and are capsule type A or D. Cross-immunity is higher between strains of the same serotype. However, despite promising results in laboratory rabbits (DiGiacomo *et al.*, 1987), protection against nasal colonization and clinical disease caused by heterologous strains is incomplete and the results of field trials using an intranasal vaccine against A:12 have been disappointing (DiGiacomo and Deeb, 1989). There is a belief among some rabbit breeders that vaccination is feasible with either an autogenous vaccine or a vaccine produced for use against pasteurellosis in other species such as sheep or cattle. Claims of success with these vaccines are difficult to evaluate.

16.5.1.12 Treatment of pasteurellosis

Treatment of pasteurellosis depends on the clinical symptoms and the type and emotional or financial value of the rabbit that is suffering from the disease. The treatment of abscesses, respiratory tract infections, dacryocystitis and vestibular disease is covered in other chapters.

16.5.2 *Staphylococcus aureus*

Staphylococcus aureus causes suppurative inflammation. The organism is frequently isolated from infected sites in rabbits. It can also cause a fatal septicaemia. Like *P. multocida,* healthy rabbits can carry *S. aureus* in the nasal cavity. It can also be isolated from the conjunctiva and skin of healthy rabbits. *S. aureus* may be isolated from cases of mastitis, ulcerative pododermatitis, rhinitis, conjunctivitis, dacryocystitis, abscesses and skin infections. It is often a secondary invader in tissues damaged by trauma or some other predisposing cause. The severity of disease is governed by host resistance and bacterial virulence (Delong and Manning, 1994). In rabbit colonies, staphylococcosis can cause serious losses.

16.5.3 *Bordetella bronchiseptica*

Bordetella bronchiseptica has been isolated from a variety of animal species including pigs, rats, dogs, cats, guinea pigs and rabbits. In rabbits, *B. bronchiseptica* appears to be relatively non-pathogenic although it has caused localized suppurative bronchopneumonia in laboratory rabbits treated with cortisone prior to nasal inoculation of the organism. *B. bronchiseptica* can cause serious upper respiratory tract infection in guinea pigs. Isolates of *B. bronchiseptica* from different species have been typed according to their bacterial sensitivity and investigations suggest that infected rabbits and guinea pigs can infect each other (Boot *et al.*, 1995). Many texts recommend that the two species should not be housed together because of the risk of cross-infection although actual reports of this are rare.

16.5.4 Tyzzer's disease

Tyzzer's disease is caused by a large pleomorphic, gram-negative, spore forming, obligate intracellular bacterium that is flagellate and therefore motile (Delong and Manning, 1994). The bacterium cannot be grown *in vitro* but can be grown in tissue culture. The bacterial genome is closely related to *Clostridium* species and, in recent years, the organism has been reclassified as *Clostridium piliforme* rather than *Bacillus piliformis* (Besch-Williford, 1997). Tyzzer's disease can affect a wide range of animals including rodents, cats and monkeys (Delong and Manning, 1994). The disease affects the caecum, intestine and liver causing acute diarrhoea and sudden death in the acute stage and intestinal fibrosis, stenosis and liver necrosis in chronic cases. The myocardium can also be affected. The disease usually occurs in weanling rabbits 6–12 weeks old but can occur at any age and is often predisposed by stress. Recent advances in tissue culture have led to development of diagnostic tests and serological testing is now possible in some countries. The presence of antibody in apparently healthy animals suggests latent infection of the intestinal tract. Stress or immunosuppression can precipitate overt disease (Delong and Manning, 1994). Transmission occurs by ingestion of spores that can survive in the environment for some time after an infected animal has been removed. Overcrowding, stress, low dietary fibre and transport predispose to clinical disease. Supportive treatment and antibiotic therapy are generally unrewarding.

16.5.5 Salmonellosis

Salmonella organisms can be carried by wild rodents that contaminate food and water. The clinical signs can range from asymptomatic carriers to diarrhoea, emaciation and death. No successful treatment has been described.

16.5.6 *Escherichia coli*

Escherichia coli is generally absent from the gut flora in rabbits. However, *E. coli* can cause enteritis, especially in suckling rabbits, and is an important cause of enteritis and death in rabbit colonies. An association has been made between colibacillosis and intestinal coccidiosis, which enhances *E. coli* proliferation. There is variation in pathogenicity between strains of *E. coli* and a large number of strains have been isolated from outbreaks of enteritis. An 'attaching and effacing' strain has been identified in the UK with reported mortality rates of 25–75% (Dannatt *et al.*, 2000). This organism attaches closely to caecal epithelial cells.

16.5.7 Clostridial enterotoxaemia

Clostridia are anaerobic gram-positive bacilli capable of producing powerful enterotoxins which can produce severe enteric disease. Clostridial enterotoxaemia is usually fatal. Small numbers of *Clostridia* spp. are normal inhabitants of the gut flora of rabbits. *Clostridium spiriforme, Clostridium difficile* and *Clostridium perfringens* can cause enterotoxaemia in rabbits (see Section 10.10.2). Weanling rabbits are most commonly affected.

Clostridium spiriforme produces an iota toxin. Glucose is required as a substrate for iota toxin formation. High dietary starch levels are believed to predispose to enterotoxaemia by causing 'carbohydrate overload' of the caecum. Residual starch that reaches the caecum can be broken down to release glucose as a substrate for iota toxin formation. This situation is more likely to occur in juvenile rabbits rather than adults. Immature rabbits do not digest starch efficiently in the small intestine, but in adult animals starch is broken down and absorbed before it reaches the caecum. In adults, enterotoxaemia is usually related to other factors such as stress or antibiotic therapy, which disrupt the caecal microflora and allow *Clostridia* spp. to proliferate.

16.5.8 Other causes of bacterial enteritis

Vibriosis and *Campylobacter* have been reported as causes of enteric disease in rabbits. A syndrome known as 'histiocytic enteritis' has been reported in Japan. Adenoviruses, parvoviruses, rotaviruses, coronaviruses and Herpes-like viruses have been isolated from outbreaks of enteric diseases of rabbit colonies. These infections are unlikely to be encountered in the adult pet rabbit. Percy and Barthold (1993) and DiGiacomo and Mare (1994) give detailed accounts of these infections.

16.5.9 Treponematosis

Treponema cuniculi is a specific pathogen of rabbits. It is a spirochaete that causes crusty, inflammatory lesions on the genitalia and face (see Plate 10). It is sexually transmitted (see Section 9.13). Young rabbits can be infected during their passage through the birth canal. The disease is also known as venereal spirochaetosis or 'rabbit syphilis'. Treponematosis is endemic in some breeding colonies and is occasionally encountered in the pet rabbit.

16.5.10 Listeriosis

Listeria monocytogenes infection is uncommon in rabbits. It is characterized by abortion and sudden death. Contaminated feed can cause outbreaks in breeding colonies. *L. monocytogenes* has a predilection for the gravid uterus in advanced pregnancy. Infection can cause abortion, stillbirths and death of the doe. *Post-mortem* signs include straw-coloured fluid in the peritoneal cavity, disseminated pale miliary foci on the liver and visceral congestion. Fibrinous exudate and ecchymosis can be seen on the serosal surface of the uterus.

16.5.11 Paratuberculosis (Johne's disease)

Paratuberculosis, caused by *Mycobacterium paratuberculosis,* affects many species, especially ruminants. It is characterized by diarrhoea, emaciation and loss of bodily condition and most animals become infected as neonates through the ingestion of contaminated milk or water. Clinical infection becomes apparent after a prolonged subclinical phase that can last for several years. Although the disease is most often reported in ruminants, monogastric animals have been infected experimentally without evidence of clinical disease. Oral infection of newborn rabbits can produce intermittent diarrhoea and granulomatous enteritis similar to that observed in cattle.

In Scotland, the high incidence of paratuberculosis in wild rabbits has been linked with a high prevalence of infection in cattle. A survey of wild rabbits revealed that 67% were infected with *Mycobacterium paratuberculosis* (Greig *et al.*, 1997). Epidemiological studies found an association between the infection in wild rabbits and a history of Johne's disease on the farms where the rabbits were caught (Greig *et al.*, 1999). *Mycobacterium avium* subspecies *paratuberculosis* was also isolated from foxes and stoats collected from affected farms (Beard *et al.*, 1999). In the wild rabbits affected with paratuberculosis, general body condition was good although a proportion of them had thickened areas of intestinal mucosa with occasional granuloma. Large numbers of intracellular acid-fast bacilli were present in the lesions.

16.5.12 Pseudotuberculosis

Pseudotuberculosis, caused by *Yersinia pseudotuberculosis*, is a common infection in rodents, especially guinea pigs. In rabbits, the disease is usually encountered in wild animals although it has been described in captive ones. Affected rabbits suffer from a wasting disease, a dull coat and occasional diarrhoea. Nodular swelling of the liver may be detected on abdominal palpation (Wood, 1978). *Yersinia pseudotuberculosis* can be isolated from faeces or caecal contents. Lesions of pseudotuberculosis include large areas of caseous necrosis in the mesenteric lymph nodes, liver and spleen. Necrosis of Peyer's patches in the small intestine and caecum may be found. The disease may also involve other organs such as the liver and spleen (DeLong and Manning, 1994). Yersiniosis is associated with vermin and control of mice and rats is required (Okerman, 1988).

16.5.13 Tularaemia

Tularaemia is an acute septicaemic disease caused by *Francisella tularensis*. It is common in wild rabbits and hares but is seldom encountered in domestic rabbits. The organism can affect many vertebrate species and has zoonotic potential. Most human cases that have been linked to rabbits have followed exposure to the cottontail (*Sylvilagus floridanus*). According to Delong and Manning (1994), there have been no reported human cases of tularaemia acquired from *Oryctolagus cuniculus*.

16.5.14 Lyme disease

Lyme disease is an acute, often recurrent polyarthritis of dogs and humans caused by a spirochaete *Borrelia burgdorferi*. It is a tick-borne disease. Cottontail rabbits (*Sylvilagus floridanus*) have been shown to have antibodies to *Borrelia burgdorferi* in areas where

Key points 16.3

- *Pasteurella multocida* is a very small non-motile, gram-negative, ovoid, coccoid or short rod that shows bipolar staining. It is aerobic and facultatively anaerobic
- *P. multocida* forms circular, convex smooth colonies on blood agar after 24 h incubation. The colonies are generally 2–2.5 mm in diameter and slightly iridescent although variations can occur. The colonies may be mucoid in appearance
- There are several serotypes of *P. multocida* that are pathogenic for rabbits. Snuffles is most frequently associated with 12:A, whereas 3:A and occasionally 3:D are more frequently associated with disease of the lower respiratory tract
- Clinical disease occurs when there is disruption of the balance between mucociliary clearance and bacterial proliferation
- Pregnancy, parturition, lactation, poor husbandry, overcrowding, stress, nutritional deficiencies, genetic predisposition and bacterial serotype can affect the course of pasteurellosis, which tends to be a greater problem in the 'colony' rabbit rather than in the adult pet rabbit
- Physical separation of rabbits by a distance of a few feet will delay transmission of infection. Fomite spread can occur
- *P. multocida* can be isolated from a number of clinical conditions of rabbits. Rhinitis, sinusitis, dacrocystitis, pneumonia, otitis media, otitis interna, abscesses and genital tract infections are all manifestations of pasteurellosis
- A deep nasal swab is required for bacteriology. Bacterial culture cannot always be relied upon because of false negative results and presence of antibiotics in rabbits that have already been treated
- Serological tests for pasteurellosis and a polymerase chain reaction (PCR) test are available in the USA
- Pasteurellosis is a major problem in colonies of rabbits. Affected animals are a source of infection to other stock. Keeping the numbers down and minimizing contact between batches of rabbits reduces transmission of disease. Stress can trigger latent infections to flare up
- Clinical disease can be minimized in infected colonies by separating newly weaned rabbits from adults and by carefully controlling the environment and reducing stress factors
- Fluctuations of temperature should be avoided with an optimum temperature maintained at 16–20°C and humidity of 50–70%. Air quality should be good with around 20 air changes per hour and preferably a filter system
- Other bacterial infections of rabbit colonies include *Staphylococcus aureus, Bordetella bronchiseptica, Clostridium piliformis* (Tyzzer's disease), *Salmonella, E. coli*, clostridial enterotoxaemia, *Campylobacter, Treponema cuniculi, Listeria monocytogenes, Pseudomonas, Fusiformis* and *Corynebacterium* spp
- Wild rabbits can be infected with *Mycobacterium paratuberculosis* (paratuberculosis, Johne's disease), *Yersinia pseudotuberculosis* (pseudotuberculosis), *Francisella tularensis* (tularaemia) and *Borrelia burgdorferi* (Lyme disease).

rabbit-feeding *Ixodes* are abundant (Telford and Speilman, 1989).

16.5.15 Non-specific bacterial infections

There are many other bacterial infections of rabbits. They are associated with stress, overcowding, injuries, reproduction, poor husbandry and intercurrent disease. Examples include *Pseudomonas*, *Fusiformis* and *Corynebacterium.*

16.6 Viral diseases

16.6.1 Myxomatosis

Myxomatosis is a fatal disease of the European rabbit (*Oryctolagus cuniculi*). It is characterized by subcutaneous swellings that exude a mucoid secretion when sectioned. Lesions occur around body orifices and on the face especially on the eyelids. Pet rabbits can contract the disease by direct contact with infected wild rabbits or via insect vectors. The disease is mainly spread by arthropods, especially the European rabbit flea *Spilopsyllus cuniculi.* In wild rabbits, outbreaks of myxomatosis wax and wane according to the virulence of the strain and the immune status of the native rabbit population.

16.6.1.1 History of myxomatosis

Myxoma virus was one of the first viruses to be discovered. It affected a group of laboratory rabbits in Uruguay in 1896 (Fenner and Fantani, 1999). In 1927, Aragao recognized virus particles in stained smears and called attention to its close resemblance with smallpox and fowlpox. Myxoma virus was later classified as a pox virus (Fenner and Ross, 1994). Brazilian workers found that the virus is transmitted mechanically by fleas and mosquitoes.

Myxomatosis is now an endemic disease of wild rabbits throughout Europe. It was first recognized in England in 1953 after it crossed the channel from France where it was illegally introduced in 1952. Prior to this, in 1952, infected rabbits had been released into the Heisker Islands in the Outer Hebrides as a deliberate experiment in pest control. Two years later, in 1954, the rabbit population was as large as ever despite the considerable mortality that resulted from myxomatosis (Fenner and Fantani, 1999). Although there were efforts to eradicate myxomatosis in the UK, the disease spread rapidly through the wild rabbit population in the summer of 1953 and was endemic by the late 1950s. The attitude to myxomatosis in the UK was different from other parts of the world. Rabbits were frequently kept as pets and there was outcry at the sight of blind, sick rabbits stumbling along roads or on commons and other public places. As a result, in 1954, it became an offence knowingly to use or permit the use of an infected rabbit to spread the disease into an uninfected population. This law was difficult to enforce.

16.6.1.2 Epidemiology of myxomatosis

Myxoma virus causes a trivial infection in its natural host, either *Sylvilagus brasiensis* (Tapeti, Forest rabbit, found in Mexico or Argentina) or *Sylvilagus bachmani* (Brush rabbit) which is native to California. In the European rabbit *Oryctolagus cuniculi*, myxoma virus causes a serious and life-threatening disease. Myxomatosisis can occur in hares but infection is rare and usually mild.

There are different strains of myxomatosis that affect wild rabbits, e.g. the Standard Laboratory (Moses) strain and the Lausanne strain, which is more virulent. The Standard Laboratory strain produces relatively flat skin lesions in contrast to the protuberant lesions produced by the Lausanne strains (Fenner and Ross, 1994). Some variants are associated with fewer and smaller skin lesions but cause massive pulmonary oedema.

In field conditions, myxomatosis is spread by insect vectors especially fleas and mosquitoes, although any insect that penetrates the skin will transmit the disease. The disease can also be spread directly between rabbits by contact or inhalation. The virus persists in hutches that have been contaminated with fluid from lesions from infected rabbits and will infect unvaccinated rabbits that are put into them. *Cheyletiella parasitovorax* can act as a vector in the spread of disease (Fenner and Fantani, 1999).

The life cycle of the insect vector affects the pattern of disease outbreaks and epidemiology of myxomatosis. Mosquitoes are the main vectors in many parts of the world. In those countries where myxomatosis is transmitted by mosquitoes, the disease spreads rapidly and is frequently encountered in pet rabbits housed in hutches. There is a high seasonal incidence. In the UK, disease outbreaks tend to remain localized with isolated pockets of infection and the disease is only sporadically encountered in pet rabbits. The difference in epidemiology is attributed to the difference in the life cycle of insect vectors. In the UK, the European rabbit flea, *Spilopsyllus cuniculi*, is the major insect vector rather than mosquito species *Aedes* and *Anopheles* spp. Even in the absence of the host, fleas can maintain infectivity throughout the winter and act as a reservoir of infection for the following year. Fleas are an effective means of transmission due to their life cycle that is synchronized with the reproductive status of the doe and results in heavy flea infestations of susceptible neonates.

Different strains of the myxoma virus show a variation in virulence. Rabbits infected with highly virulent strains die so quickly that the disease is not transmitted as readily as the less virulent strains. Environmental temperature also has an effect on mortality rates with the disease being more lethal at low temperatures. There is a genetic resistance to myxomatosis in some individuals.

16.6.1.3 Clinical signs of myxomatosis

The pathogenesis of myxomatosis follows the same pattern as other pox virus infections (Fenner and Ross, 1994). Sequential replication of the virus takes place at the inoculation site and the regional lymph node. It is followed by cell-associated viraemia and generalized infection throughout the body. The disease starts with a skin lesion, which typically develops 4–5 days after inoculation of the virus and enlarges to become about 3 cm in diameter 9–10 days after infection. The rabbit is viraemic, with virus replication taking place throughout the lymphoid system. The eyelids become thickened and eventually the eyes are completely closed by the ninth day with a semipurulent ocular discharge. Secondary lesions develop throughout the body, typically on the nares, lips, eyelids and base of the ears and on the external genitalia and anus. Aerosol infection can result in pneumonic signs, which is a feature of outbreaks in intensive farmed rabbits. This syndrome is characterized by a longer incubation period (1–3 weeks) and accompanied by lacrimation and mucopurulent nasal discharge (Fenner and Fantani, 1999). Myxomatosis is accompanied by sterility and abandonment of litters.

Myxomatosis is usually fatal due to inanation, secondary bacterial infection or in wild rabbits, predation. In rabbits that recover, inflammation of the testicles renders a buck infertile for up to 12 months (Fenner and Fantani, 1999). Very young rabbits are particularly susceptible to infection and die more rapidly than adult animals unless they have some passive immunity.

Several factors determine whether rabbits survive or die from myxomatosis and how long they live after infection. Infected rabbits mount an immune response that can be detected by *in vitro* tests about 7 days after infection and reach peak levels by about 28 days (Fenner and Ross, 1994). Antibodies persist for prolonged periods and give absolute immunity for many months. Maternal transfer of antibodies takes place and immunity lasts for 4–5 weeks in baby rabbits. Some rabbits have a genetic resistance to infection, which has limited mortality rates in outbreaks in wild rabbits. Genetic resistance to infection varies between rabbit populations and countries. British rabbits were slow to develop resistance in comparison with Australian rabbits (Fenner and Ross, 1994). A phenomenon known as 'paternal resistance' is also described. It has been discovered that bucks mating within 7 months of infection sometimes confer partial resistance to progeny born to the mated doe within the following 7 months. Speculation about some immunogenic factor in semen has been made (Fenner and Ross, 1994).

16.6.1.4 Relationship of myxomatosis with Shope fibroma virus

The viruses that cause myxomatosis are members of the *Leporipoxvirus* genus that cause fibromas in their natural hosts. The natural host of myxoma virus is not the European rabbit (*Oryctolagus cuniculi*) but the Forest rabbit (*Sylvilagus brasiensis*) or Brush rabbit (*Sylvilagus bachmani*) that are native to North or South America. Another important member of the *Leporipoxvirus* genus is rabbit fibroma virus (Shope fibroma virus), which naturally affects the cottontail (*Sylvilagus floridanus*). In the European rabbit (*Oryctolagus cuniculi*) Shope fibroma virus causes a benign fibroma.

Shope fibroma virus is endemic in cottontails in the Eastern USA. It causes fibromas that remain localized but can persist for months. In newborn or immunocompromised individuals, generalized fibromatosis can occur (Fenner and Fantani, 1999). Like myxomatosis, Shope fibroma virus is spread by insect vectors. Transmission by mosquitoes occurs more readily than in the European rabbit. In situations where cottontails and mosquitoes are common, generalized fibromatosis can occur in adults because multiple mosquito bites produce a fibroma at each site (Fenner and Fantani, 1999).

In the European rabbit (*Oryctolagus cuniculi*), fibromas caused by Shope fibroma virus regress within 3 weeks of inoculation. Abundant virus can be found in the superficial layers of fibromas caused by Shope fibroma virus in the natural host, *Sylvilagus floridanus,* in comparison with fibromas in the European rabbit (*Oryctolagus cuniculi*). Shope fibroma cannot be established as an enzootic disease in European rabbits but cross-immunity between Shope fibroma virus and myxomatosis occurs and European rabbits that have recovered from infection with Shope fibroma virus are immune to myxomatosis.

16.6.1.5 Immunization

In common with other pox viruses, dead vaccines are unlikely to be effective and so a live vaccine is required to confer resistance to myxomatosis. Live attenuated strains of myxoma virus have been used for vaccination but problems have occurred with virulence and possible immunosuppression (Fenner and Fantani, 1999). The discovery of Shope fibroma virus and its cross-immunity with myxomatosis led to the development of a live

Key points 16.4

- Myxomatosis is characterized by subcutaneous swellings that exude a mucoid secretion when sectioned. Lesions occur around body orifices and on the face especially the eyelids
- The disease is mainly spread by arthropods, especially the European rabbit flea *Spilopsyllus cuniculi.* Mosquitoes are vectors in many parts of the world
- In wild rabbits, outbreaks of myxomatosis wax and wane according to the virulence of the strain and the immune status of the native rabbit population
- Myxomatosisis can occur in hares but is rare and usually mild
- Environmental temperature has an effect on mortality rates with the disease being more lethal at low temperatures
- Myxomatosis starts with a skin lesion at the site of inoculation. The rabbit becomes viraemic with virus replication taking place throughout the lymphoid system. Secondary lesions develop throughout the body, typically on the nares, lips, eyelids and base of the ears and on the external genitalia and anus
- Aerosol infection can result in pneumonic signs, which may be a feature of outbreaks in intensive farmed rabbits
- Myxomatosis is accompanied by sterility and abandonment of litters
- Myxomavirus is a member of the Leporipoxvirus genus. It causes a trivial infection in its natural host, either *Sylvilagus brasiensis* (Tapeti, Forest Rabbit, found in Mexico or Argentina) or *Sylvilagus bachmani* (Brush Rabbit) which is native to California. In the European Rabbit (*Oryctolagus cuniculi*), myxomavirus causes a serious life-threatening disease
- Another important member of the Leporipoxvirus genus is rabbit fibroma virus (Shope fibroma virus), which naturally affects the Cottontail (*Sylvilagus floridanus*) and causes a benign fibroma in European rabbits. Attenuated Shope fibroma virus is used to manufacture vaccine against myxomatosis
- It is possible, on rare occasions, for rabbits to recover from myxomatosis. Ambient temperature affects the course of the disease with high environmental temperature increasing recovery rate (85°C)
- Antibiotics, a warm environment, good nursing and non-steroidal analgesics can be used treat myxomatosis. Corticosteroids are contraindicated due to their immunosuppressive effects. Opioid analgesics are ineffective in ameliorating signs of pain.

vaccine containing Shope fibroma virus. The present day vaccine that is available in the UK (Nobivac Myxo, Intervet) is a live, attenuated freeze-dried virus vaccine containing Shope fibroma virus grown in cell-line tissue culture.

16.6.1.6 Recovery from myxomatosis

It is possible for rabbits to recover from myxomatosis. Apart from the virulence of the virus strain, certain environmental factors affect the resistance of the rabbit to myxomatosis, i.e. intercurrent infection and environmental temperature. Ambient temperature affects the course of the disease with high environmental temperature increasing recovery rate (85°C). Antibiotics, a warm environment and good nursing can be successful and some pet rabbits have survived myxomatosis although their chances are not good. The risk of secondary problems such as gastrointestinal stasis or pasteurellosis is ever present. Non-steroidal analgesics are useful but the use of corticosteroids is contraindicated due to their immunosuppressive effects. Opioid analgesics do not appear to be effective in ameliorating signs of pain. In a study of the effect of buprenorphine on the course of myxomatosis in laboratory rabbits, there was no difference in survival time. Treated rabbits refused food and water a day earlier than untreated rabbits and had lower rectal temperatures immediately prior to death (Robinson *et al.*, 1999).

16.6.2 Viral haemorrhagic disease (VHD)

Viral haemorrhagic disease (VHD) is a highly infectious lethal disease of rabbits with a high mortality rate. It is caused by a host-specific calicivirus. VHD only affects the European rabbit *Oryctolagus cuniculi*.

The disease may be called 'rabbit haemorrhagic disease' (RHD) and the virus known as 'rabbit haemorrhagic disease virus' (RHDV). Sometimes the term 'rabbit calicivirus disease' (RCD) is used. VHD originated in 1984 in the People's Republic of China that, at that time, was the world's largest exporter of rabbit meat. A disease broke out in a colony of Angora rabbits that had recently been imported into Germany (Fenner and Fantani, 1999). Except for the suckling rabbits, all the rabbits died within a week and in less than 9 months the disease had spread over 50 000 square kilometres and reached Italy and Europe. By 1988, VHD had been reported in commercial rabbits in many countries worldwide, probably introduced through rabbit meat. In Europe, the disease spread into the wild rabbit population. In 1990, VHD reached Scandinavia. Wild rabbits in the densely populated island of Gotland became nearly extinct within 1 week (Gavier-Widén, 1996). Hundreds of rabbits were seen dead in the fields and many more died in their burrows. Pet rabbits that had been kept indoors and fed on commercial food started dying indicating that humans can act as vectors for VHD. Coincidentally, another disease, European Brown Hare Syndrome (EBHS) was sweeping through Europe. EBHS is caused by a distinctly different calicivirus.

In 1996, a non-pathogenic calicivirus was recovered from breeding rabbits in Italy that produced seroconversion and was found to protect rabbits against VHD. The virus has been isolated and identified as a calicivirus. There is evidence that this virus existed before the onset of VHD (Capucci *et al.*, 1997).

16.6.2.1 Pathogenesis of VHD

VHD is caused by a calicivirus that has a predilection for hepatocytes and replicates within the cytoplasm of these cells. Experimentally infected rabbits die 3–4 days after infection.

VHD is essentially a necrotizing hepatitis, often associated with necrosis of the spleen (see Plate 35). Disseminated intravascular coagulation produces fibrinous thrombi within small blood vessels in most organs, notably the lungs, heart and kidneys resulting in haemorrhages. Death is due to disseminated intravascular coagulopathy or to liver failure.

16.6.2.2 Epidemiology of VHD

The calicivirus that causes VHD is antigenically similar to the virus that causes European Brown Hare Syndrome. Attempts to cross-infect rabbits and hares with heterologous virus have failed to induce disease. VHD only affects the European rabbits, not cottontails or other small mammals such as chinchillas, guinea pigs, rats and mice.

VHD calicivirus can survive for long periods outside the host. Viable virus has been detected for as long as 105 days on a cloth (Fenner and Fantani, 1999). Environmental temperature is an important factor in the survival of the virus which can remain viable for 22–35 days at 22°C but only for 3–7 days at 37°C. VHD virus is spread by oral, nasal and parenteral transmission and is present in urine and faeces from infected rabbits. Contaminated foods can be a source of infection.

When VHD is introduced into a susceptible population, the mortality rate is high and can be 90–100% in rabbits over 2 months of age. Infected young rabbits survive and become immune so when the disease becomes endemic the morbidity and mortality rate falls. In wild rabbits, the disease appears to break out every second year. Insects mechanically transmit the virus in viraemic blood from one animal to another. VHD virus can survive for several weeks in carcasses and skin. Fleas, blowflies and mosquitoes are known to spread the disease (Fenner and Fantani, 1999). PCR techniques have shown that virus can be retained in the body of blowflies for up to 9 days and bushflies for 7 days. Fly 'spots' (faeces) are also infective and can contaminate pasture. Flies can travel long distances and be carried along by the wind and spread the disease far and wide. It has also been demonstrated that domestic and wild carnivores can play an important role in the epidemiology of VHD since virulent material can be collected from faecal material after experimental oral inoculation. The virus is very stable in carcasses even after freezing and thawing (Lumeij, 1997). Up until October 1996, VHD was a notifiable disease in Great Britain. It is now endemic and poses a real threat to the pet rabbit due to its resistance and ease of transmission. Deaths have been reported nationwide that have been confirmed at *post-mortem* to be due to VHD.

16.6.2.3 Clinical signs of viral haemorrhagic disease

VHD has a short incubation period of 3–4 days. The disease can be peracute with animals being found dead within a few hours of eating and behaving normally. Acute cases are quiet, pyrexic with an increased respiratory rate and usually die within 12 h. A feature of the disease is a dramatic drop in blood pressure that makes it difficult to find a vein to take blood samples or set up intravenous fluids Dying rabbits are pallid, shocked and collapsed. Haematuria, haemorrhagic vaginal discharges or foamy exudate from the nostrils may be seen. Vascular infarcts can occur within the brain and occasionally convulsions or other neurological signs are seen just before death. Agonal vocalizing and cyanosis have been described (Donnelly, 1995). The 'classic' picture is a dead rabbit in opisthotonus with a haemorrhagic nasal discharge. The occasional rabbit can recover from the acute phase, only to develop jaundice and die a few days later. Young rabbits less than 4 weeks of age remain unaffected and develop a life-long immunity if they are exposed to the disease. Unexposed rabbits become increasingly susceptible until 6–10 weeks of age when physiological resistance to the virus disappears. The physiological age immunity of young rabbits has been ascribed to the increase in hepatic transaminase production that occurs after 5 weeks of age (Donnelly, 1995). In adult rabbits, the mortality rate is high. There is no treatment for affected rabbits.

16.6.2.4 Diagnosis of VHD

VHD is suspected in any sudden death especially if more than one rabbit in the household has died. The *post-mortem* picture may be of a healthy rabbit with non-impacted food in the stomach and hard faecal pellets in the distal colon, suggesting that death was sudden. The liver is always affected, although the gross appearance may not reflect the severe histopathological changes. The liver is enlarged, friable and pale with a distinct lobular pattern (see Plate 35). The spleen is also enlarged. Haemorrhages can be found in any organ but are usually present in the lung. The trachea is often full of a foamy exudate. Haematologically, there are fibrin thrombi, lymphopaenia, a reduction in platelets and a failure of other blood clotting factors that result in multiple organ failure due to general circulatory dysfunction. Disseminated intravascular coagulation is a characteristic feature of the pathogenesis of VHD (Chasey, 1997). Histopathology confirms acute hepatic necrosis. There may be many other changes such as acute nephropathy or alveolar haemorrhage. Congestion and haemorrhages can occur in any organ due to terminal intravascular coagulation. The typical histopathological changes in the liver are usually diagnostic but there are a number of other tests that confirm the diagnosis, including hamagglutination tests and electron microscopy. Large numbers of characteristic calicivirus can be detected by electron microscopic examination of liver (Chasey *et al.*, 1995). Fresh liver is required by the laboratory. ELISA tests are also available.

16.6.2.5 Vaccination

Due to the devastating effects of VHD in China, a vaccine was quickly developed from inactivated virus obtained from the liver and spleens of infected rabbits. The immunological response to inactivated vaccines is good. VHD virus is difficult to grow in tissue culture so attenuated strains have not been produced. Virus antigen harvested from experimentally infected rabbits is inactivated with formalin or β-propiolactone to produce effective killed vaccines that are commercially available. Vaccination is advisable for all pet rabbits (see Section 3.2). At the present time, there is only one type of attenuated vaccine available in the UK (Cylap, Websters). Genetically engineered vaccines are being produced that insert the gene for the coat protein of the VHD virus into attenuated myxoma virus for simultaneous immunization of VHD and myxomatosis (Barcena *et al.*, 2000).

16.6.3 Papillomatosis

There are descriptions of two papillomaviruses that can affect rabbits. Shope papillomavirus causes a benign disease in cottontails (*Sylvilagus floridanus*) but may cause malignant neoplasms resembling squamous cell carcinomas in the European rabbit (*Oryctolagus cuniculus*). The disease occurs in the wild population of cottontails in the Eastern USA and in domestic rabbits in some American commercial units.

Shope papillomavirus is immunologically distinct from the other papillomavirus, which causes oral papillomatosis. Oral papillomatosis is manifested by wart-like growths on the ventral aspect of the tongue and on other parts of the oral mucosa. The virus is transmitted in oral secretions containing sloughed cells from the warts. Young rabbits are most susceptible and the papillomas grow slowly over a period of 6–9 months. The animals become immune at which point the base of the papilloma becomes inflamed causing sloughing of the tumour, ulcer formation and finally re-epithelialization. Oral papillomas of rabbits are not known to undergo carcinomatous transformation (Kraus *et al.*, 1984).

16.6.4 Coronavirus

Coronavirus infection in rabbits was initially described in 1968. Affected rabbits were pyrexic, developed pulmonary oedema and pleural effusion and mortality rates were high. Iridocyclitis has been associated with the disease. An analogy with feline infectious peritonitis has been made. Coronavirus has also been implicated in outbreaks of enteric disease in weanling rabbits.

The virus has not been propagated *in vitro* and it is unclear whether it is a naturally occurring pathogen of rabbits or a virus from another species adapted to rabbits in contaminated treponemal stocks (DiGiacomo and Mare, 1994). The disease was first recognized in the 1960s in rabbits inoculated with suspensions of rabbit testes containing *Treponema pallidum* (human syphilis). Subsequently the agent has been detected in *T. pallidum* infected rabbit tissue throughout the world. Coronavirus infection is used experimentally to produce a rabbit model of cardiomyopathy and has only been described in laboratory rabbits. Antibodies to the virus cross-react with human and other mammalian coronaviruses (DiGiacomo and Mare, 1994).

16.5 Mycotic infections

16.5.1 Dermatophytosis

Dermatophytosis (ringworm) is occasionally encountered in rabbits. *Trichophyton mentagro-*

Key points 16.5

- Viral haemorrhagic disease (VHD) is a highly infectious lethal disease of rabbits with a high mortality rate. It is caused by a host-specific calicivirus. VHD only affects the European rabbit *Oryctolagus cuniculi*
- The disease may be called 'rabbit haemorrhagic disease' (RHD) and the virus known as 'rabbit haemorrhagic disease virus' (RHDV). Sometimes the term 'rabbit calicivirus disease' (RCD) is used
- The causative calicivirus of VHD has a predilection for hepatocytes. VHD is essentially a necrotizing hepatitis. Death is usually due to disseminated intravascular coagulopathy
- VHD calicivirus can survive for long periods outside the host. Viable virus has been detected for as long as 105 days on cloth
- VHD virus is spread by oral, nasal and parenteral transmission and is present in urine and faeces from infected rabbits. Contaminated foods can be a source of infection
- When VHD is introduced into a susceptible population, the mortality rate is high and can be 90–100% in rabbits over 2 months of age
- VHD has a short incubation period of 3–4 days. The disease can be peracute with animals being found dead within a few hours of eating and behaving normally
- The 'classic' picture is a dead rabbit in opisthotonus with a haemorrhagic nasal discharge
- Haematuria, haemorrhagic vaginal discharges or foamy exudate from the nostrils may be seen
- Vascular infarcts can occur within the brain and occasionally convulsions or other neurological signs are seen just before death
- There is no specific treatment for affected rabbits
- Young rabbits, less than 4 weeks of age, remain unaffected and develop a lifelong immunity if they are exposed to the disease. Unexposed rabbits become increasingly susceptible until 6–10 weeks of age when physiological resistance to the virus disappears
- The typical histopathological changes in the liver are usually diagnostic
- An effective vaccine against VHD is available in the UK
- Other viruses that affect rabbits include papillomavirus, coronavirus, rotavirus, and parvovirus
- Fungal infections of domestic rabbits include *Trichophyton mentagrophytes, Microsporum canis, Dermatophilus congalensis* and aspergillosis.

phytes and *Microsporum canis* are the species most commonly described (Percy and Barthold, 1993). Lesions are usually found on the base of the ears and muzzle but can involve other areas of the body such as the paws (see Section 9.15). Asymptomatic carriers can occur. Young rabbits are most likely to be affected (Vangeel *et al.*, 2000). *Dermatophilus congalensis* has been isolated from rabbits.

16.5.2 Aspergillosis

Pulmonary aspergillotic granulomas have been described in laboratory rabbits (Percy and Barthold, 1993).

References

Allan, J.C., Craig, P.S., Sherington, J. *et al.* (1999). Helminth parasites of the wild rabbit *Oryctolagus cuniculus* near Malham Tarn, Yorkshire, UK. (Abstract). *J Helminthol.*, **73**, 289–294.

Barcena, J., Morales, M., Vazquez, B. (2000). Horizontal transmissible protection against myxomatosis and rabbit haemorrhagic disease by using a recombinant myxoma virus (Abstract). *J Virol.*, **74**, 1114–1123.

Beard, P.M., Henderson, D., Daniels, M.J. *et al.* (1999). Evidence of paratuberculosis in fox (*Vulpes vulpes*) and stoat (*Mustela erminea*). *Vet Rec.*, **145**, 612–613.

Beauvais, B., Sarfati, C., Challier, S., Derouin, F. (1994). *In vitro* model to assess effect of antimicrobial agents on *Encephalitozoon cuniculi. Antimicrob Agents Chemother.*, **38**, 2440–2448.

Besch-Williford, C. (1997). Tyzzer's disease in rabbits. In *Rabbit Medicine and Procedures for Practitioners. Program and Abstracts.* pp 113–117. House Rabbit Society Veterinary Conference, USA.

Boot, R., Thuis, H., Wieten, G. (1995). Multifactorial analysis of antibiotic sensitivity of *Bordetella bronchiseptica* isolates from guinea pigs, rabbits and rats. *Lab Anim*, **29**, 45–49.

Bywater, J.E., Kellett, B.S. (1979). Humoral immune response to natural infection with *Encephalitozoon cuniculi* in rabbits. *Lab Anim.*, **13**, 293–297.

Capucci, L., Nardin, A., Lavazza, A. (1997). Seroconversion in an industrial unit of rabbits infected with a non-pathogenic rabbit haemorrhagic disease-like virus. *Vet Rec.*, **140**, 647–650.

Chasey, D. (1997). Rabbit haemorrhagic disease; the new scourge of *Oryctolagus cuniculus*. *Lab Anim.*, **31**, 33–44.

Chasey, D., Lucas, M.H., Westcott, D.G. *et al.* (1995). Development of a diagnostic approach to the identification of rabbit haemorrhagic disease. *Vet Rec.*, **137**, 158–160.

Cox, J.C., Ross J. (1980). A serological survey of *Encephalitozoon cuniculi* infection in the wild rabbit in England and Scotland (Abstract). *Res.Vet Sci.*, **28**, 396.

Cox, J.C., Gallichio, H.A. (1978). Serological and histological studies on adult rabbits with recent naturally acquired encephalitozoonosis. *Res Vet Sci.*, **24**, 260–261.

Cox, J.C, Hamilton, R.C, Attwood, H.D. (1979). An investigation of the route and progression of *Encephalitozoon cuniculi* infection in adult rabbits. *J Protozool.*, **26**, 260–265.

Cox, J.C., Pye, D., Edmonds, J.W., Shepherd, R. (1980). An investigation of *Encephalitozoon cuniculi* in the rabbit *Oryctolagus cuniculus* in Victoria, Australia (Abstract). *J Hyg (Lond.)*, **84**, 295–300.

Cox, J.C., Edmonds, J.W., Shepherd, R.C. (1981). Toxoplasmosis and the wild rabbit *Oryctolagus cuniculus* in Victoria, Australia with suggested mechanisms for dissemination of oocysts (Abstract). *J Hyg.*, **87**, 331–337.

Dannatt, L., Gunning, R., Higgins, R. (2000). Attaching and effacing *E. coli* in rabbits. *Vet Rec.*, **147**, 524.

Deeb, B. (1993). Update for veterinary practitioners on pasteurellosis in rabbits. *J Small Exotic Anim Med.*, **2**, 112–113.

De Groote, M.A., Visvesvara, G., Wilson, M.L. *et al.* (1995). Polymerase chain reaction and culture confirmation of disseminated *Encephalitozoon cuniculi* in a patient with AIDS: successful therapy with albendazole. *J InfectDis.*, **171**, 1375–1378.

Delong, D., Manning, P.J. (1994). Bacterial diseases. In *The Biology of the Laboratory Rabbit*, 2nd edn. (P.J. Manning, D.H. Ringler, C.E. Newcomer, eds). pp 131–170. Academic Press.

Deplazes, P., Mathis, A., Baumgartner, R. *et al.* (1996). Immunological and molecular characteristics of *Encephalitozoon*-like microsporidia isolated from humans and rabbits indicate that *Encephalitozoon cuniculi* is a zoonotic parasite (Abstract). *Clin Infect Dis.*, **22**, 557–559.

DiGiacomo, R.F., Deeb, B.J. (1989). Pasteurellosis in rabbits – sequelae and vaccination. *J Appl Rabbit Res.*, **12**, 10–13.

DiGiacomo, R.F., Mare, J. (1994). Viral diseases. In *The Biology of the Laboratory Rabbit*, 2nd edn. (P.J. Manning, D.H. Ringler, C.E. Newcomer, eds). pp 171–197. Academic Press.

DiGiacomo, R.F., Garlinghouse, L.E. Jr., Van Hoosier. G.L. Jr (1983). Natural history of infection with *Pasteurella multocida* in rabbits. *J AmVet Med Assoc.*, **183**, 1172–1175.

DiGiacomo, R.F., Deeb, B.J., Bernard, B.L. *et al.* (1987). Safety and efficacy of a streptomycin dependent live *Pasteurella multocida* vaccine in rabbits (Abstract). *Lab Anim Sci.*, **37**, 187–190.

Donnelly, T.M. (1995). Emerging viral diseases of rabbits and rodents: viral haemorrhagic disease and hantavirus. *Sem Avian Exotic Pet Med.*, **4**, 83–91.

Ewringmann, A., Göbel, T. (1999). Untersuchungen zur Klinik und Therapie der Encephalitozoonose beim Heimtierkaninchen (Article in German, English summary). *Klientierpraxis*, **44**, 357–372.

Fenner, F., Fantani B. (1999). *Biological Control of Vertebrate Pests. The History of Myxomatosis – An Experiment in Evolution.* CABI Publishing.

Fenner, F., Ross, J. (1994). Myxomatosis. In *The European rabbit. The History and Biology of a Successful Coloniser.* (H.V. Thompson, C.M. King, eds). pp 205–235. Oxford University Press.

Franssen, F.F.J., Lumiej, J.T., Van Knapen, F. (1995). Susceptibilty of *Encephalitozoon cuniculi* to several drugs *in vitro*. *Antimicrob Agents Chemother.*, **39**, 1265–1268.

Fuentealba, I.C., Mahoney, N.T., Shadduck, J.A. *et al.* (1992). Hepatic lesions in rabbits infected with *Encephalitizoon cuniculi* per rectum. *Vet Pathol.*, **29**, 536–540.

Gannon, J. (1980). The course of infection of *Encephalitozoon cuniculi* in immunodeficient and immunocompetent mice. *Lab Anim.*, **14**, 189–192.

Gavier-Widén, D. (1996). Viral hepatitis of rabbits and hares in Scandinavia. In *Zoo and Wildlife Medicine*. (M. Fowler, ed.) pp 322–325, W.B. Saunders.

Greig, A., Stevenson, K., Perez, V. *et al.* (1997) Paratuberculosis in wild rabbits (*Oryctolagus cuniculus*). *Vet Rec.*, **140**, 141–143.

Greig, A., Stevenson, K., Henderson, D. *et al.* (1999). Epidemiological study of paratuberculosis in wild rabbits in Scotland. *J Clin Microbiol.*, **37**, 1746–1751.

Gustaffson, K., Wattrang, E., Fossum, C. *et al.* (1997). *Toxoplasmosis gondii* infection in the mountain hare (*Lepus timidus*) and domestic rabbit (*Oryctolagus cuniculus*). *J Comp Path.*, **117**, 351–368.

Harcourt, R.A. (1967). Toxoplasmosis in rabbits. *Vet Rec.*, **81**, 91–92.

Hollister, W.S., Canning, E.U., Viney, M.(1989). Prevalence of antibodies to *Encephalitozoon cuniculi* in stray dogs as determined by an ELISA. *Vet Rec.*, **124**, 332–336.

Hofing, G. L., Kraus, A.L. (1994). Arthropod and helminth parasites. In *The Biology of the Laboratory Rabbit*, 2nd edn. (P. J. Newcomer, D.H. Ringler, C.E. Newcomer, eds). pp 231–258, Academic Press.

Joste, N.E., Rich, J.D., Busam, K.J., Schwartz, D.A. (1996). Autopsy verification of *Encephalitozoonosis intestinalis* (microsporidiosis) eradiction following albendazole therapy (Abstract). *Arch Pathol Lab Med.*, **120**, 199–203.

Kimman, T.G., Akkermanns, J.P. (1987). *Encephalitozoon cuniculi* in a rabbit-breeding colony (Article in dutch, English abstract). *Tijdschr Diergeneeskd*, **112**, 1405–1409.

Kraus, A., Weisbroth, S.H., Flatt, R.E., Brewer N. (1984). Biology and diseases of rabbits. In *Laboratory Animal Medicine*. pp 207–237. Academic Press.

Kunstyr, I., Lev, L., Naumann, S. (1986). Humoral antibody response in rabbits to experimental infection with *Encephalitozoon cuniculi*. *Vet Parasitol.*, **21**, 223–232.

Leibenberg, S.P., Badger, V.M. (1984). Suppurative osteomyelitis in the foot of a rabbit. *J Am Vet Med Assoc.*, **185**, 1382.

Leland, M.M., Hubbard, C.B., Dupey, J.P. (1992). Clinical toxoplasmosis in domestic rabbits. *Lab Anim Sci.*, **42**, 318–319.

Lelkes, L., Corbett, M.J. (1983). A preliminary study of the transmission of pasteurella multocida in rabbits. *J Appl Rabbit Res.*, **6**, 125–126.

Levkut, M., Horvath, M., Balent, P. *et al.* (1997). Catecholamines and encephalitozoonosis in rabbits (Abstract). *Vet Parasitol.*, **73**, 173–176.

Li, T., Qiao, G.L., Hu, G.Z. *et al.* (1995). Comparative plasma and tissue pharmaockinetics and drug residue profiles of different chemotherapeutants in fowls and rabbits (Abstract). *J Vet Pharmacol Ther.*, **18**, 260–273.

Lumeij, J.T. (1997). Disease risks with translocations of rabbits and hares into, out of and within Europe. *J Br Vet Zool Soc.*, **2**, 19–25.

Lyngset, A. (1980). A survey of serum antibodies to *Encephalitozoon cuniculi* in breeding rabbits and their young (Abstract). *Lab Anim Sci.*, **30**, 558–561.

Manning, P.J., DiGiacomo, R.F., Delong, D. (1989). Pasteurellosis in laboratory animals. In *Pasteurella and Pasteurellosis* (C. Adlam, J.M. Rutter, eds). pp 264–289. Academic Press.

Morrisey, J.K. (1996) Parasites of ferrets, rabbits and rodents. *Sem Avian Exotic Pet Med.*, **5**, 106–114.

Niederkorn, J.Y., Shadduck, J.A. (1980). Role of antibody and complement in the control of *Encephalitozoon cunuculi* infections by rabbit macrophages (Abstract). *Infect Immun.*, **27**, 995–1002.

Okerman, L. (1988). *Diseases of Domestic Rabbits*. Blackwell Scientific Publications.

Owen, D.G. (1992). *Parasites of Laboratory Animals. Laboratory Animal Handbooks No 12*. Royal Society of Medicine Services Ltd.

Pakes, S.P., Gerrity, L.W. (1994). Protozoal diseases. In *The Biology of the Laboratory Rabbit*, 2nd edn. (P.J. Manning, D.H. Ringler, C.E. Newcomer, eds). pp 205–224. Academic Press.

Pattison, M., Clegg, F.G., Duncan, A.L. (1971). An outbreak of encephamyelitis in broiler rabbits caused by *Nosema cuniculi*. *Vet Rec.*, **88**, 404–405.

Percy, D.H. and Barthold S.W.(1993) Rabbit. In *Pathology of Laboratory Rodents and Rabbits*. pp 179–223. Iowa State University Press.

Petersen-Jones, S.M., Carrington, S.D. (1988). Pasteurella dacryocystitis in rabbits. *Vet Rec.*, **122**, 514–515.

Poonacha, K.B., Stamper, R.D. (1985). Encephalitozoonosis in a parrot. *J Am Vet Med Assoc.*, **186**, 700–702.

Pye, D., Cox, J.C. (1977). Isolation of *Encephalitozoon cuniculi* from urine samples. *Lab Anim.*, **11**, 223–224.

Robinson, A.J., Muller, W.J., Braid, A.L., Kerr, P.J. (1999). The effect of buprenorphine on the course of disease in laboratory rabbits infected with myxoma virus (Abstract). *Lab Anim.*, **33**, 252–257.

Sanchez, S., Mizan, S., Ritchie, B. W., Lee, M.D. (2000). Pasteurellosis in rabbits. *Compendium on Continuing Education*, **22**, 344–350.

Sobottka, I., Albrecht, H., Schafer, H. *et al.* (1995). Disseminated Encephalitozoon (Septata) intestinal infection in a patient with AIDS: novel diagnostic approaches and autopsy-confirmed parasitological cure following treatment with albendazole (Abstract). *J Clin Microbiol.*, **33**, 2948–2952.

Stiles, J., Didier, E., Ritchie, B. *et al.* (1997). *Encephalizoon cuniculi* in the lens of a rabbit with phacoclastic uveitis: confirmation and treatment. *Vet Comp Ophthalmol.*, **7**, 233–238.

Suter, C., Müller-Doblies, U.U., Hatt, J.-M., Deplazes, P. (2001). Prevention and treatment of *Encephalitozoon cuniculi* in rabbits with fenbendazole. *Vet. Rec.*, **148**, 478–480.

Telford, S.R., Speilman, A. (1989). Enzootic transmission of the agent of Lyme disease in rabbits (Abstract). *Am J Trop Med Hyg.*, **41**, 482–490.

Vangeel, I., Pasmans, F., Vanrobaeys, M. *et al.* (2000). Prevalence of dermatophytes in asymptomatic guinea pigs and rabbits. *Vet Rec.*, **146**, 440–441.

Whittaker, D. (1989). Pasteurellosis in the laboratory rabbit: a review. *Vet Ann.*, **29**, 285–291.

Wills, J. (2001). Coenurosis in a pet rabbit. *Vet Rec.*, **148**, 188.

Wilson, J.M. (1979). The biology of *Encephalitozoon cuniculi*. *Med Biol.*, **57**, 84–101.

Wood, C. (1978). The pet rabbit – veterinary problems. *Vet Rec.*, **102**, 304–308.

17

Post-mortem examination of rabbits

The procedure for *post-mortem* examination in rabbits is similar to other species. A methodical approach is required (Bivin, 1994). A preprinted checklist of findings can be useful. Initially the carcass is inspected, weighed and, if necessary, radiographed before embarking on autopsy. A ventral midline, longitudinal incision exposes the abdominal organs, which are examined systematically. The thoracic viscera are removed, paying careful attention to the larynx and surrounding structures. The head is examined and skinned, paying particular attention to the teeth, ear canals and structures of the cheek and orbit. The brain, nasal cavity and sinuses can be examined by careful removal of the parietal and nasal bone, or the bones of the skull can be preserved for further examination after cleaning. Sample collection for bacteriology and/or histopathology is important. Many diseases require histopathological confirmation.

A list of *post-mortem* findings and possible diagnoses is given in Table 17.1. Some features of *post-mortem* examination of rabbits are given in Box 17.1. Normal anatomy is illustrated by Barone *et al.* (1973).

17.1 Preparation of *post-mortem* tissue for further examination

As rabbits are used so extensively as laboratory animals, many pathologists are familiar with lagomorph histopathology. The manner in which samples are collected, fixed and submitted to the laboratory is important and

Box 17.1 *Post-mortem* examination of rabbits

- Autolysis, especially of abdominal contents takes place very quickly after death and *post-mortem* examination within 4 h is advisable, especially when intestinal disorders are suspected. Chilling the carcass in a refrigerator slows autolysis
- The fat of most rabbits is white but occasionally yellow fat may be encountered. This is a genetic condition. Affected rabbits lack a specific liver enzyme that is required to metabolize xanthophylls (Lindsey and Fox, 1994)
- It is normal for muscle tissue of rabbits to appear pale in colour
- The stomach, intestines or caecum can rupture after death. If *ante-mortem* rupture has occurred, there are signs of haemorrhage, inflammation and peritonitis
- The spleen of the rabbit is small in comparison with other species, it is normally less than 1 cm in diameter and up to 4 mm long
- The stomach should always contain some food
- The caecal contents should be soft but not fluid or impacted
- Normal rabbit urine often contains quantities of calcium carbonate sediment. Normal urine can vary in colour from yellow to orange, brown or red
- Hepatic lipidosis develops rapidly during periods of anorexia especially in obese animals. It is the end stage of many diseases
- Rabbit kidneys can show a typical pitted appearance that is caused by *Encephalitozoon cuniculi*. This can be an incidental finding.

Table 17.1 *Post-mortem* findings and possible diagnoses

Stage of examination	*Findings*	*Possible causes*	*Further information*
External examination			
External examination of skin/fur	Wounds	• Predator attack • Fight wounds from cage mate (?stress) • Recent dematting	Section 9.2
	Scale	*Cheyletiella parasitovorax*. ?associated with debility, flexibility problems or dental disease	Section 9.14.2.3
	Wet fur under chin	Salivation due to spurs on cheek teeth	Section 7.6.8
	Matted fur (especially on face and perineum)	Lack of grooming, debility, flexibility problems, dental disease, poor husbandry	Section 9.7
	Soiled, wet perineum	Urinary incontinence, uneaten caecotrophs, poor husbandry	Section 9.7.3
	Abscesses	• Dental disease • Fight wounds • Foreign bodies	Section 8.1
	Mammary development (? mastitis)	• Pregnant • Lactating • Pseudopregnant	Section 9.18
	Diarrhoea oozing from anus	• Enterotoxaemia • Enteritis (especially juveniles) • Coccidiosis (especially juveniles)	Section 10.10
External examination of limbs **NB** Ring over hock indicates a pedigree animal and gives the year of birth	Ulcerative pododermatitis	Debility, obesity, disability, poor husbandry, immobility, large breed. Can cause pain and stress	Section 9.10
	Staining and exudate on medial aspect of forepaws	Associated with rhinitis, ?dental disease, pasteurellosis, nasal foreign bodies	Section 13.2
	Swollen foot caused by occlusion of blood supply by ring	Ring too small or entrapped fur and skin debris beneath ring	Section 3.1.6
	Fractures	Predator attack or other trauma	Section 12.2
	Abscesses	• Fight wounds • Foreign bodies • Haematogenous spread	Section 8.1
Examination of head	Otitis externa	• Bacterial infection • *Psoroptes cuniculi* • Foreign body	Section 9.9 Section 9.14.2.1
	Nasal discharge: Purulent	• Rhinitis, ?Pasteurellosis • Nasal foreign body • Periapical infection • Myxomatosis	Section 13.2.1 Section 13.3 Section 8.1 Section 16.6.1
	Haemorrhagic	• Viral haemorrhagic disease (often die in opisthotonus) • Trauma or predator attack	Section 16.6.2
	Swollen eyelids	• Myxomatosis • Acute renal failure and fluid retention	Section 16.6.1 Section 14.5.3.2
	Purulent ocular discharge	• Myxomatosis • Dacrocystitis • Conjunctivitis • Conjunctival foreign body	Section 16.6.1 Section 11.6.4 Section 11.6.2
	Exophthalmos	• Trauma • Retrobulbar swellings: tumours, abscess, cysts • Glaucoma • Buphthalmia	 Section 8.1 Section 11.5.1
	Epiphora/facial dermatitis	• Dental disease • Ocular disease	Section 7.6.5 Section 11.6.3

continued

Table 17.1 *continued*

Stage of examination	*Findings*	*Possible causes*	*Further information*
Internal examination			
Examination of the stomach and small intestine. (**NB.** The stomach and intestinal contents should be examined for presence of potentially toxic substances, e.g. heavy metals or unusual plant material. Placing the contents in a bowl of water is useful)	Distended dilated stomach full of fluid/gas	• Pyloric obsruction (rare) • Intestinal obstruction, e.g. felts of hair, pulses such as dried peas or beans, tumours, cysts, abscesses, adhesions, stenosis • Terminal stages of mucoid enteropathy	Section 10.5 Section 10.9
	Impacted stomach contents, often mixed with quantities of hair (trichobezoar)	Gastrointestinal hypomotility secondary to some painful or stressful condition or situation. Usually associated with hepatic lipidosis in animals that have died as a result of the condition	Section 10.3.1
	Gastric ulceration	Associated with any condition that causes inappetance. Can rupture	Section 10.4
	Inflammation of small intestine	• Secondary to obstruction • Tyzzer's disease is associated with haemorrhage and necrosis of distal ileum (also typhlitis and focal necrosis of liver) • Intestinal coccidiosis • Enterotoxaemia (usually affects caecum but occasionally affects small intestine)	Section 10.5 Section 16.5.4 Section 10.10.1 Section 10.10.2
	Intestinal stenosis	• Previous surgery • Neoplasia e.g. lymphoma • Tyzzer's disease	Section 10.5.1 Section 10.5 Section 16.5.4
	Multiple oval cysts in mesentery	*Cysticercus pisifomis*	
Examination of caecum and colon	Ecchymotic haemorrhages on serosal surfaces, liquid, gassy contents Oedema of gut wall	Enterotoxaemia. (clostridial organisms may be seen on gram-stained smears of gut contents)	Section 10.10.2
	Impacted, dry caecal contents	• Mucoid enteropathy • Dysautonomia • Caecal impaction	Section 10.9 Section 10.8 Section 10.7
	Distended caecum with watery, light brown contents. Maybe ecchymoses and oedema enlargement of mesenteric lymph nodes	Enteritis, e.g. *E. coli*, viral infections in rabbit colonies	Section 10.10
	Ecchymoses, fibrinous exudate on serosal surface of caecum and colon	Tyzzer's disease (also pale miliary foci in liver)	Section 10.10.4
	Necrotic foci	• Hepatic coccidiosis • Salmonella • Yersinia • Tyzzer's disease • Tularaemia • Listeriosis	Section 10.10 Section 16.5
Examination of liver	Hepatic lipidosis (often accompanied by fatty infiltration of other organs, e.g. kidneys	Terminal event in a number of diseases that cause anorexia	Section 10.3.2
	Hepatomegaly	• Viral haemorrhagic disease (also splenomegaly, and haemorrhage in other organs)	Section 16.6.2

continued

		• Septicaemia	
		• Hepatic coccidiosis (also enlarged thickened bile ducts within parenchyma)	Section 10.10.1
		• Neoplasia	
		• Congestive heart failure	Section 13.6
		• Lymphoma (pale in colour)	
		• Toxoplasmosis	Section 16.4.3
	Nodules or foci	• Hepatic coccidiosis	Section 10.10
		• Salmonella	Section 16.5
		• Tyzzer's disease	
		• Yersinia	
		• Tularaemia	
		• Neoplasia	
Examination of spleen	Splenomegaly	• Viral haemorrhagic disease	Section 16.6.2
		• Septicaemia	
		• Congestive heart failure	Section 13.6
		• Toxoplasma	Section 16.4.3
Examination of kidneys	Pitted appearance	• Exposure to *Encephalitozoon cuniculi*	Section 14.5.1
	Urolithiasis	Associated with urinary tract obstruction Linked with calcium excretion	Section 14.4.5
	Calcification of renal tissue (may be seen in conjunction with mineralization of other tissues such as aorta)	• Vitamin D toxicity • Chronic renal failure	Section 14.5.2
	Fatty infiltration	Associated with hepatic lipidosis Terminal event of many diseases that cause prolonged anorexia	Section 10.3.2
	Serosal haemorrhages	• Viral haemorrhagic disease	Section 16.6.2
		• Septicaemia	
		• Toxicity, e.g. anticoagulant rodenticides, triazines	Section 12.6.1.2
	Circumscribed, white nodules	Embryonal nephroma, a benign tumour that may be found as an incidental *post-mortem* finding	Section 14.5
	Enlarged kidneys	• Septicaemia	
		• Congestive heart failure	Section 13.6
		• Neoplasia, e.g. lymphoma (pale and irregular)	
Examination of bladder and genital tract	Sediment in urine. Brown, orange or red coloured urine	Normal	Section 14.3
	Sludgy, thick viscid urine	'Sludgy urine'	Section 14.4.2
	Uroliths	Urolithiasis	Section 14.4.5
	Uterine neoplasms	Uterine adenocarcinoma	Section 14.6.6.1
	Necrotic masses in broad ligament	• Metastatic spread from uterine adenocarcinoma	Section 14.6.6.1
		• Fat necrosis	
		• Infection/granulomas associated with suture material from ovariohysterectomy	Section 15.3
	Blood filled protrusions in endometrium	Endometrial venous aneurysms	Section 14.6.6
	Dead fetuses	• Pregnancy toxaemia	Section 10.3.3
		• Metritis, e.g. listeriosis, pasteurellosis	Section 16.5.10 Section 16.5.1
	Pyometritis/abscesses	Pasteurellosis	Section 16.5.1
	Orchitis	• Fight wounds	
		• Myxomatosis	Section 16.6.1

continued

Table 17.1 *continued*

Stage of examination	*Findings*	*Possible causes*	*Further information*
Examination of heart, lungs and trachea **NB.** The larynx and nasopharynx should be examined carefully, especially if rabbits have died suddenly. Foreign bodies are common	Abnormal appearance of heart	• Cardiomyopathy • Congenital heart defects • Tyzzer's disease	Section 13.6.1 Section 13.6 Section 16.5.4
	Haemorrhagic areas in lung tissue	• Acute suppurative pneumonia, e.g. pasteurellosis • Viral haemorrhagic disease	Section 16.5.4.1 Section 16.6.2
	Pneumonia, bronchopneumonia	• Bacterial infections, *P. multocida, S. aureus* • Aspiration pneumonia • Mucoid enteropathy	Section 13.2.5 Section 10.9
	Haemorrhagic exudate in trachea	Viral haemorrhagic disease	Section 16.6.2
	Foreign material in larynx	Inhalation or penetration of hay, hair or other foreign material. May be associated with dental disease	Section 13.4
Examination of buccal cavity	Dental abnormalities	• Congenital • Due to trauma: fractured teeth or jaw • Acquired	Section 7.3
	Ulceration of soft tissue of lips, gums and buccal mucosa	• Injury from overgrown teeth • Iatrogenic injury from dental burrs or tooth clippers • Penetrating foreign bodies	Section 7.6 Section 7.10.2
Examination of structures of head after removal of skin **NB.** If the skull is not destined for further examination, the nasal bone can be removed to expose the nasal cavity and sinuses, the parietal bone removed to expose the brain and the tympanic bullae opened to examine the contents	Purulent exudate in nasal cavity	• Foreign material such as hay, seeds or plugs of hair in nasal cavity • Periapical abscesses of maxillary cheek teeth • Dilation and rupture of nasolacrimal duct • Rhinitis due to bacterial infection • Sinusitis	Section 13.3 Section 8.1 Section 11.6.4 Section 13.2.3
	Abscesses	• Dental disease • Penetrating wounds, e.g. fight wounds or from overgrown teeth • Foreign bodies, stems of hay, grass seeds	Section 8.1

influences the results that are obtained from histopathological examination. Representative samples of a range of tissues should be submitted to the laboratory, including heart, liver, kidney, spleen, lung and lymph node. Sections of grossly abnormal and normal tissue from organs such as the liver may be helpful. Organs such as the heart or brain can submitted whole, which allows the histopathologist to orientate the tissue correctly.

Autolysis of the gut is rapid in rabbits. Intestinal tissue needs to be harvested as soon as possible after death. To obtain diagnostic samples, 1–2 cm of a representative length of hollow viscera such as intestine can be opened longitudinally and pinned out on a wooden tongue depressor with the mucosal surface away from the wood. Hypodermic needles (23 g) are suitable for this procedure. The orientation of the tissue is marked on the tongue depressor in pencil before being

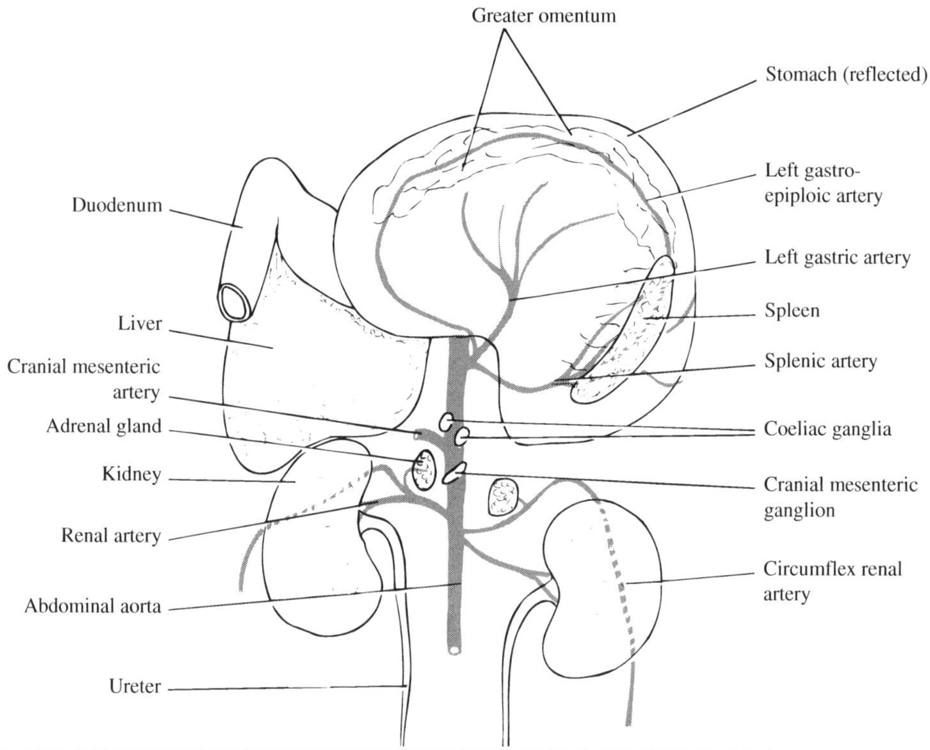

Figure 17.1. Site of mesenteric ganglia (redrawn, with permission, from Barone *et al.* 1973). The site of the mesenteric ganglia of the rabbit is illustrated. Histopathological examination of the autonomic ganglia is required to demonstrate lesions associated with dysautonomia. A detailed description of the location and removal of the ganglia is given in Section 17.3)

floated in 10% formol saline with the side with the tissue attached face-down. The container should be covered to prevent evaporation of formal saline. After at least 24 h, preferably longer, the needles can be removed and the tissue transferred to a plastic bag that is labelled, sealed, packaged in a suitable container and posted. In this way the tissue is orientated and fixed properly and the samples can be posted without risk of leakage.

Enterotoxaemia is a cause of sudden death. Anaerobic conditions in intestinal or caecal contents can be maintained by tying off both ends of a section before removal and submission to the laboratory for aerobic and anaerobic culture (Langan and O'Rourke, 2000). Alternatively, swabs of intestinal contents can be poked to the bottom of transport media to maintain anaerobic conditions.

17.2 Examination for parasites

Wet preparations of intestinal contents or faeces can be examined for protozoan cysts or worm eggs. Identification of oocysts is based on special staining techniques and morphological characteristics that are outside the remit of most practice laboratories. Flotation techniques are useful to concentrate ova and oocysts. A quick, qualitative technique is to mix the sample with saturated salt solution, centrifuge it and fill the container to the brim. A cover slip is then placed over the meniscus and left for a few minutes before it is removed and placed on a microscope slide for examination.

Intestinal coccidiosis can be found on intestinal scrapings. Impression smears can also be used to detect protozoan parasites. Migrating sporozoites of *Eimeria steidae* may be located in mesenteric lymph nodes (Owen, 1992). The node is carefully halved before being applied firmly to a clean slide, which is then air-dried and stained. *E. steidae* can also be found in bile aspirated from the gallbladder during *post-mortem* examination of affected rabbits.

17.3 Examination of autonomic ganglia

Histopathological examination of the autonomic ganglia is recommended in all rabbits that have died from intestinal motility disorders that are suggestive of dysautonomia, particularly constipative mucoid enteropathy.

Neuropathological changes can be assessed in ganglia from four sites (cranial mesenteric, caudal mesenteric, stellate and cranial cervical ganglia) and in the brain. The mesenteric ganglia are illustrated in Figure 17.1. The following description of the location and removal of autonomic ganglia is given by Katherine Whitwell (personal communication).

The ganglia are removed with the rabbit lying on its right side. The left abdominal and thoracic walls are removed. The presence of fat deposits obscures the pale ganglia. Stroking the tissue gently with the flat edge of a scalpel blade (No. 22) is a useful way of removing the soft overlying fat and exposing the ganglia. The ganglia have a firmer consistency than fat but are semitransparent. The largest and most readily located ganglion is the cranial mesenteric ganglion. The left branch of the cranial mesenteric ganglion can be found ventral and cranial to the left adrenal gland, lying on the left side of the aorta. The tiny (single) caudal mesenteric ganglion lies in the roof of the mesentery subtending the distal colon. It is long and thin and should not be confused with the friable lymph nodes that lie beneath it. The left stellate ganglion can be found by transecting the midtrachea and attached oesophagus before deflecting them to expose the tissues at the entrance to the right side of the chest, beneath the first rib. The cranial cervical ganglion is a tiny fusiform swelling within the proximal end of each sympathetic trunk at the base of the skull. The cranial cervical ganglion lies close to the slightly larger nodose ganglion that lies on the adjacent vagus nerve. The vagosympathetic trunk can be followed cranially from the midneck to locate the ganglia.

Screening for dysautonomia can only be made if an adequate sample of ganglionic tissue is obtained. Crushing artefact of tiny fragments, incomplete or incorrect sampling make it advisable to attempt to locate all four ganglia. They should be placed in a separate container from the rest of the tissues intended for histological evaluation. The cranial mesenteric ganglion can provide sufficient material on its own, if it is successfully dissected.

17.4 Examination of the head and brain

To fix the brain for histopathological investigation, a section of thin parietal bone at the base of the skull can be carefully removed to expose the brain. It is possible to nibble the bone away with volute nail clippers. Once a big enough hole is made, a midline incision through the sulcus allows formol saline to penetrate the ventricles. Prepared in this manner, the whole head can be fixed and sent to the laboratory. Alternatively, the brain can be carefully dissected away from the surrounding tissue. It is easier to remove the brain intact after it has been fixed. Brain histology can be used to confirm *E. cuniculi* infection.

Serial sections of the head can show abscesses in the tympanic bullae, cranium or nasal passages. The position of the tooth roots and their relationship with surrounding structures can also be seen. Before sectioning, the fixed head needs to be decalcified in decalcifying solution to soften the bones.

17.5 Examination of the vertebral column

Although spinal lesions may be seen radiologically, it is often worth examining the vertebral canal during *post-mortem* examination (Smith Baxter, 1975). The overlying musculature is dissected away from the vertebral column and the laminae gently removed with a pair of nail clippers. The spinal cord and associated nerves are then transected and the cord lifted out of the vertebral canal to expose the floor and any compressive or traumatic lesions. It is easier to remove the spinal cord intact if the tissues are fixed tissue prior to removal.

17.6 Preparation of the skull and other bones

Prepared skulls are invaluable to see the structure of the teeth and surrounding bone. They provide basic anatomical and pathological knowledge that is useful when treating rabbits with dental disease and for radiographic interpretation. Prepared skulls are also useful to show to clients during discussions about dental disease.

To prepare the skull, the head is first skinned and removed. An easy method of removing the soft tissue is to gently cook the skull (and/or any other bones) in a microwave, pressure cooker, slow cooker or saucepan. Bones from young animals tend to disintegrate if they are boiled for too long whereas bones from old animals take longer for the soft tissues to soften sufficiently for easy removal. A period of 8–16 h on 'low' in a slow cooker is usually sufficient. After cooling, the soft tissues are cleaned from the bones under running water over a sieve. Care is required as the teeth and lacrimal bones are easily lost. Once the soft tissues have been carefully cleaned off, the bones are dropped into warm hydrogen peroxide for sufficient time to turn white, usually 30–60 minutes. They are the rinsed in water and put in a warm place to dry. In the UK, museums and other institutions use dermestid beetles to remove soft tissues from bone. Skulls and bones that are prepared using dermestid beetles can be preserved indefinitely because all traces of decomposable tissue have been removed.

References

Barone, R., Pavaux, C., Blin, P.C., Cuq, P. (1973). *Atlas d'anotomie du lapin*. Masson et Cie.

Bivin, W.S. (1994). Basic biomethodology. In *The Biology of the Laboratory Rabbit*, 2nd edn. (P.J. Manning, D.H. Ringler, C.E. Newcomer, eds). pp 72–86. Academic Press.

Langan, G.P., O'Rourke, D. (2000). Rabbit microbiology and virology. In *Laboratory Medicine* (A.M. Fudge, ed.) pp 325–333. W.B. Saunders.

Lindsey, J.R., Fox, R.R. (1994). Inherited diseases and variations. In *The Biology of the Laboratory Rabbit*, 2nd edn. (P.J. Manning, D.H. Ringler, C.E. Newcomer, eds). pp 293–313. Academic Press.

Owen, D.G. (1992). Parasites of laboratory animals. *Laboratory Animal Handbooks No 12*. Royal Society of Medicine Services Ltd.

Smith Baxter, J. (1975). Posterior paralysis in the rabbit. *J Small Anim Pract.*, **16**, 267–271.

Index

(Main sections appear in **Bold**)